Language Disorders
A Functional Approach to Assessment and Intervention

2nd edition

Robert E. Owens, Jr.
State University of New York at Geneseo

Allyn & Bacon
Boston   London   Toronto   Sydney   Tokyo   Singapore

Acquisitions Editors: Ann Castel Davis/Kris Farnsworth
Production Editor: Patricia A. Skidmore
Photo Editor: Anne Vega
Production Manager: Pamela D. Bennett
Designer: Julia Zonneveld Van Hook
Cover Illustration: Antonio Gore, Southeast School, Columbus, OH FCBMR/DD

Library of Congress Cataloging-in-Publication Data
Owens, Robert E.
       Language disorders : a functional approach to assessment and intervention / Robert E. Owens,
Jr. — 2nd ed.
               p.   cm.
       Previously published : New York : Merrill, 1991
       Includes bibliographical references and index.
       ISBN 0-02-390271-X
       1. Language disorders in children.   I. Title
RJ496.L35O94 1995   94-17792
618.92'855—dc20   CIP

Photo credits: pp. 3, 21, 147, 263, 377, 459: Anne Vega, Prentice Hall and Merrill; pp. 63, 309: Barbara
Schwartz, Prentice Hall and Merrill; pp. 119, 183, 293, 423: Todd Yarrington, Prentice Hall and Merrill;
p. 235: Dan Floss, Prentice Hall and Merrill.

Printed in the United States of America

10 9 8 7 6 5 4   99 98

To my parents,
who have freely given of their love
and
asked for nothing in return

CONTENTS

APPENDICES

PREFACE

The second edition of *Language Disorders: A Functional Approach to Assessment and Intervention* is the result of an exhaustive compilation of studies conducted by my professional colleagues and of several years of clinical work in speech-language pathology with both presymbolic and symbolic children and adults. In this book, I concentrate on children because of the special problems they exhibit in learning language. Adults who are acquiring language, or who have lost language and are attempting to regain it, represent a much more diverse group and would be difficult to address in one text. This statement does not imply that children are a homogeneous group or that intervention with this group is easy. Any school speech-language pathologist will attest otherwise. This heterogeneity is reflected in the new Chapter 2, which describes various identifiable language impairments.

I call the model of assessment and intervention presented in this text *functional language*. This approach goes by other names, such as environmental or conversational, and includes elements of several other models. Where I have borrowed someone's model, ideas, or techniques, full credit is given to that person. I find assessment and intervention to be an adaptation of a little of this and a little of that within an overall theoretical framework. Readers should approach this text with this in mind. Some ideas presented are very practical and easy to implement, whereas others may not apply to particular intervention settings. Readers should use what they can, keeping in mind the overall model of using the natural environment and natural conversations as the context for training language. I am the first to acknowledge that I do not have a monopoly on assessment and intervention methods, nor do I pretend to have all of the answers.

Within *Language Disorders*, I have made some content decisions that should be explained. First, I have used the feminine pronoun when referring to the speech-language pathologist in recognition of the fact that most speech-language pathologists are women. I apologize to male speech-language pathologists, who should take comfort in the fact that the much-overworked masculine pronoun has been given a deserved rest. Second, I group all children with language problems, both delays and disorders, under the general rubric of *language-impaired*. This expedient decision was made recognizing that this text would not be addressing specific disorder populations except in a tangential manner. Third, I address two special cases in Chapter 11, which discusses classroom applications of the functional model, and in Chapters 12 and 13, which discuss children who are presymbolic and minimally symbolic. Chapter 11 recognizes the large numbers of speech-language pathologists who work within the public schools and the revolution in service delivery that is occurring there. Chapters 12 and 13 address a population close to my heart and to my initial clinical experiences.

The second edition of this text is updated and more inclusive than the first. Readers will find a new chapter describing different identifiable language impairments. The chapter on classroom intervention (Chapter 11) has been greatly expanded to reflect current realities in intervention services and to enhance the overall model of using the child's communicative contexts in intervention.

Finally, the second edition contains greatly expanded and enhanced sections on children with limited English proficiency and those speaking nonstandard dialects. This addition also reflects the more inclusive nature of changes within our profession and education in general.

ACKNOWLEDGMENTS

No text is written without the aid of other people. First, I thank the reviewers of this edition: Dr. Robert Ackerman, East Stroudsburg University of Pennsylvania; Dr. Lynn Bliss, Wayne State University; Dr. Darlene Davies, San Diego State University; Dr. Pamela Dutcher, Andrews University; and Dr. Judy Flanagin, University of South Dakota.

I also acknowledge the advice and counsel of Brenda Rogerson, a colleague, confidant, and dear friend of long standing; Dr. Shirley Szekeres, chair, Department of Speech Pathology and Audiology, Nazareth College; and Dr. Addie Haas, chair, Department of Communication, State University of New York at New Paltz, a constant inspiration and breath of freshness, and someone who helps me stretch my imagination and explore new possibilities. My many conference presentations and long hikes in the woods with Dr. Haas are always a learning experience and a joy. In addition, special thanks and much love to my partner, Tom Menzel, for his patience, support, and understanding. Other contributors include Dr. Linda House, chair, and Dr. Kathy Jones, both of the Department of Speech Pathology and Audiology, State University of New York at Geneseo; and Donna Cooperman, Department of Speech Pathology and Audiology, College of St. Rose. Finally, my deepest gratitude to Dr. James MacDonald, Department of Speech Pathology and Audiology, The Ohio State University, for introducing me to the potential of the environment in communication intervention.

Robert E. Owens, Jr., Ph.D.

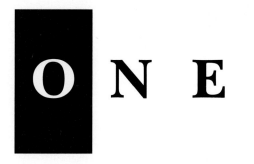

ONE

Introduction

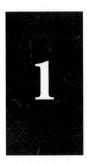

1 | A Functional Language Approach

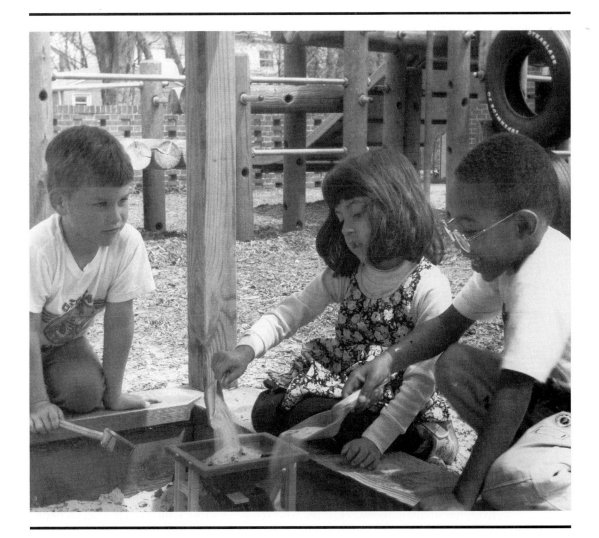

Language is a vehicle for communication, especially participation in conversations (Loban, 1979). In other words, "language is a social tool" used in communicative interactions (McLean & Snyder-McLean, 1978, p. 47). Thus, language can be viewed as a dynamic force or process, rather than as a product (Muma, 1978). The goal of speech-language intervention, therefore, should extend beyond language itself to include better communication. Newly acquired language skills should be evaluated to the extent that they enhance overall communication. Enhancing communication is the goal of a functional language approach.

A functional language approach to assessment and intervention, as described in this text, targets language as it is used or as it works for the language user as a vehicle for communication. In clinical practice, a functional approach to language impairment is a communication–first approach. The focus is the overall communication of the child with language impairment and of those who communicate with the child. As stated, the goal is better communication that works in the client's natural communicative contexts. Thus, "if the therapeutic strategy does not result in the child's acquiring a generalized communicative repertoire, we have failed (or at least have not succeeded)" (Warren & Rogers-Warren, 1985, p. 5). The speech-language pathologist needs to ensure that the language skills that are targeted and trained generalize to the everyday environment of the child. This concern for language use necessitates a new primacy for pragmatics in intervention protocols.

In short, in a functional language approach, conversation between children and their communication partners becomes the vehicle for change. By manipulating the linguistic and nonlinguistic contexts within which a child's utterances occur, the partner facilitates the use of certain structures and provides evaluative feedback while maintaining the conversational flow. From the early data collection stages through target selection to the intervention process, the speech-language pathologist and other communication partners are concerned with the enhancement of overall communication. The functional approach, therefore, is a holistic one that uses as much of the child's natural environment as possible.

Functional language approaches have been used to increase mean length of utterance and multiword utterance production; the overall quantity of communication; pragmatic skills, such as requesting, responsiveness, and initiation; vocabulary growth; language complexity; receptive labeling; and intelligibility and the use of trained forms in novel utterances in children with mental retardation, autism, specific language impairment, language learning disability, developmental delay, emotional and behavioral disorders, and multiple handicaps (Alpert & Rogers-Warren, 1984; Dyer, Williams, & Luce, 1991; Friedman & Friedman, 1980; Girolometto, 1988; Halle, Baer, & Spradlin, 1981; Hart & Risley, 1974, 1975, 1980; McGee, Krantz, Mason, & McClannahan, 1983; Nye, Foster, & Seaman, 1987; Scherer & Olswang, 1989; Schwartz, Chapman, Terrell, Prelock, & Rowan, 1985; Theodore, Maher, & Prizant, 1990; Warren, McQuarter, & Rogers-Warren, 1984; Whitehurst et al., 1991; Yoder, Kaiser, Alpert, & Fischer, 1993). Even minimally symbolic children who require a more structured approach benefit from a conversational milieu (Hart & Rogers-Warren, 1978; MacDonald & Gillette, 1982; Owens, McNerney, Bigler-Burke, & Lepre-Clark, 1987). In addition, functional interactive approaches improve generalization even when the immediate results differ little from those of more direct instructional methods (Alpert & Rogers-Warren, 1984; Cole & Dale, 1986; Halle et al., 1981; Hart & Risley, 1968; Rogers-Warren & Warren, 1985; Warren & Kaiser, 1986a).

In the past, language-training programs have focused on language form and content, with little consideration given to pragmatics or language use (Spinelli & Terrell, 1984). The typical approach to teaching language forms has been a highly structured, behavioral one emphasizing the teaching of specific behaviors within a stimulus-response-reinforcement paradigm (Fey, 1986). Thus, language is not a process but a product or response elicited by a stimulus or produced in anticipation of reinforcement.

Many speech-language pathologists prefer structured approaches because the speech–language pathologist can predict accurately the response of the child with language impairment to the training stimuli. In addition, structured behavioral approaches increase the probability that the client will make the appropriate, desired response. Language lessons usually are scripted as drills and, therefore, are repetitive and predictable for the speech–language pathologist.

The child becomes a passive learner, and active processing by the child is disregarded. The speech–language pathologist manipulates structured stimuli in order to elicit responses and dispenses reinforcement. Her overall style is highly directive (Ripich & Panagos, 1985; Ripich & Spinelli, 1985). In other words, clinical procedures are unidirectional and speech–language pathologist directed (Snow, Midkiff-Borunda, Small, & Proctor, 1984). These "trainer-oriented" approaches (Fey, 1986) are inadequate for developing meaningful uses for the newly acquired form or content.

Structured behavioral or trainer-oriented approaches that exhibit intensity, consistency, and organization have been successful in teaching some language skills to the mentally retarded (Guess, Sailor, & Baer, 1974) and to other language-impaired populations, such as children with language learning disability (LLD). Such approaches work, and the results are measured easily because the objectives are specific and discernible.

A major problem with present clinical approaches, however, is generalization from clinical to more natural contexts (Hunt & Goetz, 1988). Such generalization usually is not automatic (Spinelli & Terrell, 1984).

Lack of generalization can be a function of the material selected for training, the learning characteristics of the child, or the training paradigm. Stimuli present in the clinical setting that directly or indirectly affect the behavior being trained may not be found in other settings (Costello, 1983). Some of these stimuli, such as training cues, have intended effects, whereas others, such as the speech-language pathologist herself, may have quite unintended ones. In addition, clinical cues or consequences used for teaching may be very different from those encountered in everyday situations. This lack of natural consequences also may remove the motivation to use the behavior elsewhere.

In contrast, functional approaches give more control to the child and decrease the amount of structure in intervention activities. Indices of improvement are an increase in successful communication, rather than the number of correct responses (Marion, 1983). Procedures used by the speech-language pathologist and the child's communication partners more closely resemble those in the language-learning environment of children developing normally. In addition, the everyday environment of the child with language impairment is also included in training.

Naturally, the effectiveness of any language-teaching strategy will vary with the characteristics of the child with language impairment and the content of training (Connell, 1987a; Friedman & Friedman, 1980). For example, children with language learning disability seem to benefit more from specific language training than do other children with language impairment (Nye et al., 1987). Likewise, children with more severe language impairment initially benefit more from a structured imitative approach.

In this chapter, we explore a rationale for a functional language approach. This rationale is based on the primacy of pragmatics in language and language intervention and on the generalization of language intervention to everyday contexts. Generalization is discussed in terms of the variables that influence it. After the rationale is established, we discuss in following chapters various language impairments and assessment and intervention methods within the functional model.

PRAGMATICS

Pragmatics is the relationship between communicative partners and the form and meaning of the language being used. In short, pragmatics consists of the intentions or communication goals of each speaker and of the linguistic adjustments made by each speaker for the listener in order to accomplish these goals. Most features of language are affected by pragmatic aspects of the conversational context. For example, the selection of pronouns, verb tenses, articles, and adverbs or adverbial phrases of time involves more than syntactic and semantic considerations. The conversational partners must be aware of the preceding linguistic information and of each other's point of reference.

Pragmatics and accompanying issues of context have raised concerns about the number and type of features that speech-language pathologists should assess and train (Duchan, 1983b). An earlier interest by speech-language pathologists in psycholinguistics has led to the present therapeutic emphasis on increasing utterance length by increasing syntactic complexity. The speech-language pathologist's role has been to discover each child's individual learning strategies and to use these within the unidirectional, speech-language pathologist-directed approach mentioned previously (Snow et al., 1984). Intervention goals usually have been based on language form, with use frequently ignored. In short, the child's communicative intentions have been considered irrelevant. More pragmatic intervention goals might include communication functions, turn taking, discourse structures, and registers or styles of language.

With the therapeutic shift in interest to semantics or meaning in the early 1970s came a new recognition of the importance of cognitive or intellectual readiness but little understanding of the importance of the social environment. Most intervention approaches maintained structural behavioral teaching techniques.

The influence of sociolinguistics and pragmatics in the late 1970s and 1980s has led to interest in conversational rules and contextual factors. Everyday contexts have provided a backdrop for explanations of linguistic performance (Duchan, 1984). Of specific interest is the way individuals negotiate interactions and meanings with one another.

In working with special populations, the focus is shifting to a continuation of the communication process, rather than to treating specific symptoms of disorder (Duchan, 1982b, 1984; Frankel, 1982). Previously, for example, children's behaviors were considered either appropriate or inappropriate to the stimulus-reinforcement situation, rather than as a part of the interaction. Echolalia and unusual language patterns of children labeled as autistic, psychotic, and retarded were considered inappropriate and, therefore, were extinguished (Schreibman & Carr, 1978) or punished (Lovaas, 1977) in order to decrease their frequency of occurrence. When emphasis shifts to pragmatics and to the processes that underlie behavior, however, the child's language can be considered on its own terms (Tager-Flusberg, 1981a). In fact, echolalia and delayed echolalia seem to occur, in part, when the child does not understand or when the child expresses certain intentions (Curcio & Paccia-Cooper, 1982; Duchan, 1983a; Paccia-Cooper & Curcio, 1982; Prizant, 1983a; Prizant & Duchan, 1981).

The sociolinguistic model acknowledges not only individual differences among children but also stylistic differences within children as they interact with varying communicative partners. "The natural outgrowth of such [sociolinguistic] procedures is to involve families and teachers in training programs in which they create environments and interactive modes that are finely tuned and responsive to the communicative attempts and language competencies of [language impaired] . . . children" (Duchan, 1984, p. 67).

The traditional, or *formalist,* view of language as a composite of various rule systems, consisting of syntax, morphology, phonology, semantics, and pragmatics (Figure 1.1), may be inadequate (Prutting, 1982). This multileveled, formalist approach has given way to a *functional* model and to a more holistic approach to intervention. Language is a social tool, and, as such, considerations of language use are paramount. The formalist model is being replaced for many speech-language pathologists by one in which pragmatics is the overall organizing framework. Increasingly, speech-language pathologists are recognizing that structure and content are influenced heavily by the conversational constraints of the communication context.

This view of language has necessitated a very different approach to language intervention (Prutting, 1983). In effect, intervention has moved from an *entity approach,* which targets discrete isolated bits of language, to a *systems or holistic approach,* which targets language within the overall communication process (Norris

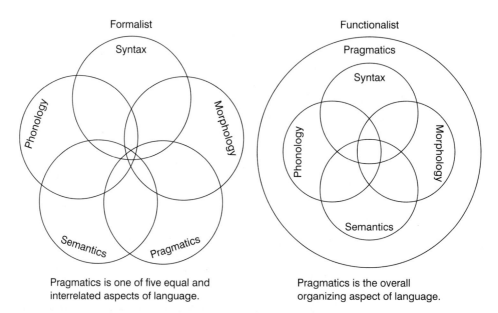

Pragmatics is one of five equal and   Pragmatics is the overall
interrelated aspects of language.   organizing aspect of language.

FIGURE 1.1
Relationship of the aspects of language

& Hoffman, 1990a). Therapy has become process, rather than product, oriented (Snow et al., 1984). Language is an integrated system used by the child to produce desired effects appropriate to the social context (Norris & Hoffman, 1990a).

The major implication of a systems or holistic approach is a change in both the targets and the methods of training (Craig, 1983; Muma, Pierce, & Muma, 1983). If, as formalists contend, pragmatics is just one of five equal aspects of language, then it offers yet another set of rules for training. Thus, there will be additional training goals, but the methodology need not change. The training still can emphasize the *what,* with little change in the *how,* which can continue in a structured behavioral paradigm.

In contrast, an approach in which pragmatics is the organizing aspect of language necessitates a more interactive conversational training approach, one that mirrors the transfer environment in which the language will be used. Therapy becomes bidirectional and child oriented, and conversation is viewed as a language-learning context (Cook-Gumperz & Gumperz, 1978; Snow et al., 1984; Waterson & Snow, 1978; Wells, 1981). Such an approach has been demonstrated to be effective (Friedman & Friedman, 1980). Thus, the conversational context becomes the teaching *and* transfer environment.

Dimensions of Communication Context

Language is more than just uttering words in linear sequence (Steinmann, 1982). Language is purposeful and takes place within a dynamic context. "We do not experience language in isolation . . . [but] in relation to a scenario, some background of persons and actions and events from which the things are said to derive their meaning" (Halliday, 1974, p. 28).

In other words, context affects form and content and may, in turn, be affected by them. *Context* consists of a complex interaction of the following eight factors (Dudley-Marling & Rhodes, 1987):

> *Purpose.* Language users begin with a purpose that affects what to say and how to say it (Knoblauch, 1980).
>
> *Content.* We use language to communicate about something. The topic of discourse will affect the form and the style.
>
> *Type of discourse.* Certain types of discourse, such as a debate or a speech, use a characteristic type of structure related to the purpose.
>
> *Participant characteristics.* Participant characteristics that affect context are background knowledge, roles, life experiences, moods, willingness to take risks, relative age, status, familiarity, and relationship in time and space (Graves, 1981).
>
> *Setting.* Setting includes the circumstances under which the language occurs.
>
> *Activity.* The activity in which the language users are engaged will affect language, especially the choice of vocabulary.
>
> *Speech community.* The speech community is that group with whom we share certain rules of language. It may be as large as the speakers of a language, such as English, or as small as two people who share a secret language of their own.
>
> *Mode of discourse.* The purpose and the relations of language users in time and space usually are determined by the mode of discourse. Speech and writing are modes that require very different types of interaction from the participants.

Within a conversation, participants continually must assess these factors and their changing relationships.

The context imposes certain responsibilities on language users in the form of an implicit contract. These responsibilities include the following six conversational and politeness maxims (Grice, 1975; Lakoff, 1973):

> *Be relevant.* Speakers are expected to stay on–topic unless they signal a topic change.
>
> *Be truthful.* The amount of truthfulness varies with the context, but each participant believes the other to be speaking the truth.
>
> *Be orderly.* Discourse must be orderly and cohesive.
>
> *Avoid ambiguity.* Speakers are expected to be as clear as possible. In turn, listeners are expected to signal when they do not understand the information transmitted.

Be brief. Speakers are expected to know their audiences and to provide no more information than needed.

Be polite. Speakers do not impose on their listeners. Instead, they observe the rules of turn taking, select the appropriate mode of address, and so on.

The actual rules observed in a conversation will depend on the agreement of the participants and on the context (Dudley-Marling & Rhodes, 1987).

The speech-language pathologist should be a master of the conversational context. Unfortunately, it is too easy to rely on overworked verbal cues, such as "Tell me about this picture" or "What do you want?" to elicit certain language structures. As simple a behavior as waiting can be an effective intervention tool when appropriate (Hart, 1985). Similarly, a seemingly nonclinical utterance, such as "Boy, that's a beautiful red sweater," can easily elicit negative constructions when directed at a child's green socks. Speech-language pathologists who know the dimensions of communication context understand these dimensions more effectively and manipulate them more efficiently.

At least five dimensions of the communication context must be considered by the speech-language pathologist (Prutting, 1982). They are the cognitive context, the social context, the physical context, the linguistic context, and the non-linguistic context.

The *cognitive context* includes the communication partners' shared knowledge about the physical world. Obviously, two individuals cannot share the same exact knowledge base. A toddler and her mother, for example, have very different knowledge bases, and yet they can communicate.

Parents adapt their behavior to the assumed knowledge level of their child. If the parents want the child to understand, they must adhere to topics that are known by the child or that differ only slightly. The child provides feedback that is used, in turn, by the parents in structuring the conversation. In the clinical setting, speech-language pathologists know much more than the client about the behavior being taught and must modify their behavior accordingly.

The *social context* includes each communication partner's knowledge of the social world. Such knowledge encompasses the communication setting, the partner, and the interactional rules used by each partner. In the clinic, the speech-language pathologist should consider each child's social skills. Preschoolers who seem unaware of the need to self-monitor and to repair their production may not have social knowledge of listener needs. The speech-language pathologist must be aware of the child's social knowledge to understand the child's behavior.

In the *physical context* are each partner's perceptions of the people, places, and objects that form that context. For example, pictures are very concrete for adults but may be very abstract for young preschoolers. The speech-language pathologist can manipulate the variables within this context to resemble more closely the transfer environment. Better still, intervention can occur in everyday settings in which the training targets are likely to occur.

The *linguistic context* consists of the verbal features that precede, accompany, and follow a verbalization and that are used by each partner for processing. For example, a question usually is followed by an answer; there is an obligation to reply.

Finally, the *nonlinguistic context* contains the nonlinguistic and paralinguistic events that surround a verbal production—that is, the activity in which the conversational partners are engaged. Some activities, such as group projects, encourage conversation; others, such as silent reading, do not. The importance of this context as a facilitator of verbal production cannot be overlooked in the clinical setting. Speech-language pathologists who focus exclusively on the linguistic context produce conversations consisting of a series of didactic or question-answer type exchanges.

Summary

"We are in an exciting era in our attempts to understand the relationships among linguistic, pragmatic, social and cognitive aspects of language behavior" (Prutting, 1982, p. 132). In the clinical setting, speech-language pathologists are becoming more aware of the effects of context on communication. How well children with language impairment regulate their relationships with other people depends on their ability to monitor context (Prutting, 1982). Given the dynamic nature of conversational contexts, it is essential that intervention also address generalization to the child's everyday communication contexts.

GENERALIZATION

One of the most difficult aspects of therapeutic intervention in speech-language pathology is generalization, or carryover to nontraining situations (Fey, 1988; Halle, 1987; Hunt & Goetz, 1988; Warren, 1988; Warren, Rogers-Warren, Baer, & Guess, 1980). For our purposes, let us consider *generalization* to be the ongoing interactive process of clients and of their newly acquired language feature with the communication environment (Figure 1.2). For example, if we are trying to teach a child the new word *doggie,* we might repeat the word several times in the presence of the family dog and then cue the child with, "Say doggie." If the child repeats the word only in this situation, he has not learned to use the word. If he says the word spontaneously and in the presence of other dogs, however, then we can reasonably assume that the child can produce the word without a model and thus has learned the word.

The factors that affect generalization may lie within the training content, the learner, or the teaching program and environment but will vary as particular aspects of the teaching situation change. If a response is to occur in a nontraining situation, then some aspects of that situation must be present in the training situation in order to signal that the response should occur. In other words, the speech-language pathologist must consider the effects of the various teaching contexts on generalization to everyday contexts.

Time and again, we speech-language pathologists bemoan the fact that although Johnny performed correctly 100% of the time in therapy, he could not

FIGURE 1.2
Generalization schematic

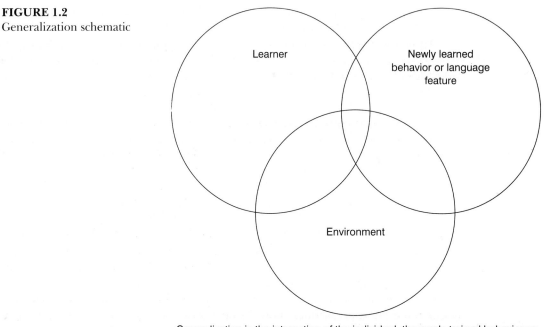

Generalization is the interaction of the individual, the newly trained behavior or language feature, and the environment. All three must be present for generalization to occur.

transfer this performance to the playground, classroom, or home. When language features taught in one setting are not generalized to other content and contexts, "the mutual [therapy] goal of communicative competence is not realized" (Rieke & Lewis, 1984, p. 41).

Failure of speech and language intervention to affect the child's everyday usage has led some professionals to conclude that "the traditional therapeutic model characterized by an adult working with a child a few minutes a day in an isolated context can never result in acceptable generalization" (Warren & Rogers-Warren, 1985, p. 5). Even though this conclusion may be overstated, it does pose the general problem: How can we get the language features trained in the therapy session to generalize to the client's other use environments?

In the past, some speech-language pathologists have used a "train and hope" strategy (Stokes & Baer, 1977), in which we have faith that the training will generalize but little influence over that possibility. This condition reflects a failure to manipulate the variables that affect generalization. Language training may not generalize because it is taught out of context, does not represent either the child's communicative functions or linguistic knowledge or experiences, and/or presents few communicative opportunities. To some extent, generalization is also a result of the procedures used and of the variables manipulated in language training. Finally, the very targets chosen for remediation may contribute to a lack of carryover.

With each client, the speech-language pathologist needs to ask: Will this procedure (or target) work in the child's everyday environment? Is there a need within the everyday communication of the client for the feature that is being trained, and do the methods used in its teaching reflect that everyday context? In a recent meeting with a student speech-language pathologist, the answer to these questions was no. As a result, we decided to forego auxiliary verb training with a middle-aged adult with mental retardation in favor of communication features more likely to be used within the client's everyday communication environment, such as ordering at a fast-food restaurant, asking directions, and using the telephone. In other words, we opted for a more functional approach that targeted useful skills in the everyday environment of the client.

Variables That Affect Generalization

Generalization is an essential part of learning. Even the young child using her or his first word must learn to generalize its use to novel content. The word *doggie* may be used with other four-legged animals. Eventually, the child abstracts those cases in which the word *doggie* is correct and those in which it is not. A Doberman, a poodle, and a stuffed collie are doggies, but a deer and a sheep are not. In short, the child is learning those contexts that obligate the use of *doggie* and those that preclude its use. Such contextual learning contributes to the underlying meaning of the word. Contexts regulate application of learned language rules (Connell, 1982).

Likewise, the young child who can say, "May I have a cookie, please?" has not learned this new utterance until it is used in the appropriate contexts. For example, it is inappropriate to use the utterance in a hardware store unless someone present has cookies. The child cannot learn all possible contexts; rather, the child learns the appropriate contextual cues, such as the presence of cookies, that govern use of the utterance.

The contexts in which training takes place influence what the child actually learns. In fact, correctness is not inherent in the child's response itself but is found in the response *in* context, as illustrated in the "May I have a cookie, please?" example. The relationship of context to learning is not a simple one, and the stimuli controlling a response may be multiple combinations of complex stimulus conditions (Goldstein, 1984).

Generalization is also an integral part of the language intervention process. Thoughts on generalization should not be left until after the intervention program is designed. Generalization is not a single-line entry at the end of the lesson plan, nor is it homework.

To facilitate the acquisition of truly functional language—language that works for the child—it is essential that speech-language pathologists manipulate the variables related to generalization throughout the therapeutic process. Table 1.1 includes a list of the major generalization variables.

Generalizations are of two broad types: *content generalization* and *context generalization*. Content is the *what* of training. Content generalization occurs when

TABLE 1.1
Variables that affect generalization of language training

Content Generalization	Training Targets
	Training Items
Context Generalization	Method of Training
	Language Facilitators
	Training Cues
	Consequences
	Location of Training

the child with language impairment induces a language rule from examples and from actual use. Thus, the new feature (e.g., plural -*s*) may be used with content not previously trained, such as words not used in the therapy situation. Content generalization is affected by the *targets* chosen for training, such as the use of negatives, and by the specific choice of *training items,* such as the words and sentences used to train negation.

Overall, the content selected for training reflects a speech-language pathologist's theoretical concept of language and of the strategies for language learning. More and more, speech-language pathologists are selecting targets that reflect use, rather than grammatical units. When grammatical units are targeted, different uses or functions for those units are essential to training.

Context is the *how* of training. Context generalization occurs when the client uses the new feature, such as the use of auxiliary verbs in questions, within everyday communication, such as in the classroom, at home, or in play. In each of these contexts are differences in persons present and in the location, as well as in the linguistic events that precede and follow the newly learned behavior. In short, generalization can be facilitated when the communication contexts of the training environment and of the natural environment are similar (Spinelli & Terrell, 1984).

Context includes an intrapersonal component unique to each individual and an interpersonal component shared by all persons in the communication setting (Spinelli & Terrell, 1984). *Intrapersonal variables* include each partner's cognitive and social knowledge or context, variables that may differ greatly across special populations. These variables, discussed previously, influence the selection of content and the individualization of program design.

Interpersonal variables include situational factors (e.g., method of training, personnel involved, training cues, reinforcement method, location and time of training, and objects present) and participant factors (e.g., conversational roles of the participants). The effects of some of these variables on generalization are discussed in detail in the following sections.

Training Targets

The very complexity of language probably makes it impossible for the speech-language pathologist to teach everything that a child with language impairment needs to become a competent communicator. Obviously, some language features must be ignored. Target selection, therefore, is a conscious process with far-reaching implications. Training target selection should be based on the actual needs and interests of each child within her or his communication environments.

The focus of instruction should be on increasing the effectiveness of child-initiated communication. Both the frequency and the sophistication of this communication can be increased through intervention (McCormick, 1986).

Language is a dynamic process that is influenced heavily by context. Thus, language features selected for training should be functional or useful for the child in the communication environment. Forms acquire real meaning only when they are used to accomplish some intention.

Generalization is also a function of the scope of the training target and of the child's characteristics and linguistic experience with the target. Language knowledge exists along a continuum from restricted or specific rules with a narrow application to broad, unrestricted rules with wide application. The scope of a training target will affect generalization. In general, language rules with broad scope generalize more easily than those with more restricted scope (Kamhi, 1988).

The scope of rule application can be a function of the way it is taught. In part, narrow, restricted teaching may reflect a behaviorist bias that reduces training targets to easily identifiable and observable units. Rules interpreted by the child as applying to a limited set of lexical items combined in a very specific manner will involve little generalization (J. Johnston, 1988a).

The child's prior knowledge of language also influences generalization. The failure of training to generalize may reflect training targets that are inappropriate for the knowledge level of the child. For example, it would be inappropriate to train indirect commands prior to the child's understanding and using yes/no questions and direct commands.

In conclusion, training targets should be selected on the basis of each child's actual communication needs and abilities, rather than on some preconceived agenda. The targets selected for training should be functional or useful in the client's everyday communication environment. We can expect optimum generalization only when the content logically flows from one training level to the next and when the client has a need and a use for this content in communication. More broad-based language rules generalize better than rules with limited scope and application.

Training Items

The actual items selected for intervention, such as the specific verbs to be used in training past tense or the sentences to be used in training negation, and the linguistic complexity of these intervention items also can influence generalization. In general, it is best if these items come from the natural communication environment of the child with language impairment. Structured observation of this environment can aid intervention programming. For example, the active child may use the verbs *walk, jump,* and *hop* frequently. It is more likely that use of the past tense *-ed* will generalize if these frequently occurring words are used in the training.

Individualization is important because of the many different use environments across children with language impairment. The child who is institutionalized may have very different content to discuss than does the child who resides at home. The interests of younger children are also very different from those of adolescents.

Targeted linguistic forms, whether word classes or larger linguistic structures, should be trained across several functions. For example, negatives used with auxiliary verbs can occur in declaratives ("That doesn't fit"), imperatives ("Don't touch that"), and interrogatives ("Don't you want to go?") and in functions, such as denying ("I didn't do it") or requesting information ("Why didn't you go?").

For optimum generalization, then, it is necessary to select training items from the child's everyday environment. In addition, these items should be trained across linguistic forms and/or functions and across linguistic and nonlinguistic contexts.

Method of Training

The training of discrete bits of language devoid of the communication context actually may retard learning and growth (Cazden, 1972; Damico, 1988; N. Nelson, 1993). In its strictest sense, the formalist construct of language as separate and autonomous components assumes little or no interaction among the linguistic units. Such fragmentation allows minute analysis units to eclipse the essential language qualities of intentionality and synergy (Damico, 1988). In other words, language use in communication is lost. Intervention that focuses on these specific, discrete, structural entities fosters drills and didactic training. These adversely affect the flow, intentionality, and meaningfulness of language (Oller, 1983). Language should be viewed holistically (J. Norris & Hoffman, 1990b; Silliman, 1993).

The training of language involves much more than just the training of words and structures. Clients should be learning strategies for comprehending language directed at them and for generating novel utterances within several conversational contexts.

Training should occur in actual use within a conversational context. Prutting (1983) states that language intervention should meet the "Bubba" criterion. *Bubba* is Yiddish for "grandmother." If we were to explain our intervention approach to our Jewish grandmother, she would reply: "Oh, I could have told you that. It just makes sense to use conversations to train. Why didn't you ask me?" In other words, the training regimen should make sense. Our intervention methodology should flow logically from our concept of language.

If language is a social tool and if the goal is to train for generalized use, then it follows that language should be trained in conditions similar to the ultimate use environment. Thus, the speech-language pathologist should modify the interactional context within which language is trained so that it closely resembles or actually takes place within the child's ongoing everyday communication environment. It is important, therefore, to view context not as a backdrop but as an ongoing process (Cook-Gumperz & Corsaro, 1976; Cook-Gumperz & Gumperz, 1978).

Discussion of the method of training leads naturally to consideration of the other contextual variables. For optimum generalization, training should occur within a conversational context with varying numbers of facilitators, cues, consequences, and locations.

Language Facilitators

"To ensure that the language trained is functional and, therefore, most likely to be generalized, language training should be conducted by those who spend the most time communicating with the child" (Warren & Rogers-Warren, 1985, p. 7). This conclusion suggests that parents, teachers, aides, and unit personnel, in addition to the speech-language pathologist, should be language facilitators because of their relationship with and the amount of time each spends with the child.

Interactional partners form communication environments for each other (McDermott, Gospodinoff, & Aram, 1976), and it is essential that the client experience newly learned language in a number of everyday communication environments. Because language is contextually variable, it will differ within the context created by the child with each communication partner. Thus, generalization depends on the number of communication partners we can involve in the intervention process (Craig, 1983). With children developing normally, the number of individuals they see during the day or week is positively correlated with the rate of language development (K. Nelson, 1973).

Language facilitators are "adults who increase the child's potential for communication success" (Craig, 1983, p. 110). Through training, these adults could maximize their teaching potential within the everyday activities of the child.

Programs that involve the child's communication partners, especially parents, produce greater gains for children than do programs that do not (Baker, Murphy, Heifitz, & Brightman, 1975; Fredricks, Baldwin, & Grove, 1974; L. Watson & Bassinger, 1974). Parents offer a channel for generalizing to the natural environment of the home (Tiegerman & Siperstein, 1984). With parent or caregiver training, both parents and teachers can function on a continuum from paraprofessionals to general language facilitators (Adler, 1988; King, 1976; McDade & Varnedoe, 1987; Owens, 1982d).

With these additional language facilitators, the traditional role of the speech-language pathologist changes. In essence, the speech-language pathologist becomes a programmer of the child's environment, manipulating the variables to ensure successful communication and generalization. To be effective, the speech-language pathologist must recognize that the child's communication partners are also clients, as well as agents of change (MacDonald, 1985). In addition, the speech-language pathologist must act as a consultant, helping each interactive dyad fine-tune its conversational behaviors.

Training Cues

Too often children are trained solely to respond to trainer cues. Goals for the child should include both initiating and responding behaviors in the situations in which each is appropriate. Therefore, the speech-language pathologist must consider training language through a great variety of both linguistic and nonlinguistic cues.

Research has demonstrated the beneficial effects of a nurturant style of facilitator behavior on children's language acquisition (Barnes, Gutfreund, Satterly, & Wells, 1983; Cross, 1978, 1984). The nurturant style is child directed or child centered, with the adult responding to child initiations. The adult encourages child utterances by subtle manipulation of the context and responds to the child in a conversational manner. A functional language approach adapts these techniques as naturally as possible to intervention.

Speech-language pathologists use conversational or linguistic techniques to facilitate child utterances or use familiar nonlinguistic routines and activities that will encourage verbal initiations by the child. The nonlinguistic context can be manipulated along a continuum from highly structured routines that can promote interactions with noninteractive children to more open-ended, less structured interactions (Duchan & Weitzner-Lin, 1987).

Contingencies

The nature of the reinforcement used in training is also a strong determiner of generalization. Edibles or social reinforcement used in training may have little relationship to the language feature being trained. For best generalization to the natural use environment, "consequences that are related directly to the language utterance and communication function made by the student should be provided" (Stremel-Campbell & Campbell, 1985, p. 266). Everyday, natural consequences are best. If the child requests a paintbrush, he should be given one, unless, of course, there is a good reason not to give it. If that is the case, then the child should not have been required to learn the request.

Weaning the child away from edible reinforcers in favor of social ones is commendable as long as the social reinforcer is likely to be found in the natural communication environment. Verbal or social training consequences such as "Good talking," encountered only rarely in the course of everyday conversations, should be discontinued as soon as possible in favor of more natural responses.

Functional approaches offer a variety of response modes that demonstrate acceptance or rejection and redirection of the child's utterance while maintaining the conversational flow. Consequences such as "Good talking" end social interaction by commenting on the correctness of the child's utterance only and leaving little that the child can say in return. Verbal responses that combine feedback about correctness/incorrectness with additional information can be both a language-learning opportunity and a communicative turn (Rieke & Lewis, 1984).

Not every utterance is reinforced in the natural environment. In the course of everyday conversations, many utterances are not reinforced. In typical language intervention, however, every utterance by the child may be reinforced. Behaviors continuously reinforced are easy to extinguish. Intermittently reinforced responses are much more resistant and more closely resemble patterns found in the real world.

Location

The location of training involves not only places but also events. For maximum generalization, language should be trained in the locations, such as the home, clinic, school, or unit, and in activities in which it is used, such as play or household chores. Children removed from familiar contexts "may be unable to exhibit their most creative uses of language" (Lieven, 1984, p. 22).

Language should be trained within the daily activities of the client (Hart & Rogers-Warren, 1978). Daily routines can provide a familiar framework within which conversation can occur (Lieven, 1982, 1984; Snow & Goldfield, 1983). The familiar situation provides a frame that allows for a degree of automatization important in the acquisition of such skills as language (Reason & Mycielska, 1982). Often called *incidental teaching,* this approach attempts to ensure that children learn and have ample opportunity to use language within naturally occurring activities (McCormick, 1986; Owens, 1982d; Warren & Rogers-Warren, 1985). Generalization increases with the similarity of the original learning situation to the transfer situation (Brown & Campione, 1984). If the conditions for training and use are the same, the need for contrived generalization strategies is alleviated.

Activity heavily influences language (Levinson, 1978), so the forms used depend to some extent on these activities. The ideal training situation is one in which the child with language impairment is engaged in some meaningful activity with a conversational partner who models appropriate language forms and functions (Staab, 1983). In this way, the child learns language in the conversational context in which it is likely to occur. It is within these everyday events that language is acquired naturally and to these events that the newly trained language is to generalize.

Within these daily events are naturally occurring communication sequences (Craig, 1983). Daily events, such as phone calls, friendly meetings, dinner preparation, and even dressing, can provide a framework for language and for language training. The frame provides a guide to help the participants organize their language and their language learning. Routines and "familiar situations may provide the child with support for the next step" (Lieven, 1984, p. 22). The speech-language pathologist can plan conversational roles and language training through the use of such daily events.

Summary

Language training should be a dynamic process of exchange that occurs during natural events in different environments and with different conversational partners (Snow et al., 1984). Reinforcement should be the intrinsic conversational success of the child. The variables relative to content and context can, if manipulated carefully, facilitate generalization of newly learned language features.

Unfortunately, in practice, generalization is too often the final step in planning client training. Instead, "communication goals and effects should be preserved and considered the first, pervasive, and most basic step in intervention planning and not some final set of generalization rules" (Craig, 1983, p. 110).

CONCLUSION

The functional approach emphasizes nurturant and naturalistic approaches (Duchan & Weitzner-Lin, 1987). The nurturant aspect requires the speech-language pathologist/facilitator to relinquish control to the child and to respond to the child's communication initiations. The naturalistic aspect emphasizes everyday events and context. Language makes sense only when used within a communication context. Thus, the speech-language pathologist must become a master in the manipulation of that context in order to facilitate communication and generalization. Language is trained while it is actually used in everyday contexts. As a result, the training generalizes.

Learning and generalization are the result of good planning based on a knowledge of the variables that affect generalization and the individual needs of each child. The content selected for training and the context within which this training takes place are both important aspects of the generalization process. The speech-language pathologist must determine the best response for the child's initiations and the best contexts for facilitating intervention targets.

Although the role of the speech-language pathologist within the functional language paradigm will change from primary direct service provider to language facilitator and consultant, she still will have primary responsibility for planning and intervention. Recognizing the need to meet these responsibilities more effectively, many professionals have proposed more functional intervention goals and procedures, such as those outlined in this text.

It is easy to deride functional approaches as offering no framework for learning, allowing the child total freedom. Yet, the approach outlined in this chapter is not one in which the speech-language pathologist and child converse with little intervention occurring. Under such conditions, there is little development on the part of the child and little generalization.

Professionals often cast a wary eye on implementation of such conversational and communication-based approaches to language intervention. The fear is that intervention will deteriorate into a "Hey, man, what's happenin'?" approach, too open-ended to be effective in changing client behavior. Although this danger does exist, it is not inherent in functional approaches. As this text progresses, we discuss assessment and training procedures that enable speech-language pathologists to maintain a teaching momentum within the more natural context of conversation.

In the following chapters, we explore language impairments, assessment, and intervention. After a discussion of language impairments, we discuss the assessment process and the collection and analysis of conversational and narrative data. In the following chapters, an intervention paradigm and various techniques are presented, along with discussion of two special applications: one to an environment (the classroom) and one with a population (children who are presymbolic and minimally symbolic).

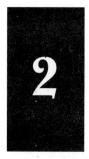

2 Language Impairments

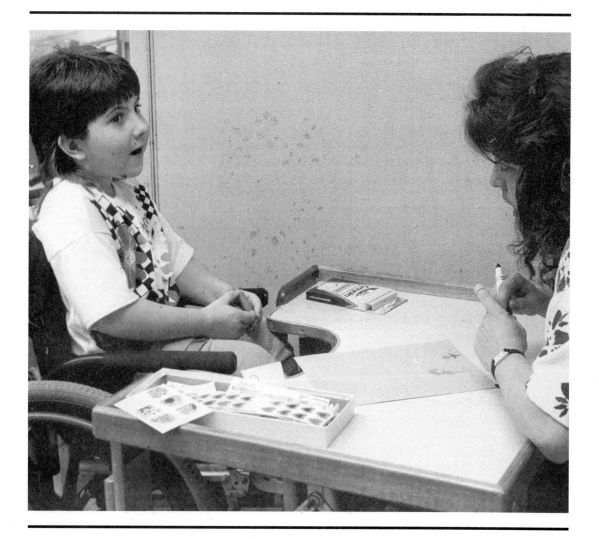

I have chosen in this text to use the term *language impairment* to refer to both language disorders and language delays. Although it may be debatable that some children with either or both are not impaired in their daily lives, the term seems inclusive and will help us avoid arguments such as whether children with mental retardation exhibit disorders or delays.

The American Speech-Language-Hearing Association, the professional organization for speech-language pathologists, defines *language disorder* as follows:

> A LANGUAGE DISORDER is impaired comprehension and/or use of spoken, written and/or other symbol systems. This disorder may involve (1) the form of language (phonology, morphology, syntax), (2) the content of language (semantics), and/or (3) the function of language in communication (pragmatics) in any combination. (Ad Hoc Committee on Service Delivery in the Schools, 1993, p. 40)

To this very language-specific definition, Bashir (1989) has added more description and causal information:

> *Language disorders* is a term that represents a heterogeneous group of either developmental or acquired disorders principally characterized by deficits in comprehension, production, and/or use of language. Language disorders are chronic and may persist across the lifetime of the individual. The symptoms, manifestations, effects, and severity of the problem change over time. The changes occur as a consequence of context, content, and learning task. (p. 181)

Bashir has added the elements of both inertia and change across time and circumstance, important elements in the definition and in intervention. Problems may persist with or without intervention but will vary with many of the factors discussed in Chapter 1.

A definition of *language delay* would be similar, but the element of immature language or a slower than average rate of development would be added. Such words as *disorder* and *deficit* would be replaced with *delay* and *immaturity*.

Our definition of language impairment also should reflect the primacy of pragmatics. One could easily argue that because language is a social tool, it does not demonstrate impairment until it is used for actual communication. In addition, I feel more comfortable saying what language impairment is not. Specifically, it is not just a difference. For our purposes, we shall consider the term **language impairment** to apply to a *heterogeneous group of developmental and/or acquired disorders and/or delays principally characterized by deficits and/or immaturities in the use of spoken or written language for comprehension and/or production purposes that may involve the form, content, and/or function of language in any combination*. Language impairment may persist across the lifetime of the individual and may vary in symptoms, manifestations, effects, and severity over time and as a consequence of context, content, and learning task. Language differences, such as those found in some individuals with LEP and with different dialects, do not in themselves constitute language impairments.

Although the fine points of a definition may seem similar to medieval arguments over the number of angels able to fit on the head of a pin, such definitions are essential to any discussion of language impairments. In attempting to clarify the definition of language impairment, we have, no doubt, raised more questions than we have answered. For example, causal factors, such as prematurity, although important, are omitted from the definition because of their diverse nature and the lack of clear causal links in many children with language impairment. In general, causal categories are not directly related to later language attributes (Lahey, 1988). Likewise, diagnostic categories, such as mental retardation, are not included for many of the same reasons. The definition also states that language differences are not disorders or delays, although the general public and some professionals often confuse them. We explore all of these issues in this chapter and those that follow.

In this chapter, I describe the most common diagnostic categories of children with language impairment. I attempt to personalize this discussion whenever possible, but readers should remember that we are examining groups of children, not individuals. For example, no one child with language learning disability may exhibit all of the characteristics ascribed to these children. In conclusion, we try to find some commonalities and differences across various disorders and explore the most common language problems seen by speech-language pathologists.

DIAGNOSTIC CATEGORIES

Many categories of disability have language components. In this section, we discuss some of these categories in detail, attempting to describe similarities and differences.

Research from children with language impairment suggests that normal language learning requires the following (J. Johnston, 1991):

1. The ability to perceive sequenced acoustic events of short duration
2. The ability to attend actively, to be responsive, and to anticipate stimuli
3. The ability to use symbols
4. The ability to invent syntax from the language of the environment
5. Enough mental energy to do all of the above simultaneously

Because language is learned naturally from another person in the course of conversation, we add an additional requirement:

6. The ability to interact and communicate with others

Many of the children described in the following section have problems in one or more of these areas. As we discuss each language impairment, readers should try to keep these abilities in mind.

There is a danger in describing categories of children and then assigning children to these categories. In general, such categories are helpful for discussion of the shared characteristics of individuals who represent the category (G. Lakoff, 1987), but the category can become self-fulfilling. Children assigned to the category then are treated as the category, not as individuals. It is important to remember that the child is not *autistic* or an *autist*, but rather is a child *with autism.*

Many children with language impairment cannot be described easily by one of the categories discussed in this chapter. Such children may have more than one primary diagnostic category or characteristics that do not fit into any category. It is important for the speech-language pathologist to remember that each child represents a unique set of circumstances and that language will vary accordingly. Language assessment and intervention likewise should be individualized.

Within each disorder category below, we limit the discussion to general characteristics, language characteristics, and possible causal factors. I have chosen not to discuss some categories because of the small numbers of children or the paucity of research data. I have omitted other categories because language disorders are tangential to the primary disorder. Finally, some categories, such as deafness, have such pervasive communication problems as to be beyond the scope of this book in their entirety.

Mental Retardation

The American Association on Mental Retardation (AAMR) defines mental retardation as a "significantly subaverage general intellectual functioning existing concurrently with deficits in adaptive behavior and manifested during the developmental period" (Grossman, 1983, p. 1). This definition, which is the result of committee decision making, needs some explanation.

Significantly subaverage means two standard deviations below the mean, a position at the extreme of the human intelligence curve. Approximately 3% of the population is below this point, which is at an IQ of 68. The definition is concerned with more than IQ, which is a measure of past learning, and considers *general intellectual functioning* plus *adaptive behaviors,* which include personal independence and social responsibility. Intelligence testing should be culture-free, and adaptive behavior should be measured against the individual's own cultural group (Mercer & Lewis, 1975). Finally, individuals with mental retardation are considered to be developmental beings, so the definition covers the period during which humans develop into adults. Only individuals who meet all of the criteria are considered to have mental retardation.

The exact number of individuals who have mental retardation is unknown. Estimates vary from 1% to 3% of the population or approximately 2.5 to 7.5 million people in the United States.

As in all disorders, severity varies across individuals, although usually little change occurs in individual severity over time. Severity usually is related to IQ, as noted in Table 2.1. Nearly 90% of the retarded population is classified as mildly retarded.

TABLE 2.1
Severity of mental retardation

Severity	IQ Range	% of MR	Characteristics
Mild	52–68	89	Usually live and work independently within the regular community. Often have families.
Moderate	36–51	6	Capable of some semi-independence at work and in residence. As adults, many work in supportive environments and live with relatives or in community residence.
Severe	20–35	3.5	Capable of learning some self-care skills and are not totally dependent. Some adults are able to work in a supportive environment and live with relatives or in community residences.
Profound	19 and below	1.5	Capable of learning some basic living skills but will require continual care and supervision. Often exhibit multiple handicaps.

Source: Adapted from Grossman, H. (1983). *Classification in mental retardation.* Washington, DC: American Association on Mental Deficiency.

Not every child with mental retardation is similar. Obviously, some difference in severity will occur, and other factors, such as amount of home support, living environment, education, type of retardation, mode of communication, and age, must be taken into account. I have worked with very social, very verbal preschoolers and adolescents with multiple disabilities and very little recognizable communication.

Language Characteristics

Language is often one of the most impaired areas for the child with mental retardation and may be the single most important characteristic of the retarded population (Ingalls, 1978). Even when compared with normally developing children of the same mental age, children with mental retardation often exhibit poorer language skills (Kamhi, 1981).

Although some of this language difference may be attributed to low intellectual functioning, this factor alone does not fully explain the phenomenon. In addition, the cognition-language relationship is an inconsistent one across individuals with mental retardation (J. Miller, Chapman, & MacKenzie, 1981). For approximately half of the retarded population, both language comprehension and production levels are similar to cognitive levels. In other words, a 6–year–old child with mental retardation might have a mental age and a language age of 42 months. In 25% of the population, both language comprehension and production are below the level of cognition. Finally, in another 25%, language comprehension and cognition are at similar levels but production is below both.

Both qualitative and quantitative differences occur between the language of children with mental retardation and children developing normally (Table 2.2)

TABLE 2.2
Language characteristics of children with mental retardation

Pragmatics	Gestural and intentional developmental patterns similar to those of children developing normally.
	May take less dominant conversational role.
	Poorer clarification skills than mental age-matched peers developing normally.
Semantics	More concrete word meanings.
	Slow vocabulary growth.
	More limited use of a variety of semantic units.
	Children with Down syndrome able to learn word meanings from exposure in context as well as mental age-matched peers developing normally.
Syntax/Morphology	Length-complexity relationship similar to that of preschoolers developing normally.
	Same sequence of general sentence development as children developing normally.
	Shorter, less complex sentences with fewer subject elaborations or relative clauses than mental age-matched peers developing normally.
	Sentence word order takes precedence over word relationships.
	Reliance on less mature forms, though capable of more advanced.
	Same order of morpheme development as preschoolers developing normally.
Phonology	Phonological rules similar to those of preschoolers developing normally but reliance on less mature forms, though capable of more advanced ones.
Comprehension	Poorer receptive language skills, especially children with Down syndrome, than mental age-matched peers developing normally.
	Poorer sentence recall than mental age-matched peers.
	More reliance on context to extract meaning.

Source: Based on Abbeduto, Davies, Solesby, & Furman (1991); Bedrosian & Prutting (1978); Bender & Carlson (1982); Bradbury & Lunzer (1972); Chapman, Kay-Raining Bird, & Schwartz (1990); Chapman, Schwartz, & Kay-Raining Bird (1988); Dever & Gardner (1970); Graham & Graham (1971); Greenwald & Leonard (1979); Ingram (1972); Kahn (1975); Kernan (1990); Klink, Gerstman, Raphael, Schlanger, & Newsome (1986); Lackner (1968); Layton & Sharifi (1979); Lobato, Barrera, & Feldman (1981); McLeavey, Toomey, & Dempsey (1982); Merrill & Bilsky (1990); Mervis (1988); Moran, Money, & Leonard (1984); Naremore & Dever (1975); Newfield (1966); Owens & MacDonald (1982); Prater (1982); Rondal, Ghiotto, Bredart, & Bachelet (1988); Rosin, Swift, Bless, & Vetter (1988); Semmel & Herzog (1966); Shriberg & Widder (1990); Vihman (1978)

(Weiss, Weisz, & Bromfield, 1986). In general, below a mental age of 10 years, children with mental retardation and those without follow similar developmental paths, although children with mental retardation seem to produce shorter, less elaborated utterances—a quantitative difference. After a mental age of 10 years, the developmental paths begin to differ more and the differences between the two groups become qualitative.

A great deal of information is available on the language of children with mental retardation, especially those with mild retardation and with Down syndrome, a chromosomal anomaly. Most of these data are summarized in Table 2.2. As mentioned, this is group data, and individual children may have language that differs greatly.

In general, the overall sequence of development of children with mental retardation is similar to that of children developing normally, although the rate is slower (Pruess, Vadasy, & Fewell, 1987). This pattern can be seen in development of intentions, role taking, presupposition, sentence forms, morphological markers, and phonological processes (Bender & Carlson, 1982; Bradbury & Lunzer, 1972; Dever & Gardner, 1970; Ingram, 1972; J. Johnston & Schery, 1976; Kahn, 1975; Lackner, 1968; Lobato, Barrera, & Feldman, 1981; McLeavey, Toomey, & Dempsey, 1982; Newfield & Schlanger, 1968; Owens & MacDonald, 1982; Shriberg & Widder, 1990). **Presupposition** is the speaker's assumption of the listener's perspective, what she or he knows and needs to know. In addition to the above, children with Down syndrome are also as skilled as their mental–age-matched peers developing normally in inferring novel word meanings and in producing these words correctly thereafter (Chapman, Kay-Raining Bird, & Schwartz, 1990).

Even when children are matched for mental age, however, children with mental retardation seem to use more immature forms than do their peers developing normally. The utterances of children with mental retardation tend to be shorter and less complex (McLeavey et al., 1982; Naremore & Dever, 1975). Similarly, phonological processes of less mature children continue to be used by more mature children with mental retardation even when these processes are unnecessary (Klink, Gerstman, Raphael, Schlanger, & Newsome, 1986; Moran, Money, & Leonard, 1984). In other words, processes will be used to simplify a word even when the child can produce the word correctly. Children with Down syndrome and mental retardation are also less skilled in requesting clarification of information and engage in more verbal perseveration than do mental–age-matched peers developing normally (Abbeduto, Davies, Solesby, & Furman, 1991; Rein & Kernan, 1989). **Perseveration** is excessive talking on a topic when it is inappropriate or previously addressed.

Conversations require the integration of all aspects of language within a dynamic context. It is possible that the difficulties noted in the language of children with mental retardation reflect problems integrating learning into ongoing events. Possibly these children are using their available cognitive energy to monitor and understand the conversation, leaving little for integration of language skills. All of us experience this phenomenon with newly acquired skills until they become more automatic. For example, children with mental retardation are capable of learning syntactic rules, and yet they tend to rely on less mature word order rules, a less mature and simpler method of interpretation (Graham & Graham, 1971; McLeavey et al., 1982; Semmel, 1967). Likewise, although capable of requesting clarification, children with mental retardation are less likely to do so within conversations (Abbeduto et al., 1991).

Finally, some children with mental retardation, especially those with Down syndrome, exhibit poorer receptive language skills than do their mental–age-matched peers developing normally (Abbeduto, Furman, & Davies, 1989; Chapman, Schwartz, & Kay-Raining Bird, 1988; Mervis, 1988; Rosin, Swift, Bless, & Vetter, 1988). The context seems particularly important for these children in aiding comprehension of both literal and figurative language (Ezell & Goldstein, 1991). As we will see in children with other language impairments, context usually can be trusted when language is incomprehensible.

Possible Causal Factors

Possible causal factors for mental retardation are many and varied, including, but not limited to, biological and social–environmental causes of retardation and language impairments, and information–processing differences related to language comprehension and production (Table 2.3). Any discussion of causality must be tempered with the recognition that for many children the cause of mental retardation is unknown. In addition, more than one causal factor may be at work. In any case, causal factors rarely are related directly to the performance level of the child in question.

Biological factors.   Biological causes may be a factor for a majority of children with mental retardation (Grossman, 1983). These include genetic and chromosomal causes, such as Down syndrome; maternal infections, such as rubella; toxins and chemical agents, including fetal alcohol syndrome; nutritional and metabolic causes, such as PKU; gestational disorders, primarily in the formation of the brain or skull; complications from pregnancy and delivery; and gross brain diseases, including tumors. In general, a strong correlation exists between biological factors and severity of retardation. Although biological causal factors may explain, in part, resultant retardation, they tell us very little about development, specifically language acquisition.

Social-environmental factors.   Social-environmental causal factors of retardation are more difficult to identify and may involve many interactive variables. Deprivation, poor housing and diet, poor hygiene, and lack of medical care can all affect adversely the development of the child although the exact effect of each is unknown and varies with each child.

It has been assumed and demonstrated in some early studies that the mothers of children with mental retardation respond less to their children because these children display only limited behaviors (Brooks-Gunn & Lewis, 1984). This reasoning has been shown to be untrue.

TABLE 2.3
Causal factors related to mental retardation (Adapted from Grossman, 1963)

Type	Examples	Characteristics
Biologic		
Genetic and chromosomal	Down syndrome (Trisomy 21)	Broad head and characteristic facial features, small stature, mental retardation
	Fragile X syndrome	Mental retardation in males, possible learning disabilities in females.
	Cri-du-chat syndrome	Catlike cry, microcephaly, mental retardation
Infectious processes	Maternal rubella	Cardiac defects, cataracts, hearing loss, microcephaly, possible mental retardation
	Congenital syphilis	Deafness, vision problems, possible epilepsy or cerebral palsy, mental retardation
Toxins and chemical agents	Fetal alcohol syndrome	Persistently deficient growth, low brain weight, facial abnormalities, cardiac defects, mental retardation
	Lead poisoning	Central nervous system and kidney damage, hyperactivity
Nutrition and metabolism	Phenylketonuria (PKU)	Reduced pigmentation, motor coordination problems, convulsions, microcephaly, mental retardation
	Tay-Sachs disease	Progressive deterioration of nervous system and vision, mental retardation, death in preschool years
	Inadequate diet	Small stature, possible mental retardation
Gestational disorders	Hydrocephalus	Enlarged head caused by increased volume of cerebral-spinal fluid, visual defects, epilepsy, mental retardation
	Cerebral malformation	Absence or underdevelopment of cerebral cortex and resultant mental retardation
	Craniofacial anomalies	Malformed skull and associated mental retardation
Complications of pregnancy and delivery	Extreme immaturity or preterm infant	Low birth weight, higher prevalence of central nervous system disorders
	Exceptionally large baby	Possible birth injury to central nervous system
	Maternal nutritional disorders	Low birth weight, higher prevalence of central nervous system disorders
Gross brain diseases	Tumors and tuberous sclerosis	Tumors in heart, seizures, tuberous "bumps" on nose and cheeks, mental retardation
	Huntington disease	Degenerative neurological functioning evidenced in progressive dementia and cerebral palsy
Social-Environmental		
Psychosocial disadvantage	Subnormal intellectual functioning in immediate family and/or impoverished environment	Functional retardation
Sensory deprivation	Maternal deprivation	Functional retardation and failure to thrive
	Prolonged isolation	

Source: Owens, R. (1993). Mental Retardation. In D. Bernstein & E. Tiegerman, *Language and communication disorders in children.* New York: Merrill/Macmillan. Reprinted by permission.

In general, maternal behavior varies with the child's language level, whether the child has mental retardation or is developing normally (Rondal, 1978). Mothers of children with mental retardation talk more to their children (Berger & Cunningham, 1983). By attributing more meaning to their children's less frequent behaviors, these mothers are able to interact more frequently (Yoder & Feagans, 1988). In short, mothers of children with mental retardation interpret more of their children's behaviors as communicative than do mothers of children developing normally.

Mothers of children with mental retardation match their verbal behavior to the child's language ability while adopting a teaching role themselves (Davis, Stroud, & Green, 1988). Within teaching situations, mothers of children with mental retardation and without both use a directive style, although mothers of children with mental retardation continue this style into play interactions. Although they exert more control in play than do mothers of children developing normally, mothers of children with Down syndrome are equally or more responsive (Tannock, 1988a, 1988b).

Control includes trying to elicit more responses from their children. Although this elicitation occurs more frequently, it does not occur at a greater rate than that of mothers of children developing normally because the mothers of children with mental retardation talk more overall to their children. When their children do not respond, these mothers often repeat their previous utterance (Maurer & Sherrod, 1987). The result is that mothers of children with Down syndrome take more turns even though their children respond more passively than do children developing normally.

Processing factors.   There may be differences in the cognitive, or information–processing, abilities of the mentally retarded population that cannot be attributed to low IQ alone (Das, Kirby, & Jarman, 1975; Detterman, 1979; Greenspan, 1979; Spitz, 1979; Stephans & McLaughlin, 1974). Children with mental retardation do not seem to process information in the same manner as mental–age-matched peers developing normally. This difference is especially critical for **learning,** which we shall define as a change in behavior that results from rehearsal. Cognitive abilities important for learning are attention, discrimination, organization, memory, and transfer. These are displayed schematically in Figure 2.1.

Each individual processes information in a somewhat different manner. These differences can be explained by structural differences in the brain and by functional or learned differences, such as the way one learned to learn or to solve problems. These learned differences influence, among other things, decisions about attending, schemes for organization, and rules and strategies for approaching new problems.

Attention.   Attention includes awareness and active cognitive processing. As noted in Figure 2.1, we do not attend to all stimuli. Attention may be momentary or may extend over time. In general, individuals with mild retardation can sustain attention as well as mental–age–matched peers who are nonretarded

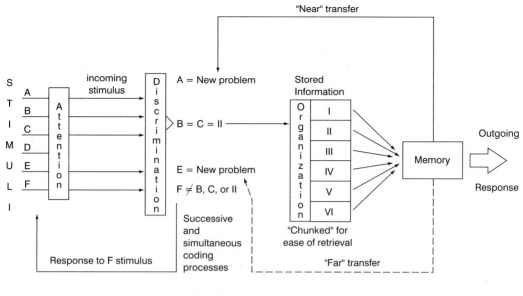

FIGURE 2.1
Schematic representation of information processing
Source: Bernstein, D., & Tiegerman, E. (1993). *Language and Communication Disorders in Children.* New York: Merrill/Macmillan. Reprinted by permission.

(Karrer, Nelson, & Galbraith, 1979). Difficulty comes for the individual with mental retardation in the scanning and selection of stimuli to which to attend.

Discrimination.   Discrimination is the ability to identify stimuli from a field of competing stimuli. Decisions are made on similarity and dissimilarity of stimuli. In Figure 2.1, Stimuli B and C are similar to each other and to other information stored previously in Area II. In general, individuals with mental retardation have difficulty identifying relevant stimulus cues (Mercer & Snell, 1977; Zeaman & House, 1979). This difficulty reflects, in part, the tendency of individuals with mental retardation to attend to fewer dimensions of a task than do individuals who are nonretarded. If the stimulus dimensions chosen are not the salient ones, the individual's ability to discriminate and to compare new information to stored information is limited. Discrimination can be taught, however, and individuals with mental retardation can apply this information to discrimination tasks as well as can individuals who are nonretarded (Ross & Ross, 1979).

In general, discrimination ability and speed are related to severity of mental retardation. The more severe the retardation, the slower and less accurate the discrimination. Persons with severe or profound mental retardation have more limited attentional capacity and are less efficient at attention allocation (Nugent & Mosley, 1987).

Organization.   Organization is the categorizing or "chunking" of information for storage and is extremely important for later retrieval. Information that is organized is more easily retrievable. Material that is unorganized or organized poorly will hinder later recall and quickly will overload memory capacity. More efficient processing requires increasingly better organization, which, in turn, leaves more room for more information (Case, 1978). Capacity for long-term storage is virtually unlimited.

In general, individuals with mild-moderate mental retardation have difficulty developing organizational strategies to aid storage and retrieval (Spitz, 1966). They do not seem to rely on mediational or associative strategies or to use them as efficiently as individuals who are nonretarded. In **mediational strategies,** a word or a symbol, such as a category name, forms a link between two entities. In **associative strategies,** one word or symbol aids in recall of another, as in "bacon and ___" or "salt and ___."

Information coming into the brain for processing enters and undergoes two types of synthesis: simultaneous and successive (Cummins, 1979a; Cummins & Das, 1978; Luria, 1975). **Simultaneous synthesis or coding** is related to higher thought, and separate elements are synthesized into groups so that all members of the group can be retrieved simultaneously. Overall meaning of language, rather than individual syntactic or phonological units, is coded. **Successive synthesis or coding** occurs in linear fashion, one at a time. Language would be processed at the unit level, rather than holistically. Both processes are used for encoding and decoding of information, both linguistic and nonlinguistic.

Individuals with mild mental retardation exhibit both types of coding (Jarman, 1978; Jarman & Das, 1977); however, these individuals may use these processes differently from individuals who are nonretarded, especially in complex tasks (Das, Kirby, & Jarman, 1979). In addition, individuals with Down syndrome seem to have greater difficulty with successive processing than do other mental–age-matched retarded individuals. This deficit may explain, in part, the poor auditory memory and expressive language abilities of individuals with Down syndrome (Burr & Rohr, 1978; Sommers & Starkey, 1977).

Transfer.   Transfer, or generalization, is the application of previously learned material in the solving of similar but novel problems or in similar but novel situations. This area of processing is especially difficult for individuals with mental retardation. Although learning may enhance performance, it does not enhance generalization (Borkowski & Cavanaugh, 1979; A. Taylor & Turnure, 1979). In general, the more severe a person's mental retardation, the weaker his transfer abilities (Bricker, Heal, Bricker, Hayes, & Larsen, 1969; N. Ellis et al., 1982; Reid, 1980).

There are two types of transfer: near and far. *Near transfer* involves only minimal changes between known information and the novel problem; *far transfer* involves substantial changes. In Figure 2.1, Stimulus A is similar enough to stored information to be considered near transfer; Stimulus E, dissimilar enough to be considered far. As might be assumed, for most individuals, near transfer is easier than far transfer. Persons with mental retardation have difficulty with both types, in part, because of an inability to detect similarities. Thus, generalization deficits may reflect discrimination and organization problems mentioned previously.

Memory. Memory involves the retrieval of previously stored information. The capacity for storage and the speed and accuracy of retrieval increases with maturity. Retrieval is limited and dependent on environmental cues; the frequency of previous retrieval; competition from other memory items, especially within the same category; and the recentness of learning. All else being equal, it is easiest to retrieve information that is frequently retrieved, has few competing memory items, has distinct environmental cues, and was learned recently.

In general, individuals with mental retardation demonstrate poorer recall than individuals developing normally. The more severe the retardation, the poorer the memory skills. Individuals with mild-moderate mental retardation are able to retain information within long-term memory as well as individuals who are nonretarded, although the retrieval process is slower (Belmont, 1967; Merrill, 1985). No doubt, organizational deficits contribute to difficulty retrieving information.

More obvious differences between the retarded and nonretarded population can be seen in short-term memory (A. Brown, 1974; Butterfield, Wambold, & Belmont, 1973; Gutowski & Chechile, 1987). Poor performance by individuals with mild mental retardation may reflect a limited use of associational strategies and organizational/storage deficits. It may be affected also by the rapid rate of forgetting found in the retarded population, especially within the first 10 seconds (N. Ellis, Deacon, & Wooldridge, 1985).

Information is retained by rehearsal. It appears that individuals with mental retardation do not spontaneously rehearse (N. Bray, 1979; A. Brown, 1974; Butterfield et al., 1973; Frank & Rabinovitch, 1974; Kellas, Ashcroft, & Johnson, 1973; Reid, 1980) and that they need more time than individuals who are nonretarded to do so (Turner & Bray, 1985).

Memory can be affected also by the type of information. Individuals with mental retardation do more poorly with auditory information than with visual (N. Ellis, Woodley-Zanthos, & Dulaney, 1989). Within auditory information, nonlinguistic signals, such as a car horn or a doorbell, are much easier for individuals with mental retardation to remember than linguistic information (Lamberts, 1981). In general, nonlinguistic signals can be recognized and recalled similarly by individuals with retardation and without. It is in the recall of linguistic information that differences become evident.

Sentence recall involves reproduction from memory and editing of the recalled text (Kintsch & van Dijk, 1978). Difficulty probably is encountered by individuals with mental retardation in the second stage (Bilsky, Walker, & Sakales, 1983).

Auditory memory deficits are exhibited more by individuals with Down syndrome than by those with other types of retardation (Marcell & Weeks, 1988). This difficulty may be related to poor echoic memory, a passive retention strategy that enables the hearer to continue to hear a sound after it has ceased (Watkins & Watkins, 1980). It seems that the echo decays more rapidly among individuals with Down syndrome than among individuals developing normally (Marcell & Armstrong, 1982).

Problems in information processing help us understand mental retardation and other disorders but do not explain these disorders. Differences may represent the cause, the result, or a concurrent problem (Leonard, 1987).

Conclusion

Generalizations about the language skills of the retarded population are complicated by the many causes of mental retardation and by different severities. Overall, language development follows a path similar to normal development but at a slower pace. Still, differences occur, such as the reliance on less mature forms and the overuse of others. These differences may reflect the information–processing difference found in individuals with mental retardation, especially in the areas of organization and memory.

Language Learning Disability

The National Joint Council on Learning Disabilities (1991) has adopted the following definition of learning disabilities:

> Learning disability is a general term that refers to a heterogeneous group of disorders manifested by significant difficulties in the acquisition and use of listening, speaking, reading, writing, reasoning, or mathematical abilities. These disorders are intrinsic to the individual, presumed to be due to central nervous system dysfunction, and may occur across the lifespan. Problems in self–regulatory behaviors, social perception, and social interaction may exist with learning disabilities but do not by themselves constitute a learning disability. Although learning disabilities may occur concomitantly with other handicapping conditions . . . or with extrinsic influences . . ., they are not the result of those conditions or influences. (p. 19)

As with other disorders, learning disability is characterized by heterogeneity. It is also important to note that the cause is presumed to be *central nervous system dysfunction,* although other conditions also may be present. The cause of learning failure is not environmental, nor is it these other accompanying conditions. Although not stated, it is assumed that children with learning disabilities have normal or near-normal intelligence.

Most children will not have all of the characteristics of learning disabilities. For example, approximately 15% have difficulty with motor learning and coordination. More than 75% have difficulty learning and using symbols (Miniutti, 1991). These children are considered to have a *language learning disability* (LLD).

The characteristics of children with learning disabilities are many and varied. In general, they divide into six categories: motor, attention, perception, symbol, memory, and emotion. Symbol difficulties are discussed under language characteristics. It should be stressed that these characteristics are not the cause of the disorder, but rather are the result of it. These characteristics interact with each other, however, so that poor attention is related to poor perception, which, in turn, affects memory.

Motor difficulties usually involve **hyperactivity,** a condition of overactivity in which children seem to be constantly in motion. Even in a camp situation in which I worked, children with learning disabilities and hyperactivity would be active all day and still evidence plenty of energy well into the night. Approximately 5% of all children have hyperactivity, but the condition is nine times as prevalent in boys as in girls (Sattler, 1988). Not all children with hyperactivity have learning disabilities, nor do all children with learning disabilities have hyperactivity. The condition is difficult to assess, especially among preschoolers, in part because of the wide range of variability (S. Campbell, 1985).

Children with hyperactivity have difficulty attending and concentrating for more than very short periods of time. Unlike children with autism who may be hyperactive at one time and hypoactive at another, children with hyperactivity are always up. Other motor difficulties may include poor sense of body movement, poorly defined handedness, poor eye-hand coordination, and poorly defined concepts of space and time.

Attentional difficulties include a short attention span and inattentiveness. Children with learning disabilities seem easily distracted by irrelevant stimuli and easily overstimulated. Other children with learning disabilities may become fixed on a single task or behavior and repeat it. This fixation is called **perseveration.** Several children with whom I have worked would repeat an utterance over and over, seemingly unaware that they were doing it.

Perception and reception are not the same. Learning disability is not a sensory or reception disorder. Perceptual difficulties are interpretational difficulties. These occur after the stimuli are received. As might be assumed, children with learning disabilities may confuse similar sounds and words, and similar printed letters and words. In addition, these children may have difficulty in *figure-ground* perception and in *sensory integration.* Figure-ground perception involves being able to isolate a stimulus against a background of competing stimuli. For example, figure-ground discrimination, on the one hand, would include being able to listen to the teacher while other things are occurring in the classroom. Sensory integration, on the other hand, involves being able to make sense of visual and auditory stimuli occurring at the same time. Each may carry part of the message. For example, gestures, facial expression, body language, intonation, and verbal language may be used to convey information. Each alone may be insufficient.

Memory difficulties include short-term storage and retrieval problems. Children with learning disabilities often have difficulty remembering directions, names, and sequences. Word-finding problems are also common.

Finally, emotional problems also may accompany learning disabilities but are not generally believed to be a causal factor. Rather, emotional problems are a reaction to or an accompaniment to the frustrating situation in which these children find themselves. Children with learning disabilities have been described as aggressive, impulsive, unpredictable, withdrawn, and impatient. Some children may exercise poor judgment, have unusual fears, and/or adjust poorly to change.

I worked with a child with learning disabilities who was afraid of shoes, a rather unusual fear. In others, poor adjustment to change may reflect dependence on routines when one has difficulty interpreting language in those contexts.

Language Characteristics

Usually all aspects of language, spoken and written, are affected in children with LLD. It should be stressed again that although these children may play the TV or radio at a loud volume, or seem to talk too loudly, or squint and rub their eyes when reading, *the problem is not sensory.* Nothing is wrong with their hearing or vision that is causing the problem. Difficulties are perceptual. This is not to say that hearing and vision problems are nonexistent among these children. Such problems can occur in any population but are not the cause of the language learning disability.

Children with LLD may have difficulty with the give-and-take of conversation and with the form and content of language (Table 2.4). Synthesizing of language rules seems to be particularly difficult, resulting in delays in morphological rule acquisition and in the development of syntactic complexity (Golick, 1976;

TABLE 2.4
Language characteristics of children with language learning disability

Pragmatics	Little problem with turn taking. Difficulty answering questions or requesting clarification. Difficulty initiating or maintaining a conversation.
Semantics	Relational term difficulty (comparative, spatial, temporal). Figurative language and dual definition problems. Word-finding and definitional problems. Conjunction (*and, but, so, because,* etc.) confusion.
Syntax/Morphology	Difficulty with negative and passive constructions, relative clauses, contractions, and adjectival forms. Difficulty with verb tense markers, possession, and pronouns. Able to repeat sentences but often in reduced form, indicating difficulty learning different sentence forms. Article (*a, an, the*) confusion.
Phonology	Inconsistent sound production, especially as complexity increases.
Comprehension	*Wh-* question confusion. Receptive vocabulary similar to that of chronological age-matched peers developing normally. Poor strategies for interacting with printed information. Confusion of letters that look similar and words that sound similar.

Source: Based on Baker, Ceci, & Hermann (1987); Bryan (1981); Catts (1986); Denckla & Rudel (1976a, 1976b); Edwards & Kallail (1977); D. Johnson & Myklebust (1967); Kail & Leonard (1986); Lieberman, Meskill, Chatillon, & Schupack (1985); Menyuk & Looney (1972); Moran & Bryne (1977); Nippold & Fey (1983); Seidenberg & Bernstein (1986); Vogel (1975); Wiig & Semel (1973, 1974, 1975, 1976); Wiig, Semel, & Crouse (1973)

Rosenthal, 1970; Wiig & Roach, 1975; Wiig & Semel, 1976; Wiig, Semel, & Crouse, 1973). In short, all areas of language are affected.

Word–finding is a particular problem found in both conversations and narratives (German, 1987), resulting in greater time needed to respond verbally (Wiig, Semel, & Nystrom, 1982). Retrieval difficulties may result in more communication breakdown (MacLachlan & Chapman, 1988), characterized by repetitions, especially of pronouns before words seemingly difficult to retrieve ("*He, he, he* . . . John was . . . "), reformulations, substitutions of indefinite pronouns (*it*), empty words (*one, thing*), delays, and insertions ("He was . . . *oh, I can't remember* . . .)(German & Simon, 1991).

Overall oral language development for children with LLD may be slow (Reed, 1986). Their language is often like that of younger children, although children with LLD may use more mature structures less frequently (Leonard, 1979). As preschoolers, these children may exhibit little interest in language, unable to follow a story or disinterested in books.

Word–retrieval difficulties may reflect the deficient vocabularies of children with LLD (Leonard, 1990; Snyder, 1984; Wiig, 1990). Young children with LLD have poor understanding of literal meanings (Rizzo & Stephens, 1981). As these children age, they experiecne difficulties with multiple and figurative meanings (R. Lee & Kamhi, 1990; Lutzer, 1988; Nippold & Fey, 1983; Nippold, Stephens, & Fey, 1983; Seidenberg & Bernstein, 1986; Wiig, 1990; Wiig & Semel, 1984).

The linguistic demands of the classroom are often well above the oral language abilities of these children. The well–documented academic underachievement of children with LLD demonstrates the link between language deficits and learning disabilities (Catts & Kamhi, 1986; Liberman, 1983). Oral language skills are the single best indicator of reading and writing success in school. Difficulty with oral language skills among children with LLD is evidenced later in written language and learning problems, called dyslexia and dysgraphia (Doehring, Trites, Patel, & Fiedorowicz, 1981; Gillam & Johnston, 1985; Maxwell & Wallach, 1984; Rubin, 1988; Stark & Tallal, 1988; Vogel, 1983).

Dyslexia is a reading disorder characterized by word recognition and/or reading comprehension abilities 2 years below the expected level due to no known emotional, environmental, intellectual, perceptual, or obvious neurological problem (Vellutino, 1979). Word-recognition problems may reflect deficits that underlie both reading and word finding (Casby, 1992; Wolf & Segal, 1992). In fact, naming and reading problems co-occur in dyslexia, indicating a relationship between the two (Ackerman, Dykman, & Gardner, 1990; Blachman, 1984; Bowers, Steffy, & Swanson, 1986; Denckla & Rudel, 1976a, 1976b; A. Ellis, 1981; Spring & Farmer, 1975; Wolf, 1979). Naming speed and reading seem independent of phonological awareness but related to each other, possibly sharing processes related to speed (Bowers & Swanson, 1991; Felton & Brown, 1990; Mann, 1984). Slower letter- and word-naming speeds may impede decoding and word-recognition processes (Wolf & Segal, 1992).

Dysgraphia is difficulty writing, especially with the motor skills involved. Obviously, writing involves much more, including the integration of linguistic, cognitive, and motor skills, thus presenting a formidable challenge to children with LLD. Writing problems among these children often persist into adolescence and adulthood (Blalock, 1981; Isaacson, 1987; Moran, Schumaker, & Vetter, 1981). Difficulties include spelling errors, word omission and substitution, punctuation, agrammatical sentences, and lack of organization (Englert & Thomas, 1987; Gerber, 1986; Wiig & Semel, 1976). These errors often reflect an underlying deficiency in syntactic and morphological knowledge (Rubin, Patterson, & Kantor, 1991). Writing difficulties become even more evident as the child progresses through school (Gerber, 1984; Poplin, Gray, Larsen, Banikowski, & Mehring, 1980).

Although reading and writing are different, certain underlying processes influence both. They are interrelated; therefore, difficulties in one are seen in the other. For example, often there is no overall organization to the writing of children with LLD. In reading, they also fail to understand the underlying organization, thus treating each sentence as separate and unrelated to the whole (Raphael & Englert, 1990; Seidenberg, 1989).

The behavior of children with LLD also demonstrates the interrelatedness of cognition and language. This relationship can be seen in analogical reasoning skills in which known concepts are used to solve novel problems. In verbal proposition (A is to B as C is to __), one type of analogical reasoning, language abilities appear to be more important than, but not exclusive of, cognitive abilities (Masterson, Evans, & Aloia, 1993). Children with LLD demonstrate difficulty with verbal analogies such as these (Kamhi, Gentry, Mauer, & Gholson, 1990; Nippold, Erskine, & Freed, 1988).

Possible Causal Factors

Several causal factors may contribute to language learning disability. Central nervous system dysfunction indicates a strong biological basis, but information processing, especially perception, is equally important.

Biological factors.   Learning disabilities occur more frequently in families with a history of the disorder and following premature or difficult birth. These facts, along with central nervous system dysfunction, demonstrate a biological link to the disorder. In addition, the use of neurostimulants, such a Ritalin, to stimulate neurotransmitters and enable children with hyperactivity to concentrate and attend further suggests a biological basis for some learning disabilities. The result is long-term academic and learning improvement (Gittelman-Klein & Klein, 1976; Rie & Rie, 1977; Rie, Rie, & Stewart, 1976; Zametkin & Rapoport, 1987).

It has been suggested that a breakdown occurs along the neural pathways that connect the midbrain with the frontal cortex. This is the area of the brain responsible for attention, regulation, and planning (Bass, 1988).

Biological factors alone are insufficient to explain the characteristics that accompany learning disability. For those, we must look to other causal factors.

Social-environmental factors.   Although our definition of learning disability precluded any environmental causality, certain environmental factors are important. The well–documented language and, in turn, interactional difficulties of children with LLD certainly will influence the child's development.

Similarly, many of the acting-out behaviors of these children are in response to the very frustrating situation of their lives. Until the disorder is diagnosed, these children are accused of not trying or of being lazy or stupid. Many of the children with whom I have worked had extremely poor self–images. Many were afraid to try anything new; others would do anything for attention and recognition, even if such recognition were negative. The successes or failures that we have as we interact with others have a great influence on our future interactions.

Processing factors. Children with LLD do not appear to function in a manner appropriate for their intellectual level. They seem unable to use certain strategies or to access certain stored information.

Children with LLD exercise poor attentional selectivity, concentrating on inappropriate or unimportant stimuli (Levine, 1987). Appropriate and important information may be screened out along with other information. These children have difficulty deciding on the relevant information to which to attend.

As mentioned previously, discrimination is extremely difficult for children with LLD. The child has difficulty deciding on the relevant aspects of a stimulus that make it similar or dissimilar to another. Children with LLD do more poorly than mental–age–matched peers on rule extraction or identification from repeated exposures (Masterson, 1993b).

Obviously, information that is poorly attended to and poorly discriminated will be poorly organized. These are children for whom the world often does not make sense, especially linguistically. Their storage categories reflect this confusion. Unlike children with mental retardation, who do not organize spontaneously, children with LLD do organize information but too inefficiently for easy retrieval.

Memory is related to storage or availability and retrieval or accessibility, distinct but related processes (Bjork & Bjork, 1992). Growth in word knowledge results in larger storage capacity by creating semantic networks in which words are related and organized. This growth occurs later and more slowly among children with LLD (Leonard, 1990; Reed, 1986; Rizzo & Stephens, 1981; Snyder, 1984; Wiig, 1990). One result is less accurate and slower retrieval by children with LLD (Garnett & Fleischner, 1983; German, 1984; Leonard, Nippold, Kail, & Hale, 1983; Wolf, Bally, & Morris, 1986).

Effective learners actively process, interpret, and synthesize information by using effective strategies to monitor and organize learning (A. Brown, 1978; Flavell, 1978). Children with LLD often fail to access or use task–appropriate strategies spontaneously (A. Brown, 1980; Sternberg & Wagner, 1982; Torgesen, 1977, 1982). These problems persist throughout adolescence and into adulthood (Alley, Deshler, & Warner, 1979; Faford & Haubrich, 1981; Gottesman, 1979).

Conclusion

Language learning disability is an extremely complex concept. Although it is relatively easy to describe the outward behaviors of children with LLD, it is very difficult to explain the underlying processes. In short, biological or neurostructural differences and functional neuroprocessing differences in children with LLD affect their ability to attend to, discriminate, and remember linguistic and other stimuli, resulting in language that may be impaired in all aspects and in all modes of transmission and reception.

Specific Language Impairment

Specific language impairment (SLI) can be characterized as "significant limitations in language functioning that cannot be attributed to deficits in hearing, oral structure and function, or general intelligence" (Leonard, 1987, p. 1). In other words, this category of language impairment has no obvious cause and seems not to affect or be affected by anatomical, physical, or intellectual problems. Unlike children with mental retardation, but similar to those with language learning disability, children with SLI exhibit language performance scores significantly lower than their intellectual performance scores on nonverbal tasks. Unlike children with LLD, children with SLI do not exhibit perceptual difficulties.

Children with SLI are a heterogeneous group in their language skills, characterized by several distinct subtypes (Aram, 1991; Aram & Nation, 1975; Stark & Tallal, 1988). In fact, SLI is characterized more by the exclusion of other disorders than on some readily identifiable trait or behavior (Leonard, 1991). This situation has complicated research, especially the selection criteria for subject selection (McCauley & Demetras, 1990). Similarly, clinical identification is difficult and is usually based on the absence of other contributing factors. This situation has led some to conclude that "for a large portion, probably the majority, of children so-classified, the category is inappropriate" (Dale & Cole, 1991, p. 80).

Even with a paucity of criteria for characterizing children with SLI, we can make certain definitive statements. Children with SLI may appear to be delayed in one aspect of language, although the language problem is not the result of delay, and children with SLI will not catch up to other children their age without intervention (Leonard, 1991). Even in their apparent delay, children with SLI are unlike children developing normally at any stage of development (J. Johnston, 1988; Leonard, 1991).

Language Characteristics

As with other language impairments, significant language differences are seen across children. The language impairment may be primarily, but not exclusively, expressive or receptive, or a combination of the two, and affect different aspects of language, although language form seems to be affected more than other aspects (Aram, 1991; J. Johnston & Kamhi, 1984; N. Nelson, 1993). In addition, the disorder changes within the individual child, especially with age. Errors seen in speech may be present also in writing (Gillam & Johnston, 1992).

In general, children with SLI have difficulty (a) extracting regularities from the language around them, (b) registering different contexts for language, and (c) constructing word-referent associations for lexical growth (Ellis Weismer, 1991; Leonard,

1987). The result is difficulty in morphological and phonological rule formation and application and in vocabulary development (Bishop, 1979, 1982; Bishop & Adams, 1992; Ellis Weismer, 1991; Rice, Buhr, & Oetting, 1992; van der Lely & Harris, 1990). Pragmatic problems result from inability to use effective forms to accomplish language intentions. Specific language problems are listed in Table 2.5.

The conversational behaviors of children with SLI compared with those of mental–age–matched peers developing normally are marked by both qualitative

TABLE 2.5
Language characteristics of children with specific language impairment

Pragmatics	May act like younger children developing normally.
	Less flexibility in their language when tailoring the message to the listener or repairing communication breakdowns.
	Same pragmatic functions as chronological age-matched peers developing normally, but expressed differently and less effectively.
	Less effective than chronological age-matched peers in securing a conversational turn. Those with receptive difficulties most affected.
Semantics	First words and subsequent vocabulary development occurs at a slower rate, with occasional lexical errors seen in younger children developing normally.
	Naming difficulties may reflect less rich and less elaborate semantic storage than actual retrieval difficulties. Long-term memory storage problems are probable.
Syntax/Morphology	Co-occurrence of more mature and less mature forms.
	Similar developmental order to that seen in children developing normally.
	Fewer morphemes, especially verb endings, auxiliary verbs, and function words (articles, prepositions) than younger MLU-matched peers. Learning related to grammatical function as in children developing normally.
	Tend to make pronoun errors, as do younger MLU-matched peers, but tend to overuse one form rather than making random errors.
Phonology	Phonological processes similar to those of younger children developing normally, but in different patterns, i.e. occurring in units of varying word length rather than in one- or two-word utterances.
Comprehension	Poor discrimination of units of short duration (bound morphemes).

Source: Based on Albertini (1980); Beastrom & Rice (1986); Bliss (1989); Brinton, Fujiki, Winkler, & Loeb (1986); Craig & Evans (1993); Craig & Washington (1993); Gallagher & Craig (1984); J. Johnston & Kamhi (1984); J. Johnston & Schery (1976); Kail, Hale, Leonard, & Nippold (1984); Kail & Leonard (1986); Khan & James (1983); Leonard (1980, 1986, 1989); Leonard, McGregor, & Allen (1992); Liles (1985a, 1985b); Loeb & Leonard (1988); Merritt & Liles (1987); Paul & Shriberg (1982); Rice & Oetting (1993); Rice, Oetting, Marquis, Bode, & Pae (1994); Watkins & Rice (1989)

and quantitative differences (Craig, 1993). Qualitative differences, such as difficulty initiating interaction and inappropriate responses, lead to increased interruptions by other children and other quantitative changes. The child with SLI is less likely to interact with other children over time as the child experiences repeated failure. As a result, children with SLI often are ignored by other children in the classroom and experience reduced interactional opportunities.

As might be expected, given the auditory processing problems of children with SLI, morphological inflections, such as past tense -ed and plural -s; and function words, such as prepositions and articles (a/the), are especially difficult (Dale & Cole, 1991; Leonard, McGregor, & Allen, 1992). These morphemes are small units of language that receive little stress or emphasis in speech. Verb endings and auxiliary verbs pose a particular problem, as does use of pronouns (Albertini, 1980; Frome, Loeb & Leonard, 1991; J. Johnston & Schery, 1976; Khan & James, 1983; Leonard, 1982). The two problems are related because pronoun selection (he vs. they) determines verb endings (walks vs. walk) (Connell, 1986a).

Language comprehension and processing are active processes in which the listener infers the meaning from the auditory message, contextual information, and stored world and word knowledge. Children with SLI do not appear to employ actively all of this available information. In general, children with SLI have difficulty constructing an integrated representation of a series of events, whether the series is presented verbally or nonverbally (Bishop & Adams, 1992). Thus, vocabulary growth—which occurs as the result of inferring meaning from repeated exposure and without direct reference or prompting from adults—will be very difficult for the child with SLI using limited active processing strategies (Rice, Buhr, & Nemeth, 1990; Rice et al., 1992).

Difficulty forming internal representations can also be seen in the play of children with SLI (Rescorla & Goossens, 1992). In general, toddlers and preschoolers with SLI exhibit less non-object play, less well developed sequential play, and fewer occurrences of symbolic play than chronological age-matched peers. The two groups exhibit equal engagement with toys and functional conversational play behavior. Overall, children with SLI develop play in the same manner as do children developing normally but at a slower pace (Roth & Clark, 1987; Skarakis-Doyle & Prutting, 1988; B. Terrell, Schwartz, Prelock, & Messick, 1984; Udwin & Yule, 1983).

Possible Causal Factors

Causes of SLI are as difficult to determine and may be as diverse as the children who have the impairment (J. Johnston, 1991; Tomblin, 1991). With such a diverse population, it is not surprising that several possible causal factors have been identified.

Biological factors.   Possible biological factors include brain asymmetry, in which language functions are located in different areas from those found in the majority of individuals, and delayed myelination, the progressive process of nerve sheathing that results in more rapid transmission of impulses (Galaburda, 1989; Hynd,

Marshall, & Gonzalez, 1991; Kinsbourne, 1981; Love & Webb, 1986). The reported adeptness of children with SLI in analyzing visual, spatial patterns is considered by some to be evidence of greater reliance on the right hemisphere of the brain (J. Johnston, 1982a). Language processing, at least linear or sequential processing, is concentrated in the left temporal lobe.

Processing factors.   Although children with SLI demonstrate normal nonverbal intelligence, they may also demonstrate cognitive impairments not exhibited on standard intelligence measures (J. Johnston, 1982a, 1988b; Kamhi, Catts, Koenig, & Lewis, 1984; Kamhi, Minor, & Mauer, 1990; Leonard, 1987). Information–processing problems of children with SLI occur in processing incoming information, in memory, and in problem solving (Ellis Weismer, 1991; Hoskins, 1979; L. Nelson, Kamhi, & Apel, 1987). Although interpretation of rapid, sequenced auditory processing, especially of linguistic information, is difficult, isolated nonlinguistic signal processing seems normal (Stark & Tallal, 1981; Tallal & Piercy, 1973a, 1973b, 1974, 1975; Tallal & Stark, 1981). Rapid, sequenced visual and tactile stimuli are also difficult to interpret (Tallal, Stark, Kallman, & Mellitis, 1981). As mentioned previously, these children do not seem to employ active processing strategies that use contextual information and stored knowledge.

Short-term auditory sequential memory and problem solving of complex reasoning tasks are also affected in children with SLI (J. Johnston & Smith, 1989; Kamhi, Gentry et al., 1990; L. Nelson et al., 1987). It is not surprising that auditory sequential memory is difficult because this is the type of information the child is having difficulty processing. Similarly, problem solving is also an active process that requires use of contextual information and prior knowledge. It should be noted, however, that when children with SLI are matched with younger children possessing the same language abilities, differences in short–term auditory memory disappear (van der Lely & Howard, 1993).

Conclusion

Much discussion has taken place concerning the viability of SLI as a separate category of language impairment. It has been suggested that SLI is not a distinct disorder category, but merely represents children with limited language abilities as the result of genetic and/or environmental factors (Leonard, 1987, 1991; Tomblin, 1991). It is possible, as some have suggested, that children with SLI represent the lowest range of normal population and not a distinct group.

Morphological difficulties seen in children with SLI may reflect the difficulty of this type of learning and the overall linguistic competence of individual children. Morphology is the language component most tied to overall language learning ability (Dale & Cole, 1991).

Even the language-nonverbal intelligence gap found in children with SLI may not be definitive. Approximately 28% of the normal population has verbal IQ scores at least 15 points below nonverbal IQ scores (Leonard, 1987). It is possible that this discrepancy is a natural and predictable variation in child language developmental delay (K. Cole, Dale, & Mills, 1990).

Some educators have suggested that SLI may not even be a useful concept, especially because clinical tools are unable to diagnose it easily and accurately (Aram, Morris, & Hall, 1993). It is possible, however, that future research will result in better methods of identification.

Autism

Autism is a disorder that is somewhat difficult to characterize because its supposed nature may be changing with the advent of new intervention, such as facilitated communication (see Chap. 13). The American Psychiatric Association (1987) defines autism as an impairment in reciprocal social interaction with a severely limited behavior, interest, and activity repertoire. The Autism Society of America further defines autism as a disorder that has an onset prior to 30 months of age and that consists of *disturbances* in the following areas (Ritvo & Freeman, 1978):

- Developmental rates and the sequence of motor, social-adaptive, and cognitive skills
- Responses to sensory stimuli—hyper- and hyposensitivity in audition, vision, tactile stimulation, motor, olfactory, and taste, including self-stimulatory behaviors
- Speech and language, cognition, and nonverbal communication, including mutism, echolalia, and difficulty with abstract terms
- Capacity to appropriately relate to people, events, and objects, including lack of social behaviors, affection, and appropriate play

As in other language impairments discussed in this chapter, children with autism are a diverse group. For example, to the best of our ability to measure, slightly more than half of the children with autism have IQs below 50, with the remainder evenly split between 50–70 and 71 and above (Schreibman, 1988).

Some of the points raised in the definition of autism need an explanation, although communication is discussed in more detail later. First, it is rare that the disorder is identified prior to 18 months of age. Therefore, descriptions of infancy are retrospective. Infants with autism have been described as either lethargic, preferring solitude and making few demands, or highly irritable, with sleeping problems and screaming and crying (Coleman & Gillberg, 1985). Usually, between 18 and 36 months, the signs become more pronounced, including more frequent tantruming, repetitive movements and ritualistic play, extreme reactions to certain stimuli, lack of social play, and communication difficulties (Freeman & Ritvo, 1984; Ornitz, Guthrie, & Farley, 1977).

In approximately 20% of the cases, parents report normal development until 24 months (Freeman & Ritvo, 1984). Early identification is often difficult because of the lack of obvious medical problems and the early normal development of motor abilities. Infrequently, onset occurs in later childhood.

Development often proceeds in spurts and plateaus, rather than smoothly. Most areas of development are affected by delay and disorder, although occasionally one area, such as mechanical or mathematical abilities, is normal or above. I have worked with children well above average in mathematics but unable to dress themselves or to participate in meaningful conversations. Motor behaviors may include toe walking, rocking, spinning, and, in extreme cases, self-injurious behaviors, such as biting, hitting, and head banging. One adolescent with whom I worked was covered with scars and scabs from self-inflicted scratches and bites. Another child pounded his head with his fist an average of more than 7,000 times in a 5-hour school day.

Hyper- and hyposensitivity to stimuli may be found in the same child. For example, loud noises may get no response from the child, while whispering results in a catastrophic response. In general, children with autism tend to prefer shiny objects, especially those that spin; things that can be twirled; and noises they produce themselves, such as teeth grinding. Children with autism seem to prefer routines and may become extremely upset with change. Individual children may have very definite preferences in taste, touch, and smell. I worked with one child whose only food preference was dill pickles. Self-stimulatory behaviors may include rocking, spinning, and hand flapping.

Relational disorders may be the most distressful aspect of autism, especially for parents (Bristol, 1988). In particular, children with autism often avert their gaze or stare emptily and lack a social smile, responsiveness to sound, and anticipation of the approach of others (Ornitz et al., 1977). Parents often are treated as "things" or, at best, no different from other people. The effect on parents can be imagined.

Language Characteristics

Communication problems are often one of the first indicators of possible autism. These may include a failure to begin gesturing or talking, a seeming non-interest in other people, or a lack of verbal responding.

Poor social interaction and poor communication skills are extremely characteristic of children with autism. The main problem is one of language and communication; speech does not seem to be difficult (Schuler & Prizant, 1987). For those who speak, speech is often wooden and robotlike, lacking a musical quality.

A significant portion of the autistic population, between 25 and 60%, remains mute or nonspeaking (Fish, Shapiro, & Campbell, 1966; Paluszny, 1979). Until recently, this lack of speech also has meant that they remained noncommunicating. This situation is changing for some, but not all, children using **facilitated communication,** an augmentative communication technique in which the child's hand is assisted as he points to different letters and spells his message.

Those children using speech and language may demonstrate immediate or delayed **echolalia,** a whole or partial repetition of previous utterances, often with the same intonation. Immediate echolalia is variable, increasing in highly directive situations, with unknown words, following an inability to comprehend, in the presence of an adult, in unfamiliar situations, in face-to-face communication with eye contact, and with longer, more complex utterances (B. Campbell & Grieve, 1978; Carr, Schreibman, & Lovaas, 1975; Charlop, 1986; Fay & Anderson, 1981; Paccia–Cooper & Curcio, 1982; Violette & Swisher, 1992). Immediate echolalia also has been found to signal agreement in some children (Prizant & Duchan, 1981). No such data are available for delayed echolalia. One child with whom I worked would repeat many of the utterances directed to him during the day as he lay in bed prior to sleep. Even though echolalia may be outgrown, other problems, especially those related to pragmatics, persist in the child's language (Lord, 1988).

In general, pragmatics and semantics are affected more than language form (Tager-Flusberg, 1981a, 1981b). The give-and-take of conversation seems to be particularly difficult. The range of communication functions is often very limited, and its development is sequential rather than synchronous, as seen in children developing normally (Wetherby & Prutting, 1984). In addition, functions may be expressed in an individualistic or idiosyncratic manner, such as saying "Sesame Street is a production of the Children's Television Workshop" for "Goodbye."

Children with autism also seem to have difficulty matching the content and form of language to the context (Swisher & Demetras, 1985). Occasionally, children will incorporate rote utterances, such as the child who says, "Attention, K-Mart shoppers" to get attention. Even those individuals who have acquired language often have peculiarities and irregularities in their communication. Specific language characteristics are listed in Table 2.6.

Although errors in language form occur in children with autism, these are not as severe as those for semantics and pragmatics. Syntactic errors that are present seem to represent lack of underlying semantic relationships (Bartolucci, Pierce, Streiner, & Eppel, 1976). Phonological development appears to follow the same sequence as that of children developing normally and not to be delayed inordinately (Bartolucci et al., 1976; Fay & Schuler, 1980). As noted previously, however, stress patterns and prosody may be affected.

Possible Causal Factors

In the past, children with autism have been classified as having an emotional-, physical-, environmental-, or health-related impairment. The cause may be any and all of these, although the primary causal factors are probably biological (Schreibman, 1988).

Biological factors.   Approximately 65% of all individuals with autism have abnormal brain patterns (DeMyer, 1975). The incidence of autism accompanying prenatal complications and fragile X syndrome and among those with a family history of autism is higher (Schreibman, 1988). All of these suggest a biological basis but do not explain the actual disorder. Other studies have found unusually high levels of serotonin, a neurotransmitter and natural opiate; abnormal development of the cerebellum, the section of the brain that regulates incoming sensations; multifocal disorders of the brain; and impairment of the neural subcortical structures with accompanying impairment in cortical development (Courchesne, 1988; Rapin & Allen, 1983; Schopler & Mesibov, 1987; Schreibman, 1988). In

TABLE 2.6
Language characteristics of children with autism

Pragmatics	Difficulty initiating and maintaining a conversation, so much shorter conversational episodes. Limited range of communication functions. Difficulty matching form and content to context. May perseverate or introduce inappropriate topics. Immediate and delayed echolalia and routinized utterances. Few gestures. Overuse of questions, frequent repetition. Frequent asocial monologues. Difficulty with stylistic variations and speaker-listener roles. Gaze aversion, seeming use of peripheral vision.
Semantics	Word-retrieval difficulties, especially for visual referents. Underlying meaning not used as a memory aid. More inappropriate answers to questions than age-matched peers.
Syntax/Morphology	Morphological difficulties, especially with pronouns and verb endings.[*] Construct sentences with superficial form, often disregarding underlying meaning. Less complex sentences than mental age-matched peers developing normally. Overreliance on word order.
Phonology	Phonology variable within individual child, often disordered. Developmental order similar to children developing normally. Least affected aspect of language.
Comprehension	Impaired comprehension, especially in connected discourse such as conversations.

Source: Based on Alpert & Rogers-Warren (1984); Baltaxe & Simmons (1983); Bartolucci, Streiner, & Eppel, (1976); Cantwell, Baker, & Rutter (1978); Lord (1988); Lord & O'Neill (1983); Lord et al. (in press); Rapin & Allen (1983); Rumsey, Rapoport, & Sceery (1985); Simmons & Baltaxe (1975); Swisher & Demetras (1985); Wetherby & Prutting (1984)

any case, brain dysfunction interferes with incoming signal awareness, perception, and integration.

Social-environmental factors.   Early studies blamed parents for autism. Parents were described variously as cold, unfeeling, and distant; their children behaved in reaction to this environment. No basis has been found for this conclusion. That is not to say that parental behavior is unimportant. Parents affect their children, and the children, in turn, affect their parents. In general, the parents interact with their children with autism at the appropriate language level.

Processing factors.   Children with autism have difficulty analyzing and integrating information (Dalgleish, 1975). When attending, they tend to fixate on one aspect of a complex stimulus, often some irrelevant, minor detail (Maltz, 1981).

In other words, responding is very overselective (Lovaas & Schreibman, 1971; Lovaas, Schreibman, Koegel, & Rehm, 1971). This fixation, in turn, makes discrimination difficult.

Overall processing by children with autism has been characterized as a "gestalt" method (Prizant, 1983b) in which unanalyzed wholes are stored and later reproduced in identical fashion, as in echolalia. In this relatively inflexible system, input is examined in its entirety, rather than analyzed into its component parts, such as "Attention K-Mart shoppers." Information usually is reproduced in a context that is in some way similar to the initial context, such as trying to gain attention. This reliance on unanalyzed wholes could account for the tendency of children with autism to repeat an agrammatical sentence, rather than to correct it as language-matched children with mental retardation will do. It is possible that children with autism depend more heavily on simultaneous language processing than on successive. Language use depends on being able to analyze language into rules and to use these rules creatively to generate more language.

The behavior of children with autism suggests that very little of the world makes sense to them. The storage of unanalyzed wholes may account for the reported behavioral problems accompanying increased stimulation (Bryson, 1970). Children with autism seem to overload quickly. Information "swallowed" whole could quickly "fill" the system.

Storage of unanalyzed wholes also might hinder memory. Children with autism reportedly are less able to use environmental cues to aid memory (Hermelin & O'Connor, 1967), possibly because those cues do not exist as separate entities in the child's memory. It is also difficult for children with autism to organize information on the basis of relationships between stimuli (Hermelin, 1978).

In addition, children with autism have difficulty transferring or generalizing learned information from one context to another (Koegel & Rincover, 1977). This difficulty reflects the inability of these children to identify the relevant contextual information.

Conclusion

As with other disorders that have been discussed, autism demonstrates heterogeneity. Great differences are found in severity, especially in communication abilities. In general, these differences affect the pragmatic and semantic aspects of language and may reflect processing difficulties such as stimulus overselectivity and storage of unanalyzed wholes.

Brain Injury

Children with brain injury are often confused with other children who have impairments, such as children with LLD, mental retardation, or emotional disorders. As a group, children with brain injury differ greatly as a result of the site and extent of lesion, the age at onset, and the age of the injury. In general, the smaller the damaged area, the better the **prognosis,** or chance of recovery. Other factors vary with the type of injury or are too complicated to generalize in a short chapter.

Brain injury in children may result from traumatic brain injury (TBI), cerebrovascular accident (CVA) or stroke, congenital malformation, convulsive disorders, or encephalopathy, such as infection or tumors. Each has different characteristics, although some similarities in language occur. Only the most prevalent types of injury are discussed here.

Traumatic Brain Injury (TBI)

Approximately 1 million children and adolescents in the United States have traumatic brain injury or TBI, a diffuse brain damage as the result of external physical force, such as a blow to the head received in an auto accident. TBIs are not congenital or degenerative. Individuals may range from nearly full recovery to a vegetative state in some very severe cases.

Deficits may be cognitive, physical, behavioral, academic, and linguistic (Ewing-Cobbs, Fletcher, & Levin, 1985; Rosen & Gerring, 1986; Satz & Bullard-Bates, 1981; Savage, 1991; Savage & Wolcott, 1988; Ylvisaker, 1986). *Cognitive deficits* include perception, memory, reasoning, and problem–solving difficulties. Such deficits may be permanent or temporary and may partially or totally affect functioning ability. Psychological maladjustment or "acting out" behaviors, called **social disinhibition,** may also occur. For example, I once evaluated a young man with TBI who kept insisting on kissing my hand. Other characteristics include lack of initiative, distractibility, inability to adapt quickly, perseveration, low frustration levels, passive-aggressiveness, anxiety, depression, fear of failure, and misperception.

Severity may range from a *mild concussion,* defined as a loss of consciousness for less than 30 seconds, to longer, more severe conditions. *Moderate TBI* is a loss of consciousness or post-traumatic amnesia for 30 minutes to 24 hours, with or without skull fracture. *Severe TBI* consists of a coma for 6 hours or longer. Severity is not directly related to the deficits mentioned above (Russell, 1993).

Variables that affect recovery are extremely independent among children with TBI (Lehr, 1989; Middleton, 1989; Savage, 1991). Statements about recovery are complicated by some of the characteristics of the population at risk for TBI. In general, this population has a lower IQ, higher social disadvantage, poorer schooling, and more behavioral and physical difficulties prior to injury than the general population (N. Nelson & Schwentor, 1990; Shaffer, Bijur, Chadwick, & Rutter, 1980). In the light of these facts, variables that affect recovery seem to include degree and length of unconsciousness, duration of post-traumatic amnesia, age at injury, age of injury, and post-traumatic ability (Dennis, 1992; Russell, 1993). In general, shorter, less severe unconsciousness, shorter amnesia, and better post-traumatic abilities indicate better recovery.

Age at time of injury is a less definitive factor because the child is developing when the injury occurs. Although younger children have less to recover, they also do not have the benefit of as much past learning as older children. Younger children may exhibit more severe and more long-lasting problems (Levin, Ewing-Cobbs, & Benton, 1984).

Age of the injury also can be an inaccurate predictor. In general, the older the injury, the less chance of change, but this aspect is complicated by the delayed onset of some deficits (Russell, 1993). Neural recovery over time is often unpredictable and irregular.

Language characteristics.   Language problems are usually evident even after mild injuries (Levin & Eisenberg, 1979a, 1979b). Pragmatics seem to be the most disturbed aspect of the language of children with TBI. This fact can be noted in narratives and in conversation (Liles, Coelho, Duffy, & Zalagens, 1989; Mentis & Prutting, 1987). Utterances are often lengthy, inappropriate, and off-topic, and fluency is disturbed (Winogron, Knights, & Bawden, 1984; Ylvisaker, 1986). Language comprehension and higher functions such as figurative language and dual meanings also may be affected.

By comparison, language form is relatively unaffected. Surface structure may be sufficient to convince the unknowing that language is relatively unimpaired. The child's language may seem appropriate and effective in school until the third or fourth grade, when he is required to analyze and synthesize (Russell, 1993). Semantics, especially concrete vocabulary, is also relatively undisturbed, although word retrieval, naming, and object description difficulties may be present (Ewing-Cobbs, Levin, Eisenberg, & Fletcher, 1987). Other characteristics are listed in Table 2.7.

TABLE 2.7
Language characteristics of children with traumatic brain injury (TBI)

Pragmatics	Difficulty with organization and expression of complex ideas. Off-topic comments. Ineffectual, inappropriate comments. Short narratives include story grammar and cohesion, as do those of normally developing peers.
Semantics	Word retrieval, naming, and object description difficulties, although vocabulary relatively intact. Automatized, overlearned language relatively unaffected.
Syntax/Morphology	Sentences may be lengthy and fragmented.
Phonology	Few phonological difficulties although there may be some dysarthria or apraxia due to injury.
Comprehension	Some problems due to inattention and speed of processing. Poor auditory and reading comprehension. Difficulty with sentence comprehension due to difficulty assigning meaning to syntactic structure. Most routinized, everyday comprehension unaffected. Vocabulary comprehension usually unaffected, except for abstract terms.

Source: Based on Butler-Hinz, Caplan, & Waters (1990); Ewing-Cobbs, Levin, Eisenberg, & Fletcher (1987); Groher (1983); Hagen (1984); Jordan, Murdock, & Buttsworth (1991); Levin, Benton, & Grossman (1982); Levin & Eisenberg (1979a, 1979b); Levin, Grossman, & Kelly (1976); Mentis & Prutting (1987); Sarno (1980); Sarno, Buonaguro, & Levita (1986); Savage & Wolcott (1988); Winogron, Knights, & Bawden (1984); Ylvisaker (1986)

Some deficits will remain long after the injury even when overall improvement is good (T. Campbell & Dollaghan, 1990; Ewing-Cobbs et al., 1987; Jordan, Ozanne, & Murdoch, 1988; Levin & Eisenberg, 1979a, 1979b). Although there is considerable variability among children with TBI, many subtle deficits remain, especially in pragmatics (Dennis & Barnes, 1990).

Possible causal factors. Obvious biological and physical factors are involved in TBI. More important is the manner in which informational processing is affected. As mentioned, children with TBI are often inattentive and easily distractible. Attention fluctuates, and they have difficulty focusing on a task (Levin, Eisenberg, Wigg, & Kobayoski, 1982).

All aspects of organization—categorizing, sequencing, abstracting, and generalization—are affected. Children with TBI seem stimulus-bound, unable to see relationships, make inferences, and solve problems (Cohen, 1991; Ylvisaker, 1986). They evidence difficulty formulating goals, planning, and achieving (Ylvisaker & Szekeres, 1989). This deficiency often is masked by intact vocabulary and general knowledge.

Finally, children with TBI exhibit memory deficits in both storage and retrieval. Long-term memory prior to the trauma is usually intact.

Cerebrovascular Accident (CVA)

Cerebrovascular accidents occur when a portion of the brain is denied oxygen, usually because of a rupture in a blood vessel serving the brain. Most frequently, damage is specific and localized. Patterns of recovery suggest that adjoining portions of the cortex augment the functioning of the damaged portion (Papanicolaon, DiScenna, Gillespie, & Aram, 1990).

CVAs usually are found in children with congenital heart problems or arteriovenous malformations. Prognosis is good (Aram & Ekelman, 1987; Aram, Ekelman, & Whitaker, 1986, 1987; Hecaen, 1983). Naturally, the variability will be great, depending on the site and extent of the lesion. Language problems often accompany left hemisphere damage.

Language characteristics. Long-term subtle pragmatic difficulties are common (Dennis, 1980; Visch-Brink & van de Sandt-Koenderman, 1984). Language form usually returns quickly, although performance may deteriorate with increased demands. Word retrieval may be extremely difficult at first, with deficits in both speed and accuracy (Aram, 1988). Language comprehension also is affected initially. Children usually recover, although higher level academic and reading difficulties may persist (Aram & Ekelman, 1988).

Conclusion

The underlying relationship between cognition and language varies with age and with the aspect of language studied. At many points in development, we are not able to describe the exact relationship. It is not surprising that we cannot fully explain the mechanisms at work when the brain is injured. Still, we can predict that vocabulary and structural rules will return more easily than higher order functions, such as conversational skills that require complex synthesis of language form, content, and use. Even those children who seem to recover may continue to exhibit long-term subtle pragmatic difficulties.

Early Expressive Language Delay

As much as 10–15% of middle-class American children may be "late bloomers," children who may not achieve 50 single words and 2-word utterances by 24 months of age (Rescorla, 1989). Most of these children will "outgrow it," and from their late start "catch up" with their peers. For the approximately 40–50% with expressive language delay (ELD), however, the problem will continue through preschool and become a more specific language problem by school age (Paul, 1989b; Rescorla, 1990; Thal, 1989). Children with ELD do not outgrow their language impairment (Fischel, Whitehurst, Caulfield, & DeBaryshe, 1988; Paul, 1989a, 1991; Rescorla, 1989; Rescorla & Schwartz, 1988; Whitehurst, Fischel, & Arnold, 1989).

Language Characteristics

In general, children with ELD exhibit substantial delays in expressive language, compared to their receptive understanding and their nonverbal intelligence (Whitehurst et al., 1991). Even so, approximately 33% of children with ELD exhibit poorer comprehension than "late bloomers" (Paul, Looney, & Dahm, 1991; Thal, Tobias, & Morrison, 1991). Specific language characteristics are listed in Table 2.8.

TABLE 2.8
Language characteristics of children with expressive language delay (ELD)

Pragmatics	Quantitative difference from chronological peers. Exhibit same range of intentions, but use fewer in interactions.
	Narrative difficulties.
	Conversational difficulties
Semantics	Vocabulary development accelerates and approaches normal after late start.
Syntax/Morphology	Rule learning difficulties.
	Morphological development similar to that of children developing normally.
Phonology	Less mature syllable structure than chronological peers— fewer consonants in repertoire.
	More consonant errors.
	Articulation errors.
Comprehension	Auditory comprehension unaffected in most children.
	Reading difficulties.

Source: Based on Paul (1991); Paul & Alforde (1993); Paul & Jennings (1992); Paul & Smith (1991); Whitehurst et al. (1991)

As might seem obvious, this language impairment manifests itself early. Children with ELD do not gesture as much as either their chronologically age-matched peers developing normally or "late blooming" peers. This lack of gestures is correlated with comprehension difficulties and a lack of vocabulary development (Bates, Thal, Whitesell, Fenson, & Oakes, 1989; Thal et al., 1991). Unlike "late bloomers," children with ELD do not use gestures to compensate for their expressive language deficits (Thal & Tobias, 1992). As children with ELD mature, their vocabulary development accelerates, but their development of language form does not (Paul & Smith 1991). Language use is also greatly affected.

Possible Causal Factors

Causal factors are difficult to identify in children with ELD because nonverbal intelligence, birth and delivery, hearing, and self help and motor skills all seem to be within normal limits (Paul, 1991). Still, some differences suggest causal factors.

Biological factors.   Although there are no obvious biological factors, the increased prevalence in families with a history of speech and language problems suggests a biological basis. In addition, the indication is strong that otitis media, or middle ear infection, may contribute to the problem, but it is not the sole cause of the language impairment (Friel-Patti, 1990; Paul, Lynn, & Lohr-Flanders, 1990).

Social-environmental factors.   Again, there are no obvious factors. Parents do report, however, that their children are overactive and difficult to manage (Paul, 1991).

Conclusion

Children with ELD are at risk for academic failure when they begin school (Aram, Ekelman, & Nation, 1984; King, Jones, & Lasky, 1982). Although they appear normal in kindergarten, children with ELD do not have the basic language skills for reading and writing in first grade (Scarborough & Dobrich, 1990). Therefore, it is important that these children be identified early and that intervention begin prior to school age.

Neglect and Abuse

Children who are neglected and abused constitute a large portion of the preschool and school-age population that, until recently, had not been identified as having distinct language problems. It is estimated by the U.S. Department of Health and Human Services (1981) that more than 1 million children are neglected or abused each year in the United States. Although these children do not constitute a clinically defined category, they do present language difficulties.

Table 2.9 presents the types of neglect and abuse that have been identified (Sparks, 1989). The effect will vary with each child (Augustinos, 1987).

TABLE 2.9
Types of neglect and abuse

Physical neglect	Abandonment with no arrangement for care, including inadequate supervision, nutrition, clothing, and/or personal hygiene, and/or failure to seek needed or recommended medical care.
Emotional neglect	Failure to provide a normal living experience, including attention and affection; and/or refusal of treatment or services recommended by professional personnel.
Physical abuse	Bodily injury, such as neurological damage, or death from shaking, beating, and/or burning.
Sexual abuse	Both nonphysical abuse, such as indecent exposure or verbal attack, and physical abuse, such as genital-oral stimulation, fondling, and/or sexual intercourse.
Emotional abuse	Excessive yelling, belittling, teasing/verbal attack, and/or overt rejection.

Source: Sparks, S. N. (1989). Speech and language in maltreated children: Response to McCauley & Swisher (1987). *Journal of Speech and Hearing Disorders, 54,* 124–126.

Neglect and abuse are extreme examples of a dysfunctional family and are a sign of the type of social environment in which the child learned language (Cicchetti, 1987; Cicchetti & Lynch, 1993; Salzinger, Feldman, Hammer, & Rosario, 1991). Although neglect and abuse are rarely the direct cause of the communication problem, the context in which they occur directly influences the child's development.

Neglect and abuse are not limited to any economic class, although incidence increases as income decreases. It is believed that the increased economic, social, and health problems and lower levels of education and employment of the poor increase the risk of maltreatment (Trickett, Aber, Carlson, & Cicchetti, 1991).

Language Characteristics

All aspects of language are affected, although it is in language use that children who are neglected and abused exhibit the greatest difficulties (Blager & Martin, 1976) (Table 2.10). In general, children who are neglected and abused are less talkative and have fewer conversational skills than their peers. Utterances and conversations are shorter than those of their peers. They are less likely to volunteer information or to discuss emotions or feelings.

In school, these children have depressed verbal language performance (Allen & Oliver, 1982; Lynch & Roberts, 1982; Oates, Peacock, & Forrest, 1984). A high correlation is found between deficient verbal and reading ability and neglect and abuse (Burke, Crenshaw, Green, Schlosser, & Strocchia-Rivera, 1989).

Possible Causal Factors

Certainly, negative social-environment factors are important in the development of language by children who are neglected and abused, but biological factors should not be overlooked. Medical and health problems among poor Americans also can contribute. Direct effect is difficult to determine because of the multiplicity of overlapping factors, especially among the poor (Fox, Long, & Langlois, 1988; McCauley & Swisher, 1987; Sparks, 1989).

Biological factors.   Neglect and abuse are not limited to poor families, but in these families or in cases of extreme neglect, biological factors also may contribute. Poor maternal health, substance abuse, poor or nonexistent pediatric services, and poor nutrition can all affect brain development and maturation (Restak, 1979). Physical abuse also may cause lasting physical or neurological damage. We do not know the long-term effects on the brain of lack of environmental stimulation.

Social-environmental factors.   Either or both parents may be neglectful or abusing, but it is the mother's or caregiver's everyday responsiveness to the child that has the most effect on language development. The quality of the child-mother attachment is a more significant factor in language development than is maltreatment and can moderate or exacerbate the effects of neglect or abuse (Gersten, Coster, Schneider-Rosen, Carlson, & Cicchetti, 1986; Mosisset, Barnard, Greenberg, Booth, & Spieker, 1990).

Several factors, including childhood loss of a parent, death of a previous child, pregnancy complications, birth complications, current marital or financial problems, substance abuse, maternal age, and/or illness, can disturb maternal attachment (Barbero, 1982). In turn, mothers may adopt two general patterns of interaction (Crittenden, 1981, 1988). Most abusive mothers are *controlling*, imposing their will on the child. As controllers, they tend to ignore the child's initia-

TABLE 2.10
Language characteristics of children who are neglected and abused

Pragmatics	Poor conversational skills.
	Inability to discuss feelings.
	Shorter conversations.
	Fewer descriptive utterances.
	Language used to get things done with little social exchange or affect.
Semantics	Limited expressive vocabulary.
	Fewer decontextualized utterances, more talk about the here and now.
Syntax/Morphology	Shorter, less complex utterances.
Phonology	Similar to peers.
Comprehension	Receptive vocabulary similar to peers.
	Auditory and reading comprehension problems.

Source: Based on Coster & Cicchetti (1993); Coster, Gersten, Beeghly, & Cicchetti (1989); Culp et al. (1991); Fox, Long, & Langlois (1988)

tions, thus decreasing the amount of verbal stimulation received by the child. *Neglecting* mothers, however, are unresponsive to their infant's behaviors because they have low expectations of deriving satisfaction from the infant. Either situation includes a lack of support for the development of meaningful communication skills with little active interaction, such as playing games, hugging, patting, or nuzzling, and little "baby talk" (Allen & Wasserman, 1985; Dietrich, Starr, & Kaplan, 1980; Hyman, Parr, & Browne, 1979; Wasserman, Green, & Allen, 1983).

The result is insecure attachment on the part of the child (Browne & Sagi, 1988; Carlson, Cicchetti, Barnett, & Braunwald, 1989; Crittenden, 1988). The child may be apprehensive in the presence of the parent and may avoid interaction to lessen the chance of hostile responses. Early stimulus-response bonds—the infant's notion that her or his behavior results in an adult reinforcing response—may be nonexistent, further depressing the child's behavior. Obviously, this is not an ideal language learning environment.

Conclusion

Only now are we beginning to understand the effect of caregiver behavior on the infant. Although it seems intuitive that neglect and abuse would cause language and communication problems, especially in language use, the data are only correlational, not cause and effect.

CONCLUSION

At this point, most students are in need of a 1–sentence summary statement that once and for all distinguishes each language impairment from the others. Unfortunately, I do not have one forthcoming. We are discussing real human beings who do not like to be placed in boxes and asked to perform in certain ways.

Still, one needs to make some sense from the wealth of information presented. At the risk of generalizing too much, let's try. At the beginning of the chapter, I cited six abilities needed for normal language development. It might be helpful to consider these in conceptualizing the language impairments discussed (Table 2.11).

Perceptual difficulties are reported for some of the disorders mentioned, but not all. Nor are they similar in type and severity. For children with SLI, on the one hand, perceptual difficulties seem to be limited to rapid, sequenced auditory stimuli. On the other hand, perceptual difficulties are the essence of language learning disability and autism. Even here the difference seems to be one of perception and sensory integration in LLD and threshold levels in autism.

Attentional difficulties also accompany several of the language impairments discussed. Again the variability is great. Children with autism are either seemingly inattentive or fixated on one, often irrelevant aspect of a stimulus. In contrast, children with TBI experience attentional fluctuations and seem to attend for only brief periods.

All of the language impairments discussed include difficulty using symbols. That is the essence of a language impairment. This difficulty varies between children with mental retardation and autism who have great difficulty with symbol-

TABLE 2.11
Language learning requirements and the difficulties of children with language impairment*

Requirements	Language Impairment						
	MR	**LLD**	**SLI**	**Autism**	**TBI**	**ELD**	**Neglect/Abuse**
Ability to perceive sequenced acoustic events of short duration	X	X	X	X	X		
Ability to attend actively, to be responsive, and to anticipate stimuli		X		X	X		
Ability to use symbols	X	X	X	X	X	X	X
Ability to invent syntax from the language in the environment	X	X	X	X		X	
Enough mental energy to do all the above simultaneously	X		X		X		X
Ability to interact and communicate with others				X			X

* Xs represent problem areas in language learning and use.

referent relationships and children who are neglected and abused who have little difficulty with language form and content.

Language is rarely taught formally. Instead, children acquire language by hypothesizing the rules from the give-and-take of conversational speech. This can be a difficult task if the child is inattentive or has difficulty perceiving language.

The requirement of having enough mental energy is a tricky one. We shall broaden the concept somewhat. Children with mental retardation may lack the mental abilities for some tasks, while those with SLI and TBI may use vital mental energy on lower level tasks, leaving little for language analysis and synthesis. The frequently reported depression of children with TBI and children who are neglected and abused also limits the cognitive energy available for language learning.

Finally, the ability to interact and communicate with others probably is affected in each of the language impairments discussed. The difficulty is in determining whether an inability to interact and communicate reflects a cause of the impairment, a result, both, or just an accompanying feature. Among at least two groups of children—those with autism and those who are neglected and abused— inability to interact seems directly related to the language impairment exhibited.

Each language impairment presents a somewhat different image. In a clinical sense, however, the important features to which a speech-language patholo- gist attends are the individual characteristics of each child, not the diagnostic category. Naming and describing a language impairment does not necessarily explain it. In addition, many children diagnosed as language impaired will not have any readily identifiable characteristics.

Implications

Language impairments are not outgrown. Even with intervention, language impairments are rarely "cured." Typically, they change and become more subtle (Wallach & Liebergott, 1984). Children with preschool language impairments continue to have trouble with linguistic and academic tasks (Aram & Nation, 1980; Hall & Tomblin, 1978; Maxwell & Wallach, 1984; Strominger & Bashir, 1977). Low achievers have persistent subtle language difficulties not evident in their syntactic structures. Reading performance is affected particularly (Hill & Haynes, 1992). As adults, children with language impairments may continue to do poorly in speech and language, although nonlinguistic skills seem normal (Felsenfeld, Broen, & McGue, 1992). With or without intervention, certain ramifications of having a language impairment affect academic performance and social acceptance.

Poor oral language usually results in poor reading and writing ability. It has been hypothesized that poor reading reflects the child's lack of language awareness skills, called metalinguistic abilities (Menyuk et al., 1991). For example, a child may be unaware of syllable or phonetic segmentation of words. This awareness is crucial for reading. These higher level language skills often are lacking in those with language impairments and may explain why the reading performance of children with ELD and SLI is poorer than might be expected.

Within the classroom, children with language impairments form a separate subgroup that interacts increasingly less with their peers developing normally (Guralnick, 1990; Hadley & Rice, 1991). One's relative communication skills influence participation. Because children with language impairments are poor communicators overall (Fey, 1986), they are increasingly ignored.

In general, a child's popularity is associated with her or his conversational skills (Hazen & Black, 1989). Children with language impairments initiate little verbal interaction, are less responsive, use more short and nonverbal responses, and are less able to maintain a conversation (Rice, Snell, & Hadley, 1991). The result is fewer interactions with others (Hadley & Rice, 1991).

Two other devices used by popular children—narration and humor—also are affected (Paul & Smith, 1993). The narratives of children with language impairments often lack cohesion, and humor is poorly used and comprehended (Bernstein, 1986; Nippold, 1985; Spector, 1990). Difficulties in one aspect of language often signal the coexistence of possibly undetected difficulties in other aspects (McNutt & Hamayan, 1984; Ruscello, St. Louis, & Mason, 1991; Shriberg, Kwiatkowski, Best, Hengst, & Terselic-Weber, 1986; Shriner, Holloway, & Daniloff, 1969; Smit & Bernthal, 1983; Whitacre, Luper, & Pollio, 1970).

Syntax and morphology are usually not aberrant, characterized more by the continued use of less mature forms (Curtis, Kutz, & Tallal, 1992; Leonard, 1987,

1988). Word formation processes, usually consisting of a free morpheme plus one or more bound morphemes, are also normal but less mature (Clahsen, 1989; Leonard, Sabbadini, Leonard, & Volterra, 1987; Leonard, Sabbadini, Volterra, & Leonard, 1988; Rom & Leonard, 1990). Similarly, phonological patterns usually reflect those of younger children (T. Campbell & Shriberg, 1982; Ingram, 1991; Shriberg et al., 1986).

Children with language impairments often continue to have poor vocabularies and poor higher level semantic skills. These include difficulties with abstract meanings, figurative language, dual meanings, ambiguity, and humor (Donahue & Bryan, 1984; Kamhi, 1987; Nippold, 1985; Spector, 1990; van Kleeck, 1984; Wiig & Semel, 1984).

Finally, language comprehension difficulties, especially at higher levels such as detection of ambiguity, may persist. These difficulties reflect the underlying language difficulties evidenced in expressive language (Skarakis-Doyle & Mullin, 1990).

Speech-language pathologists are responsible for intervening to correct some language difficulties, to modify others, and to teach compensation skills for still others. In the chapters that follow, we explore a model that proposes to do this in the most natural way possible.

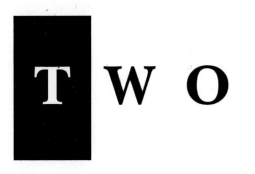

T W O

Communication Assessment

Communication Assessment of Children

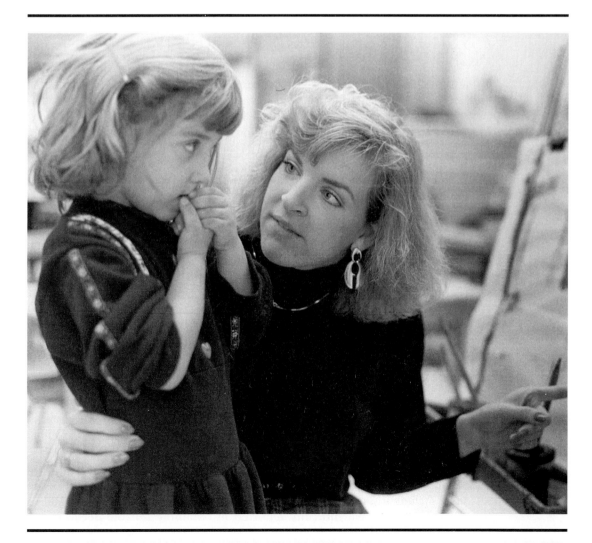

N o clear line exists between assessment and intervention. Both are part of the intervention process, and portions of each are found in the other. Ideally, assessment and measurement are ongoing throughout intervention. "In this way diagnosis becomes an ongoing process rather than a one-time occurrence at the initial evaluation" (Kamhi, 1984, p. 227). No clinical goal should be determined or modified without first obtaining data on the communication performance of the affected child.

In this chapter, we explore the differences between psychometric and descriptive assessment paradigms and describe a combined or integrative approach that attempts systematically to address the shortcomings of both approaches while describing the child's use of language in context. In the final portions of the chapter, we discuss the special difficulties found in assessment of minority children with different dialects who are limited English proficient.

PSYCHOMETRIC VERSUS DESCRIPTIVE PROCEDURES

The goals of communication assessment are to identify and describe each child's unique pattern of communication behaviors and, if that pattern signifies a language impairment, to recommend treatment, follow-up, or referral ("Preferred practice patterns," 1993). Through this process, the speech-language pathologist determines (a) whether a problem exists, (b) the causal-related factors, and (c) the overall intervention plan.

There are two major philosophical approaches to this task. The *normalist* philosophy is based on a norm or average performance level—usually a score—that society considers typical of normal functioning and that is reflected in more traditional language assessment procedures. In contrast, the *neutralist* or criterion-referenced approach compares the child's present performance to past performance and/or is descriptive in manner.

Traditional language assessment procedures heavily emphasize the use of standardized psychometric or norm-referenced tests (Craig, 1983; L. Miller, 1993; Muma, 1983). This situation is reflected in the fact that more than 100 norm-referenced language assessment tools are commercially available. Ideally, a standardized test has been given to a large number of children from various populations, has demonstrated reliability and validity, and has normative data that provide either scale score, age equivalent, or numerical score comparisons (J. Miller, 1978).

Reliability is the repeatability of measurement. More precisely, reliability is the accuracy or precision with which a sample taken at one time represents performance of either a different but similar sample, or the same sample at a different time. Factors that may affect reliability include individual change over time, sample differences, and the limited nature of the sample in size or inclusiveness. Very limited samples usually result in unstable or undependable scores. Thus, the test must include a sample large enough to be reliable yet not unwieldy. Add to these concerns the great difficulty reported in obtaining reliable performance from children, especially toddlers (Rescorla, 1991), and the magnitude of the task of producing a reliable measure is tremendous.

Test makers and users are concerned with both internal consistency and various measures of reliability. **Internal consistency** is the degree of relationship among items and the overall test. If a test has high internal consistency, children who score well overall should tend to get the same items correct, whereas those who score low should tend to perform similarly among themselves. Measures of internal consistency usually are stated as item-test or subtest-test correlations or as the correlation of passing/failing an item or subtest with passing/failing the test.

Measures of reliability include *test-retest reliability, alternate form reliability,* and *split-half reliability.* In test-retest reliability, the child is administered the same test with a time interval between each administration. With alternate forms, the child is administered equivalent or parallel forms of a measure. Finally, a test may be divided into equivalent halves. In each case, the two test scores are compared and the consistency of scores measured. This value is expressed as a reliability or correlational coefficient or as a standard error of measure. The closer the reliability coefficient to a value of 1 and the lower the standard error or standard deviation of the error scores, the more reliable is the measure.

In addition, the speech-language pathologist is concerned with the probability of two judges scoring the same behavior in the same manner, thus describing the child's behavior more accurately. As a group, scoring procedures that use a definite criterion for correct-incorrect determination, such as accepting only specific responses as correct, are more reliable than those that use scaled scoring, such as grading responses by their degree of correctness. The latter can have increased reliability if each score has definite criteria or if the tester has received specific training.

Validity is the effectiveness of a test in representing, describing, or predicting an attribute of interest to the tester. In short, it is a measure of the test's ability to assess what it purports to assess. The tester is interested in measuring all of the attribute being tested but nothing other than that attribute. For example, some tests of receptive language abilities require the child to respond verbally. Clearly, this requirement goes beyond the stated domain of the attribute being tested.

Professionals should be cautious when choosing tests. Few language screening tests, for example, meet criteria for validity or provide information to enable the speech–language pathologist to determine validity for herself (Sturner et al., 1994).

To test an abstract concept such as intelligence, test designers must select concrete tasks (Kamhi, 1993). These tasks, in turn, often become the defining features of the abstract entity supposedly measured. Thus, intelligence becomes the sum of the test tasks.

Tests are not presentations of the overall attribute or behavior, but are merely samples of that attribute or behavior. From the samples, testers make inferences about the overall attribute or behavior. If the samples are not valid measures, the inferences will be incorrect. Validity is not self-evident and must be proven. Three types of proof or evidence are criterion validity, content validity, and construct validity.

Criterion validity is the effectiveness or accuracy with which a measure predicts success. This usually is calculated as the degree to which a measure correlates with some other suitable measures of success. Finding other suitable measures can be difficult.

Content validity is the faithfulness with which the sample or measure represents some attribute or behavior. In other words, the sum of the tasks involved should define or constitute the attribute or behavior being measured. For example, a test maker or user must decide what constitutes correct and effective use of language. A valid test would assess the use or process, as well as the content of language. Measures should reflect the professional literature, research, and expert opinion on the constitution of the attribute or behavior tested. If the correspondence is good, then the test has some content validity.

Finally, **construct validity** is the accuracy with which or the extent to which a measure describes or measures some trait or construct. Professionals are interested in the accuracy and significance of results and in how precisely the measure notes individual or group differences. Construct validity usually is determined by comparing the measure with other acceptable measures of the attribute or behavior in question. This procedure is based on the assumption that the measure used in comparison is valid.

Tests or measures help the speech-language pathologist determine how the child's performance, in the form of a score, compares with that of children who supposedly possess the same characteristics (McCauley & Swisher, 1984a, 1984b). Most frequently, tests are used to determine average and less-than-average performance for decisions about the need for intervention services (Lund & Duchan, 1988).

Unfortunately, many traditional assessment procedures do not reflect current definitions of the nature of language (Craig, 1983; Ray, 1989). Although normative tests may be good for measuring isolated skills, they provide very little information on overall language use. Thus, important linguistic processes needed in conversational exchange may not be measured.

More descriptive approaches, such as language sampling, highlight the individualistic nature of the child's communicative functioning noted in language development studies. In contrast, psychometric normative testing imposes group criteria on an individual, thereby obviating an assessment of the individual (Muma & Pierce, 1981). Each method of assessment has its strengths and weaknesses, as well as possible applications within the clinical setting. These are described in the following sections.

PSYCHOMETRIC ASSESSMENT PROTOCOLS

Ideally, a test elicits a standard and representative sample of a behavior. A test is normed by using specified explicit procedures and administering the test to a sample from a specific population. As such, normed tests enable the speech–language pathologist to compare individual performance with that of a larger population. In general, norm-referenced assessment tools have the advantages of objectivity, replicability, and elimination of unwanted or uncontrolled variation (Weiner & Hoock, 1973). Tests help focus and sharpen observational skills and are particularly helpful when deciding whether a problem exists (Longhurst, 1984).

Although normed tests are potentially valid, reliable, and precise in measurement, it is difficult to find a language test that is acceptable in all three areas (Darley, 1979). In addition, normed tests do not easily accommodate cultural and individual variation, nor do they begin to provide a true picture of the richness and complexity of the child's communication behavior (Leonard, Prutting, Perozzi, & Berkley, 1978; Newhoff & Leonard, 1983). In other words, "at their best . . . tests provide an unclear picture of communication performance" (L. Miller, 1993, p. 13).

Tests are less complex than the language being assessed (Ray, 1989). Language is multidimensional, and its use individualistic, making it difficult to measure (Dale, 1980; Damico, 1988; Fillmore, Kempler, & Wang, 1979). "Attempts to assess the ability to use language on the basis of responses to items on a formal test," declared one expert, "are probably a waste of time and money for the practitioner faced with real children" (Dever, 1978, p. 19).

Test Differences

Language assessment instruments differ widely even when purported to measure the same entity. For example, both the Bankson Language Screening Test (Bankson, 1977), a rambling, multidimensional tool, and the Fluharty Preschool Speech and Language Screening Test (Fluharty, 1978) purport to identify young children with language impairments. The Bankson correlates well with ratings from Developmental Sentence Scoring (DSS) (L. Lee, 1974) of a spontaneous language sample. In contrast, the Fluharty fails to identify many children who would be classified as language-disordered on the basis of their DSS ratings (Blaxley, Clinker, & Warr-Leeper, 1983). As with other screening instruments, the Fluharty may be too insensitive to be an effective language screen (Sturner, Heller, Funk, & Layton, 1993).

Even tests that seem to be significantly correlated, suggesting an interrelationship of criterion validity, may seem less so when subtests or various portions of tests are compared. For example, the Peabody Picture Vocabulary Test-Revised (PPVT-R) (Dunn & Dunn, 1981), the Test of Early Language Development (TELD) (Hresko, Reid, & Hammill, 1981), and the Preschool Language Scale (PLS) (Zimmerman, Steiner, & Pond, 1979) are significantly correlated, although the expressive and receptive portions of the TELD separately are not (Dale & Henderson, 1987; McLoughlin & Gullo, 1984). Thus, the TELD fails to identify children with these specific problems.

Ironically, the PPVT-R and other seemingly similar vocabulary measures, such as the Picture Vocabulary subtest of the Test of Language Development-Primary (TOLD-P) (Hammill & Newcomer, 1982, 1988), the Expressive One–Word Picture Vocabulary Test (Gardner, 1979), and the Receptive One–Word Picture Vocabulary Test (M. Gardner, 1985) correlate only moderately for older preschool children (Channell & Peek, 1989).

Nor does positive correlation mean that tests are acceptable substitutions for each other. The TOLD-P does not provide a sufficient sample to allow it to substitute for the results of the PPVT-R (Friend & Channell, 1987).

Tests also can differ in their levels of difficulty. The Test of Adolescent Language (TOAL) (Hammill, Brown, Larsen, & Wiederholt, 1980, 1987, 1989), the Clinical Evaluation of Language Functions (CELF) (Semel & Wiig, 1980), and the Fullerton Language Test for Adolescents (Thorum, 1986) seem inordinately difficult, whereas the Screening Test of Adolescent Language (STAL) (Prather, Breecher, Stafford, & Wallace, 1980) identifies a more appropriate number of students (about one-fifth) as having difficulty (Lieberman, Heffron, West, Hutchinson, & Swem, 1987).

All tests are not created equal and should be researched carefully by speech-language pathologists before being used. In the following section we explore some of these differences, specifically test content, and some of the common misuses of tests. Finally, the variables that should be considered in test selection are discussed.

Content

The major criticism of existing instruments is the inadequacy of the content covered in both breadth and depth (Launer & Lahey, 1981). Great inequity also occurs with age of the child. In general, there are very few standardized measures for toddlers and adolescents and an abundance of measures for preschoolers and early school-age children (Rescorla, 1991; Scott, Nippold, Norris, & Johnson, 1992).

Two issues relative to content validity—relevance and coverage—must be addressed in test construction (Messick, 1980). **Content relevance** is the precision with which a certain aspect of language is delineated or defined. This is necessary to determine the dimensions of that aspect and its members. For example, tests of syntax may be organized on the basis of transformational grammar, R. Brown's (1973) 14 morphemes, and semantic-syntactic categories, or on no recognizable rationale. Without a framework, content items may be selected on "an unprincipled, arbitrary, and impressionistic basis" (Lieberman & Michael, 1986, p. 77).

The issue of content relevance is made more complicated by our lack of an agreed definition of language (Lahey, 1990). In addition, the child's knowledge of language, called *competence,* is measurable only as behavior or performance, which are affected by contextual variables, such as speed and complexity. Thus, poor performance may indicate an underlying deficit, a difficulty accessing the underlying system, or a problem with the testing content.

Content coverage is the representativeness with which an aspect of language is sampled. Theoretically, coverage of language features should reflect general use.

Some features may be more significant than others, although this fact can be verified only through statistical analysis. Otherwise, subtle language impairments may go undetected. For example, the Test of Language Development (TOLD) (Newcomer & Hammill, 1977), the Carrow Elicited Language Inventory (CELI) (Carrow, 1974), and the Clinical Evaluation of Language Functions (CELF) emphasize early language development while missing more subtle later developing features. A single test's rather limited sample of a child's skills is an inadequate base on which to build a sound remedial program (Lieberman & Michael, 1986).

The psychometric testing model produces data on minimal portions of behavior, thus reducing language to simple, often irrelevant dimensions that may not reflect the qualities of that language overall (Kamhi, 1993; Muma, 1983; Oller, 1979). By fragmenting language into observable and measurable features, tests may highlight skills only tangentially related to language ability. Tests tend to emphasize structural components of language because they are easy to observe. Although structured testing may reveal the child's ability to use language in one context, it reveals very little about the child's language as it is needed and used in everyday communication (P. Cole, 1982).

By isolating language performance from the conversational context, tests may be measuring skills other than those they claim to measure. In fact, "language use in isolation often bears little resemblance to language use in context" (Newman, Lovett, & Dennis, 1986, p. 31). For example, the child may use interrogatives throughout the day to obtain information, desired objects, and needed assistance but may be unable to form interrogatives in isolation when given a group of words to include. In addition, the process of the test situation may be so foreign to the child or alien to the child's everyday communication environment that it influences the language the child produces. Performance may be affected also by factors as diverse as the child's state of health on the day the test is administered, attention level and comprehension of the instructions, and perception of the test administrator.

In short, norm-referenced approaches offer "canned" assessment with little consideration for the individual needs of the child with whom they are used. The tendency is for assessment procedures to take priority over the child, with test selection based on commercial availability or clinical popularity (Duchan, 1982a; Kamhi, 1984). Tests are a priori and product oriented, offering little information on the appropriateness of the features being tested. The test results, in turn, offer little assistance in identifying individual problems and in planning intervention.

Misuse of Normative Testing

Norm-referenced tests should be used with caution. Lieberman and Michael warn, "Let the clinician beware" (1986, p. 71). The best advice is to be an "informed clinician" (Siegel & Broen, 1976) and a wise consumer. Speech–language pathologists should be mindful of the frequent misuse of these instruments (Lieberman & Michael, 1986; McCauley & Swisher, 1983, 1984b; Stephens & Montgomery, 1985), among them (a) misuse of scores as a summary of a child's performance, (b) use of inappropriate norms, (c) inappropriate assumptions based on test results, (d) use of specific test items to plan intervention goals, and (e) use of tests to assess therapy progress.

Misuse of Scores

The most frequent score used on standardized measures is the mean or average score. Test makers assume that the average score is the "normal" score. Test scores that are extreme or that represent the performance of children whose ages are at the extremes for the norming population should not be considered as reliable as more central measures.

It is important to recall that a wide scoring area about the mean, called **standard deviation,** is considered to fall within the normal range. When plotted, the total number of individuals receiving each score will form the familiar *bell-shaped curve,* represented in Figure 3.1. Approximately two-thirds of the population will score within one standard deviation on either side of the mean score. The speech-language pathologist must decide where "non-normal" occurs. If she uses only one standard deviation for separating normal from non-normal, she will find that nearly one-third of the population, approximately 16% above and 16% below, fails to fall within this range. Two standard deviations is a better index of deviancy, leaving approximately 3% of the population above and 3% below those within the normal range. A second index is the 10th percentile, the lowest 10% of the norming sample. Children who score at or below the 10th percentile are often considered to be other-than-normal.

Actually, all scores are part of the normal distribution because each is used to construct that distribution. Those at either end represent a quantitative difference in score that we term *disordered, deviant,* or *impaired.* Obviously, our boundary

FIGURE 3.1
Parameters of the normal distribution

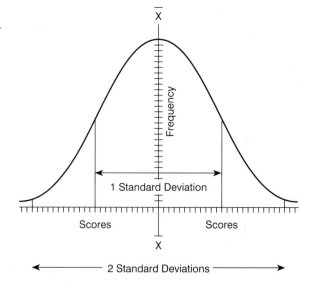

of 2 standard deviations is relative. To some extent, "our dependence on the use of numerically based assessment, evaluation, and testing has resulted in the creation of disabilities where only people with differences and individual variations exist" (L. Miller, 1993, p. 16). The speech-language pathologist must decide when the difference is so great as to impair the individual. We should remind ourselves that the 1% of the population that are blood type B-negative is not considered deviant, just different (L. Miller, 1993).

The use of scores imposes some constraints that many professionals overlook. First, numbers establish equalities and inequalities. For example, 2 is twice 1 and half of 4. It would seem, therefore, that a child with a score of 4 has twice the skill of one with a score of 2, but it measures number of responses, not quality.

Second, all test items are assumed to be equal because each has the same weight (L. Miller, 1993). If there is one item each for the verb *to be* and past tense *-ed,* they each receive the same score even though they are not of equal importance developmentally.

Beyond her concerns about numerical equalities-inequalities, the speech-language pathologist must consider the standards for comparison of children, such as chronological, mental, and language age. The exact relationship of cognition and language is unclear. Thus, even a child with matching but low mental age and language age should be considered for intervention and likely will benefit (K. Cole et al., 1990), although not all professionals agree (Lyngaas, Nyberg, Hoekenga, & Gruenewald, 1983).

Age-equivalent scores—the average or projected age of children getting a certain number of items correct—seem to be even less reliable than are other indices, such as standard scores and percentile ranks, and less sensitive to individual differences (Lahey, 1990). Of course, all of these values are only as representative as the norming population. Often, specific age-equivalent scores are determined by test makers through interpolation from the scores achieved by children at various other ages.

These scores imply some standard of performance, when in fact, there is none except the numerical score. Nor is an attempt made to describe the normal range beyond the mean score for some age. Thus, such scores are of little value in determining those who are language impaired. Often, differences of 6 months to 2 years between the age of the child and the age-equivalent score are used as evidence of an impairment (Stark & Tallal, 1981). This issue is complicated for children whose mental age is below their chronological. It hardly seems fair to compare a 6–year–old child with mental retardation to a 6–year–old who is developing normally.

The use of age-equivalent scores also can lead to erroneous assumptions about children's behavior. The equality of scores does not translate to an equality of behavior and offers an inadequate description of that individualistic behavior (Longhurst, 1984; McCauley & Swisher, 1984b). A child who achieves the same score as a younger child may not make the same kinds of errors (Lawrence, 1992). Two children with the same scores could have answered very different items correctly. In addition, all items are not of equal value even though the scores imply equality. Age-equivalent scores should be used with caution in a report and should be accompanied by some explanation of their value. Some professionals warn that such scores should never be used (Salvia & Ysseldyke, 1988).

Speech-language pathologists habitually should check the **standard error of measure** (SEm) for information about the confidence of test scores (J. Brown, 1989). Because tests are less than perfectly reliable, a certain amount of error is reflected in each score. In short, the larger the SEm, the less confidence one can have in the test's results.

The SEm can be added to and subtracted from a test score to establish a band of confidence. For example, assume that a child received a score of 75 on two different tests with confidence intervals of 2 and 6, respectively. On the first test, the child's error-free or true score is most probably 73-77; on the second, it is 69-81. The speech-language pathologist can have more confidence that the score of 75 on the first test is closer to the child's actual performance.

Larger SEm values also may mean that scores that seem very different actually overlap, as shown in Figure 3.2. Child A received a score of 81, and Child B received a score of 90. A SEm of 6 applied to each score results in an overlap. Therefore, the children's actual abilities may be much more similar than the test results indicate.

The speech-language pathologist should check the test manual to obtain the SEm. Because this information is not always available, the speech-language pathologist may wish to determine this value from Table 3.1 (J. Brown, 1989). The entering values of standard deviation and reliability coefficient usually are provided in the test manual.

Quantification of behaviors is not inherently bad. Measurement should be meaningful and functional and should reflect accurately the entity being evaluated (Kamhi, 1993). It is important that test designers define the entities being tested and provide a rationale in the test manual for the tasks selected.

Speech-language pathologists should read, understand, and evaluate the manual accompanying the test and be knowledgeable of test construction and administration (Stephens & Montgomery, 1985). The literature about a certain test should be studied thoroughly before the test is used.

Inappropriate Norms

Often, the norming sample does not represent the population with which the speech–language pathologist is using the assessment procedure (Lahey, 1990). In

FIGURE 3.2
A comparison of scores using standard error of measure

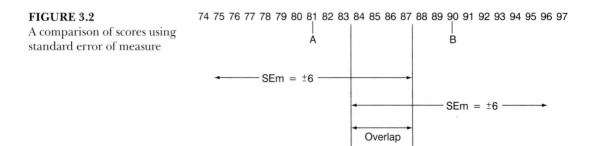

TABLE 3.1
Table of standard error of measure reliability and standard deviation values to estimate the standard error of measure (SEm)

Standard Deviation	Reliability Coefficient								
	.95	.90	.85	.80	.75	.70	.65	.60	.55
30	6.7	9.5	11.6	13.4	15.0	16.4	17.7	19.0	20.1
28	6.3	8.9	10.8	12.5	14.0	15.3	16.6	17.7	18.8
26	5.8	8.2	10.1	11.6	13.0	14.2	15.4	16.4	17.4
24	5.4	7.6	9.3	10.7	12.0	13.1	14.2	15.2	16.1
22	4.9	7.0	8.5	9.8	11.0	12.0	13.0	13.9	14.8
20	4.5	6.3	7.7	8.9	10.0	11.0	11.8	12.7	13.4
18	4.0	5.7	7.0	8.0	9.0	9.9	10.6	11.4	12.1
16	3.6	5.1	6.2	7.2	8.0	8.8	9.5	10.1	10.7
14	3.1	4.4	5.4	6.3	7.0	7.7	8.3	8.9	9.4
12	2.7	3.8	4.6	5.4	6.0	6.6	7.1	7.6	8.0
10	2.2	3.2	3.9	4.5	5.0	5.5	5.9	6.3	6.7
8	1.8	2.5	3.1	3.6	4.0	4.4	4.7	5.1	5.4
6	1.3	1.9	2.3	2.7	3.0	3.3	3.6	3.8	4.0
4	.9	1.3	1.5	1.8	2.0	2.2	2.4	2.5	2.7
2	.4	.6	.8	.9	1.0	1.1	1.2	1.3	1.3

Note: This table of standard error of measurement is based on the formula $SEm = SD \sqrt{1 - r_{11}}$ where *SD* is the standard deviation of the test scores and r_{11} is the reliability coefficient for internal consistency of the test scores.

Source: Brown, J. (1989). The truth about scores children achieve on tests. *Language, Speech, and Hearing Services in Schools, 20,* 366–371. Reprinted with permission.

this situation, the norms are inappropriate and should not be used. This situation occurs most frequently with minority or rural children or with children from lower socioeconomic groups. In these cases, local norms should be prepared by following the norming procedure described in the test manual. Some tests, such as the Test of Language Development-Intermediate (TOLD-I) and the CELF, explain this process in detail.

Incorrect Assumptions

Test scores may represent only scores and not actual differences in linguistic ability. As mentioned, it is possible for two children to receive the same score and have very different linguistic abilities. Therefore, the speech-language pathologist must analyze each child's performance on different aspects or subtests in order to obtain descriptive information. Subtest scores should be interpreted independently from each other so as not to influence their interpretation.

The speech-language pathologist also should be cautious in extrapolating global language development from scores on language tests, especially those that sample only one or two aspects of language (McLoughlin & Gullo, 1984). The PPVT is an excellent receptive vocabulary test, but it does not address other aspects of language or indicate overall language use.

Identifying Intervention Goals

A thorough description of the child's behavior is needed before the speech-language pathologist can identify areas needing intervention. Individual test items or subtests do not provide an adequate sample of that behavior. Because test items represent only a small portion of language, they do not provide enough information on which to base therapy goals. At the very least, more than one psychometric assessment procedure should be used because of the variability of some children across tests (Rizzo & Stephens, 1981; Stephens & Montgomery, 1985). The more test scores available, the more reliable the assessment. Nor will test scores describe how children function within their everyday communication environment. Only through the use of a number of assessment protocols can the speech-language pathologist hope to determine intervention objectives (Lahey, 1990). Psychometric tests are only a portion of the assessment process.

Measuring Therapy Progress

The continued use of norm-referenced tests to assess therapy progress may result in the child's learning the test, thus producing artificially high results. However, widely spaced testing or the use of different forms of the same test or of different but highly correlated tests can demonstrate changes in behavior over time (McCauley & Swisher, 1984b). Criterion-referenced tests are more appropriate for measuring individual progress.

Age-equivalent scores should not be used to measure change, however, because the scale units for items are ordinal, at best, with unequal intervals between scores (Lawrence, 1992). All items are not equal. A child whose score has changed little may have made more progress than another child whose score has changed more.

Variables in Test Selection

The speech-language pathologist should be a wise consumer of assessment materials and should base test selection on several factors. Of particular interest are test reliability and validity, discussed previously. Even language tests that meet very stringent psychometric or measurement criteria may not correlate highly or be very precise discriminators of impaired and nonimpaired language (Plante & Vance, 1994).

Other considerations in test selection include appropriateness of the test for a particular child, the manner of presentation and comprehensiveness, and the type and sensitivity of the test results. A test should be appropriate to the child's age or functioning level. In addition, the norming population should be sufficiently large and varied to include representatives of the child's racioethnic and socioeconomic background. If the child is from an identifiable minority, the speech–language pathologist should check to see whether the norming information gives data by such groups.

Appropriateness may relate also to manner of presentation. Some children perform better under certain conditions than under others. For example, children with a language learning disability can perform better if visual input accompanies the verbal. The manner of presentation may reflect the overall theoretical basis of the test. A sentence imitation test, for example, relies on auditory processing of verbal stimuli, rather than on picture cues. Other practical issues related to presentation include the number of items and the content coverage discussed previously.

In turn, too few or poorly discriminatory items can lead to less sensitive scoring, in which one question can change the child's performance score several percentage points. The type of result, whether percentage, percentile, or age equivalent, is also a practical consideration in test selection. Depending on the test, the interpretive value of such scores may be very limited.

When given a choice of information from different tests and subtests, speech–language pathologists display a remarkable similarity in the relative importance they attach to different measures (Records & Tomblin, 1994). Receptive measures, such as the TACL–R and the PPVT–R are relied on heavily. Sentence imitation and grammatical closure tasks also are preferred. Familiarity with the test procedure, overall opinion of the measure, and clinical experience are all factors in test or task selection and in the relative importance attached to data obtained from different measures.

Summary

Perceptive individuals decry overdependence on and poor interpretation of the results of testing. Although standardized tests, especially those in language, frequently have been maligned (Darley, 1979; Dever, 1978; McCauley & Swisher, 1984a, 1984b), speech–language pathologists often are required to incorporate the results of these procedures into their overall assessments. It is important for speech–language pathologists to recognize that tests are informative, but not the be-all and end-all of evaluation. Awareness of a test's shortcomings can greatly aid the interpretation of a child's performance (Stephens & Montgomery, 1985).

The issue of testing is central to the purpose of assessment. Data gathered in an assessment should be relevant to the initial clinical complaint, to the determination that a problem exists, to individual differences and individual processing, to the nature of the problem, to prognosis, to intervention implications, and to accountability (Muma, 1986). Otherwise, according to Muma, it is just a *numbers game*.

DESCRIPTIVE APPROACHES

The descriptive approach, usually based on observation and a conversational sample of the child's language, is a widely taught method of defining children's communicative abilities. Unfortunately, because of time constraints, the method is not widely used, although it is gaining favor (McCauley & Swisher, 1984b; Muma, Lubinski, & Pierce, 1982; Muma, Pierce, & Muma, 1983; Newhoff & Leonard, 1983; Rees, 1978). Descriptive approaches have the potential of allowing speech–language pathologists to regard the language process while maintaining contextual integrity and individual differences (Muma, 1986).

Spontaneous sampling alone is best used as an indicator of the child's overall language functioning, rather than as a device for noting specific language problems. More specific data can be obtained by probing the child's conversational behavior. In general, data from a language sample correlate significantly with results from elicited imitation and sentence completion tasks, although the syntactic structural patterns vary widely (Fujiki & Willbrand, 1982).

The advantages of the descriptive approach are that the speech-language pathologist can apply her own theoretical model to the assessment process and can probe and assess areas that seem most handicapping to the child (Duchan, 1982a; Kamhi, 1984). For example, the speech-language pathologist who follows a sociolinguistic model of language is free to explore the pragmatic and conversational aspects of the child's language. "By gathering clinical data and formulating and testing hypotheses based on these data, the speech-language pathologist ensures that the clinical process remains flexible and attuned to the client's changing needs" (Kamhi, 1984, p. 227). To do this, the speech-language pathologist must understand the complex interaction of constitutional—biological, cognitive, psychological, and social—and environmental forces.

The continuous speech sample has several advantages over more formal structured-response measures. Although testing reveals some information, "it reveals very little about the function, content, and form of the child's language in the various circumstances in which language is needed and employed in daily living" (P. Cole, 1982, p. 93). For example, single-word responses on a test may not be as adequate a database for phonological analysis as a longer conversational response might be, although there is some disagreement on this point (Ingram, 1976; Klein, 1984; Shriberg & Kwiatkowski, 1980). Some phonological processes, such as final consonant deletion, neutralization, stopping, and weak syllable deletion, may not be exhibited in single-word responses. Possibly these processes are the most sensitive to linguistic and extralinguistic factors found in continuous speech (Klein, 1984).

The disadvantages of the descriptive approach are (a) the level of language expertise needed by the speech-language pathologist in order to elicit and analyze the child's language, (b) the length of time needed to collect and analyze the child's language, and (c) the reliability and validity of the sample (Kelly & Rice, 1986). Although a number of descriptive protocols exist, the speech-language pathologist may not feel sufficiently well versed in all aspects of language to choose those appropriate for each child. For example, some protocols emphasize form or content, although these alone will not ensure appropriate use (Roth & Spekman, 1984a). In this situation, the speech-language pathologist may feel abandoned in pragmatics to fend for herself. For many theoreticians, the communicative value of each language event lies in the pragmatic functions of each utterance (Prutting & Kirchner, 1983). Yet, speech-language pathologists may not be comfortable with the pragmatic aspects of language. In addition, a large caseload may preclude the use of lengthy descriptive procedures. Finally, as in psychometric testing, the speech-language pathologist may not elicit a valid sample of the child's usual language usage.

Reliability and Validity

Language samples are more susceptible than standardized measures to speech-language pathologist bias (Nye et al., 1987). This problem is especially critical when such measures are used to assess intervention effectiveness. The speech-language pathologist must attempt to analyze the language sample in the most objective manner possible. Descriptions of the physical behaviors observed are generally more reliable than subjective judgments of the causes or reasons for these behaviors. One way to increase reliability is to separate the actual events from inferences based on these events and to base decisions on the data from these events (Duncan & Fiske, 1977).

Reliability across observations can be increased by taking the following three precautions (Duncan & Fiske, 1977):

1. *Define the behaviors to be observed as explicitly as possible and train observers to ensure good inter- and intra-observer reliability.* The selection of the taxonomy of behavior categories to be observed will affect the validity of the observation. For example, a taxonomy of preschool speech acts would not be appropriate for rating the behavior of adolescents functioning above the preschool range. Accuracy also can be controlled by making point-to-point comparisons between the ratings of two observers. This type of analysis helps sharpen definitions and to highlight possible areas of confusion.

2. *Make judgments on only one type of behavior at a time.* This procedure may require the use of videotaping so that a language sample can be replayed often for additional judgments on other behaviors.

3. *Do not make summation judgments while observing "on-line."* It is too easy for preconceived notions of the child to influence our interpretation. Judgments about overall behavior are best made after assessing the accumulated data. There is danger in attempting to fit the child into one of the language impairment categories mentioned in Chapter 2.

Some threats to validity are found within the sample itself. For example, preschool children vary in their attentiveness and disposition to talk moment by moment (Shriberg & Kwiatkowski, 1985). Given this condition, the possible threats to validity in a speech sample, even with older children, are **productivity,** or the amount produced; **intelligibility,** or the amount understood by the listener; **representativeness,** or the typicality of the sample; and **reactivity,** or the response of the child to differing stimuli (Shriberg & Kwiatkowski, 1985).

Productivity

The uncommunicative child or the child who produces only a few utterances will not give the speech-language pathologist a productive sample from which to work even though such a sample may reflect accurately the child's typical output. The child may have little language with which to talk. The key to greater produc-

tion is for the speech-language pathologist to plan a variety of elicitation tasks
that serve the purpose of gathering the sample (Wren, 1985).

Intelligibility

Intelligibility is the amount of agreement between what the speaker intended to
say and what the listener interpreted from the sample. If much of the sample is
unintelligible, few utterances will be suitable for analysis. In general, intelligibility
can be increased with increased speech–language pathologist control over the
content of the child's utterances. In short, the speech–language pathologist who
knows the topic can determine more easily what the child said.

Representativeness

A sample may not represent the child's typical behavior. Language samples often
are collected in an atypical context, for example, a clinical room with the speech-
language pathologist as the conversational partner. Much of the sample may be
atypical when removed from the child's typical conversational context (Roth &
Spekman, 1984b). Three issues are relative to the representativeness of the conversational sample: *spontaneity, variability of context,* and *stability of the structure/func-
tion sampled* (Muma, 1983).

Spontaneity is increased if the child is allowed to establish the topic and/or
the activity. Interesting and varied stimulus materials can provide an excellent
basis for spontaneous conversation and can elicit a variety of forms and functions.

Variability of the context and stimulus items will elicit a greater variety of
child behaviors theoretically more representative of the child's everyday behavior.
Data should be collected in a variety of settings, with a variety of partners, and on a
variety of child-based conversational topics to ensure versatility (A. Johnson, Johnston, & Weinrich, 1984). Because quantity and complexity vary with the task, no
single task will yield a representative sample of the child's language (Wren, 1985).

Unrepresentative samples may reflect other-than-normal usage by the child.
In this situation, the structures or functions sampled may vary widely from one
situation to another. Everyday situations are most likely to elicit typical use and
thus provide some stability across situations.

Some debate has concerned whether speech–language pathologists should
try to elicit typical or maximum production from the child. This debate is fueled
by the often-reported gaps between what children with language impairment are
capable of doing with their language and what they typically do (Wiig & Semel,
1976; Wren, 1981, 1982). The speech–language pathologist must decide on the
appropriate task to use. For example, storytelling tasks yield a larger average or
mean length of utterance (MLU), while picture interpretation tasks elicit greater
language quantity (Atkins & Cartwright, 1982; Stallnaker & Creaghead, 1982).

Reactivity

The child's reaction to the techniques and the materials also will affect the overall
validity of the sample produced. Sampling conditions and the nature of the content or stimuli available can greatly affect the sample. A directed condition, such

as one in which the speech–language pathologist uses a questioning technique, allows the examiner more control over the content being discussed and may, in turn, increase intelligibility (Weeks, 1971). Unfortunately, this improved intelligibility may sacrifice productivity and representativeness. In general, too much control restricts the child's output. For example, sentence-building tasks in which the child is asked to "Make a sentence with the word *X*" elicit the least typical language and very short sentences (Wren, 1985).

Words or structures divorced from dialogue, as in the previous example, require high-level metalinguistic skills to manipulate and thus are difficult for the child with language disorders. Other tasks, such as sentence repetition, sentence completion, and judgment of grammaticality, are unreliable and should not be used without a spontaneous conversational sample (Fujiki & Willbrand, 1982). Yet, even though the more open-ended conversation may be more representative, it is usually less intelligible and may be difficult for some children with language impairment. For example, children with language learning disability exhibit difficulty with conversations, as with other assessment protocols (Bryan, Donahue, & Pearl, 1981; Bryan, Donahue, Pearl, & Herzog, 1981; Donahue, 1984; Noel, 1980; Roth, 1986; Spekman, 1981).

Similarly, specific stimulus items may increase intelligibility by controlling the topics discussed. In addition, the use of these items may enable the speech–language pathologist to repeat stimulus conditions in subsequent evaluations. Again, increased intelligibility may result in decreased productivity of a variety of forms and functions and limited content. Further, the child may develop or already have a stereotypic pattern of responding to the item. For example, a doll may elicit a reduced style similar to "motherese."

The items chosen and the directions given also may affect the validity of the sample. For example, pictures can be used to elicit language, but the instructions given to the child often affect the quantity of language produced. The typical directive "Tell me about this picture" elicits less language than a more directive style (Wren, 1985), such as the following:

> I'd like you to make up a story from this picture. I want you to tell me a whole story that has a beginning and an end. Start with " Once upon a time" and tell me the whole story.

The best advice for any speech-language pathologist is to remain flexible in order to shift between different contexts and different content and to elicit the kinds of language behavior desired. "The examiner needs to have on hand a variety of stimulus materials and be skillful in identifying and discussing a range of topics of potential interest to the child whose speech is being sampled" (Shriberg & Kwiatkowski, 1985, p. 330).

Summary

Descriptive approaches are not without problems. Although they are potentially more representative of the child's everyday performance than formal testing, this potential is not guaranteed. In addition, descriptive approaches require that the speech-language pathologist have considerable knowledge of language and of the variables that affect children's language performance. Skillful manipulation of these variables by the speech-language pathologist can enhance the potential intervention value of descriptive methods.

AN INTEGRATED FUNCTIONAL ASSESSMENT STRATEGY

Adequate evaluation is one of the most difficult and demanding tasks faced by the speech-language pathologist. The goal—much more complex than providing a score or a category label—is to describe the very complex language system of the child. Each child has a unique pattern of language rules and behaviors to be revealed and described.

A number of speech-language professionals have suggested a combined assessment approach, although the exact components of each differ (P. Cole, 1982; Kelly & Rice, 1986; Klein, 1984; McCauley & Swisher, 1984b). Almost universally, speech-language professionals would agree that no single measure or session is adequate (Emerich & Haynes, 1986).

It is helpful to consider assessment procedures as existing along a continuum from formal, structured protocols to informal, less structured approaches. In general, the more structured the elicitation session, the less variety of structures and meanings expressed (J. Miller, 1978). Language elicited in more structured tasks is usually shorter and less complex, especially with younger children, than language sampled in less controlled situations (Fey, Leonard, & Wilcox, 1981; Longhurst & Grubb, 1974).

Generally, the more specific the information desired, the more structured the approach. In this way, assessments can help the speech–language pathologist sharpen and focus what was observed. Even formal tests or portions of tests can be used in an informal way as a probe of specific behavior. Naturally, normative data cannot be used when the test procedure is altered in any way.

The speech–language pathologist must consider the following seven variables in designing and implementing the assessment process (Kelly & Rice, 1986):

1. Child's chronological and functional age
2. State of child's sensory system (vision, hearing, etc.)
3. Caregiver concerns
4. Status of child's psychological functioning
5. Child's interests and materials available
6. Child's activity level
7. Child's attention span

"Judicious manipulation of these subject and setting variables facilitates elicitation of a representative sample of the child's receptive and expressive communicative functioning" (Kelly & Rice, 1986, p. 89). In general, alternation of structured and less structured tasks keeps the child's attention and provides variety and relief from the speech–language pathologist's demands. The speech–language pathologist should readily adapt the methods to the child and be mindful that the child will respond differently to different adults.

The speech-language pathologist should keep in mind the *what, why,* and *how* of assessment (J. Miller, 1978). Considering why the child is being assessed helps the speech-language pathologist clarify the purpose. This clarity, in turn, enables the speech-language pathologist to decide what specific behaviors to assess and the best evaluative methods to use. The reasons for assessment can be grouped as (a) identification of children with potential problems, (b) establishment of baseline functioning, and (c) measurement of change. Baseline functioning enables the speech-language pathologist to determine the present level of performance, the extent of the language impairment, and the nature of the problem.

The combined or integrated assessment approach provides the most thorough evaluation. A combined approach should include a questionnaire and/or caregiver interview, an environmental observation, a speech-language pathologist-directed formal psychometric assessment, and a child-directed informal assessment consisting of a conversational sample from the child. The actual components will differ with each child. Each component is discussed in the remainder of this chapter.

The data-gathering process is scientific in nature in that it must be unbiased and objective. This collection process should be precise and measurable, with very little intrusion by the speech–language pathologist's conclusions. It is important, however, not to lose the child in the mass of data, and clinical intuition is an important factor in summarizing data and in determining which aspects of language to evaluate.

At each diagnostic step, objectives should be derived from the information collected to this point. Thus, each step becomes more focused, and the possible language problems are highlighted. Figure 3.3 presents a possible stage process of collecting data toward the goal of providing recommendations for intervention or modifications in ongoing programming. At each stage, the process becomes more focused. The following discussion deals with a number of assessment steps, both formal and informal, that are aspects of an overall integrated functional model.

Questionnaire, Interview, and Referral

Caregivers—parents, teachers, and others—are central to a functional assessment and intervention process (Kelly & Rice, 1986). Teachers can be a valuable referral source and should be encouraged to be alert for children with potential language problems (Siegel, 1979). Initial caregiver involvement helps build rapport, increases the validity of the assessment results, and introduces the caregivers to the intervention process.

A caregiver interview or questionnaire can be a valuable source of initial information on client functioning and on the perceived problem from the care-

FIGURE 3.3
A model of the assessment
process

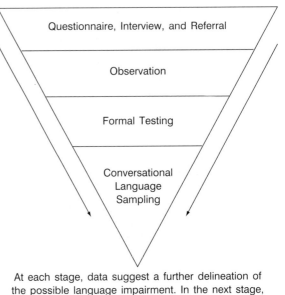

At each stage, data suggest a further delineation of
the possible language impairment. In the next stage,
the possible impairment can be more sharply defined.

giver's perspective. Caregiver expectations for the child also provide an indication of the caregiver's willingness and perceived need to work with the child.

With very young children, caregivers can be a source of information for dif-
ficult-to-test behaviors. For example, vocabulary checklists completed by parents
correlate well with other measures of vocabulary (Bates, Bretherton, & Snyder,
1988; Beeghly, Jernberg, & Burrows, 1989; Dale, 1991; Dale, Bates, Reznick, &
Morisset, 1989). In other areas of oral language, such as intelligibility, parents are
less accurate (Kwiatkowski & Shriberg, 1992).

It is best to ask questions of caregivers in a straightforward manner, with no
hesitation that might signal embarrassment or discomfort. The speech-language
pathologist avoids tag questions (e.g., "You don't . . . , do you?") that seek agreement, rather than confirmation or information. Responses are treated matter-of-
factly with little comment that might discourage the caregiver from talking. A list
of possible questions is presented in Table 3.2 (Brinton & Fujiki, 1989; Cole,
1982; Lund & Duchan, 1988; Spinelli & Terrell, 1984).

Caregiver responses should be analyzed and hypotheses formed before
deciding on the strategy for the remainder of the assessment. Potential language
problems should be researched thoroughly throughout the remainder of the
assessment process.

Observation

For the most natural interaction, the speech-language pathologist will want to
observe caregiver(s) and peer(s) with the child as conversational partners in such
everyday settings as the home and the classroom. In the classroom, the speech-

language pathologist might observe the child participating in a number of activities. This situation is not always possible. Time may not permit observation alone. In this case, the speech-language pathologist may wish to observe closely while collecting a language sample and may form tentative hypotheses for later confirmation from the analyzed sample.

If observation occurs in a more clinical setting, appropriate toys and both structured and nonstructured activities are provided for the child and conversational partner. Caregivers are encouraged to use familiar objects and the child's favorite toys or objects from home or the classroom. Ideally, the speech-language pathologist would observe the child's behavior with various communication partners. Caregivers should be encouraged to ask questions.

The speech-language pathologist should instruct caregivers to interact as typically as possible with the child. It is essential that caregivers not quiz or direct the child to perform during the observation (Cole, 1982). Optimum performance

TABLE 3.2
Interview or questionnaire format

Questions relative to language uses:
How does the child let you know items desired? What does the child request most frequently?
   What does the child do when requesting that you do something?
   When wants you to pay attention?
   When wants something?
   When wants to direct your attention?
Does the child ask for information?
How does the child express emotion or tell about feelings?
   What emotions does the child express?
Does the child make noises when playing alone? Does the child engage in monologues
   while playing? Does the child prefer to play alone or with others?
Does the child describe things in the environment? How?
Does the child discuss events in the past, future, or outside of the immediate context?

Questions relative to conversational skill:
When does the child communicate best?
How does the child respond when you say something? How does the child respond to others? Does the child interact more readily with certain people and in certain situations, and if so, with whom and when?
With whom and when does the child communicate most frequently?
Does the child initiate conversations or activities with you and with others? What is the child's most frequent topic?
Does the child join in when others initiate conversations or activities?
Does the child get your attention before saying something to you?
   How does the child do this? Does the child maintain eye contact while talking to you?
Does the child take turns when talking? Does the child interrupt? Are there long gaps between your utterances and the child's responses? Will the child take a turn without being instructed to do so or without being asked a question?
When the child speaks to you, is there an expectation of a response? What does the child do if you do not respond?

When the child responds to you, does the response usually match or is it relevant to what
    you said?
How does the child ask for clarification? How frequently does this occur?
If you ask the child for more information or for clarification, what happens? Does the
    child demonstrate frustration when not understood?
When the child asks for or tells you something, is there usually enough information for
    you to understand?
When the child tells you more complex information or relates an event or a story, is it
    organized enough for you to follow the train of thought?
Does the child have different ways of talking to different people, such as adults and small
    children? Does the child phrase things in different ways with different listeners? Is the
    child more polite in some situations?
Does the child seem confused at times? What does the child do if confused?

Questions relative to form and content:
Is the child able to understand simple directions?
Does the child know the names of common events, objects, and people in the environ-
    ment? What types of information does the child provide about these (actions, objects,
    people, descriptions, locations, causation, functions, etc.)?
Does the child seem to rely on gestures, sounds, or the immediate environment to be
    understood?
Does the child speak in single words, phrases, or sentences? How long is a typical utter-
    ance? Does the child leave out words? Are the child's sentences complex or simple?
    How does the child ask questions?
Does the child use pronouns and articles to distinguish old and new information?
Does the child use words for time, such as **tomorrow, yesterday,** or **last night?** Does the
    child use verb tenses?
Can the child put several sentences together to form complex descriptions and explana-
    tions?

Source: Compiled from Brinton & Fujiki (1989); P. Cole (1982); Lund & Duchan (1988); and Spinelli
& Terrell (1984)

is attained if the speech–language pathologist unobtrusively remains in the room
or leaves and observes from outside via observation windows or video monitors.

The style of interaction is more than just the frequency of various forms of
behavior. More important are the ways in which the child uses the various features of his interactional style. The key question is, How does the child interact
with others?

Routinized situations may provide the child with a scaffold within which
processing becomes automatized before the child is capable of more elaborate
formulation (Lieven, 1984). The speech–language pathologist needs to assess the
child's familiarity with the situation and the degree to which that situation provides a prop for the child's language. Atypical situations will not elicit typical performance.

The INREAL/Outreach Program of the University of Colorado recommends
an observation strategy called SOUL. The acronym stands for *silence, observation,*

understanding, and listening. The adult remains *silent* for periods of time, assessing the situation before talking. *Observation* of the child's play and interactions with other people occurs prior to forming hypotheses. *Understanding* is insight into the child that comes from the distillation of data collected during observation. Finally, *listening* requires total involvement by the adult and the use of responses appropriate to the functioning level of the child.

The reliability of observation is increased if the speech-language pathologist's descriptions detail as closely as possible the actual observed behavior (Duncan & Fiske, 1977). Inferences and hypotheses come later. The speech-language pathologist obtains from the caregiver interview some notion of what to observe. It is best if the observation is videotaped or audiotaped for later referral.

Table 3.3 is a list of some features that the speech-language pathologist might observe. This list is not exhaustive. Each category is discussed in some detail in Chapters 5 and 6, where we consider the analysis of a conversational sample. The purpose of observation is to note within the larger scope of interaction the language characteristics to be tested, collected, and analyzed later in the assessment.

Reliability of observation is not fortuitous. Speech-language pathologists should train together thoroughly so that their observations are as accurate and as objective as possible. This accuracy and objectivity can be accomplished by repeated observation and scoring of videotaped samples by more than one speech-language pathologist. Scoring then can be compared, discussed, and modified in light of reexamination of taped samples.

TABLE 3.3
Features to note while observing the child

Form of language. Does the child use single words, phrases, or sentences primarily? Are the sentences of the subject-verb-object form exclusively? Are there mature negatives, interrogatives, and passive sentences? Does the child elaborate the noun or verb phrase? Is there evidence of embedding and conjoining?

Understanding of semantic intent. Does the child respond appropriately to the various question forms (what, where, who, when, why, how)? Does the child confuse words from different semantic classes?

Language use. Does the child display a range of illocutionary functions, such as asking for information, help, and objects, replying, making statements, providing information? Does the child take conversational turns? Does the child introduce topics and maintain them through several turns? Does the child signal the status of the communication and make repairs?

Rate of speaking. Is the rate inordinately show or fast? Are there noticeable or lengthy pauses between the caregiver and child's turn? Are there noticeable or lengthy pauses between the child's adjacent utterances? Does the child use fillers frequently or pause before producing certain words? Are there frequent word substitutions?

Sequencing. Does the child relate events in a sequential fashion based on the order of occurrence? Can the child discuss the recent past or recount stories?

Formal Testing

In general, the role of testing is twofold: (a) to identify, by means of normative testing, the child with potential language problems, and (b) to begin a description of the child's language performance. Although screening tests may crudely address the first issue, they certainly do not address the second. Except as a tool for eliminating consideration of impairments in certain aspects of language, screening tests are of very little diagnostic value.

Within the evaluation, a change to more formal tasks might be accomplished through the use of a nonthreatening receptive task, such as the Peabody Picture Vocabulary Test-Revised (PPVT-R). Such a task allows the child to become accustomed to the speech–language pathologist's direction.

Assessing All Aspects of Language

It is important that the speech–language pathologist make a thorough assessment of all aspects of language. Only rarely is a language impairment limited to one aspect alone. Should this be the case, however, as with a high-functioning child with TBI who manifests only lingering pragmatic difficulties, testing of all aspects confirms the absence of problems and provides a holistic image of the child's language. This task may necessitate more than one session with the child and caregivers. Table 3.4 presents some of the more widely used language tests, organized by areas assessed by each. Issues relative to each aspect of language are discussed in the following section.

Pragmatics.   Very few tests are available that assess the child's conversational skills. In general, the tests are of two varieties—a storytelling format and topic discussion. In the latter, as exemplified by *Let's Talk* (Bray & Wiig, 1987; Wiig, 1982a) and the Test of Pragmatic Language (Phelps–Terasaki & Phelps–Gunn, 1992), various topics and situations are presented to the child, and he is expected to respond appropriately. In all of these test situations, the essential feature of conversational relevance is strained, and it is doubtful that a true description of the child's abilities is attained. For example, this topic discussion format makes it difficult to assess question comprehension with commercially available tests (Moeller, Osberger, & Eccarius, 1986). In general, questioning is sampled inadequately, restricted in type, and lacking in variation of communicative contexts (Parnell & Amerman, 1983).

The nature of pragmatics makes formal testing difficult. It is also difficult to establish reliable norms because such aspects of pragmatics as the amount of talking, the frequency of initiations, the type of discourse structure, and the register are situationally related. At present, it seems more appropriate to use a conversational sample to assess children's language use.

Semantics.   When does the speech–language pathologist know that a child has learned a word? Tests typically assume an all–or–nothing phenomenon in which the child either does or does not know the meaning (Crais, 1990). In reality, acquisition of word knowledge is a gradual process that may continue through the lifetime of an individual. An individual child's success or failure on a test item may be dependent on several factors, such as the type of task or the manner of cuing. Testing tasks are often contrived, decontextualized, and highly literate (Nippold, Scott, Norris, & Johnson, 1993).

Testing of semantic abilities usually is confined to picture identification, word definitions, and word categories. Of interest are the child's comprehension and production vocabularies. Comprehension vocabulary usually is measured by having the child point to a picture that best represents the word produced by the test administrator. Such tests tell the speech-language pathologist very little about the frequency of use or the depth or breadth of the child's understanding of the concept named. Comprehension of longer utterances usually is assessed by having the child follow simple commands or directives.

When a word is not fully understood by a child, he may rely on other comprehension strategies based on linguistic features, such as word order, or on nonlinguistic features, such as the position or size of the stimulus (Edmonston & Thane, 1992). These strategies are considered rarely in a formal assessment. Subsequent sampling may include probing of the strategies used. During testing, the speech-language pathologist should note behaviors, such as locational preferences in pointing responses and verbal comments that accompany responding.

Expressive or productive vocabulary usually is tested by having the child name pictures or supply a definition. Scoring may be of a correct-incorrect or scaled type. The latter allows for partially correct responses. Descriptions by the speech–language pathologist of the type of definition given by the child can be valuable in determining the maturity of the child's lexicon. Early definitions usually rely on use. These are followed in order by descriptions, use in context, synonyms and explanations, and finally, conventional definitions (Curtis, 1987).

Categorical understanding is assessed by asking the child to supply an antonym or a synonym or to name related words in a category. Between ages 5 and 9, the child undergoes a change in the organization of language, from a syntactic to a more categorical system. Thus, category membership and related words, not just simple word meaning, should be tested with all children in late elementary and high school. The Fullerton Test, the Test of Adolescent Language, and the Word Test assess definitions, figurative language, and word associations.

Word–association tasks such as naming another member of a category may be ineffectual in differentiating children with language impairment and those without (Kail & Leonard, 1986). Responses are dependent more on the familiarity of the category and the number of prototypic responses possible (Crais, 1990).

Other semantic–related tasks include giving antonyms or synonyms, stating similarities and differences, telling all one knows about a word, detecting semantic absurdities, explaining figurative language, and noting multiple meanings. Each task requires different abilities, such as determining the task demands, focusing on critical semantic dimensions, and interpreting cues, that can be complicated by word–retrieval difficulties.

TABLE 3.4
Aspects of language covered by commonly used tests

Test Name	Test Type		Aspect of Language					Mode	
	Screening	Diagnostic	Syntax	Morphology	Phonology	Semantics	Pragmatics	Receptive	Expressive
Adolescent Language Screening Test	X		X	X	X	X	X	X	X
Analysis of the Language of Learning		X	X		X	X			X
Assessment of Phonological Processes	X	X			X				X
Bankson Language Screening Test	X		X	X				X	X
Berko Test of English Morphology		X		X					X
Carrow Elicited Language Inventory		X	X	X					X
Clark-Madison Oral Language Test		X	X	X					X
Clinical Evaluation of Language Functions	X	X	X	X		X		X	X
Compton Phonological Assessment of Children	X	X			X				X
Evaluating Communicative Competence		X	X			X	X	X	X
Fullerton Language Test for Adolescents		X	X	X	X				X
Full-Range Picture Vocabulary Test		X				X		X	

TABLE 3.4, *continued*

Test	C1	C2	C3	C4	C5	C6	C7	C8	C9
Interpersonal Language Skills Assessment	X		X					X	
Language Processing Test	X			X				X	
Let's Talk Inventory for Children	X		X					X	
Miller-Yoder Language Comprehension Test		X				X		X	
Multilevel Informal Language Inventory	X			X		X	X	X	
Northwest Syntax Screening Test	X	X				X	X		X
Oral Language Sentence Imitation Diagnostic Inventory	X					X	X	X	
Patterned Elicitation Syntax Screening Test	X					X	X		X
Peabody Picture Vocabulary Test		X		X				X	
Phonological Process Analysis	X				X			X	
Test of Adolescent Language	X	X		X		X	X	X	
Test of Auditory Comprehension of Language—Revised		X				X	X	X	
Test of Language Development—Intermediary	X			X		X	X	X	
Test of Language Development—Primary	X	X		X		X	X	X	
The Word Test	X			X				X	

Many individuals, especially children with LLD or TBI, exhibit word-finding and word substitution difficulties. Little is known about word-retrieval processes, especially among children. In children, the words substituted usually share some visual attributes with the target word referent, such as saying *sheet* for *cape* and *net* for *screen*. Late elementary school children with LLD exhibit more visually related word substitution errors than do children developing normally (German, 1982). Additional word-finding substitutions found in children with LLD include functional descriptions, such as *bookholder* for *shelf* (Denckla & Rudel, 1976a, 1976b; D. J. Johnson & Myklebust, 1967).

Diagnostically, use of these word-finding strategies indicates that the child comprehends the word but has difficulty retrieving it (German, 1982). Several test protocols are provided in Table 3.5 (Snyder & Godley, 1992). Although testing may reveal a deficit in visual confrontation naming skills, such tests rarely

TABLE 3.5
Confrontational naming protocols

Test, Author(s), Date	Description
Boston Naming Test, Kaplan, Goodglass, & Weintraub, 1983	Unnormed, for adults. Records accuracy but not latency. No different contextual cues or categories.
Clinical Evaluation of Language Fundamentals-Revised, Semel, Wiig, & Secord, 1987	Normed. Word associations subtest.
Controlled Word Association Test, Benton, 1973	Unnormed for children; has adult mean score. Name in 1 minute as many words as can with a certain sound.
Word Latency Test, Rutherford & Tesler, 1971	Unnormed, uses only known items. Assesses response time.
Test of Adolescent and Adult Word Finding, German, 1990	Normed. Tests variety of contextual cues and categories. Considers frequency, familiarity, category, difficulty, response time, and accuracy.
Test of Word Finding, German, 1986, 1989	Normed. Tests variety of contextual cues and categories. Considers frequency, familiarity, category, difficulty, response time, and accuracy.
Test of Word Finding in Discourse, German, 1991	Normed. Uses pictures for narration. Assesses productivity and incidence of word-finding difficulties.
Word Naming Test, Wiegel-Crump & Dennis, 1986	Unnormed, uses picture, definition, rhyming, and category cues with words supposedly known by age 4.

Source: Adapted from Snyder, L. S., & Godley, D. (1992). Assessment of word-finding disorders in children and adolescents. *Topics in Language Disorders, 13*(1), 15–32.

indicate the nature of the deficit. Identification of the word-retrieval strategies of these children may aid in the design of remediation techniques directly related to these strategies.

One method for attaining more information from tests is a double naming technique (Fried-Oken, 1987). In this procedure, a standard naming test is administered twice. The results are examined to identify error response groups that occur once and twice. The double error group or errors that occur on both administrations require further analysis.

The speech–language pathologist administers a number of cues with the double error words to determine whether the errors are related to word-finding difficulties and to identify naming strategies. In this procedure, cues are adminis-trated in the following order (Fried-Oken, 1987):

1. *General question.* The child is asked a general, open-ended question, such as, "Can you think of another word for this?" or "What is this again?" that provides no additional linguistic information.

2. *Semantic/phonemic facilitator.* Two cues, based on additional semantic and phonemic information, are administered. The order of presentation varies, but the speech–language pathologist should record carefully the order and the response. The semantic cue describes the object's function, provides a superordinate label (categorical), or states the location. For example, if the picture shows a sofa, the speech–language pathologist might say, "It's something you sit on," "It's a piece of furniture," or "You find it in the living room." The child's response and the type of semantic facilitator should be noted.

   The phonemic cue includes the initial phoneme of the desired label ("The word starts with a /_/.") This type of cue requires certain metalin-guistic skills in order for the child to use the information.

3. *Verification.* If the child is still incorrect, the speech–language pathologist provides the correct label and asks whether the child has ever seen this object before in order to verify whether the word is in the child's reper-toire.

The child's responses and the cues are analyzed to determine the qualitative nature of the errors and the child's naming strategy. Possible naming strategies of 4- to 9-year-old children are listed in Table 3.6 (Fried-Oken, 1984).

Syntax. Syntactic testing can be extremely complicated because of the com-plexity and diversity of the syntactic system. Speech-language pathologists may wish to use entire test batteries or portions of several tests. The latter strategy is recommended for in-depth probing of potential problem areas. Appendix A offers an item analysis of several of the more widely used syntactic tests to aid speech-language pathologists in item selection. Naturally, when tests are used in a nonstandard manner or are combined with other subtests, the norms can no

TABLE 3.6
Naming strategy categories

Naming Strategy	Example
Phonological	foon/SPOON
Perceptual	lampshade/SKIRT
Semantic	tortoise/OCTOPUS
Semantic + perceptual	broom/MOP
	shirt/JACKET
Part/Whole	shoelace/SHOE
Functional circumlocution	you can play songs/PIANO
Descriptive circumlocution	it has numbers and hands/CLOCK
Contextual circumlocution	in a band/TAMBOURINE
Superordinate	food/CRACKERS
Subordinate	Shetland pony/HORSE
Unrelated perseveration	canoe/HARMONICA
	canoe/MUSHROOM
Comment	I don't know/GLOVE
No answer	10 + seconds of silence/MITTEN
Gesture	"strumming"/GUITAR

Source: Fried–Oken, M. (1987). Qualitative examination of children's naming skills through test adaptations. *Language, Speech, and Hearing Services in Schools, 18,* 206–216. Reprinted with permission.

longer be used. Results must be described accurately and interpreted in light of the tasks involved.

There is considerable variability across tests in the length of individual syntactic items, the structures tested, and the type of testing tasks used. Test items are as diverse as highly unnatural tasks such as word ordering or unscrambling, sentence assembling, and more natural tasks such as sentence combining (Nippold et al., 1993). Many mirror the highly decontextualized tasks found in school but do not reflect everyday language use.

In general, development of comprehension of syntactic forms precedes production. Thus, a thorough language assessment should include evaluation of both aspects. Although the receptive procedures used and the structures assessed vary widely across tests, the common element is that the child demonstrates understanding—usually by pointing to a picture or following directions—while producing only minimal language, if any.

Syntactic production typically is tested by using either a structured elicitation or a sentence imitation format. In structured elicitation, the child may be asked to describe a picture, following a model by the test administrator. The model sentence establishes the sentence form to be used but differs from the desired sentence by the structure being tested. In sentence imitation, the child gives an immediate repetition of the administrator's sentence.

The underlying assumption of elicited imitation procedures is that sentences that exceed the child's immediate memory span will be reproduced according to the child's own linguistic rule system, which the child must use as a processing aid. Theoretically, the child's sentence should be very similar to the one the child would produce spontaneously. Conversely, the imitated sentence should not contain any structures absent in the child's spontaneous language production.

Although elicited imitation serves as the basis of a number of diagnostic instruments (Carrow, 1974; Gray & Ryan, 1973; Zachman, Huisingh, Jorgensen, & Barrett, 1978a, 1978b) and as a portion of several other tools (Bankson, 1977; Foster, Giddan, & Stark, 1973; Hendrick, Prather, & Tobin, 1975; Mecham, Jex, & Jones, 1967; Newcomer & Hammill, 1977; Semel & Wiig, 1980), the validity of the procedure has been questioned frequently. In part, the issue in elicited imitation is one of scoring. Whereas most tests concern merely the accuracy of repetition, the Carrow Elicited Language Inventory (CELI) attempts to analyze the changes that children with language impairment make when they repeat.

The imitative procedure may underestimate, overestimate, or correctly estimate the child's actual language abilities (Prutting & Connolly, 1976). For example, although the performance of children with language impairment on elicited imitation tests can be enhanced by the addition of contextual cues, such as pictures or object manipulation (Hale-Haniff & Siegel, 1981; L. Nelson & Weber-Olsen, 1980; Weber-Olsen, Putnam-Sims, & Gannon, 1983), their imitations are still simpler than their spontaneous language production (Connell & Myles-Zitler, 1982). In part, this disparity may result from the fact that assumptions about the performance of nonimpaired children may not apply to children with language impairment (J. Miller, 1978).

Because the relationship between elicited imitation and spontaneously produced language is a very complex one, speech-language pathologists are advised to use elicited imitation results with caution and to rely on the data from spontaneous samples when the two differ (Fujiki & Brinton, 1987). Elicited imitation responses should be analyzed for the specific ways they differ from the model. Table 3.7 provides a method of scoring sentence imitation tasks that maximizes the available information for clinical use (Mattes, 1982). Each response is scored for grammatical acceptability, type of syntactic error, semantic equivalence, and quality of response.

Morphology. Morphological testing usually focuses on bound morphemes or inflections in the form of prefixes and suffixes. Most tests emphasize suffixes, such as tense markers, plurals, possessives, and comparators, because of their high usage and relatively early development. In general, children with good spoken and written language abilities have more morphological awareness and do better on tests (Anderson & Davison, 1988; Bailet, 1990; Carlisle, 1987; Fischer, Shankweiler, & Liberman, 1985; Liberman, Rubin, Duques, & Carlisle, 1985; Nagy, Anderson, Schommer, Scott, & Stallman, 1989; Snow, 1990; Sterling, 1983; Vogel, 1983; Wiig et al., 1973).

Suffixes can be divided into two types—inflectional and derivational. *Inflectional* morphological suffixes indicate possession, gender, and number in nouns; tense, voice, person and number, and mood in verbs; and comparison in adjec-

TABLE 3.7
Elicited language analysis procedures

		Format		

Student's Name: _____

Birthdate: _____   Examiner: _____   Test Date: _____

Test Item #	*Instructions:* Record the child's responses in the spaces below. Score responses in terms of grammatical acceptability, syntactic usage, vocabulary usage and response quality by placing a check mark in the boxes which most accurately describe the response.	Grammatical Acceptability	Correct: Identical	Correct: Nonidentical	Substitution Error	Deletion Error	Insertion Error	Modification Error	Word Sequence Error	Non-Attempt Error	Equivalent in Meaning	Related in Meaning	Unrelated in Meaning	Delayed Response	Self-Corrected Response	Perseverative Response	Comments
			Syntactic Usage on Structure Tested								Vocabulary			Response Quality			

The child's elicited imitation is written in the appropriate column at the left. Omissions, substitutions, changes in meaning and the like are noted by marking the appropriate column. The errors and target structures can be recorded under the comments column, such as "Omit past tense -ed" or "Change passive voice to active." Such analysis may help delineate unlearned structures and the cognitive-linguistic knowledge base.

tives and do not change the part of speech of the base (Fromkin & Rodman, 1984). For example, a noun can be made plural with the addition of the *-s* marker, but the noun remains a noun. Inflectional suffixes are applied conventionally by syntactic rule.

The second, larger category, derivational suffixes, is ignored in most tests. *Derivational* suffixes have a smaller range of application and many more constraints and irregularities than inflectional suffixes. Application may be unpredictable, as with *-tion,* which can be added to some but not all nouns, or may be somewhat unclear in meaning, as in *apart**ment.*** More than 80% of such multimorpheme words do not mean what the constituent parts suggest (Nagy & Anderson, 1984; White, Power, & White, 1989). The development of derivational suffixes is not as clearly understood as that of inflectional suffixes but seems related to oral

TABLE 3.7, *continued*

Response Categories

Grammatical acceptability. Child's response is a complete and grammatically correct sentence.

Syntactic usage on structure tested. The manner in which the grammatical structure tested is produced.

A. *Correct production: identical sentence frame.* Child's response is an identical word-for-word reproduction of the model.

B. *Correct production; nonidentical sentence frame.* The grammatical structure being tested is produced correctly, although the sentence frame differs from the model.

C. *Substitution error.* The child substitutes an inappropriate grammatical form for the structure being tested.

D. *Deletion error.* The child inappropriately omits the grammatical structure being tested.

E. *Insertion error.* The child inserts the grammatical structure being tested within a sentence frame where it is inappropriate.

F. *Modification error.* The child produces a modification of the grammatical structure being tested that is not acceptable in any context (ex. *him's, ain't, it's is*).

G. *Word sequence error.* The child produces the grammatical structure being tested in an appropriate position within the response.

H. *Non-attempt error.* Performance can not be evaluated (ex. *I don't know*).

Vocabulary usage. Manner in which the child's response relates semantically to the stimulus sentence.

A. *Equivalent in meaning.* Although the specific vocabulary used by the child is not identical to the model, the response is identical in meaning.

B. *Related in meaning.* The child produces a response which is partially related to the meaning of the model. The child may omit essential elements or modify vocabulary.

C. *Unrelated in meaning.* The child produces a nonmeaningful response or one that is unrelated to the model.

Response quality.

A. *Delayed correct response.* The child produces a correct response which is nonimmediate, requires a repetition of the model, or is produced after hesitation during response.

B. *Self-corrected response.* The child self-corrects an incorrect response without prompting by the examiner.

C. *Perseverative response.* The child produces a response that resembles that used on a previous test item but inappropriate for this item.

Source: Mattes, L. (1982). The elicited language analysis procedure: A method for scoring sentence imitation tasks. *Language, Speech, and Hearing Services in Schools, 13,* 37–41. Reprinted with permission.

language production abilities, reading level and exposure, derivational complexity, and metalinguistic awareness (Carlisle, 1987, 1988; Derwing, 1976; Derwing & Baker, 1979; Fisher et al., 1985; Jaeger, 1984; Meyerson, 1978; Nagy & Anderson, 1984; Nagy, Anderson, & Herman, 1987; Nagy, Herman, & Anderson, 1985; Templeton, 1980; Tyler & Nagy, 1987; Wysocki & Jenkins, 1987).

The two most common expressive test formats for morphology are *cloze,* or sentence completion, and sentence imitation. Most cloze procedure test items give the root word and require the child to respond with the root plus a suffix, as in *teach-teacher*. Tests use either actual words or nonsense words. The rationale for nonsense words is that their use will not bias performance by previous exposure. In general, tests using nonsense words, such as the Berry-Talbott Developmental Guide to the Comprehension of Grammar (Berry & Talbott, 1977), are more difficult for young children (Channell & Ford, 1991). Children with mental retardation or LLD have greater difficulty than children developing normally with nonsense word tests. Other tasks might include judgments of relatedness of words, such as *hospital* and *hospitable*, ability to deduce meaning from component parts, and ability to form words in different and changing linguistic contexts (Moats & Smith, 1992).

Although several tests have morphological portions or subtests (See Table 3.4), most have too few items and too narrow a scope to provide much valuable information (Moats & Smith, 1992). Prefixes and derivational suffixes are included on only a few tests, such as the Clinical Evaluation of Language Fundamentals (Semel, Wiig, & Secord, 1987), the Fullerton, and the TOAL-2.

Phonology.   Assessment of phonological functions should provide information on severity of the impairment; direction for intervention; baseline data on all phonemes, all error patterns; and overall intelligibility (Hodson, 1992). Error pattern determination may require at least 10 productions of each target phoneme and structure. Commonly used sampling techniques for phonological analysis include spontaneous labeling of pictures and objects (Fisher & Logemann, 1987; Fudala, 1970; Goldman & Fristoe, 1986; Hodson, 1980; Klein, 1984; Templin & Darley, 1969), conversation and narration (Shriberg & Kwiatkowski, 1980), and imitation (Weiner, 1979). Different methods of collection yield different results in the amount and type of errors produced (Andrews & Fey, 1986; Garrett & Moran, 1992; J. Johnson, Winney, & Pederson, 1980). Labeling tasks produce the greatest variety and allow for the greatest speech–language pathologist control of phonological contexts. In addition, the known targets increase the speech–language pathologist's ability to analyze unintelligible utterances (Hodson, 1980; Paden & Moss, 1985).

Ease of identification and caseload constraints would suggest that speech–language pathologists apply an initial strategy in which articulation test results are analyzed for phonological processes when a phonological disorder is suspected (Haynes & Steed, 1987; Klein, 1984). For example, the Khan-Lewis Phonological Analysis (Khan & Lewis, 1986) might be used to reanalyze the results of the Goldman-Fristoe Test of Articulation (Goldman & Fristoe, 1986). The potential user of the Khan-Lewis should note that it may be too sensitive to overall difference but not sensitive enough to levels of severity (Garn-Nunn, 1992).

Most articulation tests sample each sound once in each of the positions in which it appears in words. Other appearances are not scored. By carefully transcribing each word spoken in the test, however, the speech–language pathologist can increase the database and have additional productions to analyze for possible phonological processes. Table 3.8 is a form to use with the Goldman-Fristoe. Blank spaces on this table are used to note those phonological processes demonstrated by the child. The processes are explained in the table. Developmental information is included in Appendix B. Speech-language pathologists must be cautious with such results, however, because the number of sounds in error is not the full measure of severity or unintelligibility (Grunwell, 1987; Shriberg & Kwiatkowski, 1982).

Imitation tasks may offer a compromise between efficiency and thoroughness. Several studies have found a positive correlation across single-word free

TABLE 3.8
Phonological analysis of articulation test results

Name _____

Age _____

Date _____

Goldman-Fristoe Items	Ø Initial C	Ø Final C	Apicalization	Stopping	Assimilation	Fronting	Backing	Labialization	Voicing Change	Ø Syllable	Gliding	CC(C) Substitution	CC(C) Reduction		I	M	F
house			■			■					■	■	■		h		s
telephone					■			■			■	■			t	f	n
cup				■							■	■	■		k		p
gun			■			■		■			■	■	■		g		n
knife			■			■					■	■	■		n		f
window	■		■		■					■	■	■	■		w	n	X
wagon	■		■				■				■	■	■		w	g	n
wheel	■		■							■	■	■			w		l
chicken			■		■		■				■	■	■		tʃ	k	n
zipper			■	■							■	■	■		z	p	ɚ
scissors			■	■							■	■	■		s	z	z
duck			■		■	■					■	■	■		d		k
yellow	■		■		■	■				■	■	■	■		j	l	X
vacuum				■		■					■	■	■		v	kj	m
matches					■						■	■			m	tʃ	z
lamp			■			■					■	■	■		l		mp
shovel			■	■							■	■			ʃ	v	l
car											■				k		
rabbit											■	■	■		r	b	t
fishing					■						■	■	■		f	ʃ	ŋ
church			■	■	■						■	■	■		tʃ		tʃ
feather		■	■	■		■					■	■	■		f	ð	ɚ
pencils				■		■					■	■	■		p	s	lz
this/that				■							■	■			ð		s,t
carrot						■				■	■				k	r	t
orange	■																ndʒ
bathtub			■							■	■	■	■		b	θ	b
bath											■	■			b		θ
thumb											■	■			θ		m
finger		■	■		■	■				■	■	■	■		f	g	ɚ
ring			■			■				■	■	■	■		r		ŋ
jumping			■			■					■	■	■		dʒ	p	ŋ
pajamas						■					■	■	■		p	dʒ	z
plane				■		■				■	■	■			pl		n
blue				■		■				■	■	■			bl		X
brush				■		■					■	■			br		ʃ
drum				■		■					■	■			dr		m
flag											■	■			fl		g
Santa Claus			■								■	■			s	kl	z
Christmas											■	■			kr	s	s
tree			■	■		■			■		■	■			tr		X
squirrel			■	■		■					■	■			skw		l
sleeping						■					■	■			sl	p	ŋ
bed				■							■	■	■		b		d
stove											■	■			st		v

TABLE 3.8, *continued*

Phonological process definitions

ØInitial C Initial consonant deletion occurs when the initial consonant of a target word is omitted in the child's production. Example: /bot/ goes to [ot]

ØFinal C Deletion of final consonant occurs when a target word ending with a consonant is produced with that final consonant omitted. Example: /bot/ goes to [bo]

Apicalization In apicalization a labial consonant is replaced by a tongue-tip consonant. Example: /fud/ goes to [sud]

Stopping The process of stopping involves the replacement of a fricative, affricate or semi-vowel with a stop consonant. Example: /sop/ goes to [top]

Assimilation Assimilation refers to the influence that speech sounds can have on the production of other speech sounds. Thus if a speech sound changes to be more like another speech sound in its near environment, assimilation has occurred. The assimilation can be to other speech sounds that precede or follow the changed phone. Example: /fit/ goes to [pit] because of the influence of the stop /t/.

Fronting Fronting occurs when a velar stop or palatal affricate or fricative is replaced by an alveolar speech sound. Example: /kap/ goes to [tap]

Backing The process of backing occurs when an anterior consonant is replaced by a velar or glottal consonant. Example: /to/ goes [ko]

Labialization Labialization involves the replacement of a tongue-made articulation with a speech sound made with one or both of the lips. A common instance is the replacement of /θ/ with /f/. When the sound change only occurs in the presence of a labial consonant it is a form of assimilation.

Voicing Change Voicing change occurs whenever a speech sound changes in its voicing feature. The addition of voicing is marked by a plus sign (+). Devoicing is marked by a minus sign (–).

ØSyllable Syllable deletion can occur only in polysyllabic words. Typically, the unstressed syllable is deleted. Example: /patedo/ goes to [tedo]

Gliding Gliding entails the replacement of a liquid with a glide. Example: /lo/ goes to [wo]

CC(C) Substitution/Reduction In this process a two- or three-member cluster has a member substituted or deleted. Typically, the marked member is the one substituted for or deleted. Example: /stov/ goes to [tov] or /blu/ goes [bwu]

Source: Lowe, R. (1986). Phonological process analysis using three position tests. *Language, Speech, and Hearing Services in Schools, 17,* 72–79. Reprinted with permission.

speech and imitation samples and across connected speech and sentence imitation samples (Haynes & Steed, 1987; Paynter & Bumpas, 1977; Siegel, Winitz, & Conkey, 1963). After testing, the speech-language pathologist can collect and analyze conversational samples in order to revise her hypotheses and to plan intervention (Andrews & Fey, 1986).

Only about 20% of intelligibility is related to the percentage of correct sounds (Bishop & Edmundson, 1987; Shriberg et al., 1986). Intelligibility is more affected by error patterns; language variables, such as syllable shape, grammatical class, and stress; and prosody-voice features (Shriberg & Kwiatkowski, 1982).

Tests tend to separate phonological production from these underlying psycholin-guistic processes of discourse (Morrison & Shriberg, 1992). Therefore, conversational sampling is essential, along with an analysis of segmental errors and suprasegmental and language variables (Kwiatkowski & Shriberg, 1992).

Speech in conversation contains more speech sound errors (Dubois & Bernthal, 1978; Klein, 1984) and more clinically significant results (Andrews & Fey, 1986) than speech sampled in isolated words. Single-word production tasks do not correlate well with the results of connected speech analysis (Dubois & Bernthal, 1978; Shriberg & Kwiatkowski, 1980; Simmons-Miles, 1983). Thus, speech–language pathologists may miss some significant clinical information by concentrating only on production in isolated contexts. Most professionals agree on the need for more than single-word test performance because of coarticulation and the need to assess in the use context of ongoing conversation (Daniloff & Moll, 1968; Haynes, Haynes, & Jackson, 1982; Panagos, Quine, & Klich, 1979; Schmauch, Panagos, & Klich, 1978).

Test Modification

As mentioned previously, tests can be modified to provide the information desired by the speech-language pathologist. For example, the speech-language pathologist may wish to test a child's pronoun use in depth. No test is available that adequately assesses only these structures. The speech-language pathologist might construct her own assessment tool from portions of other tests. This type of locally prepared test may be very useful for thorough assessment. Obviously, individual test standards of administration have been violated and the norms would be invalid. Occasionally, published tests include subtest norms. In this case, a subtest on pronouns may be administered in its entirety as directed in the instructions, and the norming information would be applicable.

Test administration may be modified also for the special child who cannot perform as required or for further investigation of the child's response strategies. For example, use of pictures or repetition of instructions may enhance the performance of some children. It is important to remember that nearly all tests are designed for children developing normally. The child with mild retardation and cerebral palsy is at a very distinct disadvantage when being tested. In such cases, description of the child's ability will be much more useful for intervention than a score or age equivalent. Adherence to prescribed test procedures is more likely to result in a measure of the special child's limitations.

Testing procedures may be modified through the use of multiple sessions, increased time to respond, and increased trials. For children with attentional difficulties, the speech-language pathologist might enlarge materials, use a penlight or pointer, highlight certain information, verbally remind the child to attend, or have the child repeat the test cue. It has been my experience that children with mental retardation do not respond well to the tiny pictures used in the Denver Developmental Scale. Larger pictures result in increased responding.

The performance of children with motor problems, autism, or LLD might be affected also by visual or auditory distractions, placement of materials, temperature, lighting, light and dark contrasts, and positioning. Children who perseverate may need to be reminded that the correct answer is not always the same. Children with short-term memory problems may need to repeat cues or to have cues broken into easily processible units.

Finally, children with TBI may need a longer time to respond. The speech-language pathologist also should test beyond base and ceiling scores to identify "islands" of learning. Other modifications for these children may include reduction of distractions, different response modes, enlarged print and reduction of print per page, simplified instructions, substituting multiple choice questions to facilitate recall, giving multiple examples, providing breaks when fatigue is evident, and darkening lines or print in visual displays (Russell, 1993).

Sampling

Conversational sampling has the potential for providing the most accurate description of the child's language as it is actually used in conversational exchange. Although sampling usually includes freeplay and unstructured conversation, it also may include structured conversation and probing of language features noted in observation and testing. In the next several chapters, we discuss the best ways to maximize the information from this source through design of collection situations and analysis methods.

Conclusion

There is no one way to assess the language of children with language impairments. A combination of interviewing, observation, testing, and sampling/probing offers a holistic approach that can incorporate not only the child but also significant others and familiar communication contexts. As you will see in the final section, these aspects of language assessment are especially important when assessing the language of minority children.

CHILDREN WITH LIMITED ENGLISH PROFICIENCY AND DIFFERENT DIALECTS

More than 35 million speakers of minority language live in the United States. This number includes many Hispanic Americans or Latinos and Asian Americans and some Native Americans for whom English is a second language. In addition, a portion of working-class African Americans use Black English, a nonstandard dialect of American English. Nationally, approximately 7 million children speak English as a second language. In New York state, more than 130 languages are represented in the schools (Heberle, 1992).

In many large cities, more than 50% of the school population is minority children. Minority children have a greater dropout rate, are less successful in school, are overrepresented in programs for the disabled, and are underrepresented in programs for the gifted. The primary reason for children with LEP being referred for possible special education placement is difficulty with English (Damico, 1991b).

Unfortunately, in the United States, minority children often live in poverty. This status usually means a higher incidence of teen pregnancy, poor prenatal care, drug and alcohol abuse, low birth weight, poor nutrition, childhood illness and injury, and communication disorders. In addition, the demographics of immigration have changed recently to include many more immigrants from economically poor countries with poorer educations and few of the high literacy skills demanded by the United States' changing economy (Heberle, 1992). The differences are both linguistic and cultural.

Within the minority language population is a continuum of proficiency in English (ASHA Position Paper, 1985), including bilingual English proficient, limited English proficient (LEP), and limited in both English and the minority language. Individuals who are *bilingual English proficient* are proficient in both English and their native language. Still, they may have a language impairment in English. It is important that the speech-language pathologist be able to distinguish between a disorder and a dialectal difference that is the result of interaction of the native language and English. The speech-language pathologist must appreciate the rule-governed nature of the native language and know the contrastive features of the native language. Elective speech and language services may be provided to individuals who are bilingual English proficient and who desire more standard production of English. It is important for the speech-language pathologist to remember, however, that native dialects are not disorders.

Individuals who are **limited English proficient** (LEP) are proficient in their native language but not in English. Assessment and intervention should be conducted in the native language as mandated by federal law (PL 94-142 and PL 95-561), legal decisions (*Diana v. Board of Education,* 1970; *Lau v. Nichols,* 1974; and *Larry P. v. Riles,* 1972), and state educational regulations. Adequate service delivery by the speech-language pathologist requires native or near native fluency in both languages and ability to describe speech and language acquisition in both languages, to administer and interpret formal and informal assessment procedures, to apply intervention strategies in minority language, and to recognize cultural factors that affect service delivery to the minority language community (ASHA Position Paper, 1985). For the remainder of the text, we shall use the term *LEP* to refer to children learning English as their second language. Other children will be specified as needed.

Finally, those with limited proficiency in both English and the native language are truly communicatively handicapped. Language testing should establish language dominance and the most appropriate language for intervention (ASHA Position Paper, 1985). One error often made by inexperienced speech-language pathologists is to assume that the native language (L_1) is dominant. Young children may loose L_1 as they begin to acquire a second language (L_2), which in this case is English.

State of Service Delivery

Although the demographics of the United States are changing, the overwhelming majority of speech-language pathologists will continue to belong to the majority culture for the foreseeable future (Shewan, 1988). Approximately one in three speech-language pathologists has some bilingual clients, but more than 80% of these professionals do not feel confident in their abilities to serve these clients (Shewan & Malm, 1989; O. Taylor, 1989). Inadequacies include a lack of academic preparation and experience, unfamiliarity with the language and/or culture, and a lack of appropriate assessment tools (Adler, 1991).

Lack of Preparation and Experience

Most academic programs offer little preparation for working with minority children through either coursework or practicum. Until this deficiency changes, it is the responsibility of each speech-language pathologist to educate herself through continuing education. The following are some ways to interact more with culturally diverse populations:

> Work alongside a bilingual speech-language pathologist as her "assistant."
>
> Take a foreign language course and/or a course in cultural diversity.
>
> Join cultural organizations and attend cultural festivals.
>
> Become a Big Brother or Big Sister or volunteer to work with culturally diverse youth.
>
> Volunteer in organizations such as Habitat for Humanity.
>
> Join organizations, such as National Coalition Builders Institute, that foster cooperation and understanding.
>
> Join church groups that foster interactions with inner-city churches.
>
> Go out of your way to introduce yourself to individuals from others cultures.

Each speech-language pathologist should remember that when she enters the environment of another cultural group, she is a guest and should act accordingly. Members of the majority culture sometimes expect members of minority cultures to accept them with open arms. My experience has been that there is a period of adjustment in which mutual trust is built. Only then does acceptance begin to grow. It is sometimes difficult for members of the majority to remember that they are here to learn, not to teach, at least not initially.

Unfamiliarity with Language and Culture

Becoming familiar with another culture and another language requires shedding many preconceived notions and becoming culturally aware. This requirement is followed by education about particular languages and cultures and about language development among children with LEP and children with different dialects. It is extremely difficult to become fluent in a second language as an adult or from classroom instruction. Therefore, one method for the speech-language pathologist to overcome her linguistic deficits is to use language interpreters. This alternative is discussed at the end of this section.

Growth of awareness.   All aspects of our lives are overlaid by culture. It affects our institutions and the way we act and think. **Culture** is a shared framework of meanings within which a population shapes its way of life. It is neither static nor absolute, but has been shaped by the population's history and evolves as individuals constantly rework it and add new ideas and behaviors. It includes, but is not limited to, history and the explanation of natural phenomenon; societal roles; rules for interactions, decorum, and discipline; family structure; education; religious beliefs; standards of health, illness, hygiene, appearance, and dress; diet; perceptions of time and space; definitions of work and play; artistic and musical values, life expectations, and aspirations; and communication and language use.

Each culture has a unique outlook. It is essential for the speech-language pathologist to recognize that culture is pervasive and diffused throughout her own life. Culture forms the basis for her values and worldview. Therefore, culture influences the way she views individuals from other cultures.

Speech-language pathologists from the majority culture in the United States typically have Euro-centered standards. These standards will influence each speech-language pathologist's decisions about language impairment, although these standards may not apply among individuals from other cultures. For example, Vietnamese culture is much more tolerant of speech and language diversity than is American majority culture. Likewise, the Navajo culture values a quiet, introspective persona, which may seem withdrawn by American majority standards.

Words and concepts also are related culturally. For example, the word and the concept *crib* are not found in Korean. Table 3.9 offers other examples of cultural variants. Although the speech-language pathologist cannot know all cultures, she can become increasingly culture sensitive. It is important for her to respect other cultures and to recognize that no one culture is the standard. American majority culture is not the cultural prescriptor (N. Anderson, 1991).

Cultural sensitivity requires not only recognition of one's own culture but also examination of cultural notions held as "truths." Many traditional notions of the American majority culture, especially those involving poverty and ethnicity or race, are inappropriate. The poor are not one big homogeneous group, and cultural stereotypes of this type should be rejected (Adler, 1973; N. Anderson, 1991; Coleman & Rainwater, 1978). The overall organization of the family and home, the education level of the mother, and the amount and type of stimulation a child receives is more important for overall development than socioeconomic status (Adler, 1990; Helton, 1974).

The following are guidelines for interacting with clients from different cultures (Taylor, Payne, & Anderson, 1987):

1. Each encounter is a socially situated communicative event subject to cultural rules governing such events by both participants.
2. Children perform differently under differing conditions because of their unique cultural and linguistic backgrounds.
3. Different modes, channels, and functions of communication may evidence differing levels of linguistic and communicative performance.
4. Ethnographic techniques and cultural norms should be used for evaluating behavior and making determinations of language impairment.

TABLE 3.9
Cultural variants that may influence assessment

Concept	Majority American Culture	Cultural Differences*
Achievement	Emphasis on competition and success. Define self by accomplishments. *To the victor go the spoils.*	Cooperation and group spirit. Accept status quo. Manual labor respected.
Age	Youth is valued.	Elders are revered. Growing old is desirable.
Communication	Casual, direct eye contact, loud voice acceptable. Silence means attentiveness. Emphasize verbal.	Respectful, avoid eye contact, loudness for anger. Silence means boredom. Non-linguistic and paralinguistic important.
Control	Free will.	Fate.
Education	Universal, formal, verbal. Key to social mobility. Teacher is authority. Classroom passivity rewarded. Reflective, analytical. Tests are part of learning.	Formal for few. Entrance into mainstream society. Elders, peers, and siblings are teachers. Active, physical learning. Spontaneous, intuitive. Testing not integral.
Family	Nuclear, small, contractual partnership, child centered.	Extended, kinship important, more varied, elder or parent centered. Male or female dominated.
Gender/role	Relative equality.	Males independent, pampered. Females have many home responsibilities.
Individuality	Individual makes own life. Stress self-reliance.	Humility, anonymity, deference to group.
Materialism	Acquisition, symbol of success and power.	Excessive accumulation is bad, status ascribed.
Social interaction	Noncontact, large interpartner distance. Large group of friends desired.	Contact, physical closeness. Kinship more important than friends.
Time	Governed by clock and calendar, punctual, value speed, future oriented. Time is money. Scheduled.	Enjoy the present, can't change future. Little concept of wasting time. Flexible.

Note: * No specific culture.
Source: Compiled from Alamanza & Mosley (1980); Chamberlain & Medinos-Landurand (1991); Goldman & McDermott (1987); Gollnick & Chinn (1983); Mehrabian (1972); S. Seymour (1981)

5. Possible sources of conflict in assumptions and norms should be identified prior to an interaction and action taken to prevent them from occurring.

6. Learning about culture is ongoing and should result in constant reevaluation and revision of ideas and in greater sensitivity.

This new awareness should lead to a recognition that "assessment is a subjective process that is highly influenced by the socio-political, cultural, and linguistic context" (Chamberlain & Medinos-Landurand, 1991, p. 112). In fact, to make sense of our behaviors, we must view them against the background of culture.

Education in language, culture, and language development. Just sensitivity is not enough. The speech-language pathologist must educate herself about the dialects, languages, and cultures of the individuals she serves and about the process of dialect and second-language learning.

Typically, speech-language pathologists make two common errors in evaluating the language of minority children. Either children are identified incorrectly as having a language disorder, or those with a disorder are missed. For example, African American children from rural Alabama who speak the Black English dialect common to that area continue to delete final consonants beyond the age at which middle-class white children do (Haynes & Moran, 1989). The speech-language pathologist who is unaware of this difference might conclude, incorrectly, that these children exhibit a phonological disorder.

Dialects and languages. It is not possible to learn all of the dialects or languages one might encounter, especially in large metropolitan areas. Therefore, each speech-language pathologist should attempt to learn the contrastive influences between other languages and dialects and Standard American English. Common phonologic, syntactic, and morphologic contrasts are found in Appendix C. Speech-language pathologists also can learn high-usage words and forms of greeting in the language served.

Children in the United States who are bilingual Spanish-English or who use Spanish only may perform very differently even from each other (K. Wilcox & McGuinn-Aasby, 1988). These differences may reflect U.S. regional differences, country of origin, dialectal, or socioeconomic differences (M. Norris, Juarez, & Perkins, 1989).

Cultures. The breadth of cultural diversity is beyond the scope of this text. Suffice it to say that each speech-language pathologist should become familiar with the cultures that she serves. Reading and observation are both essential methods of learning. The speech-language pathologist must remember that cultures are not monolithic and that there is much heterogeneity, especially in the Hispanic American population. Of particular importance are the child-rearing practices, family structure, attitudes toward language impairment and intervention, and communication style. Variants of communication style include nonlinguistic and paralinguistic characteristics, such as eye contact, facial expression, and gestures; intercommunicant space and the use of silence and laughter; pragmatic aspects, such as roles, politeness and forms of address, interruption rules, turn taking, greeting and salutations, the ordering of conversational events, and appropriate topics; and the use of humor (Fasold, 1990; Hymes, 1974; Saville-Troike, 1986; O. Taylor, 1986b). It is best if the speech-language pathologist is somewhat cautious at first, until she has a sense of cultural expectations.

Cultures differ in their beliefs about health, disability, and causation. A great deal of discomfort may surround disorder and intervention. Some families will be surprised by the extent of their expected role in intervention. Speech-language pathologists should avoid assumptions or preconceived notions about cultural attitudes.

Dialect and second-language learning.   An in-depth discussion of dialect and second-language learning is beyond the scope of this chapter, but we shall explore the highlights. Not all children with different dialects are the same. Each child's language will differ with the specific dialect spoken and the maturity of language and dialect development. Although data are limited, we know that children learning Black English, the dialect spoken by some inner-city and Southern rural African Americans, show only minimal evidences of their dialect by age 3. Earlier development is closer to the middle-class standard described in most development texts. By age 5, however, most Black English forms are being used, at least in part.

In general, second-language learning is more difficult than first-language learning, which for most children is fairly effortless. A language assessment must distinguish between those errors that reflect this difficulty and those that represent a language impairment.

Most children are sequential bilingual learners: The first language (L_1) has reached a certain level of maturity before acquisition of the second language (L_2) begins. Sequential learning may maximize the interference between the two languages. **Interference** is the influence of one language on the learning of another. For example, the English /p/ is difficult for Arabic speakers but not for Spanish speakers. I have great difficulty with the Spanish *cion* ending because of my use of the French *-tion*. Interference in simultaneous bilingual acquisition seems to be only minimal (Genesee, 1988).

The monolingual "age-stage" model of development is inappropriate when describing second-language learning (Roseberry & Connell, 1991). Likewise, rate of learning is a poor index because of the many variables that affect second-language learning.

Preschool children will have an immature L_1 prior to acquisition of L_2. The result may be "semilingualism," in which the child fails to reach monolingual proficiency in either language (Skutnabb-Kangas & Toukomas, 1976). The child may be delayed in development of L_1 after exposure to L_2 if the second language is dominant in the culture. This situation is rarely considered in language assessments (Langdon, 1989). In general, competence in L_2 is related to the maturity of L_1 (Cummins, 1976, 1979b, 1980, 1984). The more mature the child's use of L_1, the easier it is to learn L_2 (Jacobson, 1985; Skutnabb-Kangas & Toukomas, 1976).

Initially, the child in preschool may be silent for a while on exposure to L_2. Although the child appears to have a language impairment, this is not the case. It takes time for the child to decipher the linguistic code (Kessler, 1984; Schiff-Myers, Coury, & Perez, 1989). Older children possess metalinguistic skills that aid in this deciphering process.

School-age children may appear to have a language learning disability. The decontextualized language of the classroom may be especially difficult. If exposure to L_2 does not occur until after age 6, it may take 5 to 7 years to acquire age-appropriate cognitive and academic skills (Cummins, 1980). The result is that in the United States, many children have never fully developed L_1—often Spanish—

and are deficient in academic use of English (L₂) (Pacheco, 1983). L₁ may exhibit arrested development or be lost if it is not used, if it is not valued by the child, discouraged by the parents, or considered less prestigious, as in the United States (Conklin & Lourie, 1983; Cummins, 1980; Lambert, 1981; Tosi, 1984).

Factors that affect L₂ competency are individual characteristics, such as intelligence, learning style, positive attitude about one's self, one's own native language, and the target language, extrovertism and a feeling of control, and a lack of anxiety about L₂ learning; and home and community characteristics, such as parental and community attitudes and the level of literacy in the home (Naiman, Frolich, & Stern, 1975; Oller, Baca, & Vigil, 1978; Pinsleur, 1980; Stevick, 1976; Tucker, Hamayan, & Genesee, 1976; Weinstein, 1984). Low socioeconomic status alone is not a negative factor but may be paired with poor literacy or poor L₁ use in the home and/or little opportunity to converse one-on-one with mature L₁ users who can label environmental entities and events and thus help the child form a conceptual base (K. Nelson, 1985).

When compared to adults learning L₂, children show a greater readiness to learn, are more perceptive of sounds, are less subject to interference from L₁, and learn through sensory activity within the immediate context (Hamayan & Damico, 1991; Krashen, Long, & Scarcella, 1979). Adult learning is verbal and abstract, emphasizing rule learning; children form their own abstractions of the rules from context. Children tend to acquire "chunks" of language, usually high-usage phrases, with conscious rule learning becoming more important after age 9 (Hamayan & Damico, 1991). Although children usually do not learn L₂ faster or more easily than adults, they eventually outperform them (Genesee, 1987; Krashen et al., 1979; Snow & Hoefnagel-Hohe, 1978). Children are more likely to take risks.

In general, L₁ forms a foundation for the learning of L₂. What the child knows from one language is transferred to the other. This may be general knowledge about sentence construction and parts of speech or similar language processes if the languages are similar. Of course, interference also can occur, but its effects are usually minimal (Dulay & Burt, 1980; Madrid & Garcia, 1985; Millford & Hecht, 1980; Wolfram, 1985; L. Young, 1982). A poor base in L₁ usually leads to difficulties in L₂.

Languages other than English are devalued in the United States. This is the result of racial and ethnic discrimination and has resulted in a bilingual educational policy that sends a very clear message on the relative value of English (Schiff-Myers, 1992). The result is weakened linguistic and ethnic ties. The most common educational paradigm is a transitional bilingual program in which the child receives 2 or 3 years of bilingual education prior to placement in a monolingual English classroom. The not-so-subtle message is that English is better. Long-term maintenance programs that attempt to continue use and development of L₁ are rare (Schiff-Myers, 1992). A period of even 3 years is insufficient for the child to attain academic proficiency in English.

It is important that the speech-language pathologist recognize the process of sequential bilingual acquisition. This is a dynamic process; the child's language is changing. At times a child may exhibit behaviors similar to those of children with LLD. Performance may vary widely within and across children. Therefore, language assessments need to be tailored individually to each child (Dulay, Burt, & Krashen, 1982; Hamayan & Damico, 1991; Hyltenstam, 1985).

Overcoming bias in an assessment.   The goal of a communication assessment with children with LEP is to differentiate difficulties that result from experiential and cultural factors from those that are related to language impairment (Damico, 1991b). Both cultural and linguistic factors influence performance in an assessment (Chamberlain & Medinos-Landurand, 1991). These may lead to misinterpretations and miscommunication. The speech-language pathologist must be careful not to stereotype behavior and draw incorrect and unfair conclusions. For example, Latin American children may seem uncooperative and inattentive, when, in fact, their behavior signifies different concepts of time, body language, and achievement.

The speech–language pathologist can avoid biasing data interpretation by asking the following questions (Damico, 1991b):

1. Are there other variables, such as limited exposure to English, infrequency of error, testing procedural mistakes, extreme test anxiety, or contextual factors, that might explain the difficulties exhibited with English?
2. Are similar problems exhibited in L_1?
3. Are the problems exhibited related to second language acquisition or dialectal differences?
4. Can the problems exhibited be explained by cross–cultural interference or related cultural phenomena?
5. Can the problems exhibited be explained by any bias effect related to personnel, materials, or procedures that occurred before, during, or after assessment?
6. Is there any systematicity or consistency to the linguistic problems exhibited that might suggest an underlying rule?

The speech-language pathologist should interpret the child's performance in light of the intrinsic and extrinsic biases inherent in the assessment process (N. Miller, 1984). Intrinsic biases, such as knowledge needed and normative samples, are part of the test, while extrinsic biases, such as sociocultural values and attitude toward testing, reside in the child.

Language use patterns of both the child and the speech-language pathologist and the language learning history of the child also may influence the assessment. Communication and interactive style are culture bound.

Bias can be overcome by addressing cultural and linguistic influences in a 4-step process (Chamberlain & Medinos-Landurand, 1991):

1. Recognize and identify variables that might affect the assessment.
2. Analyze tests and procedures for content and style.

3. Take variables into account and change procedures.

4. Teach test-taking strategies.

The speech-language pathologist should be mindful that each child's level of acculturation will differ with the age of the child and the extent of exposure to both cultures (Berry, 1980).

Use of interpreters. The accuracy of testing with children with LEP may be increased by using interpreters who speak the child's primary language (Watson, Omark, Gronell, & Heller, 1986). When an interpreter is not available, family members can aid the speech–language pathologist.

Minority children—both bilingual and dialectally different—perform significantly better with familiar examiners (Fuchs & Fuchs, 1989). This finding suggests the use of interpreters familiar with both the language and the culture of the child and his caregivers. In addition, it suggests that consistency is important, that interpreters should be staff members.

The American Speech-Language-Hearing Association (ASHA) has recommended the use of interpreters with speakers of minority language when the speech-language pathologist does not meet the recommended competencies for providing services for clients with LEP, when the language spoken by the client is uncommon in the geographic area, and when no trained professionals with competency in that language are readily available. The use of interpreters can improve significantly the assessment process (Crago & Annahatak, 1985; Godwin, 1977; Marr, Natter, & Wilcox, 1980; Perlman, 1984).

The speech-language pathologist must recognize the limitations of the process and must select and train the interpreter carefully. They must work together as a team with mutual respect. Three factors seem critical in the use of interpreters—selection, training, and relationship to the family and community (N. Anderson, 1992; Chamberlain & Medinos-Landurand, 1991; Randall-David, 1989).

Selection. Selection should be based on the potential interpreter's linguistic competencies, ethical and professional competencies, and general knowledge and personality (Chamberlain & Medinos-Landurand, 1991). The potential interpreter should possess a high degree of proficiency in both L_1 and English, be able to paraphrase well, be flexible, and have a working knowledge of developmental, educational, and communication terminology.

Ethical and professional competencies should include an ability to maintain confidentiality, a respect for the feelings and beliefs of others and for the roles of professionals, and an ability to maintain impartiality. Confidentiality is especially important if the interpreter is a resident of the immediate geographic area served. It is also important that the interpreter understand her or his personal abilities and limitations and the limitations of the position.

Finally, it is very desirable for the potential interpreter to have a knowledge of child development and educational procedures. Personal attributes include flexibility, trustworthiness, patience, an eye for detail, and a good memory.

Training.   Training must include the critical factors of assessment and intervention, including procedures and instruments or tools (N. Anderson, 1992). The interpreter must understand the importance of exact translation from L_1 to L_2 and the reverse.

Preassessment training includes the requirements of a thorough assessment and the specific test protocols, including technical language (Figueroa, Sandoval, & Merino, 1984). Rapport-building strategies and questioning techniques also should be taught.

Prior to each evaluation, the speech-language pathologist and the interpreter should review each case and the assessment procedures; practice pronunciation of the name, introductions, questioning, and nonlinguistic aspects of the interaction; and discuss the topics to be introduced. During the evaluation, the interpreter will interact with the child and caregiver(s) while the speech-language pathologist records the data. In the post-assessment interview with caregivers, the interpreter will convey the results.

Relationship with family and community.   Prior to the assessment, the interpreter should try to get to know the caregiver(s) and child. It is very important that the interpreter convey the confidentiality of the proceedings, especially if the interpreter is from the community. During the assessment, the interpreter is to translate exactly. The speech-language pathologist can aid this process by keeping interactional language simple and use of professional jargon to a minimum. It is the interpreter's responsibility to ensure that the caregivers thoroughly understand the process and the results and recommendations.

Conclusion.   Working through interpreters is difficult and does not address some of the other problems in assessment with children with LEP. The following list contains suggestions for working successfully with an interpreter (Lynch & Hanson, 1992; Randall-David, 1989). The speech-language pathologist should:

1. Meet regularly and keep communication open and the goals understood.
2. Have the interpreter meet with the child and caregiver(s) prior to an interview to establish rapport and to determine their educational level, attitudes, and feelings.
3. Learn proper protocols and forms of address in the native language.
4. Introduce herself to the family, describe roles, and explain the purpose and process of the assessment.
5. Speak more slowly and in short units, but not more loudly.
6. Avoid colloquialisms, abstractions, idiomatic expressions, metaphors, slang, and professional jargon.
7. Look directly at the child and caregiver(s), not at the interpreter. Address remarks to the caregiver(s).
8. Listen to the child and caregivers to glean nonlinguistic and paralinguistic information. What is not said may be as important as what is said.

9. Avoid body language or gestures that may be misunderstood.

10. Use a positive tone that conveys respect and interest.

11. Avoid oversimplification and condescension.

12. Give simple clear instructions and periodically check the family's and child's understanding.

13. Instruct the interpreter to translate the client's words without paraphrasing.

14. Instruct the interpreter to avoid inserting her or his own word or ideas in the translation or omitting information.

15. Be patient with the longer process inherent in translation.

Although these suggestion will not ensure success, they may lessen some friction that potentially could disrupt effective delivery of services.

Lack of Appropriate Assessment Tools

We can expect the performance of minority children to be affected by cultural differences and the performance on formal tests to reflect these differences (Oller, 1979). Likewise, negative listener or tester attitude affects children, causing poor performance. The result is lower expectations and inappropriate referral or classification (Brophy, 1983; Cummins, 1986; Rodriguez, Prieto, & Rueda, 1984).

Few, if any, nonbiased standardized language tests are available for evaluating children who are bidialectal and bilingual (Bernstein, 1989). Tests are typically unique to one culture or language. In two judicial decisions regarding placement of Mexican American and African American children in classes for the retarded (*Diana v. State Board of Education*, 1970; *Larry P. v. Riles*, 1972), the courts ruled that judgments made on the basis of responses to tests whose norming populations are inappropriate for these children are discriminatory.

Many of the tests widely used in speech-language pathology (Carrow, 1973, 1974; Kirk, McCarthy, & Winfield, 1968; L. Lee, 1971; Mecham et al., 1967) are normed on population samples with a disproportionately high number of middle-class white children. For example, older versions of the Peabody Picture Vocabulary Test (PPVT) have been shown to yield lower scores for lower socioeconomic groups and for middle-class African American children (Adler & Birdsong, 1983; Cazden, 1972; Kresheck & Nicolosi, 1973; Wolfram, 1983).

Error analysis suggests that some test items may be culturally biased against African American children. On the revised PPVT, African American children do more poorly than the norming population. Error patterns suggest that the children do not know the words and that the score spread is too narrow to be revealing (Washington & Craig, 1992).

In general, poor performance leads to lower expectations (Adler, 1990). It is inappropriate to compare children with LEP to native speakers of English. The use of chronological norms is especially questionable, given the great variety in developmental rate among minorities (H. Seymour, 1992). The child with LEP does not have language similar to a native speaker of English of a certain age. The problem becomes deciding which standard to use (Lahey, 1992).

The following five guidelines should be considered prior to using standardized tests with minority children (Musselwhite, 1983):

1. What is the relationship of the norming population and the client? Are enough minority children included to give a fair representation? Are separate norms used for different minority groups?

2. What is the relationship of the child's experience and the content areas of the test? Items using farm content, for example, may have little relevance for children in the inner city.

3. What is the relationship of the language and/or dialect being tested and the child's language and/or dialect dominance? This issue is critical in determining language impairment. The determining factor should be the child's ability to function within her or his own linguistic or dialectal community (Iglesias, 1986).

4. Will the language of the test penalize a nonstandard child by use of idiomatic or metaphoric language?

5. Is the child penalized for a particular pattern of learning or style of problem solving?

American English standardized tests can be used with modified procedures to enhance performance. Modifications may aid the speech-language pathologist in describing the child's language and communication skills. Obviously, the scores from such testing would be invalid and should not be reported.

Dual sets of norms—those from the test and locally prepared ones—can be used to compare the performance of minority children to that of the standard group and of their peer group (Musselwhite, 1983), but they must be used cautiously (H. Seymour, 1992). The test, however, is still in Standard American English. It seems more appropriate to measure the child's performance in his dialect and compare this performance to that of other children also using that dialect (H. Seymour, 1992). Unfortunately, we have very little data on this development and even fewer tests.

Parents, who presumably speak the same dialect, may be used as referents when very few normative data are available (Terrell, Arensberg, & Rosa, 1992). A language test can be given to both the parent and the child. Once the speech-language pathologist has gathered enough data, she can compare the child's performance with that of the adult. Assuming the adult has no language impairment, child-use that reflects parent-use but that differs from Standard American English would represent a dialectal difference, not a disorder. For example, omission of final plosives would result in omission of the regular past tense marker *-ed*. Just testing the child, the speech-language pathologist might assume that the child does not have past tense, when in fact, this is a dialectal characteristic. Parental omission would confirm a dialectal difference.

Some tests, such as the Preschool Language Scale (PLS) (Zimmerman et al., 1979) and the Test of Auditory Comprehension of Language (TACL) (Carrow–Woolfolk, 1985), have been normed on population samples from different languages, such as children speaking English and Spanish, by using English and a Spanish translation. Results of translated tests must be used very cautiously because they assess structures important for speakers of English and ignore those of the other language. For example, *hitting* something with a stick in English is *sticking* in Spanish, but that verb is not used when *hitting a ball.* In Spanish, one cannot *stick a ball.*

The standardized norms from such translated tests could be used to identify children with language differences. Children who exhibit language disorders relative to their peer group could be identified by use of the peer group norms.

Even this procedure may bias some results, given the diversity of some populations, such as Hispanics. Norms for all speakers of a language fail to consider dialectal variations in that language. Other variables, such as socioeconomic status, family grouping, length of time exposed to English, and quality of L_1 used at home, affect the child's performance. Locally prepared norms may be more appropriate.

The speech-language pathologist is encouraged to use language tests designed for and normed on a population that reflects the child's background. She should be proficient in L_1 and familiar with its variations or use the expertise of an interpreter. Appendix D contains a partial list of commercially available tests for children who are bidialectal and bilingual.

An Integrated Model for Assessment

Current methodology in language assessment has been described as a "discrete point approach" (Acevedo, 1986; Day, McCollum, Cieslak, & Erickson, 1981; Mattes & Omark, 1984) in which language is treated as an autonomous cognitive ability divided into many components (Damico, 1991b). Language is not viewed as holistic; rather, it is separate from environmental variables and context. We addressed this issue earlier in the chapter.

It is not surprising that several speech-language pathologists have suggested an integrated approach similar to the one presented in this chapter, one that uses the child's natural environment and that depends on descriptive analysis, rather than on normative test scores. Language and communication are not static, divisible, and autonomous, but dynamic, synergistic, and integrative (Damico, 1991b). Such an assessment would focus on the functional or use aspects of language and on flexibility of use.

The overall question would be: "Is this child an effective communicator in this context?" The criterion is not norm-referenced, but "communication-referenced" (Bloom & Lahey, 1978), with the speech-language pathologist determining the indices of proficiency.

As mentioned earlier in the chapter, data would be collected in natural settings (Iglesias, 1986). The child would converse with his natural conversational partners, parents, teachers, and peers.

As in the integrated, functional approach mentioned earlier, assessment would begin with data gathering. This collection process might include screening all children for other than English and for nonstandard dialectal use. This step could be followed by referral information from classroom teachers on children experiencing academic difficulty (Chamberlain & Medinos-Landurand, 1991). Early intervention may prevent difficulties or inappropriate classification later (Garcia & Ortiz, 1988). A teacher checklist of the child's language functions, a questionnaire, and/or caregiver interview might follow.

In addition to verifying demographic information, the speech-language pathologist should observe the child in the classroom and with peers and care-givers. Of interest is the child's language use, academic strengths and weaknesses, and learning style.

Data collection and observation would be followed by testing and language sampling. Sampling should include a wide variety of settings and activities to increase the accuracy of the language sample collected (Bernstein, 1989). Parents can be trained to listen to their child, to observe language use, and to discuss linguistic interactions (Erickson & Omark, 1981). Appendix E provides a form for reporting the myriad data essential to a fair, unbiased evaluation of children with LEP and children with different dialects (Adler 1991).

Children with LEP.   The data collection stage is particularly important with children with LEP. Many variables affect second-language development and are of interest. In addition, seemingly simple information such as age is culturally dependent and can greatly affect determinations of impairment.

Language assessments should occur where the child and the caregivers are most comfortable. Parents, especially recent immigrants, may speak little or no English. A properly trained interpreter can be very helpful in obtaining needed information. Occasionally, older siblings have sufficient English skills to answer questions or to translate for their parents. Table 3.10 contains possible questions to be asked in an interview.

Observation should occur in several settings with different conversational partners, topics, and activities. This tactic will give the speech-language pathologist some idea of the extent of bilingualism and possible language and communication difficulties.

The languages used in testing and the manner of their presentation differ with each child and the purpose of the evaluation. Testing in both L_1 and English seems essential for assessment of language impairment. In fact, federal law requires bilingual testing before such determinations are made (Ambert & Dew, 1982). Successive testing in the stronger language, followed by the weaker, results in the best performance (Pollack, 1980), especially for young children with monolingual L_1 homes (Krashen & Biber, 1988), although simultaneous testing may be best for children who exhibit poor competence in both languages or who speak a combined L_1-L_2 language, such as "Spanglish" (Cummins, 1986).

Normative testing should be supplemented by probing. Dynamic tasks, such as narration, conversation, and teach–test, are appropriate and de–emphasize

TABLE 3.10
Interview questions for children with LEP or children with different dialects

Demographic

How long has the family been in the United States?

In which country were the parents born?

From which country did the family immigrate?

How much contact does the family have with their native country?

* How long has the family been in this community?

Is the family connected to a large community from their native country?

Is there any plan to return to the native land to live?

Family

* How old is the child?

* Which family members live in the household? Number of siblings?

* Are other individuals living in the household?

In what cultural activities does the family participate?

* Who is primarily responsible for the child? (Primary caregiver?)

* Who else participates in caregiving?

* Approximately how much time do the child and caregiver spend together on a typical day?

* With whom does the child play at home?

* How much education do family members have? In what language?

Childrearing

* Are there scheduled meals?

* What types of foods usually are eaten?

* Is there an established bedtime?

* Does the child misbehave? How? How is the child disciplined? Who disciplines?

Are any television shows (radio shows, videos) in the native language? If so, how often does the child watch such shows?

* Are stories read or told to the child? If so, in what language? How often?

* Are there books, magazines, or newspapers in the home? In what language?

grammar in favor of ability to communicate and learn (Butler, 1993; Damico, 1991b).

One method of testing or probing that circumvents the speech-language pathologist's inability to speak the native language and the affects of delayed English acquisition is the *invented rule* (Connell, 1987c; Roseberry & Connell, 1991). For example, an invented rule might state that /i/ is added to a noun to mean a portion of that noun, as in book and book-/i/. This procedure can be taught through modeling and can be tested with novel objects. Modeling would be a two-step process:

"This is X, X," as the speech-language pathologist points.

"This is X-/i/, X-/i/," as the speech-pathologist points.

This would be repeated several times with a few items as the child repeats the speech-language pathologist's production of the noun and the noun plus /i/. Testing would follow a cloze procedure:

TABLE 3.10, *continued*

* At what age did the child begin school?
* Has the child attended school regularly?
* How many schools has the child attended?
  What language has been used in the classroom?

Attitudes and perceptions

* Is blame assigned for the child's problems or condition? To whom or what?
* How does the family view intervention? Is there a feeling of helplessness?
  How does the family view Western medical practices and practitioners?
  Who is the primary provider of medical assistance and information?
* From whom does the family seek assistance (organizations and individuals)?
* What are the general feelings of the family when seeking assistance?
* Does one family member act as the family spokesperson when seeking assistance?
* How is the child expected to act toward parents, teachers, or other adults? Adults
    toward the child? Are there any restrictions or prohibitions, such as the child not
    making eye contact or not asking questions?
* How important are English language skills?

Language and communication

  What language is spoken in the home? Between adults? Between caregivers and the
    child? Between the children? When playing with neighborhood friends? Other care-
    givers and the child?
  How much English is used in the home?
  What language is used in community activities, such as church, Girl Scouts, and team
    sports?
  At what age did the child begin to learn English? Where and how?
* At what age did the child say the first word? Use two-word utterances?

---

* Applicable to both LEP and dialectally different children.

Source: Compiled from N. Anderson (1991); Chamberlain & Medinos-Landurand (1991); Mattes & Omark (1984); Schiff-Myers (1992); Wayman, Lynch, & Hanson (1990)

"This is Y, Y. This is __."

Again the speech-language pathologist would point to pictures illustrating the meaning. Of interest is whether the child can abstract a language rule and then apply it to novel situations, certainly an important skill for language learning.

Children with different dialects.   Naturally, the speech-language pathologist will want to gather similar data about the child with a different dialect. Possible interview questions are contained in Table 3.10. Observation and testing are similarly important.

Family and community members can aid the speech-language pathologist in assessing performance, especially in the language sample (Bleile & Wallach, 1992; T. Campbell & Dollaghan, 1992). In one study, African American Head Start teachers were asked to judge children with poor speech and those with normally developing speech (Bleile & Wallach, 1992). The poor speech samples were analyzed and a set of community standards derived.

Similar but more stringent *social validation* (Wolf, 1978) has been accomplished by using direct magnitude estimates (DME) of subjective judgments. In DME, stimuli are scaled by assigning numerical values to them on the basis of their relative magnitude along some continuum. Each stimulus—in this case, a speech sample—is rated against a standard stimulus. Raters listen to several children and score them against a taped speech standard. For stability of scoring, at least 10 listeners are required (Stevens, 1975). Scores could range from 1-7 or 1-10. Composite scores can be converted mathematically to standard scores, such as 0-100 with 50 as the mean. Thus, the performance of a single child can be compared over time to measure improvements and can be compared with others by using the same dialect to assess overall performance.

Summary

Despite the incredible difficulties inherent in assessing children with LEP and children with different dialects, there is hope. The same integrated, functional methodology proposed for native speakers of English can be used with some modifications with these children as well. With sensitivity, unbiased administration of testing, and sampling within the everyday context of the child, a fair assessment can be accomplished.

CONCLUSION

Too often, a battery of readily available tests, given to every child regardless of possible language impairment, passes for thorough assessment. As with intervention, assessment procedures must be designed for the individual client. Standardized tests are only a portion of this process. Language tests are aids to the speech–language pathologist. They cannot "substitute for informed clinical judgment" (Siegel, 1975, p. 212).

A thorough assessment includes a variety of procedures designed to heighten awareness of the problem and enables the speech-language pathologist to delineate more clearly the language abilities and impairments of the child. For training to be truly functional, a thorough description of the child and the child's language must be made.

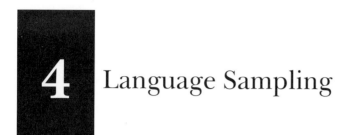

4 Language Sampling

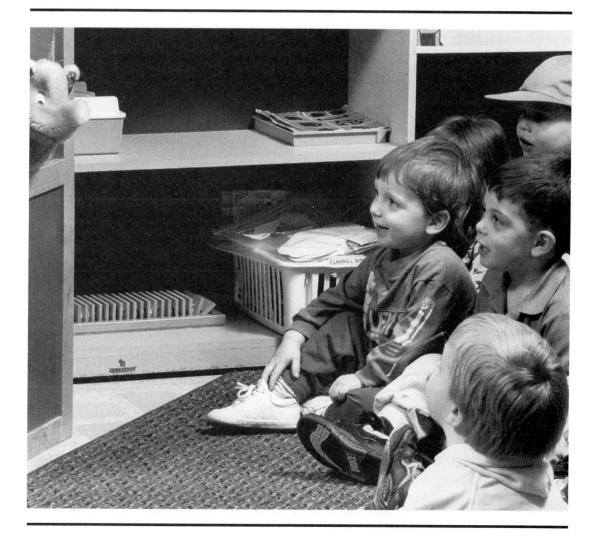

The testing context is a noncommunication one. Although tests are good for assessing global change, they miss many small or subtle behaviors. Language sampling provides more specific information for planning intervention because it includes both the content and context of language use (Blau, Lahey, & Oleksiuk-Velez, 1984). If the goal of language intervention is generalization to the language used by the child in everyday situations, it is essential that the speech-language pathologist collect a language sample that is a good reflection of that language in actual use.

Good language samples do not just occur. They are the result of careful planning and execution. The speech-language pathologist can design the assessment session so that the context fits the purpose of collecting the desired sample. The result is usually a combination of free conversation sampling and some evocative techniques.

The speech-language pathologist must make several decisions before collecting the sample. After studying the interview, observational, and testing results, decisions must be made relative to the context, participants, materials, and conversational techniques to be used. It should be remembered that "there is no way to 'make' children talk . . . [the speech-language pathologist] can only make them want to talk by creating a situation in which there is a reason to talk and an atmosphere that conveys the message that . . . [the speech-language pathologist is] interested in what they have to say" (Lund & Duchan, 1988, p. 23). In this chapter, we cover the planning, collection, recording, and transcription of conversational samples.

PLANNING AND COLLECTING A REPRESENTATIVE SAMPLE

Several issues are of importance when planning and collecting a language sample. Among the most prominent are the representativeness of the sample and the effect of conversational context. In addition, collection of several language forms and functions may require the use of evocative techniques. All of these issues are important for children with language impairments and also for children with LEP and with different dialects.

Representativeness

Representativeness can be addressed by ensuring spontaneity and by collecting samples under a variety of conditions. Spontaneity can be achieved if the child and the conversational partner engage in real conversations on topics of interest to the child. To ensure spontaneity, the speech-language pathologist can follow the (LCC)³ formula for (a) *less clinician control*, (b) *less clinician contrivance*, and (c) *a less conscious child* (Cochrane, 1983).

The speech-language pathologist's control of the context should be weak so as not to restrict the child's linguistic output in quantity or quality. Although there is some indication that speech-language pathologist style has little effect on gross measures, such as MLU and Developmental Sentence scores (J. Johnston, Trainor, Casey, & Hagler, 1981), more subtle measures may be affected to a greater degree. Control devices, such as the use of questions and selection of topics, may cause the child to adopt a passive conversational role.

Not all children will participate freely in such exchanges, and other, more structured approaches may be required. In general, the speech-language pathologist can elicit longer and more complex language from young children with picture interpretation tasks than with imperatives or story recapitulation (Atkins & Cartwright, 1982). In storytelling, the use of pictures can enhance the length and complexity of the sample, especially if the speech-language pathologist gives cues, such as "Tell me a story about this picture. Begin with 'Once upon a time.'" The least spontaneous condition involves the specific linguistic tasks of answering questions or completing sentences. The effects of each technique will vary with each child. The speech-language pathologist can relinquish some control by placing these tasks within a less formal or play format.

The sample will be less contrived if the speech-language pathologist follows the child's lead and adopts the child's topics for conversation. More contrived situations, such as "Tell me about this picture" or "Explain the rules of Monopoly," do not elicit spontaneous everyday speech. The most contrived situation occurs when the speech-language pathologist relies on a tried-and-true, never-fail list of standard questions for all clients, regardless of age, gender, or interests.

Finally, if the child is less conscious of the process of producing language, the sample will be more spontaneous. Asking the child to produce sentences containing certain elements, for example, makes the linguistic process very conscious and may be very difficult, especially out of context. Although a child may not be able to produce a sentence with *has been* on demand, the same child may be able to relate the story of the three bears with "Someone *has been* sleeping in my bed." The former task requires metalinguistic or abstract linguistic skills that may be beyond the child's abilities.

The child's caregivers can offer suggestions to the speech-language pathologist on contexts to help obtain a representative sample. It may be desirable for caregivers to serve as partners, especially with young children. After the sample has been collected, caregivers can review the data and comment on the typicality of the child's behavior.

A Variety of Language Contexts

The sampling environment can contribute to representativeness if there is a variety of contexts, including various settings, tasks, partners, and topics. Context is dynamic and complex, and the effects are very individualistic (Gallagher, 1983). One child may respond well to a certain toy and partner, while another child does not. Yet, the effect of context is rarely considered in language assessment. Contextual variables include the task or purpose of the activity, the opportunities to use language, the extent of ritualization in the event, the amount of joint attending, and the responsivity of the partner (Coggins, 1991).

The task itself, as previously noted, can affect both the number and length of the conversational interactions (Conti-Ramsden & Friel-Patti, 1987). For example, young children are more referential, attempting to focus the listener's attention, in free play, and are more information seeking in book activities (C. Jones & Adamson, 1987). Similarly, parents are influenced by context and engage in more conversation when playing with dolls than they do with cars and trucks (O'Brien & Nagel, 1987).

The opportunities to use language will vary and may need to be provided (Carpenter, Mastergeorge, & Coggins, 1983; Wetherby & Prutting, 1984). Although elicitation tasks may work for older children, they may not be effective with toddlers (Coggins, Olswang, & Guthrie, 1987).

Two aspects of context are structure and predictability (Bain, Olswang, & Johnson, 1992). *Structure* is the amount of adult manipulating of materials and evoking of particular utterances. *Predictability* is the familiarity of the overall task and materials. In general, children will produce a greater frequency and diversity of language features in low-structure situations and more new features in predictable ones (Bain et al., 1992). Free play sampling contexts have both low structure and predictability. Possibly in such low-structure contexts, children assume that the adult knows very little about the situation. In restrictive, planned contexts, children may assume that the adult knows more, and thus the children say less.

Routinized events or routines provide mutually understood and conventionalized interactions (Ninio & Wheeler, 1983). In routines, the partner provides order for the child who, in turn, depends on the partner's cuing. This informal, predictable structuring allows for the child's maximum participation by providing scripts (Platt & Coggins, 1990). **Scripts** are linguistic and nonlinguistic patterns that accompany routines, such as "How are you?—Fine, thanks. How are you?" Scripts reduce the amount of cognitive energy required for the child to participate. In general, children produce fewer topics and fewer contingent utterances in "low-script" or unfamiliar contexts (Conti-Ramsden & Friel-Patti, 1987).

An attentive, responsive partner will elicit more language from the child. In joint or shared attention situations, children produce more extended conversation and are best able to determine the meanings and intentions of the partner (Snow, Perlman, & Nathan, 1987; Tomasello & Farrar, 1986; Tomasello & Todd, 1983). Similarly, timely responses by the partner increase the child's understanding. There may be as little as a 1-second interval after a young child's utterance when he can perceive the contingency of the partner's following utterance (P. Roth, 1987).

As stated, the child's performance will vary with the amount of contextual support. This variability is important in considering intervention targets and methods (Coggins & Olswang, 1987; Olswang, Bain, & Johnson, 1990).

Variety ensures that the sample will not be gathered in one atypical situation. Instead, variety can reflect a sampling of the many interactional situations in which the child functions. Although variety is desirable, it is not always practical, especially in the public school setting. Audiotapes collected by the parent or teacher can provide an acceptable substitute.

Settings and Tasks

The best context is a meaningful activity containing a variety of elicitation tasks. In general, the child who is more familiar with the situation will give the most representative sample.

As mentioned, familiar routines provide a linguistic and/or nonlinguistic script that guides the child's behavior. For young children, play with familiar toys and partners is one of these routine situations. Language is a natural part of many routine events.

The speech-language pathologist needs to decide whether the child's typical or optimal production is desired. For example, storytelling without picture cues yields a large MLU from preschoolers but does not elicit the quantity of language associated with picture interpretation or explanation tasks. This decision on type of production is critical because children with language impairment often perform below their linguistic knowledge level.

Settings should not be too contrived. Familiar, meaningful situations with a variety of age-appropriate and motivating activities provide greater variety and thus are more representative (Kunze, Lockhart, Didow, & Caterson, 1983; F. Roth & Spekman, 1984b). Good settings for preschoolers include the free play mentioned earlier, snack time, and show-and-tell. School-age children can be sampled during group activities, class presentations, conversations with peers, and field trips. Generally, the child involved in some activity produces more language than the child who is watching others or conversing about pictures. It is better if the sample consists of two different settings in which different activities are occurring.

The challenge for the speech-language pathologist is to find a collection technique that strikes a balance. Too highly structured methods often are not representative (Connell & Myles-Zitler, 1982; Fujiki & Brinton, 1987; Lahey, Launer, & Schiff-Myers, 1983). Free play, although low in structure, may be time–consuming and result in variable unreliable data. It has been suggested that for older children, an interview technique is an effective alternative (Dollaghan, Campbell, & Tomlin, 1990). For 8– to 9–year–old children with SLI the interview technique yields more and longer utterances, more complex language forms, more temporal adjacency and semantic contingency, and more reliable, less variable results than free play (Craig & Evans, 1992).

Conversational sampling should be authentic and functional (Damico, 1993). Authenticity comes from the use of real communication contexts in which the participants convey real information (Crystal, 1987; Damico, Secord, & Wiig, 1992; Douglas & Selinker, 1985; Seliger, 1982; Shohamy & Reves, 1982). Functional sampling is most concerned with the success of the child as a communicator. Success can be measured by effectiveness in transmitting meanings, fluency or timeliness, and appropriateness of the message form and style in context (Damico, 1991a; Kovarsky, 1992).

The materials used should be interesting, age appropriate, and capable of eliciting the type of language desired. Interest can be piqued if the child is allowed to choose from a preselected group of toys or objects. Parents also can bring the child's toys from home in order to increase the validity of the sample (MacDonald, 1978a).

In general, children around age 2 respond well to blocks, dishes, pull and wind-up toys, and dolls. Children around age 3 prefer books, clothes, puppets, and such toys as a barn with animals or a street with houses and stores. These toys encourage role playing and language production. Kindergarten and early elementary school children respond best to toys with many pieces and to puppets and action figures. Finally, older children usually converse without the use of objects and can be encouraged to talk about themselves and their interests or to provide narratives. Narratives, a special type of language production, are discussed in Chapter 6.

If certain language features are desired by the speech-language pathologist, she must increase the probability of their occurrence. With school-age children, discussion of absent referents, rather than conversations based on pictures or toys in context, yields more mature language as measured by clause structure complexity, the ratio of hesitations-to-words, and grammatical and phonemic accuracy (Masterson & Kamhi, 1991).

The selection of clinical materials can affect the pragmatic performance of young children by modifying the physical context in which the sample is collected (Gallagher, 1983; Wanska, Bedrosian, & Pohlman, 1986). This selection is especially important, given the current emphasis on the use of play in pragmatic assessment and intervention (Craig, 1983; McCune-Nicolich & Carroll, 1981). When no toys are present, children are more likely to initiate memory-related topics (Bedrosian & Willis, 1987).

The speech-language pathologist should consider the nature of the toys to be used in a play assessment (Wanska et al., 1986). For example, toys with construction properties, such as Legos, Play Doh, or clay, might be used to determine whether the child can remove the conversation from the present. Such toys are more likely to elicit more displaced topics, especially as objects are being constructed (R. Chapman, 1981).

On the other hand, toys that encourage role play might be used to elicit more verbalizations or vocalizations for objects, events, and actions. Compared with construction-type toys, a toy hospital elicits more discussion of the here and now and more fantasy topics, and is more conducive to sociodramatic play and verbal representations of events and actions (Wanska et al., 1986).

Toys also may assist in eliciting specific linguistic structures. For example, children are more likely to produce spatial terms in play with objects than in conversation (Washington & Naremore, 1978). Object movement and manipulation can serve as nonlinguistic cues for the child. Because children's cognitive knowledge and linguistic performance of spatial relationships may differ markedly, manipulation of toys can aid the speech-language pathologist in assessing the child's comprehension (Cox & Richardson, 1985; Harris, Morris, & Terwogt,

1986). The toys and positions should be varied so as not to suggest answers to children (Messick, 1988).

Conversational Partners

Because the speech-language pathologist is interested in the child's use of language, the unit of analysis becomes the conversational dyad of the partner and the child and their interactive behaviors in a given context (Prutting & Kirchner, 1983). The dyadic context enables the speech-language pathologist to view the child's communication within the applied situation of the natural environment (Tiegerman & Siperstein, 1984).

Conversational partners are carefully selected and instructed in their role. It is especially important to use familiar conversational partners with children under age 3 because these children often respond poorly to strangers. Parents of young children or children with acknowledged disabilities may need special instruction to avoid having their children "perform." Uninstructed parents may feel compelled to quiz their child or to have their child recite stereotypic verbal routines such as nursery rhymes to enhance the child's linguistic output. The problem with such recitations is that they may have little to do with the conversational abilities of the child.

In general, it is best to involve the parent or caregiver and the child in some activity. Caregivers can be instructed to talk about what they and the child are doing. As mentioned, toys such as doll houses, action figure play sets, farms and towns, and puppets encourage interaction and role play.

Familiar conversational situations are chosen as well to attain the most typical spontaneous sample with the child conversing as naturally as possible. Interaction may involve one adult or child or a small group of children engaged in sharing, playing, or working in the home or the classroom.

The child should be assessed across several familiar persons with different interactive styles because of the effect that conversational partners—either individually or in small groups—have on the child's verbal output (Miranda & Donnellan, 1986; Prizant & Rentschler, 1983). For example, peer interaction usually involves more equal status between participants than do adult-child interactions (Mishler, 1975; Youniss, 1980). Adults tend to guide and control the topic when conversing with children, whereas child-child conversations are presumably more equal (Bloom, Rocissano, & Hood, 1976; R. Chapman, Miller, MacKenzie, & Bedrosian, 1981). As one might expect, these two conditions result in very different interactive styles for the child. If two children are talking, the adult should leave the room because children who are unsure of the situation will defer to the adult and thus skew the data.

The language performance of children below age 3, of minority children, and of children with LLD may deteriorate in the presence of an authority figure such as an unfamiliar adult. This does not mean that the speech-language pathologist cannot act as a conversational partner. In many ways, the speech-language pathologist is the best conversational partner because of her knowledge of language and of interactions.

The speech-language pathologist and all other participating adults need to be mindful of the inherent problems in adult-child conversations and act to reduce the authority figure persona. The adult can accomplish this by accepting the child's activity, agenda, and topics and by participating with the child. With young children, participation may necessitate using the floor for play.

The speech-language pathologist as the conversational partner can set the tone of the interaction by being nondirective, interest*ing*, interest*ed*, and responsive. She should respond to the content of the child's language, not to the way it is said. At this point, the purpose is to collect data, not to change behavior. Our goal is *collecting, not correcting*.

The speech-language pathologist can manipulate the situation skillfully to probe for a greater range of information (Spinelli & Terrell, 1984). Initially, interaction may be dampened because the speech-language pathologist is not the child's usual communication partner. Therefore, it is important for the speech-language pathologist to get acquainted slowly and in a nonthreatening manner. This task is best accomplished by meeting the child on his terms through play and by following the child's lead.

The speech-language pathologist possesses the clinical skill to elicit a variety of functions, introduce various topics, and ask questions about experiences. Role play, dolls, and puppet play provide information about the child's event knowledge in a range of situations. There is the potential to elicit a greater variety of language than might be possible when the child and parent communicate.

The best way to attain a semblance of equal authority is for the speech-language pathologist and the child to engage in a play interaction. Instead of being directive, the speech-language pathologist comments on their ongoing shared activity.

Children who are reluctant to talk to adults may be more willing to interact with a puppet or a doll. I have found that small animals, such as guinea pigs, make excellent communication partners for children. After explaining to the child that she must leave to run a short errand, the speech-language pathologist introduces the guinea pig and asks the child to talk to it so that it will not get lonely. The child should be observed and his language recorded while the speech-language pathologist is absent.

Despite conventional wisdom, neither the race of the conversational partner nor the race depicted in stimulus materials seems to affect language performance as measured by response length and response latency (H. Seymour, Ashton, & Wheeler, 1986). This is not to say that all children, particularly minority children, will be unaffected. Speech-language pathologists should be aware of potential difficulties and should approach each child with an open mind. Racial incompatibilities should not be expected, but the speech-language pathologist should be conscious of this potential.

Topics

Children have a wide variety of interests, and the conversational partners must be careful to enable the child to talk about them. Children are more spontaneous and produce more language when they are allowed to initiate the topics of discussion.

The speech-language pathologist should be prepared to shift topics as readily as activities. Therefore, the speech-language pathologist must be conversant in topics of interest to children, such as school activities, holidays, television programs, fads and fashions, and rock music.

Summary

Child variables, such as recent past experience and mood, can greatly affect language sampling because the child is often the initiator in this protocol and because there are few performance constraints (Hess, Sefton, & Landry, 1986; Klee & Fitzgerald, 1985). To get the most representative sample possible, therefore, the speech-language pathologist should use familiar situations, persons, and tasks or topics. Representativeness is enhanced if the conversational sample is collected in more than one setting, with different conversational partners and tasks or topics in each.

It may be helpful to think of interactional situations along a continuum from relatively nondirected or free to more controlled or scripted (Coggins, 1991; Shriberg & Kwiatkowski, 1985). Such toys as a dollhouse, a farm, action figures, bubbles, or dress-up clothes are rather open-ended, especially when the partner has suggested, "Let's talk and play with these things." Books or color-forms offer more control and can be used to elicit particular words, forms, and narratives. Familiar routines, such as doing the dishes, also can be used, along with such cues as "What are you going to do now?" to elicit more specific behavior. Interviews, picture labeling, and responding to questions offer the most control but at the sacrifice of spontaneity and representativeness. These latter techniques are more appropriately considered evocative techniques used to elicit specific behaviors.

Table 4.1 presents contextual variables that can be manipulated in an assessment to influence a child's performance. Each variable can be modified to offer minimal or maximal contextual support (Coggins, 1991).

TABLE 4.1
Continuum of contextual support

Variable	Minimal contextual support	Maximal contextual support
Nonlinguistic		
Interaction	Naturalistic	Contrived tasks
Materials	No toys or props	Familiar and thematic
Interactor	Clinician	Mother/caregiver
Activities	Novel	Event routines
Linguistic		
Cuing	Indirect model	Elicited imitation

Source: Coggins, T. E. (1991). Bringing context back into assessment. *Topics in Language Disorders,* *11*(4), 43-54. Reprinted with permission.

Evocative Conversational Techniques

Although the sample should represent the everyday language used by the child, free samples may have limitations, such as low frequency or nonappearance of certain linguistic features and conversational behaviors (F. Roth & Spekman, 1984b). Absence or low incidence does not mean the child does not possess these features or behaviors. Therefore, it may be necessary to supplement the sample with evocative procedures specifically designed to elicit them. Test protocols also might be modified to obtain more structured samples (Thomas, 1989).

The speech-language pathologist may need to plan both the linguistic and nonlinguistic contexts for elicitation of various functions and forms. At first, some procedures may seem stiff and formal, even forced. Initially, the speech-language pathologist may need to role–play the sampling situation and memorize conversational openers and replies. Once familiar with the many ways of eliciting a variety of functions and forms, she can relax and use the techniques more naturally as opportunities arise within the interaction.

Specific tasks that are within the child's experience also can be used to elicit specific language forms (F. Roth & Spekman, 1984b). This approach allows a broad range of pragmatic functions to occur (Kunze et al., 1983). For example, a mock birthday party can be used to elicit plurals, past tense, and questions (Wren, 1985). The speech-language pathologist might elicit plurals by saying the following:

> Today is X's birthday. Let's have a party. What are some things we'll need? (Or, Here are some things we need. What are these?)

The pathologist can use plates, spoons, glasses, candles, presents, and so on. Thus, the child's utterances are placed within some context. Within the same situation, past tense might be elicited by dropping dishes and asking what happened or by reviewing whether you did everything to get ready ("Okay, now tell me what *you* did to get ready for the party. *I* washed the dishes"). Finally, questions can be elicited by a party game variation of Ask the Old Lady (Brown, 1973).

> Let's play a question game. This is X (puppet, doll, action figure). I want you to ask X some questions about his birthday party. I wonder how old he is. You ask him.

The child may need a demonstration before being able to complete the question task.

Our interest in generalization of intervention to everyday use necessitates an interest in the pragmatic organizational framework of the sample. Some areas of interest include the intentions of individual utterances, the presuppositions or the inferential behavior of the speaker in forming the message to the assumed needs of the listener, and the social organization of the discourse that maintains the dialogue (F. Roth & Spekman, 1984a). Specific procedures and activities can be used to elicit a variety of communication intentions, examples of presupposition, and the underlying social organization of discourse within a variety of situations. Table 4.2 lists examples of situations that each elicit a variety of language functions. In addition, the speech-language pathologist is interested in ways to

TABLE 4.2
Situations with the potential to elicit a variety of language functions

Dress-up
Playing house or farm
Dolls, puppets, adventure or action figures
Farm set or street scene
Simulated grocery store, gas station, fast-food restaurant, beauty parlor
Role playing
Playing school
Acting out stories, television shows, movies
Imaginary play
Simulated TV talk show

elicit various semantic and syntactic features. These elicitation techniques are presented in the following section.

Intentions or Illocutionary Functions

Illocutionary functions are the intentions of each utterance. Most utterances clearly demonstrate the speaker's intent. For example, "I would like a cookie, please" clearly demonstrates a desire or request for some entity. Likewise, "What time is it?" demonstrates a desire for information. However, the relationship is not always so obvious. "What time is it?" might be used as an excuse. For example, the speaker who does not wish to do something and knows that time is limited might use this utterance to establish the time factor for other people.

> Well, I don't know . . ., it's getting late. What time is it? (Reply) Oh, well, I really better be going.

Utterances also may express more than one intention. For example, the speaker might respond to a piece of art with, "What do you call that *thing*?" Here, the speaker requests information and also makes an evaluation.

A number of existing taxonomies of communication intentions can be applied to the language sample. Table 6.5 presents some illocutionary taxonomies that have been used clinically with child language samples. It is best to determine the range of functions expected for the child's developmental level before organizing activities to try to elicit these intentions. Guidance regarding the intentions expected at certain ages is presented in Table 6.6.

Similar to the previous example of asking a child to produce a sentence with *has been*, asking the child to form a question about a certain topic or to make a statement out of context may require metalinguistic skills beyond the child's abilities. The following are a broad range of intentions and accompanying activities that may elicit language functions or intentions within a conversational or situational context (Creaghead, 1984; Kunze et al., 1983; F. Roth & Spekman, 1984b):

Answering/responding.   The speech-language pathologist asks the child a variety of questions while engaged in play ("Where shall we put the houses?" "Who is that?" "What's in his hand?"). Notice the type of question and the expected response.

Calling/greeting.   The speech-language pathologist leaves and reenters the situation, role–plays people entering and leaving a business, calls on the telephone, or uses dolls, puppets, or action figures to elicit greetings. If she turns away from the child with a favorite toy, the child also may call.

Continuance.   Continuance is turn filling that lets the speaker know that the listener is attending to the conversation. Typical continuants include "uh-huh," "yeah," "okay," and "right." These can be observed throughout the session. The speech-language pathologist notes when the child seems to rely on this function, rather than contribute anything new or relevant to the conversation.

Expressing feelings.   The speech-language pathologist models feeling-type responses throughout the play interaction. Dolls, puppets, or action figures are described as having certain feelings and the child is asked to help. For example, she could say, "Oh, Big Bird is sad. Can you talk to him and make him feel better?"

Hypothesizing.   The speech-language pathologist poses a physical problem for the child, such as, "How can we get everyone to the party on time?" or, "How can we get Leonardo out of the cage?" The child proposes solutions to the problem.

Making choices.   The speech-language pathologist presents the child with alternatives, such as, "I don't know whether you'd rather have a peanut butter sandwich with jelly or fluff."

Predicting.   In sequential activities, the speech-language pathologist can ponder, "I wonder what will happen now" or, "I wonder what we'll do next."

Protesting.   The speech-language pathologist can elicit protesting by putting away toys or taking away snacks before the child is finished. She also can hand the child something other than what he requested.

Reasoning.   The speech-language pathologist attempts to solve a problem, such as, "I wonder why the boy ran away" or, "I wonder what we did wrong."

Repeating.   The speech-language pathologist should note the amount of repetition of self and of the partner. This can take the form of empty comments in a conversation in which the child adds no new information, for example:

ADULT:	Did your class go to the zoo yesterday?
CHILD:	Yeah, zoo.
ADULT:	What did you like best? The monkeys?
CHILD:	Monkeys.
ADULT:	Monkeys are my favorite too. They're so funny.
CHILD:	Monkeys funny.

Replying. The speech-language pathologist should note occasions when the child responds to the content of what she has said without being required to do so. This behavior is one of the mainstays of conversation as each speaker builds on the comment of the previous speaker.

Reporting. Reporting can include several functions.

Declaring/citing. While engaged in an activity, the child spontaneously comments on the present action. The speech-language pathologist models this behavior ("Car goes up the ramp") but does not attempt to cue a response because declaring/citing is a spontaneous function. She also can engage in unexpected or unusual behavior and await the child's comment.

Detailing. The speech-language pathologist presents the child with two objects of different size or color. If the child takes one and says nothing, the speech-language pathologist models ("I'll take the little one" or "Here's a green truck") and presents other objects later. The speech-language pathologist does not attempt to cue a response because detailing is a spontaneous function.

Naming/labeling. The speech-language pathologist presents a novel object or points to pictures in a book and remarks, "Oh, look." If the child does not label the object or picture, the speech-language pathologist models the response ("Look. A clown") and goes on. The child may do so on subsequent exposure to other novel objects. The speech-language pathologist does not cue a response because labeling is a spontaneous function.

Requesting assistance/directing. The speech-language pathologist presents interesting toys that require adult help to open or use. For example, she can place objects in clear plastic containers or drawstring bags that require help to open, give the child one portion of a toy while keeping the other on a shelf, or let windup toys run down. The pathologist makes such comments as, "I wish we could play with this; it would be fun," "Oh, we could use more parts," or "Gee, we need to fix that." In another situation, the child helps two puppets or dolls solve a problem in which one will not share a special toy with the other. The speech-language pathologist also can present the child with situations that require a solution, such as taped scissors, pencils with broken points, toys with missing pieces, or paints without brushes. During interactions the speech-language pathologist should note self-directing or self-talk accompanying play. This behavior can be modeled.

Requesting clarification. This intention can be elicited when the speech-language pathologist mumbles or makes an inaccurate statement.

Requesting information. The speech-language pathologist places novel but unknown objects in front of the child. Naming the object correctly is labeling, and the speech-language pathologist should confirm. If the child labels incorrectly, the speech-language pathologist says, "No, it's not an X" or "No, can you guess what it is?" The responses "What's that?" or "What?" and those with rising intonation ("Frog?") should be considered requests for information.

The speech-language pathologist also might direct the child to use an object not in the situation or not in the expected location. If modeling is required, the speech-language pathologist can ask a question, such as, "Do you have the scissors?" When the child answers negatively, she can direct the child by saying, "Ask Sally if she does."

Requesting objects.   The speech-language pathologist exposes the child to enticing objects or edibles that are just out of reach.

Requesting permission.   The speech-language pathologist hands an interesting object to the child and says, "Hold the X for me." The technique is more effective if the speech-language pathologist uses a nonsense name for the object. The speech-language pathologist then awaits a response from the child, such as, "Can I play with X?" or just, "Play X?" The child also may request information, such as, "What's it do?"

An even more effective technique is to keep the object hidden in an opaque box. The speech-language pathologist peeks into the box, names the object, shows pleasure, and then closes the box. The speech-language pathologist might tell the object that it can come out to play when someone wants to play with it. If necessary, the speech-language pathologist can use a puppet to model the requesting behavior desired.

Creaghead (1984) has developed an elicitation protocol that targets several communication intentions and conversational devices within two different structured activities. Table 4.3 presents an outline of the two protocols. The speech-language pathologist uses each protocol as a script to elicit the intentions and devices.

Some intentions are responsive in nature, for example, answering a question or following a directive or request for action. In addition to the child's production level of such requests, it is helpful to know the child's level of response (F. Roth & Spekman, 1984b).

With responsive functions, the speech-language pathologist must not interpret noncompliance as noncomprehension. The child simply may not want to comply or may choose to ignore the request. The speech-language pathologist first should be certain that the child can perform the behavior requested. The ages at which children comprehend different levels of requests are listed in Table 4.4.

It might be helpful for the speech-language pathologist to use two children in an ask-and-tell situation so that each child can act as a model for the other. In a similar manner, the speech-language pathologist and child can switch roles as questioner (or director) and respondent.

These are just a few suggestions for eliciting a variety of communication intentions. In summary, the speech-language pathologist must consider the type of intentions displayed, their forms, the means of transmission, and the social conventions that affect these means. For example, some situations may call for the use of nonverbal means; others may not.

TABLE 4.3

Elicitation protocol for communication intentions and conversational devices

Test Procedures—Format 1	Test Procedures—Format 2
As child enters the room—check GREETING	As child leaves the room—check CLOSING
Have cookies and crackers in jar within child's view but out of reach—check REQUEST FOR OBJECT	Give the child and yourself a piece of paper and tell him to draw "mumble"—check REQUEST FOR CLARIFICATION
Hand child the tightly closed jar containing the cookies—check REQUEST FOR ACTION (help opening the jar)	After clarifying, do not give him a crayon—check REQUESTING AN OBJECT
Ask child, "How do you think we can get the jar open?"—check HYPOTHESIZING	Ask the child if he wants a red or blue crayon—check MAKING CHOICES
Say "Do you want 'mumble'?"—check REQUEST FOR CLARIFICATION	Put on big glasses and then show the child a picture of a person and call it a dog—check COMMENTING ON OBJECT and DENIAL
Ask the child if he wants peanut butter or jelly on his cracker—check MAKING CHOICES	Ask the child, "Do you want to play with 'mumble'?"—check REQUEST FOR CLARIFICATION
Hand the child the opposite of what he chose—check DENIAL	Tell the child to get the telephones, which are not in sight—check REQUEST FOR INFORMATION
Put the peanut butter and jelly on the table. Ask the child, "What are we going to do now?"—check PREDICTING	Ask the child, "What are we going to do?"—check PREDICTING
Tell the child to put peanut butter or jelly on the cracker—check REQUEST FOR OBJECT (knife)	The tester calls the child, then the child calls the tester on the telephone—check GREETING and CLOSING
Tell the child to get the knife, which is not in sight—check REQUEST FOR INFORMATION	Hold a conversation with the child. During this, make a remote-controlled toy move. The toy should be out of the sight of the tester and covered with a cloth—check COMMENT ON ACTION
Put the peanut butter and/or jelly on the cracker and eat it. Get out extra big toothbrush and pretend to brush teeth—check COMMENT ON OBJECT	Ask the child, "What happened?"—check DESCRIBING EVENT
Hold a conversation with the child. During this, pull invisible string so that rag doll falls off the table—check COMMENT ON ACTION	Ask the child, "What do you think is under the cloth?"—check HYPOTHESIZING
Ask the child, "What happened?"—check DESCRIBING EVENT	Ask the child, "Why did it move?"—check GIVING REASON
Ask the child, "Why did it fall?"—check GIVING REASON	Make the toy move briefly—check REQUEST FOR ACTION
During conversation—check ANSWERING, VOLUNTEERING TO COMMUNICATE, ATTENDING TO THE SPEAKER, TAKING TURNS, ACKNOWLEDGING, SPECIFYING A TOPIC, CHANGING A TOPIC, MAINTAINING A TOPIC, GIVING EXPANDED ANSWERS	During conversation—check ANSWERING, VOLUNTEERING TO COMMUNICATE, ATTENDING TO THE SPEAKER, TAKING TURNS, ACKNOWLEDGING, SPECIFYING A TOPIC, CHANGING TOPIC, MAINTAINING A TOPIC, GIVING EXPANDED ANSWERS
Stop leading the conversation and be silent—check ASKING CONVERSATIONAL QUESTIONS	Stop leading conversation and remain silent—check ASKING CONVERSATIONAL QUESTIONS
Request clarification—check CLARIFYING	

Note: These protocols may be used as suggested scripts for efficient elicitation of several communication intentions and conversational devices.

Source: Creaghead, N. (1984). Strategies for evaluating and targeting pragmatic behaviors in young children. *Seminars in Speech and Language, 5,* 241–251. Reprinted with permission.

TABLE 4.4
Age and comprehension of
requests

Age in years	Comprehension
2	I need a _____.
	Give me a _____.
3	Could you give me a _____?
	May I have a _____?
	Have you got a _____?
4	He hurt me. (Hint)
	The _____ is all gone. (Hint)
4½	Begin to comprehend indirect requests: Why don't you _____ or Don't forget to _____. Mastery takes several years.
5	Inferred requests in which the goal is totally masked are now comprehended. In this example, the speaker desires some juice: Now you make breakfast like you're the mommy.

Source: Adapted from Ervin–Tripp, S. (1977). Wait for me roller skate. In S. Ervin–Tripp & C. Mitchell–Kernan (Eds.), *Child discourse* (pp. 165–188). New York: Academic Press.

Presuppositional and Deictic Skills

Whereas intentions are noted at the individual level, other linguistic aspects, such as presupposition and deixis, underlie the entire conversational interaction. **Presupposition** is the speaker's assumption about the knowledge level of the listener and the tailoring of language to that supposed level. **Deixis** is the interpretation of information from the perspective of the speaker. When a speaker says, "Come here," this must be interpreted as a point close to the speaker, not as a point with reference to the listener. Deictic terms include, but are not limited to, *here/there*, *this/that*, and *come/go*.

Presuppositional and deictic skills can be assessed in *referential communication tasks* (F. Roth & Spekman, 1984b). In referential tasks, one partner describes something or gives directions to the other partner, who is usually on the other side of an opaque barrier or unable to see the speaker (see Figure 4.1). Variations include blindfold games or telephone conversations. As a rule, preschoolers perform better if describing real objects rather than abstract shapes. Deixis can be elicited by using object-finding tasks in which the child directs the conversational partner toward a hidden object.

In these tasks, the speech-language pathologist must be alert to the use of direct/indirect reference. In direct reference, the speaker considers the audience and clearly identifies the entity being mentioned. Indirect reference typically follows direct reference and refers to entities through the use of pronouns or such terms as *that one*. The child with poor presuppositional skills may use indirect reference without prior direct reference.

Additional presuppositional information can be gathered by varying the roles, topics, partners, and communication channels available in the sampling situation. Roles can be varied so that the child has an opportunity to act as listener and speaker. Assessment of both roles is essential. For example, the child with LLD generally will ask few questions for clarification even when he has little understanding of what has been said. As speakers, these children make limited use of descriptors, provide very little specific information, and are less effective than children developing normally.

The choice of topics also can influence presuppositional behavior and provide for a variety of role taking. Children can be asked to describe events about which the speech-language pathologist or partner is ignorant (e.g., a family outing). In this situation, the child must determine the amount of information necessary for the listener to understand the topic. The partner who asks the child to explain something that the partner already understands violates the principle that communication should make sense. There is no sense in explaining something that someone already understands.

As the number of communication channels decreases, the speaker is forced to rely more heavily on the remaining ones. For example, the use of a telephone requires the speaker to rely almost exclusively on the verbal communication channel. This situation is a challenge even for the nonimpaired language user. Imagine how difficult it would be to teach someone over the phone to tie a shoelace.

While gathering the language sample, the speech-language pathologist can manipulate channel availability systematically. During play, the pathologist can look away and then ask the child to describe what he or she is doing. Barrier games or blindfold games with the child in charge also may elicit interesting information. Role-playing with the telephone is more realistic.

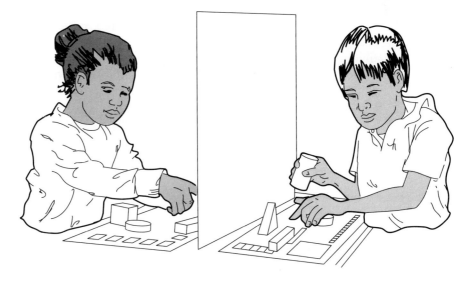

FIGURE 4.1
Barrier tasks

The use and nonuse of barriers will permit such verbal-only and verbal-plus communication. If the listener provides no feedback in verbal-only communication, the speaker must take an extremely active role in the conversation. In addition, barrier activities require listeners to adapt the speaker's perspective.

Several other activities can be used to elicit presuppositional skills. Of interest is whether the child can encode the most informative or uncertain elements in a situation. In general, human beings tend to comment on entities and events that are new, changing, or unexpected. In the sampling situation, novel items can be introduced into repetitive activities. The speech-language pathologist must attend to the child's behavior to see whether the child refers to the novel stimulus.

I know of one clinic where a kitten is abruptly introduced into the sampling situation. The speech-language pathologist says nothing but waits to see whether the child will comment and in what manner.

In general, young children with language impairment encode novel information less frequently than do children developing normally. Older school-age children with language impairment tend to use more pronouns with less identification of the referent than do children developing normally.

Pictures or objects, identical except for one element, can be used. The child can be asked to explain how the two differ. Hide-and-seek with objects can be used to assess comprehension and expression of deictic terms as the speech-language pathologist and child direct each other to find the objects.

Games and stories can elicit indirect/direct reference. For example, a story can be told and then questions asked to elicit indefinite and definite articles and/or nouns and pronouns. The child also can retell a story to a second child who has not heard it. Any portion of extended discourse, such as describing a movie, explaining how to accomplish a task, or telling a story, will be valuable clinical data (F. Roth & Spekman, 1984b).

The speech-language pathologist is interested in the lexical items used and also in the ambiguity of the referent. Of interest is the number of times the child mentions the referent by name or by the use of pronouns. Some children overuse the referent name, whereas others rely on the pronoun without sufficient return to the referent name to avoid confusion.

Finally, role-playing activities with very specific situations also can be helpful. The child in the following situation faces very definite behavioral constraints.

> Imagine you and a friend are trying to find a drinking fountain. You see a man coming down the street. While your friend remains seated on a park bench, you try to find out about the fountain. I'll be the man. What would you say? (Child responds.) Now, I'm your friend. What would you tell me?

Discourse Organization

Discourse has internal organization. For example, a telephone conversation has a recognizable pattern, as does the telling of a personal event. The social organization of discourse can be assessed within familiar activities that provide a scaffolding for dialogue (F. Roth & Spekman, 1984b). The speech-language pathologist may be interested in the amount of social and nonsocial speech. For example, preschool children frequently engage in nonsocial monologues in play, in contrast to older children, who participate more in dialogues or in social monologues. This change signals a growing awareness of the social nature of speech and language use. Among children with mental retardation, acquisition of conversational rules is related more closely to social-experiential factors, such as chronological age, than to expressive language ability as measured by average utterance length (Leifer & Lewis, 1984).

The speech-language pathologist can provide opportunities for the child to initiate conversation, to take turns, and to repair in response to self-feedback or the feedback of others in different situations. Turn taking may need to begin at a physical level with some reticent children. In conversation, the speech-language pathologist might even say, "Now it's your turn," and point to the child initially. By failing to respond to the child or by responding inappropriately, mumbling, failing to establish a referent, misnaming, or providing insufficient information, the speech-language pathologist may elicit contingent queries or requests for clarification from the child.

Semantic Terms

Relational terms, such as *in front of, more/less,* and *before/after,* are especially difficult for children with LLD and other language disorders. These children often use comprehension strategies that have several implications for assessment (Edmonston & Thane, 1992). For locational terms, these strategies may include probable location, physical properties of objects, and preferred location. Adjectival relational words, such as *big* and *little,* may be comprehended by using either a preference for amount or word synonymity. With temporal terms, strategies may include sequential probability and order-of-mention or main-clause-first.

It is easier for children to comprehend locational terms and to follow locational instructions when familiar objects are combined in familiar, predictable, or probable ways (Grieve, Hoogenraad, & Murray, 1977). Levels of comprehension can be determined by using the usual or "normal" context or a "contextually neutral" context in which object placement is not so predictable (Duchan, 1980; Lund & Duchan, 1983).

The physical properties of an object can influence responding (M. Bernstein, 1984). The child's rule may be, Containers are for *in,* and surfaces are for *on.* Containers can be turned on their sides by the speech-language pathologist and used for both *in* and *on.* Other objects may be used with different terms (Edmonston & Thane, 1990).

Some objects are fronted or have an obvious front, while others are not. This characteristic affects comprehension and production of such terms as *in front of* and *behind.* In general, these terms are easier to use with fronted objects than with nonfronted objects (J. Johnston & Slobin, 1979; Kuczaj & Maratsos, 1975). In addition, some young children interpret *behind* to mean *hidden from view by,* so they will place a small object correctly with large nonfronted objects (J. Johnston, 1984). Obviously, *in front of* and *behind* must be assessed with fronted and non-fronted, small and large objects (Edmonston & Thane, 1992).

With deictic terms, young children may employ a child-centered or speaker-centered strategy, preferring that location as the referent (E. Clark, 1978; Wales, 1986). Contrastive terms, such as *here/there*, used with different speakers may be useful (Tanz, 1980).

Quantitative terms, such as *more/less, long/short*, and *big/little* may be interpreted by using a preference for greater amount strategy in which the child usually chooses the largest one when in doubt. Assessing both words in different contexts and in different word order may help the speech-language pathologist understand the child's errors.

Similarly, height of the objects used affects comprehension of such words as *big, tall, top, young*, and *old* (E. Clark, 1980; Coley & Gelman, 1989; Harris et al., 1986; Hobbs & Bacharach, 1990; Kuczaj & Lederberg, 1977; Sena & Smith, 1990). Preschoolers often equate *big* with *tall* and *little* with *short height* (Ravn & Gelman, 1984). Objects can be placed so that their heights are similar by using stands of different heights.

Children also use a strategy in which they interpret contrastive terms to be synonymous or assign the meanings of big and little to similar terms (Bartlett, 1976; Carey, 1978; Clark, 1979). In the latter, *big* becomes synonymous with *tall, wide*, and *thick*. Object dimensions can be controlled so that the widest objects are not always the biggest overall.

Finally, temporal sequential terms, such as *before* and *after*, may be interpreted by using a most probable, order-of-mention, or main-clause-first strategy. In the most probable strategy, the child trusts experience. Among preschoolers, this is the most widely used strategy with familiar, real-world sequences (Carni & French, 1984; French & Nelson, 1981; Keller-Cohen, 1987; Trosborg, 1982). Order-of-mention or the first action mentioned occurred before the second is also popular among preschoolers, while children over age 5 often use the main-clause-first strategy in which the main clause of the sentence is assumed to have occurred first. Use of sequential terms as prepositions, as in *after she painted*, rather than as a conjunction, as in *she did X after she did Y*, and one event sequence, also as in *after she painted*, may reduce the effect of these strategies on performance. Longer utterances may be used to demonstrate such strategy use.

Language Form

The speech-language pathologist can manipulate the context to elicit particular forms. For example, the objects and the verbal routines chosen for play may contain several examples of phonemes desired for a phonological analysis.

Specific syntactic forms, such as verbs, and morphological markers, such as regular past tense *-ed*, also can be elicited in creative ways. Some illocutionary functions or intentions discussed previously in this chapter, such as requesting information, have specific linguistic forms. A few elicitation methods for specific structures are listed in Table 4.5 (Crais & Roberts, 1991).

TABLE 4.5
Elicitation of some language features

Feature	Elicitation Technique
Prepositions	Hide objects and have the child try to guess their location.
Nouns, verbs, etc.	Ask specific *Wh-* type questions: *What's that?* for nouns. *Where's X?* for prepositions. *What's John doing?* or *What did (will) Mary do?* for verbs. *How does Carol feel?* or *How did Martin do X?* for adjectives and adverbs.
Plural *-s* marker	Play games with many parts, such as Mr. Potatohead or Color-forms and have the child request desired pieces (*I want the ears.*)
Adjectives	Use similar objects of different sizes and colors. Ask child, *What do you want?*
Possessive pronouns	Play dress-up and ask, *Whose dress is this?*
Subjective pronouns	Play I Spy (*I spy something and he's big.*)
Yes/no questions	Play Twenty Questions and I Spy.
Wh- questions	Play Hide-and-Seek and other guessing games (*What's in the bag? Where's the ball?*)

Source: Crais, E. R., & Roberts, J. (1991). Decision making in assessment and early intervention planning. *Language, Speech, and Hearing Services in Schools, 22,* 19–30.

Language Sampling With Minority Children With LEP

It is even more important that the language of children with LEP and minority children be collected in several different contexts (Damico, 1991b; Iglesias, 1986). Code switching and differing language and dialect use in context is extremely important information for determining the effectiveness of the child as a communicator.

Sampling should occur in monologue and dialogue situations in both languages or dialects. Monologue activities might include static, dynamic, and abstract tasks (G. Brown, Anderson, Shillcock, & Yule, 1984). Static tasks describe relationships among objects in the context and might include directing others to perform a task or describing entities by location, size, shape, or color. Dynamic tasks describe changes over time as in narration. Finally, abstract tasks might include opinion-expressing tasks, such as arguing or justifying.

Dialogue situations should include a variety of partners because of the special constraints that each imposes on the child. The classroom is especially important because of the academic difficulties these children may encounter.

In each context, the conversational partner should pose communication problems for the child. Change and problem solving encourage communication and enable the speech-language pathologist to determine the effectiveness of the child as a communicator. In addition, such situations can offer clues to the learning style of the child (Iglesias, 1986).

RECORDING THE SAMPLE

There is no ideal length for a conversational sample. Length varies with the purpose of collection (Bloom & Lahey, 1978; Crystal, Fletcher, & Garman, 1976; L. Lee, 1974). For example, a 50-utterance sample may be adequate for lexical evaluation because it will contain 73–83% of the lexical information found in a 100-utterance sample (K. Cole, Mills, & Dale, 1989).

In the light of the constraints of the clinical sample, 50 or 100 child utterances are considered adequate, providing there is some variety of setting, partners, tasks, or topics and that other data collection methods are used. At least two different samples should be included (K. Cole et al., 1989).

Occasionally, children fall into repetitive patterns of responding, such as naming pictures in a book. This kind of activity provides very little variation in the child's behavior. It is best either to limit this type of interaction or not to use it for analysis. If, on the other hand, the child frequently exhibits perseverative or stereotypic patterns, they should be recorded for analysis, saved for supporting data, or commented on in the assessment report.

The sample is recorded permanently by using videotape, audiotape, event transcription, or a combination of these (F. Roth & Spekman, 1984b). Taping is essential because the interaction must be reviewed repeatedly for information.

Although videotaping can be intrusive and expensive, especially the initial equipment purchase, it yields the best data for describing the verbal and nonverbal behaviors observed. The alternatives to videotaping are not as reliable and thus increase the variability in the behavior recorded. Even if videotape is used, the speech-language pathologist may find a simultaneous audiotape helpful for transcribing the speech and language portion. The following recording methods are listed in order of decreasing desirability:

1. Simultaneous videotaping and audiotaping
2. Simultaneous audiotaping with pathologist descriptions of nonlinguistic behaviors recorded in one and the linguistic interaction in the other
3. Simultaneous audiotaping and written data recording on time sheets (see Table 4.6). Having more than one observer may help ensure that no behaviors are overlooked and may increase the reliability of description of those that are observed. Writing data as the interaction progresses is extremely tedious but necessary.

It is important that different data collection methods begin at the same time for later transcription. This should be accomplished as unobtrusively as possible. A cough or some similar signal can alert observers that recording has begun.

TRANSCRIBING THE SAMPLE

The conversational sample is transcribed as soon after recording as possible. This timeliness ensures that the speech-language pathologist brings to the task as much memory of the situation as possible.

TABLE 4.6
Time form for recording the nonlinguistic context

Time (sec.)	Child's Behavior	Partner's Behavior	Other	Minute ___2___
0				
.				
.				
.				
10				
.	Looks at partner			
.				
.	Points to truck			
.				
20				
.				
.	Reaches for truck			
.		Hands truck		
.				
30				
.				
.				
.	Pushes car			
.				
40	Looks at partner			
.				
.	Points to gas station			
.				
.		Moves car to gas station		
50		Moves car to gas station		
.				
.				
.				
.				
60				

The format of the transcript varies with the purpose of the assessment. For example, there is little need to transcribe the partner's utterances if the speech-language pathologist is interested only in phonological analysis. For most other purposes, however, the type of format shown in Table 4.7 is suggested.

The use of computerized analysis programs, such as SALT, requires a consistent transcription format (J. Miller, Freiberg, Rolland, & Reeves, 1992). This format will include not only the utterances but also the symbols for the program to aid it in identifying morphological markers and syntactic categories. Usually, multiple analyses can be performed without reentering the transcript or with

TABLE 4.7
Transcription format

			Minute ___2___
Time (sec.)	**Child's Utterances**	**Partner's Utterances**	**Nonlinguistic**
0			
.			
.		What do you need now?	
.			
10			
.	Can I have the truck?		C. looks at partner
.			
.			C. points to truck
.			
20		Which one?	
.	That one.		
.			C. reaches for truck
.		Oh, the red one.	P. hands truck
.		Okay.	
30		Now can we go on	
.		vacation?	
.			
.	Bro-o-om		C. pushes car
40	We need gas first.		C. looks at partner
.			
.			C. points to gas station
.		Well, then…	
.		I'll drive my car	P. moves car to gas
50		over, too.	station
.			C. moves car to gas
.			station
.		What else do we need?	
.	Gotta get soda and		
60	chips.		

only minor changes to accommodate different transcription conventions and analytic capabilities (Long, 1991).

The speech-language pathologist transcribes the linguistic behavior of both the child and the conversational partner, along with the nonlinguistic behaviors of each. Phonetic transcription can be used if there is concern about use of phonological rules. The timesheet format in Table 4.7 enables the speech-language pathologist to evaluate delays or latencies on the part of the child.

All of the child's utterances, including false starts, nonfluencies, and fillers, are transcribed. Although these linguistic elements may not be used for calculation of average or mean utterance length, they are extremely important in determining language and communication difficulties.

All utterances of the conversational partner(s) also are transcribed. These are important in assessing the manner and style of the conversational partners. The speech-language pathologist is interested in the amount of control and the amount of talking exhibited by the partner.

Determining utterance boundaries is often difficult. This is not an exact science, and the artistry of the speech-language pathologist is needed at this point. An *utterance* is a complete thought that is divided from other utterances by sentence boundaries, pauses, and/or a drop in the voice. Table 4.8 contains examples of utterance boundaries.

TABLE 4.8
Utterance boundaries

A sentence is an utterance.
    Mommy went to the doctor's tomor . . . yesterday.

Run-on sentences with *and* should contain no more than one *and* joining clauses.
    We went in a bus and we saw monkeys and we had a picnic and we petted the sheeps and one sheep sneezed on me and we had sodas and we came home.

    Utterances:
    1. We went in a bus and we saw monkeys.
    2. (And) we had a picnic and we petted the sheeps.
    3. (And) one sheep sneezed on me and we had sodas.
    4. (And) we came home.

    Other complex or compound sentences should be treated as one utterance.
    He was mad because his mommy spanked him because he broke the lamp and spilled the doggie's water.

Imperative sentences are utterances.
    Go home.

Pauses, voice drops, and/or inhalations mark boundaries.
    Eat (pause and voice drop) . . . chocolate candy.
        Two utterances: Eat. Chocolate candy.
    Eat (momentary delay) . . . chocolate candy.
        One utterance: Eat chocolate candy.

Situational and nonlinguistic cues help to determine boundaries.
    Eat (hands plate to partner insistently) . . . chocolate candy (points to candy dish).
        Two utterances: Eat. Chocolate candy.
    Want (reaches unsuccessfully) . . . mommy (turns to look).
        Two utterances: Want. Mommy.
    Want mommy (reaches unsuccessfully).
        One utterance: Want, mommy.

The linguistic context also helps.
    Partner: Well, what do you want?
    Child: Candy (pause) . . . you get it.
        Two utterances: Candy. You get it.

Declaring sentences to be utterances is easy. Most of what is said, however, is not in complete sentence form. For example, the response to a question often omits shared information and might consist of such responses as "No," "Cookie," and "Okay." Each of these is a complete utterance. Longer responses, such as "No, later" or "No, let's go later," are also single utterances. This determination might change if the child were to respond with a pause and a drop in the voice after "No." "No (pause and drop voice). Let's go later." Now there are two utterances.

Partial sentences or phrases, nonfluent units, and run-on sentences are even more difficult. A partial sentence might consist of the child pointing to an object and saying, "Doggie." This would count as an utterance. In the following exchange, the child makes an internal repair:

PARTNER: I like to play mommy.
CHILD: No, you not . . . me the . . . you baby.

The entire unit is an utterance and will be analyzed in different ways by using all or part of what the child said.

For run-on sentences, the speech-language pathologist can follow the general rule that allows two clauses to be joined together in a sentence. In the following example, sentence/utterance boundaries have been marked as they might be on a transcript:

[I went to the party, and we ate pizza] [(and) We played games, and I won a prize] [(and) We had cake and ice cream.]

Division can be aided by the child's pauses and breath patterns. Children in the late preschool years often make long strings of clauses with *and* meaning *and then*. Counting these as a single utterance inflates the mean utterance length. Once the sample is transcribed, it can be analyzed.

CONCLUSION

Collecting a representative language sample that demonstrates the child's diverse abilities is a difficult task. Careful planning and execution are required, as are exacting methods of recording and transcription. Although these procedures may seem difficult and time-consuming initially, they can be accomplished easily and relatively quickly with practice. A properly planned and executed sampling and a thorough transcription will yield an abundance of linguistic and nonlinguistic information.

Guides for collecting a language sample include the following:

■ Establish a positive relationship with the child before recording the language sample.

■ Reduce your authority figure persona to ensure more participation by the child. A child is more likely to respond naturally with someone who is an equal.

- Be unobtrusive while collecting the sample so that the child is less conscious of the process.

- The conversational partner should keep talking to a minimum. Although speech-language pathologists abhor a vacuum, when possible they should wait out the child.

- Avoid yes/no questions and constituent questions that require only a one-word response from the child. Ask process rather than product questions.

- Follow the child's lead in play and in the selection of topic. Determine the child's interests before beginning the collection process. Select those materials at the child's interest level that are likely to stimulate interest.

- If the child does not talk or responds in a very repetitive or stereotypic manner, model responses for the child or have another person model.

Only through sampling the child's linguistic abilities in a conversational context can the speech-language pathologist gain insight into how the child's language works for the child. This is the first step in designing intervention that is relevant to the child and thus more likely to generalize.

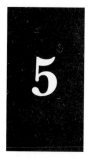

5

Analysis Across Utterances and Partners and by Communication Event

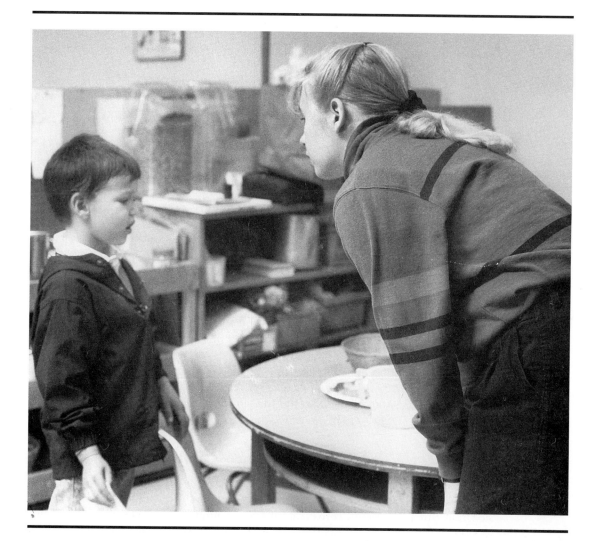

anguage is a complex symbol system, and the analysis methods used with a conversational sample reflect this complexity. For this reason, analysis of a language sample should not be a fishing expedition for possible problems. Language analysis is best used to explore certain aspects of the child's behavior brought into question through other data collection methods. If a language disorder exists, it can be confirmed by descriptive analysis of a sample of the unique language pattern of the child with language impairment.

Traditional analysis has focused exclusively on the utterance or sentence as the unit of analysis. Although this type of analysis is appropriate for many language features, it may not be the best way to assess behaviors that transcend these units. For example, an analysis of a child's use of pronouns necessitates crossing utterance boundaries in order to describe the child's introduction of new information and reference to old or established information that may have been introduced by the child or the conversational partner.

To analyze language only at the utterance level is to miss many of the child's language skills, especially those aspects that govern cohesion and conversational manipulation. For example, pronoun analysis is very different when analyzing for case or person at the utterance level and when evaluating use of reference and cohesion within a conversation. Only by going beyond individual utterances can the speech-language pathologist gain an understanding of the child's use of the many language skills possessed (Biber, 1986; Scott, 1987).

In this chapter, we explore analysis across utterances and partners and by communication event, noting the adjustments the speaker must make to meet conversational demands. These analyses are suggested when the speech-language pathologist suspects difficulties. Obviously, the many types of analysis mentioned in this chapter would be too numerous to examine and too time-consuming to perform with every child. Because little normative information is available on conversational skills, analysis at these levels is largely descriptive. Table 5.1 presents some types of analyses possible across utterances and partners and by communication event.

It is important for the speech-language pathologist to remember that many of the language features discussed in this chapter are dependent on the behavior of the partner and vary with the situation and the culture of the child and the conversational partner (Crago & Eriks-Brophy, 1992). The stimuli and reinforcers and the child's response to each, the conversational roles of each partner, and the type and amount of communication are contingent on cultural values. Tasks should be culturally relevant with functional, meaningful, culturally appropriate language. Sampling results should be analyzed with cultural variability in mind.

ACROSS UTTERANCES AND PARTNERS

Analysis at the utterance level reveals much about the child's discrete, finite language skills but may obscure the child's knowledge of the "big picture," the cohesion that threads through conversations. Some linguistic devices serve this cohesive purpose, and larger units than the utterance must be analyzed to assess their

TABLE 5.1
Types of analysis beyond the utterance

Across Utterances and Partners
Stylistic Variations
   Register
   Interlanguage and Code Switching
   Channel Availability
Referential Communication
   Presuppositional Skills
     Content and Method
     Linguistic Devices: Deictics, Definite and Indefinite Reference
Cohesive Devices
   Reference: Initial and Following Mention
   Ellipsis
   Conjunction
   Adverbial Conjuncts and Disjuncts
   Contrastive Stress

By Communication Event
Social versus Nonsocial
Conversational Initiation: Method Frequency and Success Rate
Topic Initiation: Method, Frequency, Success Rate, and Appropriateness
Conversation and Topic Maintenance: Frequency and Latency of Contingency
Duration of Topic: Number of Turns, Informativeness, and Sequencing
Turn taking: Density, Latency, and Duration
   Overlap: Type, Frequency, and Duration
   Signals
Conversation and Topic Termination
Conversational Breakdown
   Request for Repair: Frequency and Form
   Conversational Repair
     Spontaneous versus Listener-Initiated
     Strategy and Success Rate

---

development. Other devices vary across whole conversations, and one sample may be very different from another.

Stylistic Variations

The style of talking, whether formal, casual, or varied in other ways for the situation, usually does not change utterance by utterance. Rather, it is a manner of talking with a specific language partner or in a specific situation. Different styles also may be seen in role play. The speech-language pathologist is interested in the different styles used by the child in the various samples collected.

As early as age 4, children use a different style of talking when they address younger children learning language. This style resembles *motherese* or *parentese*, the stylistic changes made by parents when they address these same younger children. Mature language users have a variety of styles at their disposal and can switch styles with little effort. Such variation requires the speaker to consider the listener and the situation and the resultant requirements on the speaker.

Register

Stylistic code switching, the move from one style to another, must be judged against the age, gender, and language ability of the speaker and the listener. Styles differ according to role-taking characteristics, dialectal variations, amount of politeness, and conversational control.

Conversational roles can be established by the topics chosen, vocabulary (*dear, sir, honey*), pronunciation, and the discourse style selected. Usually, the more dominant partner takes longer turns and asks more questions. The degree of politeness also varies. In general, speakers are more polite when in the less dominant role or when requesting something that belongs to or is controlled by the other partner, who may be unlikely to grant the request. One politeness vehicle is the indirect request that does not directly state the desired consequence. Examples are, "Can you close the window?" and the more indirect, "Do you think it's cold in here?"

Children with LLD often fail to use styles based on differing situational variables. Data suggest these children do not adjust to different speakers or may adjust in different ways from children developing normally. Children with LLD may fail to recognize the characteristics of different settings. The child with language impairment may not be able to discriminate dominant from nondominant roles and the language form that goes with each. The most frequent problems with register include providing insufficient information for the listener, not knowing when to make a statement, asking inappropriate questions, giving insufficient reason for the cause and effect of a situation, and not adjusting register to the speaker (A. Johnson et al., 1984).

It may be especially difficult for the child with LLD to express feelings and emotions. These expressions may be very direct and negative. The speech-language pathologist studies the sample to determine the stylistic variations present. The value of collecting language samples in two very different but client-appropriate situations is apparent. The speech-language pathologist should look for modifications in politeness, intimacy, and linguistic code based on the age, status, familiarity, cognitive level, linguistic level, and shared past experience of the listener (F. Roth & Spekman, 1984a). Of interest is the attention the child gives to the listener's characteristics. In addition to noting stylistic variations, the speech-language pathologist looks for inappropriate styles—those that are too formal, too casual, or include excessive swearing.

The speech-language pathologist might note features such as differing utterance length with various partners. Other variations include vocabulary and topic. More subjective indices include intonational patterns and the use of attention getting and maintaining devices.

Interlanguage and Code Switching

With children with LEP, it is important to establish patterns of language use in both L₁ and L₂ (Hamayan & Damico, 1991). Two possible patterns are called interlanguage and code switching. **Interlanguage** is a combination of the L1 and L2 rules, plus ad hoc rules from neither or both languages (McLaughlin, 1977; Selinker, Swain, & Dumes, 1975). This "hybrid" language varies among children and within the individual child across situations (Tarone, 1988). Usually, interlanguages are transitional in nature, although some features may stabilize as a permanent form, especially if there is little motivation to change (Schumann, 1978; Vigil & Oller, 1976). Predictable patterns should be identified during observation and sampling. Of interest are the rules used by the child and any situational variables.

Linguistic **code switching** is the shifting from one language to another within and/or across different utterances (Sanchez, 1983). A complicated, rule-governed behavior, code switching does not signal poor language skills, although it may be used by children when they have inadequate L2 skills (Auer, 1984; Genesee, 1984; McClure, 1981; Penalosa, 1981; Poplack, 1982). As with interlanguage, code switching is influenced heavily by contextual and situational variables (Sanchez, 1983; Sprott & Kemper, 1987). For example, the Spanish-speaking storyteller might use English when referring to Anglos, and Spanish when referring to Latinos. Code switching usually occurs to enhance meaning, emphasize a change of topic, and convey humor, ethnic solidarity, and attitudes toward the listener (Hamayan & Damico, 1991).

The speech-language pathologist should note uses of interlanguage and code switching, along with sampling variables such as the situation and the partner(s). It is especially important to identify patterns that may impede the transmission of meaning or interrupt communication.

Channel Availability

Some individuals enjoy talking on the telephone. I am not among them. In part, this lack of comfort may reflect the pressure placed on the speaker to be very explicit with language in this situation. Nonlinguistic channels are unavailable.

Most children below age 11 experience less communication success when they do not visually share the communication environment (F. Roth & Spekman, 1984a). As the number of channels decreases, the child with a language impairment should have increasing difficulty communicating. In fact, children with language learning disabilities often have great difficulty if forced to rely solely on the verbal channel. The speech-language pathologist should note in the sample the relative success of the child's communication efforts as the number of channels varies.

Referential Communication

Referential communication is the ability of a speaker to select and verbally identify the attributes of an entity in such a way that the listener can identify the entity accurately (Bowman, 1984). To succeed, the speaker must be able to determine what information the listener needs, deliver that information in a specific manner, make comparisons, and use feedback on message adequacy and breakdown.

Referential communication includes directions, explanations, and descriptions. These are three essential aspects of classroom discourse, and their impairment may contribute to the academic difficulties of children with language learning disabilities (Donahue, 1985).

Presuppositional Skills

As noted in Chapter 4, presupposition is the speaker's assumptions about the context and about the listener that modify the manner and content of the speaker's utterance (A. Johnson et al., 1984). The speaker must take the conversational perspective of the listener(s) and determine what information to communicate and its form.

From early on, informativeness is a characteristic of communication. Even toddlers tend to code information that is maximally informative, thus talking about things that are new, different, and changing. For most children, the receptive and expressive ability to consider a partner's perspective is established by age 10 (Sonnenschein & Whitehurst, 1984). Although both comprehension and production require understanding of the critical features needed, production also requires knowing how and when to provide information. At age 10, children with LLD have poor referential skills and are less likely to adjust to the listener (Knight-Arest, 1984), more likely to provide ambiguous information (Spekman, 1981), and less likely to supply enough overall information (Noel, 1980). In addition, although children with LLD seem to understand directions given by others, they take longer to comply than do age-matched children who are non-LLD (Feagans & Short, 1986) and have great difficulty giving adequate instructions.

The speech-language pathologist should be alert to the informativeness of the child's utterances and to the social context. The following questions can be applied to the sample (F. Roth & Spekman, 1984a):

- What does the child choose to encode in the situation?
- Does the child encode what is novel or merely comment on what is already given?
- Does the child encode new information gesturally or linguistically?
- Are messages informative, vague, or ambiguous?
- Are different referents clearly established?
- Does the child talk differently about things present and things not?

What is coded and how.   Conversations usually contain information that is novel and informative. The speech-language pathologist is interested in whether the child adds to the conversation or only comments on what is given. In the following exchange, the child takes a turn but adds nothing of substance to the conversation.

PARTNER:	Wasn't that a great baseball game on TV last night?
CHILD:	Yeah, great game.

PARTNER:	What a great home run in the top of the ninth; I didn't expect Cincinnati to pull it out.
CHILD:	Great home run.
PARTNER:	I think they'll probably go on for the pennant. How about you?
CHILD:	Pennant.

If this sounds like the conversation of someone who doesn't know the topic well enough to comment, that may be partially correct. The child may not be able to identify the topic. Frequent repetition may indicate a semantic (word retrieval), processing, or pragmatic (not sure of the contextual demands) problem. Other children with language impairment may make vague or ambiguous contributions or use empty words, such as *one* and *thing*.

Noninformative language can take several forms (Nicholas, Obler, Albert, & Helm-Estabrooks, 1985). Table 5.2 presents forms and examples seen in children with language impairment. These types of noninformative language may be especially useful when rating the language of children with TBI and LLD. The speech-language pathologist can rate utterances to determine the strategy used by the child.

Linguistic devices.   Several linguistic devices are used to mark informativeness, including deictics and direct/indirect reference (F. Roth & Spekman, 1984a). Both of these devices can be used to note referents internal or external to the conversation; other cohesive devices, listed in Table 5.3 (Halliday & Hasan, 1976), establish relations entirely within the discourse.

Deictics.   As noted in Chapter 4, deictic terms are linguistic elements that must be interpreted from the perspective of the speaker in order to be understood as the speaker intended. The use of deixis is based on the *speaker principle,* in which the referential point shifts as speakers change, and on the *distance principle,* in which referents are coded by their distance from the speaker.

TABLE 5.2

Types of non-informative language

Empty phrases (common idioms, such as *and so on,* and *etcetera excetera*)
Indefinite terms and highly nonspecific nouns (*one, thing, that*)
Deictic terms (*this, that, here, there*)
Pronouns without antecedents
Comments on task instead of stimulus
Neologisms (*Oh, you know the one that you fly in*)
Paraphrases
Repeated words or phrases
Personal value judgments about the stimulus (*That's pretty dumb*)
Use of *and* alone
Conjunctions *but, so, or,* and *because* alone

Source: Adapted from Nicholas, M., Obler, L. K., Albert, M. L., & Helm-Estabrooks, N. (1985). Empty speech in Alzheimer's disease and fluent aphasia. *Journal of Speech and Hearing Research, 28,* 405-410.

TABLE 5.3
Cohesive devices used in English

Relation	Explanation	Example
Reference	Initially, the entity is named and may use the indefinite article (*a/an*). Subsequent mention may use a pronoun, words such as *this, that,* and *one,* or use the definite article (*the*) with the noun.	*John* went looking for a *car. He* found *one* in the city. I want to buy *a coat,* but *that one* I saw last night is too expensive.
Ellipsis	Subsequent sentences omit redundant or shared information.	Who *ate all the cookies?* I did. (Eat all the cookies) I would like to *make a phone call.* May I? (Make a phone call)
Conjunction	Conjunctions join clauses to express additive, causal, and other relationships.	We went to the circus, *and* I saw elephants. John's angry *because* I drank his soda.

Source: Adapted from Halliday, M., & Hasan, R. (1976). *Cohesion in English.* London: Longman.

Words with deictic meanings appear in several word classes, including personal pronouns (*I/me* and *you*), demonstrative adjectives (*this, that, these,* and *those*), adverbs of time (*before, after, now,* and *then*), adverbs of location (*here* and *there*), and verbs (*come* and *go*). The child's behavior, especially the errors, should be analyzed to determine confusion or overreliance on one principle or one aspect of a principle.

Definite and indefinite reference.   The mature language user is able to mark specific (definite) and nonspecific (indefinite) referents by manipulation of definite (*the*) and indefinite (*a/an*) articles. The speaker must consider what the listener knows about the topic under discussion.

Article use can be especially difficult for the child with language impairment. In part, this difficulty may reflect the use of articles also to mark new and old information. The tendency for children with language impairment is to overuse the definite article. Each article can be analyzed for appropriate referential use.

Cohesive Devices

Conversational *cohesion,* how language hangs together, can be a useful analysis tool (Halliday & Hasan, 1976). Cohesion can be expressed through syntax and vocabulary, for example, a pronoun or a demonstrative, such as *this* or *that,* to refer to the referent, which was identified previously in the conversation. *Conjoining,* the connection of phrases, clauses, and sentences through the use of such conjunctions as *and, because,* and *if,* also is used for cohesion. The major cohesive devices used in English are listed in Table 5.3.

The most frequent problems of cohesion relate to providing redundant information, deleting necessary information, using unclear and ambiguous reference, sequencing old and new information, and marking old and new information with articles and pronouns (A. Johnson et al., 1984). In short, errors usually reflect including or excluding too much information or confusing new and old information.

Reference

Reference is a linguistic device used continuously in conversation to keep information flowing and to designate new and old information. In the process, new information is stated clearly and then subsequently implied by the referral to it as old information, one utterance presupposing the other. Some children with language impairments, such as children with autism, have difficulty marking new and old information (McCaleb & Prizant, 1985).

The speech-language pathologist must note the method of introducing new information and the use of following mention. Speakers should ensure that listeners can determine easily noun-pronoun relationships. This investigation requires looking beyond traditional utterance level analysis.

Initial mention.   In initial mention, mature speakers establish mutual reference clearly, especially if the entity mentioned is not present. Generally, the referent name is stressed and preceded by the indefinite article (*a/an*). The referent often is placed at the end of the sentence, the most salient position. The following are examples of the introduction of new information:

> Did you see *John at the party*?
>
> We went to a *circus* yesterday.

In addition, referents that are present may be pointed to or handled. Young children tend to rely more on these nonlinguistic behaviors to establish new referents.

Children with LLD or autism have difficulty with new information (McCaleb & Prizant, 1985; Rees & Wollner, 1981). As speakers, they may not identify new information for the listener, assuming that the listener "just knows" what the speaker is thinking. As listeners, these children may have difficulty identifying the new information but will ask few questions to clarify. "These children often do not know what they do not know" and thus cannot inquire about it (J. Stark, 1985). With increasing language skills, the child is able to be more specific linguistically.

Children with word-finding difficulties or poor vocabularies may use empty words, such as *that, one,* or *thing,* that do not help clarify the referent. These children may rely on the immediate context and use pointing to specify the referent their nonspecific vocabulary failed to identify.

Following mention.   In following mention, previously identified referents often are moved to the initial position in the sentence and may be referred to by the use of the definite article (*the*) or a pronoun. This referral to previously cited information is called **anaphoric reference.** Pronoun use is appropriate when the referent is unambiguous or clearly identified. The pronoun should be in close proximity so that there is no confusion as to which noun it refers.

The speech-language pathologist is interested in the way the child introduces new information and refers to that information later. Also of interest is any confusion with article and pronoun use. Pronouns and a method of recording the child's use are included in Table 6.14. It is not uncommon for the preschool child or the child with LLD to introduce new information with, "She did it," leaving the listener to determine who *she* is and what *it* is.

Ellipsis

Ellipsis is a process in which redundant information is omitted. For example, the response to "What do you want?" is "Cookie," which omits the shared information "I want."

Elliptical fragments are used frequently to keep the conversation moving smoothly and rapidly, but they are missed if linguistic analysis concentrates solely on full sentences. Children with language impairment may not realize that information is shared or may assume that it is shared when it is not. Either assumption interferes with the flow of conversation. For example, the child might repeat, "Cookies, cookies, cookies," until someone asks, "What about cookies?" to which the child responds in surprise, "I want some," having assumed that the *I want* was shared.

Conjunction

Conjunctions, such as *and, then, so,* and t*herefore,* are used to connect thoughts. Although preschool children have several conjunction-type words in their vocabularies, they rarely use them to join clauses. Even kindergarten children will over-rely on *and,* which becomes an all–purpose conjunction. In addition, *and* often is used to mean *and then* when giving a sequence of events. A developmental progression for conjunctions is given in Table 6.16.

Just as conjunctions can be analyzed at the utterance level because of their use in linking clauses, conjunctions can be analyzed across utterances, as in the following exchange.

PARENT: We had a great day at the zoo. I liked the monkeys best.
CHILD: *And* feeding the deer babies.

Analysis at the level of the child's utterance alone would miss the child's considerable skill.

Adverbial Conjuncts and Disjuncts

Adverbial conjuncts and disjuncts are conversational devices used for cohesion. *Conjuncts* are intersentential forms that express a logical relationship, such as the conjunctions *then* or *so.* Conjuncts are of two types: *concordant,* such as *similarly, consequently,* and *moreover,* and *discordant,* such as *nevertheless, rather,* and *in contrast.* *Disjuncts* are used to comment on or to convey the speaker's attitude toward the topic and include words and phrases such as *honestly, frankly, perhaps, however, yet, to my surprise, it's obvious to me that,* and the like.

Conjuncts and disjuncts develop rather late in childhood and, therefore, may be good measures of adolescent language. Growth is "slow and protracted" (Nippold, Schwarz, & Undlin, 1992, p. 108). By age 12, children use only an average of 4 conjuncts per 100 utterances (Scott, 1988a). In contrast, adults average 12 conjuncts per 100 utterances. Children between ages 6 and 12 use conjuncts infrequently and rely most frequently on *then, so,* and *though* (Scott, 1984a). Adolescents use the same conjuncts but also use *therefore, however, rather,* and *consequently* most accurately in both their reading and writing (Nippold, Schwarz, & Undlin, 1992). Comprehension seems to be better than production although similar (Nippold, Schwarz, & Undlin, 1992; Scott & Rush, 1985).

The conjunct *then* can be used to signal both continuity and discontinuity in adolescent and adult language (Halliday & Hasan, 1976; Segal, Duchan, & Scott, 1991). Initially, children use *then* to mean *next,* joining clausal information. Later, *then* is used to focus on ideas presented previously, in contrast to *now,* which signals that new ideas will be presented on some topic.

In mature narratives, *then* is used approximately 20% of the time to mark discontinuity by indicating a shift (Duchan & Waltzman, 1992). This shift might be to (a) a different discourse type, as in conversation to narration or the reverse, (b) a new scene or location, (c) a different character in a narrative, or (d) a new perspective. Use of *then* seems dependent on the use of other conjuncts, such as *anyway, meanwhile, whatever,* and *now.* Narratives, discussed in Chapter 7, offer insight into conjunct use.

Contrastive Stress

Contrastive stress or emphasis can be used to negate or correct the message of a conversational partner. For example, if one speaker said, "Kathy brought cookies," the other might correct, "*Mary* brought cookies." Again, the speech-language pathologist must transcend the traditional utterance-level analysis.

COMMUNICATION EVENT

Communication event, a term coined by Roger Brown (1973) and modified by others, can represent an entire conversation or a portion thereof that includes one topic. For purposes of our discussion, we use the larger definition and include within it a conversation that comprises one or more topics.

Usually, a shared or negotiated agenda(s) occurs within a conversation. Utterances within the event support this agenda. The teenager who wants to be granted a privilege, such as getting to use the family car, is polite, and each utterance supports this agenda.

Conversations may be too open-ended for some children unfamiliar with the process or unable to decipher the code. The child may be unclear about the pur-

pose of conversation and her or his role in it. Much of this difficulty can be alleviated by using familiar conversational partners and situations and by following the
child's lead. Younger children and those with a language impairment may need
events with more definite beginnings and ends, such as putting together a puzzle.

The social organization of discourse consists of the two roles of speaker and
listener. The effective communicator has the ability to function in and contribute
to the conversation by assuming responsibility for both roles. Assessment variables that might measure a child's ability to participate effectively are the amount
of socialized speech and the child's adaptive style; conversation and topic initiation, maintenance, and termination and the completeness, relevance, and clarity
of the child's behavior; on-topic exchanges and turn taking; and conversational
repairs (James, 1989; Lund & Duchan, 1988; Prutting, 1983; F. Roth & Spekman,
1984a).

Analysis occurs at two levels: the molar and the molecular (Prutting, 1983).
At the *molar level*, the speech-language pathologist evaluates each behavior for
appropriateness or inappropriateness within the conversational context. Inappropriate behaviors may indicate problem areas for further assessment. At the *molecular level*, the speech-language pathologist is interested in the *frequency, latency,
duration, density,* and *sequence* of the child's behaviors (Prutting, 1983).

Frequency data will reveal inordinately high- or low-frequency features and
information on the range of features. *Latency,* or the span of time when an individual does not engage in behavior, is also important. Pauses and hesitations may
reveal difficulty decoding the preceding utterance or forming a response. *Duration* is the length of time that the child and the partner are engaged in a certain
behavior, such as conversational gaze or conversational turns by both partners.
Density is the number of behaviors within a certain period of time. Of interest are
the density of different conversational topics or specific linguistic structures, such
as questions. *Sequence* includes the order of events within a topic or conversation.
The child exhibiting difficulty with sequencing of a conversation may not understand the rules of conversational participation.

Decisions of appropriateness may be facilitated through the use of a modified ethnographic technique similar to that used in anthropological studies.
Using an expository form of writing, the speech-language pathologist attempts to
describe each child utterance with reference to form, content, and use, discourse
relations, code switching, learning and cognitive style, and the partner's arrangement and selection of nonlinguistic strategies, materials, and procedures (Constable, 1992). Thus, each utterance is given a reference frame in which to judge
appropriateness. Table 5.4 provides a sample of a dialogue and the accompanying ethnographic analysis. Ethnographic techniques are especially important
when assessing children with LEP or with different dialects.

Social Versus Nonsocial

Social speech is speech addressed explicitly to and adapted for a listener. It is characterized by explicitness and clarity, repairs of breakdowns, and an obligation for

TABLE 5.4
An example of ethnographic analysis

Language Sample	Ethnographic Analysis
CHILD: What's that?	Child does not seem to know the identity of an object and inquires as to its name with an appropriate *wh-* question
PARTNER: That's a "Thing-a-majibit."	addressed to the partner. The partner supplies an appropri-
CHILD: What it do?	ate answer but does not elaborate. The child seeks such elab-oration by asking a second *wh-* question in which he omits the auxiliary verb. Other sentence elements are included in
PARTNER: What do you think it does?	the proper adult word order. The partner does not answer
CHILD: On the table.	the question but responds with a second *wh-* question in order to have the child guess at the function from its appear-ance. The child responds inappropriately to the partner's
PARTNER: YES, on the table. What about "On the table?"	question, either ignoring the content of the question or mis-comprehending the meaning of the *wh-* word. The partner does not pursue the question by restating or reformulating it. Instead, the partner confirms the child's utterance and asks a
CHILD: On the table.	third *wh-* question incorporating the child's utterance. Again, the child does not respond to the content of the partner's question but repeats the previous utterance with no addi-tional information to aid the partner's understanding.

the listener to respond. Social communication includes dialogues and social monologues addressed to a listener or uttered for the mutual enjoyment of both the speaker and listener, such as rhyming and poetic nonsense. The speaker adapts the explicitness of the message for the listener and repairs breakdowns. The speaker's message is delivered as if the speaker expects a listener response.

In contrast, *nonsocial speech* is not addressed explicitly to a listener, and the listener has no obligation to respond. Nonsocial communication is usually for the speaker's own enjoyment and often consists of asocial monologues. An important measure of communication is the percentage of the child's utterances or the amount of total talk time that can be characterized as social (F. Roth & Spekman, 1984a).

Although preschoolers produce many asocial monologues, the amount of time spent in this type of production decreases with age. School-age children developing normally produce very little nonsocial speech. In general, children's communication becomes more interpersonal as they mature, with girls more likely to use language cooperatively (D. Cooper & Anderson-Inman, 1988). Boys are more likely to show domination and control, to interrupt and insult, and to play practical jokes. Older adolescents are more concerned for the wants and feelings of others, compromise and reach mutual agreement more, and are more concerned for long-term consequences in their communication than are younger adolescents or children (Selman, Beardslee, Schultz, Krupa, & Podorefsky, 1986).

Conversational Initiation

The most efficient way to initiate a conversation is to gain the listener's attention, greet the listener, and clearly state the topic of conversation or some opener, such as, "Guess what happened to me yesterday?" or "Where have you been? I haven't seen you in ages." Openers set the tone of the conversation and the subsequent turns. Opening and closing a conversation is one of the pragmatic problems most frequently encountered in children with language impairment (A. Johnson et al., 1984). Children with autism initiate very little conversational behavior—even less than other children with language impairments (Loveland, Landry, Hughes, Hall, & McEvoy, 1988). Of clinical interest is how the child initiates the conversation and how successful he is in having the conversation continue (F. Roth & Spekman, 1984a).

Method

It is best to get the listener's attention before initiating a conversation. This usually is accomplished by eye contact and a greeting. The child with language impairment may begin without any greeting or may interrupt an ongoing conversation with, "Hey." Some children use the same opener repeatedly (e.g., "Guess what?"), whatever the conversational context. Data may need to be collected over a wide variety of situations to discern a pattern. Role play can be used to determine the child's knowledge of conventional openers.

Frequency and Success Rate

Children who are withdrawn or unsure of the conversational expectations may initiate conversations only rarely. Instead, they adopt a more passive, responsive role. In contrast, other children may interrupt frequently and attempt to initiate conversation indiscriminately. Of interest to the speech-language pathologist is the density of initiations, or the number of initiations over a given time. Obviously, this figure will change with the situation. For children, lunchtime, recess, and group projects may be appropriate forums in which to collect such data.

The success rate of children in initiating conversations is also significant. Although children may attempt to begin conversations frequently, they may be ignored or mocked, depending on the audiences they choose. Each of us has experienced the "cold shoulder" at least once. Children who are socially inappropriate may experience more than their share.

Topic Initiation

Once a conversation has been initiated, the participants negotiate the topics that will be discussed. **Topic** can be defined as "the proposition or set of propositions or subject matter about which the speaker is either providing or requesting new information" (Bedrosian, 1988, p. 270). This negotiation process begins with one partner introducing a topic; the other partner agrees to adopt that topic by commenting on it, disagrees by changing the topic, or ends the conversation. Mature speakers identify the topic clearly by name and, if in the immediate context, by pointing. Preschool children and those with language impairments rely more on nonlinguistic cues, such as pointing to and holding or shaking objects.

In general, children with language impairment are less adept than both their age-matched and language-age-matched peers in their ability to direct the conversation by introducing topics (Donahue, 1983). This lack of ability might reflect difficulty introducing topics clearly and/or these children's limited lists of potential topics (Bedrosian, 1985; Dollaghan & Miller, 1986).

Method

An effectively initiated topic is identified clearly in order to establish mutual regard. As mentioned, the speaker may point, look at, and/or state the topic. Generally, the speaker provides information the listener needs to identify referents and their relationships. Topics are negotiated between speakers, and, even when explicitly stated, topics are based on the shared assumptions of each participant.

In general, the less sure the speaker is that the listener knows the topic, the longer the speaker will take to introduce it. The more mature speaker is adept at presupposing the prior knowledge of the listeners. In return for the introduction, listeners assure speakers that they understand, or they ask for clarification when they do not understand.

Topics typically are changed by stating a new one. Older elementary school children, adolescents, and adults increasingly use a conversational technique called *shading*, in which the conversation is steered from one topic to a closely related one. Adult conversations only occasionally contain very disparate topics.

The child with language impairment may not establish topics, preferring to adopt those of others. If the child does introduce topics, there may be little or no background information to aid the listener (Brinton & Fujiki, 1992). The child with language impairment may have a very restricted set of conversational or topic openers or may rely on a stereotypic utterance (e.g., "Guess what?"). Children with emotional difficulties may continue some internal conversation with the assumption that the listener has been privy to this information. As mentioned previously, children with word-finding difficulties or poor vocabularies may rely on nonspecific nouns, such as *one* or *thing*. Nonspecific verbs, such as *do* and *get*, also may be used frequently.

The child's responses to the openers of others may be nonexistent or non-contingent/off–topic. The child may not be able to identify the topic or to determine what response is required to the partner's opener.

Both the linguistic and nonlinguistic aspects of the sample should be analyzed. The nonlinguistic aspects regulate the linguistic ones and are significant in the regulation of turn initiation and termination, topic choice, and interruptions (Argyle & Cook, 1976; Craig, 1979; Duncan, 1974; Prutting, 1982).

Frequency and Success Rate

As with conversational initiation, the density and success rate of topic initiation are noteworthy. In general, less dominant speakers will introduce fewer topics and will be less successful in having their topics adopted by their partners. Lack of success also may indicate problems with topicalization, such as establishing and commenting on, marking changes in, and maintaining the topic for a sufficient length of time (A. Johnson et al., 1984). Related factors to be evaluated are the articulation clarity, degree of completeness, and form of the topic statement; social adaptation of the child's language style; degree of content relevance to the ongoing activity and to listener interests; use of eye contact; and physical proximity (F. Roth & Spekman, 1984a).

Appropriateness

The appropriateness of a topic is determined by the context. Some topics, such as the weather, are always appropriate, whereas others, such as age, income, or sexual behavior, are appropriate only in limited contexts. Each of us has favorite topics. We tend to talk about what we know.

The speech-language pathologist is interested in determining the child's favorite topics and in assessing their appropriateness in context. Although some topics will work in one context, they are inappropriate for others. Some children with language impairment have only limited topics or perseverate on a few regardless of the context.

Conversation and Topic Maintenance

Once a topic is introduced, speakers comment on that topic, each sentence reflecting the general discourse topic. In effective conversations, the participants seem to adhere to four principles: stay on topic, be truthful, be brief, and be relevant (F. Roth & Spekman, 1984a).

Each partner depends on the *contingency*, or relatedness of a response to the preceding utterance. Each response should add new information on the topic. The topic must be mentioned frequently enough to enable both participants to recall it as the conversation progresses, because the topic becomes less specific with subsequent reference.

Topic continuance may be signaled by maintenance devices, such as *Now, Well, And then, In any case, Next, So, I (you, we, they)* (did something). Some devices, called *continuants*, maintain the conversation but add little if any new information. Examples of this behavior are *yeah, uh-huh,* and *okay* when used as a signal that the listener is paying attention. Other maintenance devices are repeating a portion or all of the previous utterance.

Children with language impairments tend to engage in fewer and shorter interactions than do children developing normally. The most frequent pragmatic problems for children with language impairment include terminating sentences, connecting discourse, listening and responding to the speaker, knowing when to take a turn, and knowing how to ask and answer questions (A. Johnson et al., 1984).

Although there is little difference between the turn-taking skills at the one-word level of children with language impairment and those without, a disparity occurs and widens as language becomes increasingly more complex (S. Foster, 1985; Prelock, Messick, Schwartz, & Terrell, 1981; Reichle, Busch, & Doyle, 1986). Children with autism may not respond to initiations, while other children with language impairment may overuse turn-fillers or acknowledgments ("Uh-huh") to keep the conversation going (Bedrosian, 1988; Brinton & Fujiki, 1989; Dewey & Everard, 1974).

Frequency of Contingency

Contingent or semantically contingent utterances relate to or reflect the meaning of the prior utterance. One example of contingency is the topic of an utterance. Thus, a contingent utterance maintains the topic of the previous utterance and adds to it in some way. For example, in response to the utterance, "We went to Captain Jake's for dinner last night," a second speaker might make the contingent remark, "Oh, did you enjoy the food?" A noncontingent remark would be, "My uncle lives on a farm."

Assume for a moment that the name of the restaurant in the previous example was Uncle Jake's. In this situation, the child's remark, "My uncle lives on a farm," although off–topic, does have some link to the previous sentence. If these links can be identified, there may be a pattern that will reveal the child's processing strategy.

In general, children with language impairment are less responsive than are their age-matched peers developing language normally (Rosinski-McClendon & Newhoff, 1987; L. Siegel, Cunningham, & van der Spuy, 1979). This low level of responsiveness may reflect a history of unsuccessful communication. Often, these children respond to questions with stereotypic acknowledgements (*uh-huh, yeh*) and with nonspecific requests for clarification (*what, huh*) (Fey et al., 1981; Rosinski-McClendon & Newhoff, 1987; L. Watson, 1977).

The frequency of contingent behaviors by the child and the caregiver is of interest. The child who exhibits few contingent utterances may prefer to initiate new topics frequently (Prutting, 1983). The speech-language pathologist notes the percentage of the child's utterances that are on–topic, the relevance of the child's questions, and the child's nonverbal responses, such as following directions or looking at something that was mentioned.

A large percentage of off-topic responses may indicate a semantic disorder characterized by difficulty in identifying the topic of discussion. A listener's ability to identify a topic subsequently affects comprehension of comments made about that topic.

The speech-language pathologist should look for underlying contingency that may not be readily obvious. Children with LLD may assume that their partners know the underlying relationship and, therefore, may only include unshared information.

Of particular interest are the child's responses to questions. Such responses should be appropriate to the question and factually correct. For example, the question, "Why is he eating?" might elicit the following responses from different children:

1. Food.
2. Because.
3. He has to.
4. So he won't be hungry.
5. He's hungry.

The first answer is functionally inappropriate although functionally accurate. It does not answer the question, but tells what the man is eating. The second and third responses are appropriate but too brief to be accurate. The fourth and fifth answers fulfill appropriateness and accuracy criteria.

If an answer does not fulfill both requirements, it is in error and may indicate any number of possible breakdowns in the communication process. I have seen a child with severe emotional disorder who gave extremely inappropriate replies to emotional or personal questions, although her responses to factual questions were usually both appropriate and accurate.

A child with language impairment may not understand what the questioner or the question requires or may not realize that a reply is required. The question form and the specific *wh-* question type also may be confusing.

In general, recognition and delivery of the general kind of information required develops prior to the ability to respond with the accurate information. Some *wh-* question forms seem easier than others (Parnell & Amerman, 1983; Parnell, Patterson, & Harding, 1984). Three groupings, from easiest to most difficult, are as follows:

Easiest	What + be, which, where
	Who, whose, what + do
Most difficult	When, why, what happened, how

This order suggests a hierarchy for analysis and intervention. In addition, it is easier for children to respond to questions referring to objects, persons, or events within the immediate setting.

Various semantic question prompts can be used to facilitate production of the child's inadequate responses (Blank, Rose, & Berlin, 1978). The child's responses to these prompts can provide useful information for intervention. Table 5.5 presents a procedure for comparing the efficacy of various prompts in eliciting appropriate and accurate responses from the child. A plus sign (+) indicates appropriate or accurate responses; a minus sign (–) indicates inappropriate or inaccurate ones (Parnell et al., 1984).

Latency of Contingency

When the child makes contingent responses, there should be little delay or latency between his turn and the preceding speaker's turn. Gaps between the turns of mature speakers are brief or nonexistent (Sacks, Schegloff, & Jefferson, 1974). Research has indicated that the average amount of time needed for two adults to switch from one speaker to the next is half a second or less.

TABLE 5.5
Score form for the efficacy of various question prompts

Prompt Type	Strategy Description	Prompt Effectiveness (+, –)		Comments
		Appropriate	Accurate	
Standard focusing phrase with repetition	*Listen to the question* signals the student that a response was in error. Direct student's attention to the repetition; highlights content			
Model example with related content	Use another adult or child in context to model correct response. Then ask child, same form, new content			
Analogous examples	*What are alligators covered with?*—No response. *Seals are covered with fur. What are alligators covered with?*			
Visualization of relationships	*How are an apple and a cookie alike?* No response. Draw semantic feature chart:			

	bakes	eat	grows on tree
apple	+	+	+
cookie	+	+	–

Prompt Type	Strategy Description	Appropriate	Accurate	Comments
Relevant comparison yes/no	*What does a hockey player need?* No response. *Does a hockey player need skates?* Yes. Good. *What does he need?*			

The child's inadequate responses can be modified by using question prompts. Successful responses following a prompt are recorded as a + under both the *appropriate* and *accurate* columns.
Source: Moeller, M., Osberger, M., & Eccarius, M. (1986). Cognitively based strategies for use with hearing-impaired students with comprehension deficits. *Topics in Language Disorders, 6*(4), 37–50.

 Preschoolers and children with language impairment may allow long gaps to develop without any of the apparent embarrassment found among adults when there are long unfilled pauses. A noticeable latency prior to the child's response may indicate word-finding difficulties. Frequently, the linguistically more mature partner will fill in for the child, an act that also violates the rules of turn taking.

 Latency is an important measure for both contingent and noncontingent utterances, whether adjacent or nonadjacent. Delay may be evident in the adjacent utterances of a child with word-finding difficulties as well. Adjacent utterances are spoken as sequential behaviors by the same speaker. A nonadjacent utterance crosses conversational turns and is an utterance or turn of one partner

TABLE 5.6
Definitions and examples of utterance pairs

Types	Definitions	Examples
Contingent	The utterance of one speaker is based on the content, form, and/or intent of the other speaker.	S₁: What do you want for lunch? S₂: Peanut butter. S₁: I hope I don't miss my plane. S₂: Don't worry. Every flight is delayed.
Noncontingent	The utterance of one speaker is not based on that of the other.	S₁: What do you want for lunch? S₂: Gran'ma gots a new car.
Adjacent	Utterances spoken sequentially by the same speaker.	We went to the zoo. I saw monkeys and elephants. But my favorite part was petting the sheeps.
Nonadjacent	Utterances spoken sequentially by different speakers. The utterances may be contingent or noncontingent.	S₁: Here comes the school bus. S₂: Yukk, I was hoping he'd get a flat tire. (Contingent)

followed by an utterance or turn of the other. Definitions and examples of these categories are presented in Table 5.6.

Duration of Topic

A topic is sustained as long as each conversational partner cares to continue and can contribute relevant information. The number of turns taken on a topic is a function of the particular topic and partners involved, the conversational context, and the conversational skill of each participant.

Number of Turns

The speech-language pathologist is interested in the number of turns taken by the child and the partner on a given topic and in the manner of changing topic. In general, a greater number of turns will occur in an adult-child conversation if the child, rather than the adult, initiates the topic. Topics that are sustained longer than others may suggest the child's interest or knowledge or both.

Below age 3, children rarely maintain a topic for more than two turns (Bloom et al., 1976). In general, preschoolers take very few turns on a single topic unless enacting scenarios, describing events, or solving problems (Schober-Peterson & Johnson, 1989). More turns generally will be produced when the preschool child is directing the partner through a task or when the child is telling a story. Although the number of turns increases slightly with age, a great increase does not occur until mid-elementary school.

Informativeness

Each turn should add to the conversation by confirming the topic and contributing additional information. Children who have difficulty identifying the topic or determining what is expected of them conversationally may repeat or paraphrase old information, overuse continuants, or circumlocute. Circumlocution occurs when the child is unable to identify the topic or retrieve needed words and thus talks around the topic in a nonspecific manner. The speech-language pathologist can rate each utterance for its contribution to the topic being discussed.

Sequencing

Once a topic is introduced, a sequence of conversational acts follows. In general, more specific information is introduced until a natural termination or a change in topic occurs. Answers or replies follow questions; comments or questions follow comments. New information is introduced and later referred to as old information. A lack of sequencing may indicate a semantic disorder or a pragmatic disorder characterized by a lack of presuppositional abilities.

Topic Analysis Format

Several topic analysis formats have been proposed (Bedrosian, 1979, 1982, 1988, 1993; Mentis & Prutting, 1991). Each addresses different aspects of topic initiation, maintenance, and change. These are presented in Table 5.7. Topic initiation analysis may include the type of topic, the manner of initiation, the subject matter and orientation, and the outcome. Topic maintenance analysis may consider the type of turn and the ability of the client to further the conversation with the addition of new conversational information.

Topic Initiation

Topic initiations occur when the topic of discussion is changed in some way. Following utterances that are part of that topic express concepts subsumed by that topic. Each new topic and directly related utterances can be identified on the transcript.

Type of topic.   Each topic could be rated according to its novelness. Some children have a limited range of topics in their repertoire. Possible rating categories

TABLE 5.7
Analysis aspects of topic

Topic Initiation
    Type of Topic
    Manner of Initiation
    Subject Matter and Orientation
    Outcome
Topic Maintenance
    Type of Turn
    Conversational Information

may include *new, related, reintroduced,* and *consecutive* (Bedrosian, 1979, 1982, 1988, 1993; Mentis & Prutting, 1991). New topics would be those appearing in the conversation for the first time and not linked to the immediate preceding topic (Keenan & Schieffelin, 1976). Related topics would be linked directly to the previous topic. Reintroduced topics would have appeared in the conversation previously but prior to the immediate preceding turn (Keenan & Schieffelin, 1976). Finally, consecutive topics consist of two or more topics initiated in a turn with no opportunity for the listener to maintain the preceding topic or the first of the consecutive ones to be introduced. In addition, the speech-language pathologist could check with the caregivers to determine whether any of the topics introduced by the child are habitual ones. Table 5.8 presents examples of different types of topic initiation.

Manner of initiation.   The manner of topic initiation might include *coherent changing, noncoherent changing, shifting,* and *shading* (Bedrosian, 1979, 1982, 1988, 1993; Mentis & Prutting, 1991). Coherent changing occurs when one topic is terminated and a following topic's content is not derived from the immediate preceding topic. Noncoherent changing occurs with the absence of topic termination and/or an utterance signaling transition to a new topic. Shifting occurs when the topic being discussed serves as a source for a new topic. Shading differs from shifting in that shading is a change of focus on the same topic, rather than a discrete topic change (Schegloff & Sacks, 1973). Table 5.9 presents the different manners of initiation.

TABLE 5.8
Types of topics initiated

Topic Type		Example
New	PARTNER:	Uh-huh, and what else did you see at the zoo?
	CHILD:	**Mommy got a new car.**
Related	PARTNER:	I like monkeys too. What else? Were there any clowns at the circus?
	CHILD:	**I don't like clowns. They're scary.**
	PARTNER:	Clowns are scary? Why do you think clowns are scary?
Reintroduced	CHILD:	And Ernie spilled s'ghetti all over Bert.
	PARTNER:	Was Bert angry?
	CHILD:	Uh-huh. And. . .and Ernie. . .And Ernie laughed.
	PARTNER:	Poor Bert. That would be yukky. What else happened on *Sesame Street?*
	CHILD:	Big Bird and Little Bird singed a song.
	PARTNER:	Can you sing it for me?
	CHILD:	Uh-huh. **I don't like s'ghetti on me.**
Consecutive	PARTNER:	Oh, tell me the story.
	CHILD:	Okay. This little girl. . . . **Can you come to my birthday party? I got a new bike yesterday. Do you live here?**

TABLE 5.9
Manner of topic initiation

Manner of Initiation		Example
Coherent Changing	CHILD:	And he chased the dinosaur away.
	PARTNER:	What a great story. Anything else to tell?
	CHILD:	**I have a new baby.**
Noncoherent Changing	CHILD:	Let's have toast for breakfast.
	PARTNER:	Let me fix it.
	CHILD:	Those are supposed to go down.
	PARTNER:	You do this one, and I'll do the other one.
	CHILD:	**I'm gonna have a bowl of. . .What's that? I think it's a fireman hat. I wanta be a fireman.**
	PARTNER:	May I wear it?
Shifting	PARTNER:	There, I'm gonna make some eggs?
	CHILD:	I don't like eggs.
	PARTNER:	No, why don't you like eggs?
	CHILD:	**I want some..some juice. I like juice.**
	PARTNER:	What kind of juice do you want?
Shading	PARTNER:	Let's have toast.
	CHILD:	Where's the toaster?
	PARTNER:	I'll cook the toast.
	CHILD:	**I'll butter it. Where's the knife**?
	PARTNER:	You have to find the knife.
	CHILD:	It too sharp for toast.

Subject matter and orientation.   The *subject matter* is the content of the topic initiation. Two broad analyses might consist of judgments of appropriate versus inappropriate topics for the communication context. Orientation might include topics about self, a shared experience or interest with the listener, or a topic seemingly unrelated to the listener or a shared interest. If the topic is always the speaker or always unrelated, then serious communication problems may exist.

Outcome.   Outcomes may be rated as successful or unsuccessful (Calculator & Dollaghan, 1982). Success is dependent on the manner of initiation, the subject matter, and the form of the initiation. A command or demand form of topic initiation is probably not a good one to encourage conversational interaction. Success occurs when the conversational partner acknowledges the speaker's topic in some way, responds, repeats, agrees or disagrees, or adds information to maintain the topic. Nonsuccess includes no response, an interruption, initiation of a new topic, or a request for repair.

Topic Maintenance

Topic maintenance would be analyzed in all turns subsequent to topic initiation. Each turn can be analyzed in two ways on the basis of the continuous or discontinuous nature of the turn and on its informativeness.

Type of turn. Turns may be classified as continuous or discontinuous on the basis of their linkage or nonlinkage to the initiated topic (Table 5.10) (Bedrosian, 1985, 1993; Keenan & Schieffelin, 1976). Continuous turns include responses to requests or questions; acknowledgements, such as *uh-huh, okay,* and *yeah;* partial, whole, or expanded repetitions; appropriate emotional responses, including laughter and crying; topic incorporation, such as the addition of more information or a request for more; shading; agreement or disagreement; and a request for repair (Bedrosian, 1985). Discontinuous turns—ones not linked to the current topic—include topic initiations; off-topic responses, monologues; and evasion, including use of silence.

Analysis includes the frequency and range of each type of turn and the average number of turns per topic. The percentage of continuous versus discontinuous turns also would be valuable data (Bedrosian, 1993).

Conversational information. Turns might be analyzed for the extent to which they contribute to the development of the topic by adding relevant, novel information (Mentis & Prutting, 1991). Those adding new information include topic incorporation, such as unsolicited conversational replies that add more information or requests for new information, and answers and replies to questions that contain new information. Other turns, such as acknowledgments; requests for repair; partial, whole, or expanded repetitions; responses to requests or questions that do not contain new information; emotional responses; and agreement or disagreement, add no new information to the conversational exchange. Problematic turns include word searching, incoherent utterances, ambiguous utterances, and incomplete turns. Examples of conversational information rating are included in Table 5.11.

The speech–language pathologist can calculate the percentage of turns contributing novel information and thus furthering the topic. Other types of turns

TABLE 5.10
Continuous and discontinuous turns

Type of Turn		Example
Continuous	PARTNER: CHILD:	What's that? **A cowboy hat.**
	PARTNER: CHILD:	Put it on. **No, it's too hot for a coat.**
	PARTNER: CHILD:	We have to make some bread for dinner. **Okay, I'll help.**
Discontinuous	PARTNER: CHILD:	Do you want to hold the baby? **I'll eat my cupcake now.**
	PARTNER: CHILD:	What else happened at school? **I don't like my baby brother.**

TABLE 5.11
Informativeness of turns

Informativeness		Example
New information	PARTNER: CHILD:	Where's Mary? **She's sick today.**
	PARTNER: CHILD:	We're going to the zoo tomorrow. **Monkeys live in the zoo.**
No new information	PARTNER: CHILD:	And cowboys ride horsies too. **Ride horsie.**
	PARTNER: CHILD:	Let's play with the stove. **What?**
Problematic	PARTNER: CHILD:	What should we play now? **A. . .a. . .with a. . .a. . .with a . . .you know.**
	PARTNER: CHILD:	Who's your teacher? **At school.**

may indicate possible problem areas. Specific strategies used by children should be investigated by analyzing the form of the utterances being used.

Summary

The topic analysis categories presented in this section overlap and are not always mutually exclusive. More than one turn type and informativeness category may be present in a turn. A possible analysis format is presented in Table 5.12. It is important that each type of analysis gives the speech-language pathologist an additional tool for sorting the child's language data.

Turn Taking

Turn taking is an excellent vehicle for evaluating the interactional framework of the listener and speaker. The unit of analysis is the dyad and the interaction, rather than the individual behaviors of the child (Prutting, 1982).

The rules of turn taking (Sacks et al., 1974) specify that if only two participants are involved, both have speaking turns. In general, children's conversations consist primarily of this nonsimultaneous talking pattern (Craig & Washington, 1986). If more than two are involved, however, no participant is guaranteed a speaking turn. There is usually only one speaker at a time. If two or more speak simultaneously, all but one withdraw. Children with emotional disabilities may interrupt the speaker before the turn has ended, may ask and answer their own questions, and may take another speaker's turn (Rees & Wollner, 1981).

The listener pays attention to the speaker and demonstrates this behavior by turning toward or looking at the speaker, not interrupting, and/or acknowledging that she or he has heard and understood the speaker. Eye contact among children with LLD and emotional disturbances is often fleeting or nonexistent.

TABLE 5.12
Possible format for rating topics and turns

Categories	Turns																		Total	% of Total
	1	2	3	4	5	6	7	8	9	10	11	12	13	14	15	16	17	18		
Topic Initiation																				
Type of topic																				
New																				
Related																				
Reintroduced																				
Consecutive																				
Manner of initiation																				
Coherent change																				
Noncoherent change																				
Shifting																				
Shading																				
Subject matter																				
Appropriate																				
Inappropriate																				
Orientation																				
Self																				
Shared																				
Unrelated																				
Outcome																				
Successful																				
Unsuccessful																				
Topic Maintenance																				
Type of turn																				
Continuous																				
Discontinuous																				
Conversational information																				
New information																				
No new information																				
Problematic																				

The minimum number of turns to complete an exchange is three. The person who begins the exchange must have a second turn before an interaction has occurred, for example:

SPEAKER 1:   We just returned from Florida.
SPEAKER 2:   Oh, did you go to Disney World?
SPEAKER 1:   No, we were in Fort Lauderdale.

Each full conversational turn consists of three elements: an acknowledgment of the preceding utterance, a contribution by the present speaker, and an indication that the turn is to be shifted. In the preceding example, the previous turns are acknowledged by *oh* and *no*. Indications of turn allocation may consist of questions (as with Speaker 2), intonational markers, and pauses.

Transitions across speakers are orderly, occurring at transition points signaled by the participants. For example, the speaker will look at or address the listener when about to change a turn. The listener may look away, gesture, become restless, or emit an audible sigh when desiring a turn. A really anxious listener may cut off the last few syllables of the speaker's turn without disrupting the topic. Children with language impairment often do not use these subtle turn indicators and miss their signal value when used by others (Rees & Wollner, 1981).

Finally, the speaker who wishes to continue a turn may increase the speed or intensity of talking and continue through the transition point. If overlap occurs and interferes with understanding, the speaker "repairs" the misunderstood portion.

The speech-language pathologist can mark the transcript as turns 1-2-3 for each exchange. Of particular interest are eye contact, turn allocation signaling, and the location and cause of exchange breakdown. In addition, the frequency, variety or range, and consistency of the child's communication are noted. In other words, the child should initiate, add to, and terminate exchanges. Within each turn, the speech-language pathologist notes the presence or absence of the three aspects of a full turn and the average amount of time spent in a turn (F. Roth & Spekman, 1984a). The speech-language pathologist also can examine the effects of adult behaviors on the child's conversational turns and later can help adults develop more facilitative styles.

Turns may be classified as *oblige, comment,* or *response* (Coelho, Liles, & Duffy, 1991). An oblige is initiated by the speaker and demands a response. In contrast, a comment is initiated by the speaker but does not require a response. A response is a reply to either an oblige or a comment. The percentage of each category may indicate active and passive speakers, those that initiate and those that respond.

All responses to obliges can be analyzed further as *adequate, adequate-plus, inadequate,* and *ambiguous* (Shadden, 1992). Adequate responses give only the information requested; they are appropriate for the request. Adequate-plus responses give more than requested, while inadequate do not give enough. Inadequate responses may be invalid, irrelevant, or insufficient. Ambiguous responses are unclear. Examples are given in Table 5.13.

Density

The speech-language pathologist is interested in the density of turns within each conversation and on various topics. A low density may indicate that the child's conversational partner dominated the conversation by taking very long turns, relinquishing them to the child only occasionally, or that the child was very reticent. Children with autism may take relatively few verbal turns, thus leaving the partner to fill the void (Loveland et al., 1988). In contrast, if the child talked for lengthy turns, the density also would be low because the listener would have little chance to reply.

TABLE 5.13
Types of turns

Turn Type	Example
Oblige	Do you want some cookies? What time is it? What's that?
Comment	I really love to ski. I saw horses in the parade.
Response to comment	(Comment: This dessert is great!) It's an old family recipe.
Response to oblige	(Oblige: How old are you?)
Adequate	I'm 25.
Adequate plus	I'm 25, and I have a masters degree.
Inadequate	I go to college.
Ambiguous	None of your business. Guess.

Latency

The speech-language pathologist can summarize the overall contingent and non-contingent latencies of the child. Whereas the average adult-to-adult turn changes within about half a second, the child may be slightly slower to react. Longer periods and/or the continual use of fillers and interjections may indicate difficulties with topic identification or word finding.

Duration of Turns

There is no ideal length for a turn, although most listeners know when a turn has continued for too long. We all know at least one incessant talker who does not know when enough has been said. A child who talks incessantly may be exhibiting a semantic disorder of not knowing what information is needed to close the topic, a pragmatic disorder of not knowing the mechanisms for closing a topic, or a processing problem of not being certain what information was conveyed.

The speech-language pathologist is interested in the average length of the child's and the partner's turns. Different situations, partners, and topics may yield clinically significant differences in the length of these turns.

Type of Overlap

Most turns will be nonsimultaneous (Craig & Evans, 1989). However, overlap or simultaneous speech can be very revealing. In general, overlap is of two types: *internal* and *initial* (Gallagher & Craig, 1982). Sentence internal overlaps are used to complete the other speaker's turn and secure a turn. This ability requires a high level of pragmatic-linguistic knowledge. The child with a language impairment may interrupt internally but in a way that indicates a lack of understanding of this process. The child may add new information or change the topic, rather than complete the other speaker's utterance (Craig & Evans, 1989).

Sentence initial overlaps result when the listener interjects between sentences to secure a turn. This interjection may occur when the listener is unsure of the speaker's intention to continue or when the listener wants to gain a turn at speaking. Continual overlaps of this type may indicate a breakdown in turn taking as a result of the behavior of one or both partners. In contrast, a low incidence of interrupting, as noted among children with SLI, may indicate passivity or an inability to initiate a "turn grab" (Craig & Evans, 1989).

Frequency of overlap.   Although it may seem counterintuitive, data indicate that, as a group, children with language impairment exhibit less simultaneous speech in their conversations (Craig & Evans, 1989). Although children with language impairment may be responsive, they tend to be passive in initiating interaction or turn taking (Fey & Leonard, 1983).

Duration of overlap.   The adult rules for turn taking state that when an overlap in turns occurs (when two speakers speak at once), one speaker will withdraw. Young children or children with language impairments may continue to talk or try to outshout their partners. Some children withdraw habitually. The speech-language pathologist must determine whether the child in question is more likely to withdraw or to continue talking.

How Signaled?

Changes in turn are signaled very subtly. The child with language impairment may miss such signals. Occasionally, such a child will respond only to questions, knowing that in this situation a response is required. Other children lack a basic understanding of the expectation to reply within a conversation. Still others cannot decipher the language code efficiently enough to respond.

Conversation and Topic Termination

Conversations or topics are ended when no new information is added. In the case of a conversational termination, the topic is not changed. As with the opening of a conversation, there are often adjacency pairs, such as "Bye, see ya"—"Have a nice day" or "Thank you"-"You're welcome."

Preschool children or those with language impairment may end the conversation abruptly when they decide it is over, occasionally just "turning tail" and exiting the conversational context. Children with LLD may not prepare the listener for the termination of the conversation by signaling with body language—for example, becoming restless, looking away, or looking at a watch. In the opposite extreme, children with LLD or emotional disorder may be unable or unwilling to end the conversation and may perseverate or continue to ask questions that have been answered already.

Topics usually are terminated by shifting to another related topic. For more mature language users, this process is accomplished by *shading,* in which the speakers shift to another aspect of the topic or to a closely related topic, as in the following exchange:

SPEAKER 1:	I biked along the canal path yesterday.
SPEAKER 2:	Oh, I love to bike there at this time of year.
SPEAKER 1:	I didn't know you bike. What sort of bike do you have?
SPEAKER 2:	I have an inexpensive 12-speed.
SPEAKER 1:	I have a 10-speed . . .

The original topic of the canal bike path slid into the topic of bicycles.

Whether topics are shaded or are changed abruptly, there is normally some continuity, and the new topic is stated clearly. When there is little left to discuss on a given topic, the conversation shifts. The speech-language pathologist notes the method the child uses to terminate and change topics and to terminate conversations.

Conversational Breakdown

In essence, the entire analysis of the language of the child with language impairment is an attempt to find where the child is ineffectual, where he fails to communicate. It is important for the speech-language pathologist to determine where these breakdowns occur and how the child attempts to repair them (Audet & Hummel, 1990). The speech-language pathologist should try to determine the number of conversational breakdowns and describe the cause of breakdown, the repair attempt, the repair initiator, the repair strategy, and the outcome (F. Roth & Spekman, 1984b).

Requests for Repair

Requests for repair or contingent queries signal the listener's attentiveness or understanding and skill in addressing the point of conversational breakdown. Conversations may be maintained by use of contingent queries, such as *Huh? What?* and *I don't understand.* Such requests for repair maintain the conversation by indicating the point of breakdown, obligating the speaker to clarify, and specifying the appropriate form for that clarification.

The type of repair request varies with the linguistic maturity of the speaker and with the information sought. In general, young children use unspecific requests, such as *Huh?* and *What?* More mature speakers try to specify the information desired, as in the following exchange:

SPEAKER 1:	"We went to the zoo and saw monkeys in big cages."
SPEAKER 2:	"What was in the cages?" (Or "Where were the monkeys?" "Where did you go?")

Requests for repair may seek repetition of the preceding utterance, confirmation, or clarification.

Appropriate requests for repair and responses by the conversational partner demonstrate an awareness of the cooperative nature of conversation. Not only must the child attend to the partner's message, detect misunderstandings, and initiate an appropriate request, but she or he also must possess the knowledge and willingness to use clarification strategies to aid the partner's comprehension (Dollaghan, 1987a; Donahue, 1984).

The child who continually responds with *Huh?* or *What?* may not be attending to the conversation or may have difficulty understanding. In the classroom, such children may rely on routines to make the world understandable. In this case, the child often may look around at the other children for assurance before performing the expected behavior.

The speech-language pathologist is interested in the degree to which the child requests additional information toward maintaining the conversation and in the form of these requests. These conversational mechanisms can be triggered in conversation by the speech-language pathologist's garbling or confusing the message. This can be accomplished by mumbling, failing to establish the topic, or providing insufficient information or confusing instructions.

The child with language impairment may be unaware that communication breakdown has occurred. The speech-language pathologist can hypothesize about the child's awareness of misunderstanding and confirm the hypothesis through manipulation of utterances addressed to the child. In general, children first gain awareness of breakdowns caused by unintelligible words. The order of awareness to breakdown may be as follows (Dollaghan & Kaston, 1986):

Unintelligible word

Impossible command

Unrealistically long utterance

Unfamiliar word

Question or statement without an introduction and ambiguous, inexplicit, and open-ended statements

Frequency and form.   In general, preschool children and those with language impairment, such as those with LLD, tend to blame themselves, rather than the speaker, for misunderstanding (Meline & Brackin, 1987). Thus, these children use fewer requests for repair than might be expected, especially given the greater likelihood of communication breakdown (Brinton & Fujiki, 1982; Donahue, 1984; Donahue, Pearl, & Bryan, 1980; R. Lee, Kamhi, & Nelson, 1983). The requests produced tend to be less specific, reflecting the difficulty encountered with these forms. In short, as listeners, children with LLD do not accept the responsibility to signal miscomprehension, even when taught the procedures for doing so (Donahue, 1984). Instead, these children assume that the speaker will be unambiguous, informative, and clear.

Children's repair strategies can be assessed in different contexts, such as familiar topics, unfamiliar topics, and contrived pragmatic violations by the speech-language pathologist (Moeller et al., 1986). The child's attempts to repair can be recorded on a form such as that shown in Table 5.14. Checks in the appropriate spaces would signal the child's attempts to repair and clarify.

Although there are no norms for the frequency of repair requests, general guidelines do indicate a change in both the frequency and type of contingent query with age. The earliest requests for repair are repetitions of the partner's utterance with rising intonation (*Doggie go ride?*) or neutral requests for repetition (*What?*). With age, requests become more specific and increase in frequency, although both vary according to the conversational partner. With an adult partner, 24- to 36-month-olds use approximately 7 requests an hour, and 54- to 66-month-olds use approximately 14 (Fey & Leonard, 1984; Gallagher, 1981). When the partner is a familiar peer, the mean rate for 36- to 66-month-olds is 30 per hour (Fey & Leonard, 1984; Garvey, 1977). Obviously, there is greater likelihood of misunderstanding when two preschool peers communicate.

TABLE 5.14
Record of requests for repair

Clarification Skills	Familiar Topic	New Topic	Contrived Pragmatic Violation
Fails to seek clarification			

Indicates nonunderstanding
—nonverbally
   puzzled expression
   shrugs shoulders
—verbally
   asks for repetition
   says/signs *What?*
   I don't understand
   I don't remember			

Indicates inability to answer
   I don't remember
   I don't know the word for it
   I can't explain it			

Requests specific clarification
   What did you say about
      the _____?
   What does _____ mean?			

A pattern of clarification requests may evolve as the speech-language pathologist records the number of requests by type and by conversational context of the familiar or new topic, or contrived violation. Contrived errors or violations can be used to elicit requests for clarification.

Source: Moeller, M., Osberger, M., & Eccarius, M. (1986). Cognitively based strategies for use with hearing-impaired students with comprehension deficits. *Topics in Language Disorders, 6*(4), 37–50.

Conversational Repair

Conversational repair may be spontaneous or in response to a request for repair. Preschool children spontaneously repair very little. Even in first grade, children spontaneously repair only about one-third of their conversational breakdowns. Young children or children with language impairment often do not attempt to repair communication breakdowns. Children with unintelligible speech may find their repairs as unintelligible as their initial attempts.

Most 10-year-olds are able to determine communication breakdown and repair the damage (Lempers & Elrod, 1983). Although children with LLD at that age can identify faulty messages, they do not seem to understand when to use these skills (Donahue et al., 1980). By age 2, most children respond consistently to neutral requests for clarification (Gallagher, 1977, 1981; Tomasello, Farrar, & Dines, 1984), although they are more likely to respond if the conversational partner is an adult, rather than another child. Two-year-olds also tend to overuse "yes" and thus confirm interpretations even when incorrect, possibly because nonconfirmation requires clarification. By age 3 to 5, children respond correctly, even to specific requests, about 80% of the time regardless of the partner (Anselmi, Tomasello, & Acunzo, 1986; Garvey, 1977).

Repair can provide valuable information about communication breakdowns. Breakdown can occur for a number of reasons, including lack of intelligibility, volume, completeness of information, degree of complexity, inappropriateness, irrelevance, and lack of mutual attention, visual regard, or mutual desire (Garvey, 1975; Keenan & Schieffelin, 1976). In general, children with language impairments experience a greater number of breakdowns than do age-matched peers who are non-LLD (Fey, Warr-Leeper, Webber, & Disher, 1988; MacLachlan & Chapman, 1988).

Repairs usually focus on the linguistic structure (E. Clark & Andersen, 1979) or on the content or nature of the information conveyed (Garvey, 1977). They may use extralinguistic signals, such as pointing, to clarify. These strategies are not mutually exclusive. In general, successful outcome is related to the explicitness and appropriateness of the repair strategy chosen.

When the child repairs spontaneously, the nature of the original error and the repair attempts should be noted. The speech-language pathologist scans the transcript for all fillers, repetitions, perseverations, and long pauses. All of these may indicate word-finding difficulties on the child's part. The original error or repair attempt may be based on any number of relationships with the intended word or phrase, as noted in Table 5.15.

Spontaneous versus listener-initiated.   The speech-language pathologist is interested in the percentage of conversational repairs that are self- or listener-initiated. Usually, listeners signal a breakdown with facial expression, body posture, and/or a contingent query.

Strategy.   Immature speakers usually respond to listener-initiated requests for repair by restating the previous utterance. First graders and younger children will

TABLE 5.15
Relationship of word-finding errors and repair attempts to the intended word

Association	Example
Definition	*the thing you cook food on* for *stove*
Description	*the long skinny one with no legs* for *snake* *book holder* for *bookend* *fuzzy* for *peach*
Generic (less specific)	*do* for more specific verb *hat* for *cap, bonnet, scarf,* etc. *thing* or *one* for name of entity
Opposites	*sit* for *stand*
Partial	*ball . . . big ball . . . red ball* for *big red ball*
Semantic category	*stove* for *refrigerator* (both are *appliances*)
Sound	*toe* for *tie* (initial sound similar) *goat* for *coat* (rhyme)

repeat only once in response to a request before becoming irritated. By second grade, children usually are willing to repeat twice before becoming angry. Continued requests also may result in children providing additional information, although children with language impairments seem less flexible in the use of this strategy (Brinton, Fujiki, & Sonnenberg, 1988).

More mature speakers usually give additional information or reformulate, rather than repeat the utterance. Using their presuppositional skills, such speakers may hypothesize about the supposed point of breakdown and supply more information on this specific area. When requested to clarify, children with language impairment tend to respond less frequently and with less complex responses than do their peers developing normally (Brinton & Fujiki, 1982; Brinton, Fujiki, Winkler, & Loeb, 1986). The responses of children with language impairment lack flexibility and usually consist of repetition with little new information included to aid comprehension. Children developing normally seem to have a greater range of repair strategies at the same age (Brinton et al., 1988). The 10-year-old child with LLD is more likely to repeat, rather than reformulate, unsuccessful utterances (Feagans & Short, 1986).

The speech-language pathologist should prepare a list of the various types of contingent queries and use them in conversation with the child. Of interest is the child's rate of responding to various requests and the nature of the child's response (Fey et al., 1988).

Frequency of success.   The speech-language pathologist is interested in how successfully the child identifies breakdowns, repairs them spontaneously, and follows listener requests. In general, children with language impairment make more inappropriate responses to listener requests than do age-matched peers (Brinton et al., 1988). The responses of the listener enable the speech-language pathologist to determine the child's success.

CONVERSATIONAL PARTNER

Language does not occur in a vacuum. Children converse with many conversational partners, both at home and in school. Each partner helps form a dynamic context in which the child communicates and learns.

Parent-child interactions offer an example of a communication process finely attuned to the language skills of the child (Snow, 1979). Thus, the adult-child dyad represents a highly individualized learning exchange based on the interactional styles and skills of the two communicators (Lieven, 1978).

Variables that affect language learning are complexity, semantic relatedness, redundancy, maternal responsiveness, and reciprocity. In general, maternal linguistic complexity seems to be related to the language learner's level of comprehension.

Semantically related utterances provide a contingency-based language learning experience. The topic and subsequent content usually are derived from the child. Approximately 68% of the mother's speech is related directly to the child's verbal, vocal, and nonverbal behavior (Cross, 1977; Snow, 1977a).

The mother's input tends to be highly redundant because it relates to ongoing contextual occurrences and attempts to explain, clarify, and comment on the child's experiences and behavior. In addition, the caregiver may repeat content several times in different forms.

Consistent maternal responsiveness teaches children that their responses and behavior have a predictable effect (Beckwith, Cohen, Kopp, Parmelee, & Marcy, 1976; Bradley & Caldwell, 1976). One valuable lesson the child learns is that communication and communication partners are predictable.

These caregiver-child exchanges are reciprocal in that the child is treated as a full conversational partner and allowed to gain early conversational experience (Bateson, 1975; Stern, 1971; Stern, Jaffee, Beebe, & Bennett, 1975). Even infants are treated as full conversational partners by their mothers.

There is indication that some mothers of children with language impairment provide input that is not regulated by their children's level of understanding, and thus it is significantly longer and more complex than their children's level of comprehension (Tiegerman & Siperstein, 1984). The MLU may be near that found in adult-adult communication and may include complex structures such as indirect directives, embedded constructions, and *how/why* questions (Buium, Rynders, & Turnure, 1974; Tiegerman & Siperstein, 1982).

The proportion of utterances of mothers of children with language impairment that are related semantically is lower than that reported for mothers of children developing normally (Tiegerman & Siperstein, 1984). In addition, the form of these utterances may be highly restricted, providing the child with a limited variety of input. Because few of the maternal utterances are related semantically, there is little redundancy. Instead, mothers discuss events in the past or future and objects or events not present within the immediate shared context.

Children with language impairment may have little effect on the conversational interaction, and their verbal and nonverbal behaviors may be ignored. Mothers may persist in introducing new topics, reflecting this non-child-centered approach. Mothers of children with language impairment may be more dominant in conversations than are mothers of children developing normally, and they may initiate conversation and use directives more frequently (Loveland et al., 1988). In short, these interactions often lack the qualities of language-learning conversational exchanges.

There is a wide range in parents' ability to interpret their children's utterances correctly (Kwiatkowski & Shriberg, 1992). When a child's utterances are unintelligible to a parent because of numerous phonological errors, the parent is more likely to use facilitative strategies, such as maintaining the topic or recasting the child's utterance (Conti-Ramsden, 1990; P. Yoder & Davies, 1990). Thus, the parent takes control of the topic, allowing little opportunity for the child to initiate (H. Gardner, 1989).

Especially when working with preschool children, the speech-language pathologist should observe the conversational behavior of the primary caregiver and determine the language learning contributions. Utterances can be rated as to semantic relatedness, redundancy, and reciprocity. From these data, the speech-language pathologist can comment on the overall teaching environment provided by the caregiver's utterances and behaviors.

CONCLUSION

A language sample is a rich source of information on the child and conversational partner's language abilities. Analysis may be accomplished at the individual utterance level, across utterance and across partner, and by conversational event. Analysis should not be attempted unless the speech-language pathologist has a good understanding of the child's language and of the caregivers' concerns. Then a language sample would be analyzed to examine the portion of that language in question. A conversational sample can be the best example of a child's actual language use in context.

Utterance-level analysis is more appropriate for language form. Analysis of larger units, such as turns and topics, gives the speech-language pathologist information on the use of language in context and answers questions about the efficacy of the child's language use to communicate.

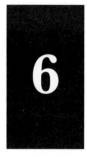

6 Analyzing a Language Sample at the Utterance Level

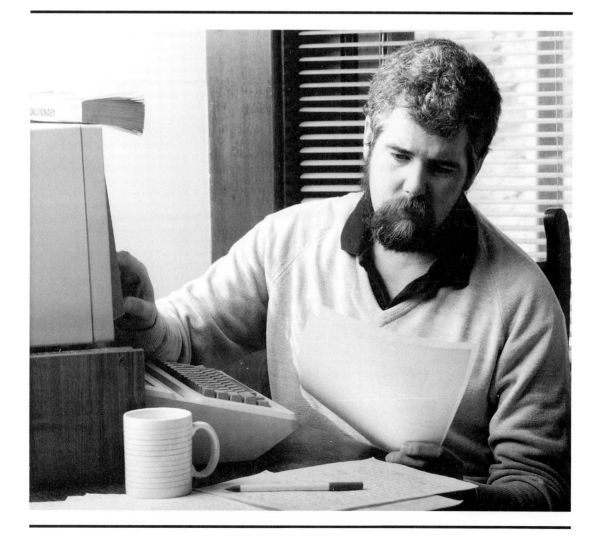

T ypical or traditional language sample analysis has concentrated almost exclusively on language form within each utterance. In this chapter, we consider a broad analysis of language that can be accomplished easily within utterances by noting significant aspects of use, content, and form. These aspects are outlined in Table 6.1. In Chapter 5, we discussed analysis across utterances and partners and by conversational event. This three-tiered—across utterances and partners, by conversational event, and within utterances—analysis method seems appropriate for describing the interactive qualities of language use within the context of conversation. Language is not a "unitary construct," but rather multidimensional. It is the responsibility of the speech-language pathologist to describe the unique character of each child's language.

Each utterance can be analyzed within use, content, and form categories following a variety of analysis formats (A. Johnson et al., 1984; Lund & Duchan, 1988). Individual utterances can yield the frequency and range of various features. Some data will be descriptive, whereas other data will be more normative. This situation reflects the research information available and the type of analysis desired.

TABLE 6.1

Analysis at the utterance level

Use
  Disruptions
  Illocutionary functions and intentions
    Frequency and range
    Appropriateness
    Encoding
Content
  Lexical items
    Type-token ratio
    Over-/underextensions and incorrect use
    Style and lexicon
  Word relationships
  Semantic categories
  Intrasentence relationships
  Figurative language
  Word finding
Form
  Quantitative measures
    Mean length of utterance
    Mean syntactic length
    T-units and C-units
  Syntactic and morphologic analysis
    Morphologic analysis
    Syntactic analysis
      Noun phrase
      Verb phrase
      Sentence types
      Embedding and conjoining
    Computer-assisted language analysis
  Phonologic analysis

A number of computer-assisted and unassisted language sample analysis methods are available. Several are listed in Table 6.2. Although each method yields different data, none presents a total picture of a child's language. In general, the more normative the results, the less descriptive and prescriptive, and vice versa. A few of the more widely used analysis methods are described in Appendix F. A generic analysis method might borrow useful portions from several of these.

LANGUAGE USE

Much language use data can be gleaned from analysis with units larger than the individual utterance. Within conversations, topics, and turns, however, the speech-language pathologist can analyze the breakdowns in communication noted in these larger units. She also can analyze the functions or intentions of individual utterances.

Disruptions

Communication breakdown or disruption can occur for many reasons. The latency noted in Chapter 5 is one type. The amount and type of disruption will vary with the language task, topic, and partner(s). In general, more breakdowns occur in narration than in conversation. In addition, the longer the utterance, the more breakdowns present (MacLachlan & Chapman, 1988). Children with language impairments experience more disruptions than children without.

The frequency of disruptions is inversely related to subjective impressions of communicative competence (Damico, 1985a; Damico & Oller, 1980; Silliman & Leslie, 1983). In addition, disruptions can be a valuable clue to a child's process of forming an utterance and to the level of cognitive and linguistic demands made on the speaker (Dollaghan & Campbell, 1992; Sabin, Clemmer, O'Connell, & Kowal, 1979). Obviously, this type of analysis is not needed for all children with language impairments but may be helpful for those with word-finding problems or with "tangled," slow, or too long utterances.

Analysis requires that the speech-language pathologist transcribe all words and word portions and all speechlike vocalizations. Pauses of 2 seconds or more also should be noted. Pauses should be obvious on a timed transcript format, as suggested in Chapter 4. All **mazes** should be identified. Mazes are language segments that, like physical mazes, disrupt, confuse, and slow the movement—movement of the conversation in this case. Mazes may consist of silent pauses, fillers, repetitions, and revisions. Typical syntactic analysis occurs after most mazes are eliminated.

Analysis steps may consist of the following (Dollaghan & Campbell, 1992):

1. Identify disruptions by the categories in Table 6.3.
2. Determine the overall frequency of disruption and the frequency for each category. Each occurrence counts as one disruption. Frequency can be calculated per 100 unmazed words. Examples are included in Table 6.4.

TABLE 6.2
Language sample analysis methods

Unassisted Methods

Pragmatics

Adolescent Conversational Analysis (Larson & McKinley, 1987)

Assessing Children's Language in Naturalistic Contexts (Lund & Duchan, 1993)

Clinical Discourse Analysis using Grice's (1975) framework (Damico, 1991a)

Language functions (Boyce & Larson, 1983; Gruenewald & Pollack, 1984; Prutting & Kirchner, 1983, 1987; Simon, 1979, 1984)

Syntax/Morphology

Assessing Children's Language in Naturalistic Contexts (Lund & Duchan, 1993)

Assessing Language Production in Children: Experimental Procedures (J. Miller, 1981)

Developmental Sentence Analysis (L. Lee, 1974)

Guide to Analysis of Language Transcripts (Stickler, 1987)

Language Assessment, Remediation, and Screening Procedure (Crystal, Fletcher, & Garman, 1976, revised 1981)

Language Sampling, Analysis, and Training: A Handbook for Teachers and Clinicians (Tyack & Gottsleben, 1977)

Phonology

Assessing Children's Language in Naturalistic Contexts (Lund & Duchan, 1993)

Assessment of Phonological Processes (Hodson, 1980)

Natural Process Analysis (Shriberg & Kwiatkowski, 1980)

Procedures for the Phonological Analysis of Children's Language (Ingram, 1981)

Narratives

Narrative level (Applebee, 1978; Larson & McKinley, 1987)

Story grammar analysis (Garnett, 1986; Hedberg & Stoel-Gammon, 1986; F. Roth, 1986; Westby, 1984, 1992; Westby, VanDongen & Maggart, 1989)

Classroom-based

Classroom script analysis (Creaghead, 1992)

Curriculum-based language assessment (N. Nelson, 1989, 1992)

Descriptive assessment of writing (Scott & Erwin, 1992)

Computer-assisted

Syntax/Morphology

Automated LARSP (Bishop, 1985)

Computerized Profiling (Long & Fey, 1988, 1989)

DSS Computer Program (Hixson, 1985)

Lingquest 1 (Mordecai, Palin, & Palmer, 1985)

Parrot Easy Language Sample Analysis (PELSA)(F. Weiner, 1988)

Pye Analysis of Language (PAL)(Pye, 1987)

Systematic Analysis of Language Transcripts (SALT)(J. Miller & Chapman, 1985)

Phonology

Computerized Assessment of Phonological Processes (CAPP)(Hodson, 1985)

Computer Managed Articulation Diagnosis (Fitch, 1985)

Computerized Profiling (Long & Fey, 1988, 1989)

Interactive System for Phonological Analysis (ISPA)(Masterson & Pagan, 1989)

Lingquest 2 (Palin & Mordecai, 1985)

Process Analysis 2.0 (F. Weiner, 1985)

Program to Examine Phonetic and Phonologic Evaluation Records 4.0 (PEPPER)(Shriberg, 1986)

Pye Analysis of Language (PAL)(Pye, 1987)

3. Compare the frequencies to the rough normative data for school-age children and adolescents that follows:

> Mean performance per 100 unmazed words: Fewer than two pauses of 2 or more seconds duration; fewer than two repetitions; fewer than one revision; fewer than one orphan (see Table 6.3); fewer than six disruptions overall

4. Note variation in different communication situations.

Scoring and analysis will require training and practice. Reliability can be attained with repeated practice by two or more speech-language pathologists working side by side.

Illocutionary Functions or Intentions

At the individual utterance level, pragmatic analysis can describe the illocutionary functions or intentions expressed and understood. The frequency and range

TABLE 6.3
Disruption analysis categories

Categories	Transcription	Definition & Example
Pauses		
Filled	Place in ( )	Conventional, but nonlexical, one-syllable filler vocalizations.
		Example: *(um), (er), (a-a-a)*
Silent	Colon & seconds	Silent interval of 2 seconds or more.*
		Example: *Then we* **:3** *Then we went home.*
Pause strings	( ) & silent marker	Silent and filled pauses in succession.
		Example: *So he (a-a-a-)* **:4** *he (a-a-a-)* **:3** *he*
Repetitions		
Forward	[RPF]	Repetition of incomplete linguistic unit which is then completed.
		Example: *Mom said we,* **Mom said we could go too.** [RPF]
Partial	[RPP]	Repetition of incomplete unit with no completion.
		Example: *So we did eat fast,* **did eat.** [RPP]
Exact	[RPE]	Repetition of previously complete unit.
		Example: *Mom said you have to go home,* **you have to go home.** [RPE]
Backward	[RPB]	Repetition with additional word(s) inserted prior to repetition.
		Example: *We went to,* **I mean, we went to school.** [RPB]
Revisions		
Purposes		
Correct error	[RVE]	Revision to correct overt incorrect information.
		Example: *We saw monk. . .***horses.** [RVE]

TABLE 6.3, *continued*

Add information	[RVA]	Revision to add more information for better comprehension. Example: *And this man he gonna cut. . .**he was a doctor** [RVA]. . .cut open...*
Delete information	[RVD]	Revision to delete information for better comprehension. Example: *She had cows and horses on. . .**no, just cows** [RVD] on her. . .*
Unknown	[RVM]	Revision for unknown or mysterious reason. Example: *She gave the cookies to the kids, **to them kids.** [RVM]*
Domain affected		
Lexical	[L]	Change in vocabulary. Example: *She love my puppies, **kitties.** [L]*
Grammatical	[G]	Change in syntax or morphology. Example: *She love, **loves** [G] my puppies*
Phonological	[P]	Change in phonology or articulation. Example: *She woves, **loves** [P] my puppies.*
Multiple	[M]	Change in more than one domain. Example: *She wove, **loves** [M] my puppies.*
Orphans		
Single phoneme or string	[OP]	Seemingly unrelated stray sound(s). Example: *Then man **b-b-b** [OP] go to. . .*
Word(s)	[OW]	Seemingly unrelated stray word(s). Example: *He take, **eat,** [OW] dog for a walk.*
Word(s) & phoneme(s)	[OS]	Seemingly unrelated stray word(s) and phoneme(s). Example: *I **b-b-boy** [OS] walk every day.*

* 2 seconds is an arbitrary length. Adult pauses are much shorter (Brotherton, 1979; Goldman-Eisler, 1968).
Source: Adapted from Dollaghan, C. A., & Campbell, T. F. (1992). A procedure for classifying disruptions in spontaneous language samples. *Topics in Language Disorders, 12*(2), 56–68.

of these intentions can be compared with those of other children of the same age. The appropriateness and form of these intentions are also of interest. Although there is little normative data on the sophistication of intention form, each intention can be analyzed for its form and means of transmission.

In adolescence, language is extremely important in peer group identification and personal self-worth (Cooper & Anderson-Inman, 1988). The underlying language difficulties of many children with language impairment result in pragmatic deficits (Donahue & Bryan, 1984; Lapadat, 1991).

Frequency and Range

Very little normative data are available on the frequency and range of intentions (F. Roth & Spekman, 1984a). This paucity reflects the contextual variability of

TABLE 6.4
Sample of disruption analysis

PARTNER: Do you help your parents at home?
CHILD: My daddy, my daddy **[RPE]**. . .:03 I help my daddy with, my daddy to
            work.**[RVE][G]**
PARTNER: Oh you help your dad? What do you do?
CHILD: He work in, outside **[RVA][L]** in a garden.
PARTNER: What do you do in the garden?
CHILD: Pull weeds and pick **(um)** matoes, tomatoes **[RVA][P]**.
PARTNER: Um-m, I love tomatoes. I have tomato plants in my garden, too. What else
            do you do?
CHILD: I do the leave stuff, the leave stuff with the **[RPP]**. . .:02 oh, you know
            [RPB]. . .:03 the thing that go like this and the leaves.
PARTNER: You rake the leaves.
CHILD: Yeah, and I sit, no, jump **[RVE][L]** and my sister.
PARTNER: You jump on your sister?
CHILD: Yeah, in the leaves, in the pile of leaves **[RVA][G]**.

---

intentions and the lack of agreement by professionals on the intentions expressed at various ages. Intentions are heavily influenced by and heavily influence the conversational context.

A number of taxonomies of illocutionary functions are available, reflecting different ages and contextual situations (R. Chapman, 1981; Dore, 1974, 1976; Owens, 1978; Prutting, Bagshaw, Goldstein, Juskowitz, & Umen, 1978; Rodgon, Jankowski, & Alenskas, 1977). I have attempted, in Tables 6.5 and 6.6, to equate these functions and to demonstrate possible changes over time. The speech-language pathologist may wish to develop a taxonomy based on one or a combination of the taxonomies presented.

The range of intentions changes with age, becoming wider and more complex with increasing age. In addition, with maturity, the child may express multiple intentions within a single utterance. Thus, the more mature speaker's ability to express different functions is more flexible. With maturity, the speaker discusses more emotions and feelings, including such phrases as "I think . . . ," and provides justifications.

After selecting the most comfortable taxonomy or combination of taxonomies, the speech-language pathologist rates each utterance of the child and conversational partner for the intentions expressed. Of interest are the conditions under which each intention occurred, possible environmental cues, and the discourse demands, such as the type of discourse (dyad, group) and nature of the task (motor, verbal, visual, or tactile) (Audet & Hummel, 1990).

The normative data available, though only limited, do demonstrate that within a conversation, partners use a wide range of intentions; no intention predominates unless warranted by the situation. The nonimpaired child will initiate conversation and reply to the initiations of the partner, seek information and provide it, ask for assistance, and volunteer information. In contrast, some chil-

TABLE 6.5
Illocutionary functions of children

Early Symbolic (Below age 2)	Symbolic (Age 2–7 years)
Dore (1974), Halliday (1975), Owens (1978)	R. Chapman (1981), Dore (1986), Folger & Chapman (1978)
Requesting action	Requests (for)
	Action
Form: Command, demand	Form: Question, command, embedded command, indirect request, suggestion
	Permission
Regulation	Regulation
Protesting	Protesting
	Rule setting
Requesting information	Requesting information
	Form: Choice (yes/no), product (what, which, who . . .), Process (how, why . . .)
Replying	Replying
Continuants	Acknowledgments
	Qualifications
	Agreements
Comments	Comments
	Assertives
Naming	Identifications
	Descriptions
Personal feelings	Personal feelings

dren, such as those with autism, may initiate communication only rarely and respond with minimal replies (Loveland et al., 1988).

Occasionally, adults or children fall into perseverative patterns of communicating, for example, the parent who constantly quizzes her or his child to name the pictures in a book or the child who keeps repeating a pleasing or tantrum phrase. Perseverative behavior can skew the data and allow one type of intention, such as answers, to predominate. These patterns should be noted during conversational sample collection, and the situations gently changed. The use of different situations and different partners may ensure a better distribution of intentions.

Some children, such as the incessant questioner, use only a limited range of illocutionary functions. If this behavior persists across a number of situations and partners, the speech-language pathologist can be reasonably certain that this narrow range of functions represents the child's typical behavior. A number of situations can be used in an attempt to elicit a variety of illocutionary functions.

Appropriateness

A very narrow intentional range may indicate inappropriate use of language. Although some contexts may require the almost exclusive use of one type of function, most conversational exchanges include a wide variety of intentions. The

TABLE 6.5, *continued*

Declarations	Statements
	Reports
	Evaluations
	Attributions
	Explanations
	Hypotheses
	Reasons
	Predictions
	Declarations
	Procedurals
	Choice makings
	Claims
Answers	Answers
	Providing information
	Form: Choice, product process
	Clarification
	Compliance
	Conversational organization
Calling/Greeting	Attention getters
	Speaker selection
	Rhetorical questions
	Clarification questions
	Boundary markers
	Politeness
	Exclamations
Repeating	Repetitions
Practicing	Elicited imitations

As children become older, they add new functions and continue to diversify those they already possess.

question of appropriateness must be judged against other factors, such as age, race or ethnicity, region of the country, socioeconomic status, gender, and, most important, the communication context.

The language sample can confirm the caregiver's observation that "John seems to ask questions all of the time, even when he knows the answers." Although the observation may not be unfounded, only data from the language sample can offer concrete proof.

The child who responds inappropriately may not know the linguistic context and may need more contextual cues. For example, children with language impairment have more difficulty responding to *wh-* questions than do children developing normally (Parnell, Amerman, & Harting, 1986). These children have more difficulty with both the accuracy and the functional appropriateness of their answers. Analysis of both of these types of errors is discussed in the section on contingency in Chapter 5. In general, children with language impairment fail to recognize the request for information inherent in questions. Even relatively sim-

TABLE 6.6
Intentions and age of mastery

Within Brown's Stage I (MLU 1.0–1.99)	
(Usually prior to 24 months)	Answering/Responding
	Continuance
	Declaring/Citing
	Denying
	Making choices
	Naming/Labeling
	Protesting
	Repeating
Emerging within Brown's Stages II and III (MLU 2.0–3.0)	
(Usually between 24–36 months)	Calling/Greeting
	Detailing
	Predicting
	Replying
	Requesting assistance/Directing
	Requesting clarification
	Requesting information
	Requesting objects
After Brown's Stage III (MLU 3.0 +)	
(Usually after 36 months)	Expressing feelings
	Giving reasons
	Hypothesizing

Sources: Carpenter & Strong (1988); Owens (1978)

ple *What + be* questions are difficult when they concern nonimmediate or non-contextual referential sources. Thus, analysis of the context within which *wh-* questions are asked is as important diagnostically as the analysis of the variety of *wh-* questions produced and comprehended.

Encoding

Intentions can be analyzed by using a means of transmission format, such as verbal/vocal/nonverbal (F. Roth & Spekman, 1984a). The transition from linguistic through paralinguistic to nonlinguistic can be used to describe a hierarchy of competency or effectiveness based on the child's developmental level. The non-linguistic context and behaviors of the conversational partners must be transcribed to make this information available.

In general, the child with poor linguistic skills will rely on other means of communicating intentions. Although some very sophisticated information can be communicated nonlinguistically, as in the popularly named *pregnant pause,* less mature language users tend to depend on nonlinguistic and paralinguistic means more than do mature users. As with the various intentions expressed, a range of transmission means should be exhibited by the child and partner.

If the child uses an augmentative form of communication, that form should be specified even more and might include physical manipulation of an object, physical manipulation of a partner, gestures, and sign or other augmentative device. Two children described as nonverbal may have very different means of communicating their intentions.

CONTENT

The understanding of word meanings and word relationships is affected by many factors, such as age, gender, and regional and racial/ethnic differences. To know a word is to know more than just a definition. It means the child understands that word's relationship to similar words of meaning and sound and to words of an opposite meaning and understands the semantic class into which the word can be placed.

Meaning extends beyond the word, however, and larger units of analysis, such as the phrase or the sentence, also must be considered. The *performative* is the deep structure meaning and intent of the utterance from which the form flows. What is said—for example, "Don't hit me"—may be very different from the intended message, which might be "Go away, I don't understand what you want."

Obviously, all of this information cannot be ascertained from a brief language sample. Word understanding can be assessed by playing games like Simon Says or by directing the child through a series of tasks. The speech-language pathologist can make statements in which words obviously are used incorrectly in order to judge the child's reactions. Word games that solicit definitions or antonyms also can provide valuable information. Sorting and categorization tasks can be part of a play situation and can provide information on the child's ability to categorize and classify. The child can be asked to name the members of a category or to deduce the category name from a list of members. The speech-language pathologist can play the "fool" and make ridiculous comparisons ("A mouse is bigger than an elephant") or silly pairings ("The comb goes between his toes") to gauge the child's reactions.

Vocabulary abilities are strongly related to reading comprehension (Curtis, 1987; Nagy & Herman, 1987). The child with semantic difficulties also may exhibit academic failure.

Children with language impairments and with language learning disabilities usually do not have difficulty with referent-symbol tasks, such as those represented by the Peabody Picture Vocabulary Test. These children may have difficulties, however, with double meanings, abstract terms, synonyms, and nonliteral interpretation (Nippold & Fey, 1983; Seidenberg & Bernstein, 1986; Wiig, 1982a, 1982b). In addition, the physical setting can be especially important for children with language impairment because they depend much more on the context for support than do children developing normally. The child may understand a word only given certain physical situations.

Initially, word meanings are learned by a process called *fast mapping*, in which a hypothesized meaning is assigned to a word on first meeting. In general, children learn new words after only one exposure by forming an initial, albeit partial, understanding based on the linguistic and nonlinguistic contexts (G. Miller & Gildea, 1987; R. Sternberg, 1987). This meaning gradually is refined or replaced with use over time.

Children with language impairments and those who are developing normally seem to learn word meanings in this fashion, although some children with language impairment, such as those with TBI, may require more subsequent exposures than do children developing normally (Keefe, Feldman, & Holland, 1989; Rice et al., 1990). Another difficulty for children with language impairment is related to recall of the phonological shape or pattern of new words (Dollaghan, 1987b). This problem also may reflect the generally slower recall rate reported for children with language impairment (Sininger, Klatzky, & Kirchner, 1989).

Lexical Items

Obviously, there are several levels of semantic analysis relative to individual words and relations between words and larger units. At the word level, the child demonstrates individual word meanings and word classes. Several questions arise relative to word use and range of meanings and relationships.

Norms are difficult to establish, especially for older school–age children and adolescents because of the individualistic nature of lexical growth. In addition, increases in vocabulary occur at a slow and steady pace into adulthood. School-age children and adolescents exhibit semantic development in the following areas (Scott et al., 1992):

Comprehension of literate verbs, such as *interpret* and *predict* (Astington & Olson, 1987)

Comprehension of textbook terms, such as *invertebrate* and *antecedent* (Nippold, 1988b)

Comprehension of adverbs of magnitude, such as *slightly* and *unusually* (Bashaw & Anderson, 1968)

Comprehension of adverbial conjuncts, such as *meanwhile* and *conversely* (Nippold, Schwarz, & Undlin, 1992) (see Chapter 5 for discussion)

Comprehension of sarcasm based on its linguistic aspects, as well as intonation (Capelli, Nakagawa, & Madden, 1990)

Comprehension of slang terms used by peers, such as *grotty* (E. Nelson & Rosenbaum, 1972)

Comprehension of complex proverbs (Nippold, 1988b)

Comprehension of complex metaphors (Nippold, 1988b)

Explanation of infrequently occurring idioms, such as *to vote with one's feet* (Nippold & Rudzinski, 1993)

Explanation of ambiguous messages

Definition of abstract concept words, such as *courage* and *justice* (McGhee & Bidlack, 1991)

Type-Token Ratio

The **type-token ratio** (TTR) is the ratio of the number of different words to the total number of words. The number of different words (NDW) in a sample of fixed length is strongly correlated with age and indexes semantic diversity (J. Miller, 1991). Significantly lower values than those in Table 6.9 might suggest retrieval problems or poor vocabulary.

The total number of words (TNW) in fixed samples also increases steadily with age and is a general measure of verbal productivity (J. Miller, 1991). For example, 3–year–olds use 205 words in 50 utterances, while 8–year–olds use 379 (Templin, 1957). Although a general measure of ease of language use, TNW also is affected by other factors, such as motor ability and word retrieval. Values of TNW are listed for a 20–minute sample in Table 6.9.

As a quantitative measure, TTR has had a checkered past of professional acceptance. This uncertainty reflects recognition that the value may vary widely with the language sample size. In general, less variability is found across larger samples of 350 words or more (Hess et al., 1986). Multiple settings and more representative samples would yield theoretically more stable values, although there may be great situational variability for an individual child (Hess, Haug, & Landry, 1989).

Children between ages 2 and 8 demonstrate TTRs of 0.42 to 0.50 (Klee, 1992; Templin, 1957). Children who receive values greater than 0.50 have greater variability and flexibility in their language, whereas those below 0.42 tend to use the same words over and over again. Very low values may indicate perseverative or stereotypic behavior, word retrieval problems, or restricted vocabulary. Children with LEP also may score lower because of their lack of English vocabulary.

A low value may indicate overreliance on words with broad application but unspecified meaning (empty words), such as *thing* and *one*. Children with poor vocabularies or word-finding difficulties may use empty words, rather than more specific words that are not at their disposal.

Two spontaneous language profiles emerge from the samples of children with word-finding problems (German, 1987). Some children exhibit word-finding difficulties both on structured naming tasks and in spontaneous samples. They exhibit reformulations, time fillers, empty words, repetitions, starters, and grammatical errors. Other children with language impairment exhibit these behaviors only on structured naming tasks, although they produce relatively less language in spontaneous samples than do children developing normally.

Mature speakers should possess a variety of words for describing sensory experiences, such as sight (*clearly*), sound (*loud*), smell (*stunk*), and feelings (*happy, tired*). They should be able to describe the environment in terms of time (*at five o'clock*) and location (*in front of*). Entities should possess physical qualities, such as shape (*sort of round*), size (*big*), number (*two, many, few*), substance (*metal, wood*), and condition (*new, ragged*). There should be terms for relationships, such as comparisons (*bigger than, as big as*) and qualifications (*nearly, not quite, only, enough*); and verbs for describing actions (*run, jump, eat*), states (*am, is, are*), and sensory processes (*feel, hear, see*). Finally, the speakers should be able to describe causation (*because . . .*) and motivation. As noted previously, these terms develop slowly. The full range is characteristic of the mature speaker.

Deictic terms, or terms that must be interpreted from the perspective of the speaker (e.g., *here, there, this, that, come, go*), offer a special problem for the child with language impairment. The shifting reference that occurs with each speaker change contributes to the child's difficulty. Children with LLD, autism, or emotional disturbances may lack either the listener or speaker perspective. These children also may refer to themselves by name and may echo the utterances of others.

Over-/Underextensions and Incorrect Usage

The speech-language pathologist should note all inaccurate uses of words that indicate some variation between the child's meaning and the conventional one. In general, meanings mature from the personal experiential ones found in preschool children to the shared conventional ones of adults.

Some children use words incorrectly because they do not know the shared conventional definition. Others use word substitutions that are incorrect. For example, a recent letter from a young adult with language learning disability included the following:

> I wish I could write as good as you. You know where to put paragraphs and how to use punctuality right.

Because I am usually late, I assume he meant *punctuation.* Further testing by the speech-language pathologist can reveal the basis of the child's substitutions. The child may miss the target word slightly, as in the above example, or may have word-finding difficulties, resulting in word substitutions.

Children with LEP may use L₂ words in either very restricted or overextended ways. Restricted use may be limited to specific features of a word or to word-for-word transfer. In the latter, for example, the English *for,* which is *pour* in French, might be used only where *pour* would be used.

Style and Lexicon

Children begin to use different styles of talking relatively early. Analysis across utterances and partners might highlight a conversational style shift. These changes can be analyzed further for the vocabulary used in different styles.

Slang is a casual manner of spontaneous conversation among peers and is important for adolescents (Finegan & Besnier, 1989; Hyde, 1982; Leona, 1978). Used appropriately, slang separates adolescents from children and adults and establishes group identity and solidarity (Cooper & Anderson-Inman, 1988). Certain vocabulary—*rad, grotty, bad*—is characteristic of adolescent slang. Word meanings change quickly and are invented often by youth (Chapman, 1987). Knowledge of slang vocabulary increases with age, with boys knowing more terms for vehicles and money and girls for clothing, boys, and unpopular individuals.

The adolescent with language impairment may seem odd in peer situations because he underuses or overuses adolescent slang or uses it inappropriately. Although difficult to assess because of its changing nature and subgroup use, slang is, nonetheless, extremely important. In brainstorming sessions, teens developing normally can suggest vocabulary targets.

The child's literate vocabulary, consisting of words primarily used in common academic contexts, is also important. A good, literate lexicon is needed to achieve academic success, especially among adolescents (Nippold. 1993). Possible lexical items are *analyze, criticize, deduce, define, infer, interpret, predict, remember,* and *understand*. Classroom teachers can suggest other useful literate terms.

Word Relationships

Each word in a language is related to other words in ways that account for the richness of that language. These relationships consist of word associations (e.g., *salt and pepper* or *king and queen*), synonyms, antonyms, and homonyms. Some of these associations are expressed in the conversational sample, whereas others need to be probed by the speech-language pathologist. These associations reflect underlying cognitive organizational strategies.

Semantic Categories

Semantic categories, such as agent, action, and location, are the earliest word classes children use. Indeed, most of the early language development of toddlers is concerned with semantic units.

Several categorization schemata attempt to describe the semantic classes of young children and adults (R. Brown, 1973; Chafe, 1970; Clancy, Jacobsen, & Silva, 1976; Fillmore, 1968; Leonard, Bolders, & Miller, 1976). Table 6.7 is a composite of these semantic category schemata. The speech-language pathologist is interested in the range of semantic categories expressed by the child.

Semantic knowledge, or the underlying concepts about properties of entities, may be a better framework than linguistic form for the assessment of children with nonstandard dialects (Wolfram & Christian, 1976). The adequacy of the semantic knowledge of these children often is questioned on the basis of the form of their language, despite evidence of the universal nature of semantic representation in such categories as action, state, location, and possession (Blake, 1984; P. Miller, 1982; Stockman & Vaughn-Cooke, 1983). It is assumed, incorrectly, that nonstandard speakers acquire concepts later than do speakers of dialects closer to Standard American English (SAE).

The developmental trends are very similar and suggest guidelines for assessment of the semantic features of nonstandard speakers (Stockman & Vaughn-Cooke, 1986). By age 30 months, working-class, nonstandard speakers use mostly two-word combinations and encode several semantic categories, such as existence, action, location, state, negation, attribution, notice, intention, and recurrence. These guidelines can be used to help identify nonstandard-speaking children who may need clinical intervention.

TABLE 6.7
Semantic categories

Semantic Function	Description	Example
Action	The predicate expresses action with a transitive or intransitive clause.	We *grew* pumpkins and squash. (Transitive) She *gave* us a dollar. (Transitive) He *swims* daily. (Intransitive)
State	The predicate makes a statement about the way things are with a transitive, intransitive, or equative clause.	I *want* a hot fudge sundae. (Transitive) Tigers *look* fierce. (Intransitive) She *is* tall. (Equative) My sister *is* now at Harvard. (Equative)
Agent or Actor	Animate instigator of action. Sometimes inanimate, especially if natural force. Usually the subject but may also be passive complement.	*Mike* threw the ball. *Termites* destroyed our cabin. *Wind* blew down the trees. The *cat* chased the dog. The dog was chased by the *cat*.
Instrument	Usually refers to the inanimate object used by the actor to effect the action stated in the verb. The actor is usually not stated but may be. The instrument function may also be adverbial, as in *on his drum*.	The *axe* split the wood. The building was erected by a *crane*. She used the *baseball bat* with great skill. The shaman kept rhythm on his *drum*.
Patient	The entity on which an action is performed. The patient may be a direct object in transitive clauses or the subject in intransitive clauses.	Mike threw the *ball*. *The lighthouse* withstood the hurricane.
Dative	The animate recipient of action. Usually the indirect object but may also be the direct object if it does not undergo any action but receives something.	Father bought *mother* a bouquet of roses. Our mascot brought *us* good luck. He built a treehouse for his *daughter*. I loved that *movie*.
Temporal	Fulfills the adverbial function of time in response to a *when* question. May also be the subject of a sentence or a complement.	I'll see you *later*. We'll meet at *four o'clock*. *Then,* I'll know. *Tomorrow* is a holiday. *Tuesday* will be our first meeting. It is *time to leave*.
Locative	Fulfills the adverbial function of place in response to a *where* question. May also be the subject of a sentence or a complement.	Some of us looked *in the old log*. I knew it was right *here*. *Chicago* is indeed a windy city. *Our house* has three bedrooms.
Manner	Fulfills the adverbial function of manner in response to a *how* question.	We stalked the big cat *carefully*. He worked *with great skill*.
Accompaniment	Fulfills the adverbial function of *with X* in response to *with whom* or *with what* questions.	He swam *with his sister*. She left *with Jim*. He hunted *with his dogs*.
Empty subjects	Serve a grammatical function.	*It* was sunny. *There* may be some rain.

Source: Adapted from Chafe (1970); Dever (1978); Fillmore (1968)

Intrasentence Relationships

In addition to an interest in the child's word meanings and relationships, the speech-language pathologist investigates other relationships expressed in the sentence through the use of conjunctions, negatives, and prepositions (Lund & Duchan, 1988), and various sentence forms, such as passive voice.

Four types of conjunctive relations are expressed in conjoined sentences (Bloom, Lahey, Hood, Lifter, & Fiess, 1980): additive, temporal, causal, and adversative.

In the *additive* form, two clauses with no dependent relationship simply are joined to one another. In the sentence "John ate pie, and Mary drank coffee," neither event depends on the other for its existence.

In the *temporal* form, one clause depends on the other to precede or follow or occur at the same time, as in "I'm going out and I'm taking a very long walk" or "I'll rake the leaves while you finish painting the trim." Practically, a person cannot take a long walk while still indoors. Other examples establish the temporal relationship more clearly, as in "I'm going to the store before I go to the party."

Causal conjoining implies a dependency in which one clause is the result of the other, for example, "I went to the party because I was invited." The preschool child may use *because* alone or at the beginning of a clause, as in "Cause I want to," although true causal conjoining occurs much later (see Table 6.16).

Finally, in *adversative* conjoining, one clause contrasts with information in the other, as in "I read the article, but I was unimpressed." One clause opposes or negates the other.

Negatives may be expressed in several ways and develop at different stages. The four mature negative forms include (a) *not* and *-n't*, (b) negative words, such as *nobody* and *nothing*, (c) the determiner *no* used with nouns, and (d) negative adverbs, such as *never* and *nowhere* (Klima & Bellugi, 1973). Again, the more mature language user should have a variety of forms. Those used by the child can be compared with the developmental data available in Table 6.16.

Prepositions are some of the hardest working and most versatile English words. They can be used to mark location (*in the box*), time (*in a minute*), or manner (*in a hurry*), and to fill adjectival and adverbial functions. These small, often unstressed words may be misinterpreted or misunderstood by children with language impairment. A strategy they use is overreliance on one form. As mentioned previously, the speech-language pathologist examines the sample for the breadth of use.

In general, children with language impairment exhibit difficulty interpreting sentences in which the information might be interpreted in a reverse manner (van der Lely & Harris, 1990). For example, a passive sentence, such as "The cat is chased by the dog" might be interpreted incorrectly as "The cat chased the dog" by using a subject-verb-object interpretation strategy. Children with language impairment have difficulty interpreting the grammatical functions of words and integrating grammatical and semantic information.

Figurative Language

Nonliteral meanings used for effect are more characteristic of school-age and adult language than of preschool language (Nippold, 1988a; Nippold & Martin, 1989). Examples include metaphors, similes, idioms, and proverbs. For the purposes of analysis, jokes and puns also can be considered figurative language. Figurative language occurs frequently in oral conversation and written texts. Interpretation of idioms is highly correlated with reading ability.

Children as young as 3½ are able to comprehend some idioms, especially the more literal ones (Abkarian, Jones, & West, 1992). In general, literal interpretation decreases with increasing age. Individual interpretive ability is related to each person's world knowledge (Winner, 1988). For example, *smooth sailing* has more meaning for the child who has some boating experience.

Idioms occur frequently in the classroom. There may be as many as four figures of speech per speaking minute (Pollio, Barlow, Fine, & Pollio, 1977). Teachers use idioms in approximately 11% of their utterances, while third– to eighth–grade reading programs contain idioms in approximately 6.7% of their sentences (Lazar, Warr-Leeper, Nicholson, & Johnson, 1989).

Idioms differ greatly in their difficulty of interpretation. In general, more familiar and more transparent or guessable idioms are easier. The child's language experience appears to be a key factor in interpretation (Nippold & Rudzinski, 1993).

The speech-language pathologist considers the range of figurative language used. Some children overrely on well-worn phrases and expressions, with little knowledge of their actual meaning. Such expressions as these can be probed by the speech-language pathologist to determine the child's actual knowledge.

Comprehension and production of idioms might be analyzed on the basis of *decomposability* of the idiom. Decomposable or analyzable idioms can be broken easily into their component parts. For example, *pop the question* or *let off steam* can be broken into components that each contribute to the overall meaning, as follows:

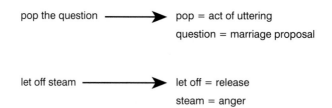

Nondecomposable idioms, such as *kick the bucket,* are difficult to break into components.

Comprehension depends on the child's intuition about the internal semantics of the idiom. In general, young children are better able to interpret decomposable idioms than nondecomposable. Third and fourth graders do equally well on both types in context. If no contextual information is available, these children also are better able to comprehend decomposable idioms (Gibbs, 1991).

Analysis of figurative language is especially important for children with LEP. Idiomatic expressions may be interpreted literally and/or based on cultural interpretation.

Word Finding

Word-finding difficulties are an impaired ability to generate a specific word that is evoked by a situation, stimulus, sentence context, or conversation (Rapin & Wilson, 1978). In Chapter 3 we discussed a method of probing for word-finding difficulties and strategies. In Chapter 5 we noted that latency may signal such difficulties. Other symptoms include frequent pauses, repetitions, circumlocutions, fillers, nonspecific words, frequent pronouns, and high usage of cliches and routinized expressions, such as *you know* (Bates et al., 1988; Snyder & Godley, 1992). Inaccurate naming may be analyzed by using the strategies presented in Table 3.6.

Several intrinsic and extrinsic variables affect word-retrieval skills. Intrinsic variables include the frequency of occurrence of the word, familiarity with the word, age of acquisition, category, and degree of abstractness. In general, more frequently used, more familiar, earlier learned, and less abstract words are easier to retrieve (Leonard, Nippold, Kail, & Hale, 1983; Milianti & Culliman, 1974; Stowe, 1988). Words from large prototype categories, such as fruits and vegetables, are easier to retrieve than those from well–defined categories, such as months, based on a small set of specific features (Armstrong, Gleitman, & Gleitman, 1983). In actual use, categories overlap and relative importance for naming will vary (Bretherton & Bates, 1984; Fried-Oken, 1984; Snyder, Bates, & Bretherton, 1981).

Extrinsic variables include the context, syntactic requirements, type of stimulus and manner of presentation, priming, and use of categories. In general, sentence contexts are easier than picture ones, which, in turn, are easier than definitions (Rudel, Denckla, Broman, & Hirsch, 1980). Formulation of more difficult sentences, however, interferes with word recall, probably because of the greater cognitive energy needed to form the sentence (Wolf, 1984). Priming results when preceding words aid recall (Balota & Duchek. 1989; Ceci, 1983; Glass & Holyoak, 1986; Kail, Hale, Leonard, & Nippold, 1984). Finally, use of subordinate categories can aid word recall (Ceci, 1983; Kail et al., 1984).

The effect of these variables can be very important and difficult to assess in a language sample. It is important, therefore, to use familiar partners, topics, and situations to facilitate retrieval.

FORM

Language form includes syntax, morphology, and phonology or the means used to encode the intentions of the speaker. Even though most language analysis methods concentrate on this aspect of language, very few normative data are available. The task is partially normative and partially descriptive, involving both quantitative and qualitative analysis. Several available analysis methods are described in Appendix F.

Quantitative Measures

Quantitative measures include mean length of utterance (MLU), mean syntactic length (MSL), T-units and C-units, and the density of sentence forms. Each is discussed in some detail.

The speech-language pathologist must be cautious with all word and morpheme counts. Careful editing of utterances is required so that interjections, false starts, and the like are not included in the count. Circumlocutions, or talking around an unretrievable word, actually may increase the length of the child's utterances. It is recommended that the speech-language pathologist follow consistent rules for counting. For example, incomplete words, nonessential repetitions, revisions not containing a complete thought, unintelligible words and phrases, and fillers might be offset in brackets and not counted. These structures are retained, however, for later analysis.

Mean Length of Utterance

Mean length of utterance is the average length in morphemes of the speaker's utterances. Up to an average of 4.0 MLU is a good measure of language complexity. Not all linguists agree (Crystal et al., 1976; J. Johnston & Kamhi, 1984; Klee & Fitzgerald, 1985). In general, there is less variability in MLU below 4.0 (Rondal, Ghiotto, Bredart, & Bachelet, 1987). This mean is reached by the nonimpaired child at around age 4, but MLU continues to increase with age. At lower MLUs, new structures added to the child's utterances increase the complexity of those sentences. After this level of development, much of the growth in complexity is the result of internal reorganization of utterance form, rather than addition of new structures. This explanation of the relationship between length and complexity is extremely simplified, and there are many related factors.

To calculate MLU, the speech-language pathologist divides the language sample into utterances. It is best not to include in analysis the portions of conversation that occurred while the child was adjusting to the partner or to the situation. The number of morphemes in each utterance is counted and totaled for the entire sample. Rules for counting morphemes on the basis of the order of development with nonimpaired children are included in Table 6.8. Brief rationales for these rules are included where appropriate.

The total number of morphemes is divided by the number of utterances from which it was derived to determine the MLU. This value then can be compared to the age data in Table 6.9. It is obvious from this table that a wide variability and a wide range of ages are considered within the normal range. Even so, the need to collect a typical sample is very important. If data have been collected in two or more settings, the MLUs from each can be compared to assess the stability of the overall data.

Although age and MLU are correlated as shown in Table 6.9, some interesting data suggest cautious acceptance of this correlation. First, the relationship of rate of MLU and age change is not a constant, as seen in Table 6.9. Second, language impairments are not necessarily evidenced by delays in MLU as might be expected (Klee, Schaffer, May, Membrino, & Mougey, 1989).

TABLE 6.8
Rules for counting morphemes relative to preschool and older children

Structure	Example	Count Psch.	Count Sch.	Rationale
Each recurrence of a word for emphasis	No, no, no.	1 each	1 each	
Compound words (2 or more free morphemes)	Railroad, birthday	1	2+	Compound words learned as a unit by preschoolers
Proper names	Bugs Bunny, Uncle Fred	1	2+	Proper names, even those with titles, learned as a unit by preschoolers
Ritualized reduplications	Choo-choo, Night-night	1	1	
Irregular past tense verbs	Went, ate, got, came	1	2	Verb tense learned as new word by preschoolers, not as *verb +ed*
Diminutives	Doggie, horsie	1	2	Phonological form CVCV easier than CVC for preschoolers and does not denote smallness
Auxiliary verbs and catenatives	Is, have, do; gonna, wanna, gotta	1	1+	Preschoolers do not know that such words as *gonna* are *going to*
Contracted negatives	Don't, can't, won't	1–2	2	Because negatives *don't, can't* and *won't* develop before *do, can,* and *will,* count as one until the positive form appears. Then count the negative forms as two morphemes.
Possessive marker (-'s)	Tom's, mom's	1	1	
Plural marker (-s)	Cats, dogs	1	1	
Third-person singular present tense marker (-s)	Walks, eats	1	1	
Regular past tense marker (-ed)	Walked, jumped	1	1	
Present progressive marker (-ing)	Walking, eating	1	1	
Dysfluencies	C-c-candy, b-b-baby	1+	1+	*Count only the final complete form.
Fillers	Um-m, ah-h	0	0	

* In the example "I want can . . . I want can . . . I want candy," only the last full production is counted, being 3 morphemes.

TABLE 6.9
Quantitative measures of language

Age in Months	MLU	*Range of Mean MLU	**MSL	**TNW (20 min.)	**NDW (50 utt.)
18	1.1	1.0–1.2			
21	1.6	1.1–1.8	2.7	240	36
24	1.9	1.6–2.2	2.9	286	41
27	2.1	1.9–2.3	3.1	332	46
30	2.5	2.4–2.6	3.4	378	51
33	2.8	2.7–2.9	3.7	424	56
36	3.1	3.0–3.3	3.9	470	61
39	3.3	3.2–3.5	4.2	516	66
42	3.6	3.3–3.9	4.4	562	71
45	3.8	3.4–4.3	4.7	608	76
48	3.9	3.6–4.7	4.9	654	81
51	4.1	3.7–5.1	5.2	700	86
54	4.3	3.9–5.8			
60	4.4	4.0–6.0			
108	8.8	7.2–10.4***			

TTR (type-token ratio) changes little with age but is in the range .45–.5 for 2– to 9-year-olds.

* Combined data from four different studies (Klee, Schaffer, May, Membrino, & Mougey, 1989; J. Miller, 1981; Scarborough, Wyckoff, & Davidson, 1986; Wells, 1985)
** MSL (mean syntactic length), TNW (total number of words) and NDW (number of different words) extrapolated from tables in Klee (1992).
*** From J. Miller, Freiberg, Rolland & Reves, 1992.

Mean Syntactic Length

Mean syntactic length (MSL) is the mean length in words of all utterances of two words or more—those utterances with some internal grammar. This measure eliminates all one-word responses, such as yes/no answers. MSL seems to correlate more strongly than MLU with age (Klee & Fitzgerald, 1985). Values for MSL are listed in Table 6.9 (Klee, 1992).

T-units and C-units

Expressive language syntax of older children and adolescents can be measured in **T-units** (minimal terminal units) (K. Hunt, 1970), consisting of one main clause plus any attached or embedded subordinate clause or nonclausal structure (discussed in the following section). Thus, the unit has shifted from the utterance to the sentence in its shortest allowable form. Any simple or complex sentence would be one T-unit, but a compound sentence would be two or more. For example, the sentences "I want ice cream" and "I want the one that is hidden in the blue box" each constitute one T-unit with varying numbers of words and clauses. "I want the ice cream in the picture, and he wants a shake" consists of two main clauses and thus two T-units. Examples of T-units are given in Table 6.10.

TABLE 6.10
Examples of T-units and C-units

Sentence Structure	Example	Number of T-units and C-units
Simple — one clause	They watched the parade on TV.	1 T-unit, 1 C-unit
Complex — embedded clause	Washington has the horse I want.	1 T-unit, 1 C-unit
Compound — conjoining of two or more clauses	*They went to the movie,* but *I stayed home.* *Mom went to work, I went to school,* and *my sister stayed home.*	2 T-units, 2 C-units 3 T-units, 3 C-units
Partial sentences		
Elliptical answers	(Who went with you?) Marshon.	1 C-unit
Exclamations	Oh, wow!	1 C-unit
Aphorisms	A penny saved.	1 C-unit

The T-unit is more sensitive than MLU to the types of language differences seen after age 5, such as phrasal embedding and various types of subordinate clauses (O'Donnell, Griffin, & Norris, 1967). Throughout the school years, a slow but regular increase occurs in sentence length in both oral and written contexts.

Children's language then can be described in words per T-unit, clauses per T-unit, and words per clause. A gradual and progressive increase in words and clauses per T-unit and in words per clause in spontaneous speech occurs with increased age throughout childhood and adolescence, although the values change only gradually during early school years (Table 6.11) (Klecan-Aker, 1985; Scott et al., 1992).

TABLE 6.11
T-units and C-units by age and grade

Units	Age 6	Grades 3-4	Grades 6-7	Grade 9	Grades 11-12
Words/T-unit					
Spoken		7.8	9.7		11.4
Written		9.5	9.4-11.8		10.6-13.3
Words/C-unit					
Oral			9.82	10.96	11.7
Written			9.04	10.05	13.27
Clauses/T-unit					
Spoken	1.26	1.31	1.5		1.5
Written		1.3	1.6		1.6-1.8
Subordinate Clauses/C-unit					
Spoken			.37	.43	.58
Written			.29	.47	.6
Words/clause					
Spoken	7.14	7.75			

Source: Scott, C. M., Nippold, M. A., Norris, J. A., & Johnson, C. J. (1992, November). *School–age children and adolescents: Establishing language norms.* Paper presented at the Annual Convention of the American Speech–Language–Hearing Association, San Antonio, TX.

To calculate these values, the speech-language pathologist divides the sample into sentences, each equaling one T-unit. The number of words and clauses then can be determined for each and divided by the number of T-units to calculate an average. The words per clause can be determined similarly.

It should be noted that the type of conversational task will influence some T-unit measures. Information-giving tasks increase the words and clauses per T-unit. In addition, at this level of development, T-unit values can be misleading because complexity and length are not directly related. For example, among adolescents, phrases may be used in place of subordinate clauses for conciseness, suggesting greater syntactic sophistication (Nippold, 1993). These include participial phrases (***Working until midnight,*** *John missed his bus*), infinitive phrases (*Candace was not afraid* ***to use the computer for typing her assignment***), and gerund phrases (***Seeing your photos*** *convinced us that we should go to Puerto Rico*) (Scott, 1988b).

A variance of the T-unit is the **C-unit** (Loban, 1976). C-units are similar to T-units but also include incomplete sentences in answer to questions (Table 6.10). C-unit values are given in Table 6.11.

The length increase in C-units is primarily through the increased use of low frequency structures. These include post-noun modifiers, such as apposition structures (*Mary* ***my instructor*** *showed us . . .*) and prepositional phrases (*The man* ***in front*** *is . . .*), complex nominals (***Dogs and cats*** *can . . .* or ***Rules such as stop on red*** *are . . .*), and elaborated verb tensing, such as modal auxiliaries (***could*** *have been*), perfect aspect (***had been*** *working*), and passive voice (*The window* ***was broken by*** *a fly ball*). Analysis of these structures might accompany calculation of C-unit values.

Syntactic and Morphologic Analysis

Many disordered populations experience difficulty with syntax and morphology. For example, children who are mildly-to-moderately behaviorally disordered seem to have word-order difficulties (Camarata, Hughes, & Ruhl, 1988).

It should be noted that some utterances defy analysis, such as those containing contrasting stress used to negate. For example, one speaker might say, "Penny went," only to be corrected by the other speaker with "*Mary* went." At a syntactic level, these two sentences would appear to be similar.

Morphologic Analysis

The speech-language pathologist is interested in intraword development, as well as in sentence development. With preschool children, she will want to analyze Brown's 14 morphemes as suggested by J. Miller (1981). These are listed in Table 6.12. Other morphemes, such as pronouns, also may be of interest. Older children may use a variety of morphological prefixes and suffixes. A list of the more common prefixes and suffixes is included in Appendix G.

Correct usage of Brown's 14 grammatical morphemes can be a clinical aid for establishing the developmental stage of preschool children (J. Miller, 1981). Table 6.12 presents the morphemes by stage of mastery, the stage in which each morpheme is produced correctly by children in 90% of the obligatory contexts.

TABLE 6.12

Brown's 14 morphemes and age of mastery

Stage of Mastery	Morpheme	Example	Age Range of Mastery* (in months)
II	Present progressive-*ing*, (no auxiliary verb)	Mommy driv*ing*.	19–28
	In	Ball *in* cup.	27–30
	On	Doggie *on* sofa	27–30
	Regular plural -*s*	Kitti*es* eat my ice cream.	24–33
		Forms: /s/, /z/, and /Iz/	
		Cats (/kæts/)	
		Dogs (/dɔgz/)	
		Classes (klæsIz/), *wishes* (/wIʃIz/)	
III	Irregular past	*Came, fell, broke, sat, went*	25–46
	Possessive *'s*	Mommy*'s* balloon broke.	26–40
		Forms: /s/, /z/, and /Iz/ as in regular plural	
IV	Uncontractible copula (verb *to be* as main verb)	He *is*. (response to "Who's sick?")	27–39
	Articles	I see *a* kitty.	28–46
		I throw *the* ball to daddy.	
	Regular past -*ed*	Mommy pull*ed* the wagon.	26–48
		Forms: /d/, /t/, and /Id/	
		Pulled (/pʊld/)	
		Walked (/wɔkt/)	
		Glided (/g l aI d Id/)	
	Regular third person -*s*	Kathy hit*s*.	26–46
		Forms: /s/, /z/, and /Iz/ as in regular plural	
V+	Irregular third person	*Does, has*	28–50
	Uncontractible auxiliary	He *is*. (response to "Who's wearing your hat?")	29–48
	Contractible copula	Man*'s* big.	29–49
		Man *is* big.	
	Contractible auxiliary	Daddy*'s* drinking juice.	30–50
		Daddy *is* drinking juice.	

* Used correctly 90% of the time in obligatory contexts.

Source: Adapted from Bellugi (1964); R. Brown (1973); J. Miller (1981)

The percentage correct value is determined by dividing the number of correct appearances by the total number of obligatory contexts. In obligatory contexts, the child might use the morpheme correctly, make an error substitution, or omit the morpheme. Table 6.13 presents selected portions of a language sample and the calculation of percentage correct for the regular plural marker.

The percentage correct yields only limited data. More descriptive information can be gained. For example, the speech-language pathologist who calculated only the

TABLE 6.13
Calculating percentage correct for plural

Utterance	Correct	Incorrect	Type of Error
2. Want more cookies.		x	
3. Three cookie.		x	Not marked
4. No, one big cookies.		x	Marked singular
22. Dogs.	x		
27. Give the pencils to me.	x		
28. I want two pencils.	x		
31. You color the foots.		x	Marked irregular
40. What blue crayons?	x		
TOTAL	5	3	

$$\text{Percentage correct} \;=\; \frac{\text{Total of correct}}{\text{Total of correct + incorrect}} \;=\; \frac{5}{8} \;=\; 62.5\%$$

percentage correct for past tense *-ed* still would not know whether errors were related to nonuse of *-ed* where required or to use of *-ed* on irregular past tense verbs. The pronoun error analysis format in Table 6.14 offers guidance for analysis with other forms.

After calculating percentage correct, the speech-language pathologist can attempt to describe the child's stage of language development. This process is not an exact science. Rarely is the determination clear-cut or is one and only one stage identified.

Morphological markers are applied to word classes. For example, the past tense *-ed* marker is confined to verbs. Therefore, the speech-language pathologist should also note word classes in which errors occur. Occasionally, errors are confined to only one word class, such as verbs. Nouns would be affected by such markers as plural regular and irregular, possessive, and articles. Verb markers include third person singular, past tense regular and irregular, present progressive, modals, *do* + verb, copula (*am, are, is, was, were*), and perfective (*have* + *be* + verb). Finally, adjective and adverb markers include, but are not limited to, comparative and superlative and adverbial *-ly*.

Pronouns offer a special case of morphological analysis because of the complex nature of the underlying semantic and pragmatic functions. If the child's strategy is "when in doubt, use the noun," then it will be difficult to find errors in pronoun substitution (Haas & Owens, 1985). More in-depth analysis is required, possibly similar to that presented in Table 6.14. The types of errors made reveal the underlying rules that the child is using.

When analyzing the oral and written language of school-age children and adolescents, the speech-language pathologist will want to note the scope of prefix and suffix use. In addition to inflectional suffixes, such as plural *-s* and past tense *-ed*, derivational suffixes also should be analyzed. These suffixes, more common in written than in oral language, are used to change word classes, as in adding *-er* to a verb such as *teach* to create the noun *teacher*. The two most common derivational changes are from verbs to nouns and from verbs to adjectives (Scott, 1984a, 1988b).

TABLE 6.14
Possible pronoun analysis method

Sub-analysis of Incorrect Responses

Stage	Pronoun	Correct	Incorrect	Total	Percent Correct	Substitution: Case	Substitution: Gender	Substitution: Person	Substitution: Number	Omission	Ambiguous Referent	Overuse of Nominal
I (MLU: 1.0–2.0)	I											
	me											
	my											
II (MLU: 2.0–2.5)	it (subj.)											
	it (obj.)											
III (MLU: 2.5–3.0)	you (subj.)											
	your											
	she											
	them											
	he											
	we											
	her (poss.)											
IV (MLU: 3.0–3.75)	his											
	him											
	you (obj.)											
	us											
	they											
	our											
V (MLU: 3.75–4.5)	its											
	myself											
	yourself											
	her (obj.)											
	their											
Post V (MLU: 4.5+)	herself											
	himself											
	ourselves											
	themselves											
	TOTAL											

Comments:

Note: Pronouns, arranged by stage of acquisition, are scored as correct or incorrect, although the total and percent columns are initially left blank. Incorrect pronoun use is then analyzed as a substitution or omission error. Substitution may be multiple, as when *she* is used for *his*, demonstrating substitutions of case and gender. When this step is completed, the sample is checked to ensure that the referent has been clearly identified for each pronoun and that the child has not overused the referent name in place of a pronoun. These are also errors, and once noted, they should be added to the incorrect total on the left. When this step is completed, the total and percent correct columns can be completed.

Children With LEP and Different Dialects

The speech-language pathologist should be mindful of dialectal and bilingual variations. Even though a child omits a morphological ending, it cannot be assumed that the child does not understand or is not able to produce the morpheme. For example, children who speak Black English may omit some word endings for phonological reasons. Others may be omitted because they are redundant, such as the plural *-s* when the noun is preceded by a number as in *ten cent*. The bidialectal or bilingual child's abilities must be established by the testing of both the marker and the concept associated with it.

The only standard for comparison of children's performance is the communication community of each child. A child's language is impaired to the extent that he or she is unable to communicate effectively in that community. Two errors that occur in language assessment are (a) mistaking dialectal variations for disorders and (b) overlooking disorders mistakenly assumed to be dialectal variations. In general, dialectal variations develop by age 5, with few noticeable at age 3 (Battles, 1990).

The most frequent morphological errors of speakers with LEP are presented in Table 6.15. Morphological markers often are omitted or overgeneral-

TABLE 6.15
Frequent morphological errors of speakers with LEP

Morpheme	Type of Error	Possible Explanation
Articles	Omission or overgeneralization of *the*	Articles are used infrequently in many languages.
Auxiliaries and modals	Omission	Many languages do not have auxiliary verbs and rely on verb markers.
Contractions	Omission	Unstressed forms often omitted; a phonological error.
Copula	Omission	Unstressed forms often omitted.
Gerund	Omission of *-ing* ending	Many languages do not have this form.
Plural *-s*	Omission or error in agreement, as in *many tree*	Unstressed forms often omitted; used when other languages mark by adjective.
Possessive *-s*	Omission or overgeneralization	Many languages use the *possession of possessor* form.
Prepositions	Substitution errors	Very complex system in English; multiple meanings of words.
Pronouns	Substitution errors, noun-pronoun agreement errors	Most languages do not have as many pronouns as English.
Regular past *-ed*	Omission or overgeneralization	Unstressed forms often omitted.
Third person *-s*	Omission or overgeneralization	Exception to English rule of no person or number markers.

ized. Some Spanish speakers lump English syllables together, decreasing intelligibility. A Cuban friend calls me "Bobowens." This chunking may cause small units such as morphemes to be de-emphasized.

Syntactic Analysis

Analysis also is accomplished at the intraclausal and clausal levels. For this type of analysis, it is best to exclude imitations, short answers to questions, and stereotypic or rote responses because these types of utterances are not usually clinically significant.

For analysis purposes, it is helpful to separate sentences and nonsentences. Sentences are grouped as declarative, negative declarative, imperative, negative imperative, interrogative, and negative interrogative. Sentences can be grouped for further analysis by length or structure. For example, declarative sentences can be categorized as subject-verb, subject-verb-object, subject-verb-complement, and multiple clauses, either embedded or conjoined. The form of the preschool child's sentences can be compared with some normative data, such as those in Table 6.16, to best determine the child's stage of development, although descriptive data are also valuable. The speech-language pathologist should note intrasentential noun and verb phrase development, sentence types, and embedding and conjoining. These and other sentence analyses are especially important for school-age children and adolescents.

The speech-language pathologist can use Table 6.16 in a comparative fashion. For example, let us assume that the child said, "I want a big doggie." The noun *doggie* has been expanded by the addition of an article and an adjective. This noun phrase occurs in the object position of the sentence. Expansion of the noun phrase in the object position is an example of structure occurring at Stage II and above, according to the intrasentential column of Table 6.16. The verb is unelaborated, as is the subject noun. These represent structures at the Stage I level or above. No further analysis is needed for sentence type.

The child with LEP may not exhibit difficulty in a sentence-by-sentence analysis. Analysis of connected speech beyond the sentence may provide more insight. Word order errors and cohesive difficulties become evident in analysis of units larger than the individual sentence.

Noun phrase. Noun phrase elaboration is assessed by describing the number and variety of noun phrase elements. Analysis of noun phrases is especially appropriate for children functioning at a late childhood or adolescent level. The order of the elements within the noun phrase is relatively fixed, although the order of development is not so definite. The noun function is obligatory, and the other modifiers are nonobligatory. In order of mention within the noun phrase, the elements are initiator(s), determiner(s), adjectival(s), noun, and post-noun modifier(s) (Crystal et al., 1976; Dever, 1978). Some or all of these elements may be present in the noun phrase, as shown in Table 6.17. Some elements may be used in combination, whereas the use of others is more exclusive.

Initiators consist of a small core of words that limit or quantify the phrase that follows. Examples are *only, a few of,* and *merely.* Most of these words can serve

TABLE 6.16
Preschool language development and Brown's stages

Stage	Approx. Age	Sentence Types	Intrasentential/Morphology
Early I (MLU 1-1.5)	12-21 mos.	Single words. *Yes/no* questions use rising intonation. *What* and *where.* *Negative + X.* Semantic word-order rules.	Pronouns *I* & *mine.* Isolated nouns elaborated as *Art./Adj. + Noun.* Serial naming without *and.*
Late I (MLU 1.5-2.0)	21-26 mos.	*S + V + O* appears. Negative *no* and *not* used interchangeably. *Yes/no* question form is *This/that + X?*	*And* appears. *In* & *on* appear.
Early II (MLU 2.0-2.25)	27-28 *mos.*	Wh- question form is *What/where + noun?* *To be* appears as main verb.*	Present progressive (*-ing*), no aux. verb mastered by 90%. Pronouns *me, my* & *it, this* & *that.* Nouns elaborated in object position only [*(Art./Adj./Dem./Poss.) + Noun*].
Late II (MLU 2.25-2.5)	28-29 mos.	Basic *SVO* used by most. Negative element (*no, not, don't, can't* interchangeable) placed between noun and verb.	*In/on* & plural *-s* mastered by 90%. *Gonna, wanna, gotta, hafta* appear.
Early III (MLU 2.5-2.75)	30-32 mos.	*What/where + N + V?* Inversion in *What/where + be + N?** *S + aux. verb + V + O* appears. Aux. verbs include *can, do, have, will.*	Pronouns *she, he, her, we, you, your, yours* & *them.* Noun elaboration in the subject & object position [*Art. + (modifier) + Noun*]. Modifiers include *alot, some* & *two.* Select irregular past (*came, fell, broke, sat, went*) & possessive (*-'s*) mastered by 90%.

also as adverbs. The speech-language pathologist must be careful to identify the accompanying noun phrase.

    Determiners come in many varieties and include, in order of mention, quantifiers; articles, possessive pronouns, and demonstratives; and numerical terms, such as *two, twenty,* or *one hundred. Quantifiers* include such words as *all, both, half, twice,* and *triple.* In combination with initiators, determiners can yield *nearly all, at least half,* and *less than one-third. Articles* include common forms, such as *the, a,* and *an.* Possessive pronouns include *my, your,* and *their. Demonstratives* serve as articles but are interpreted from the perspective of the speaker as in *this, that, these,* and *those.*

    In order of appearance, *adjectivals* consist of nouns marking possession, as in *mommy's sock,* ordinals, such as *first, next,* and *final;* adjectives, such as *little, big,* and *blond;* and nouns used as descriptors, as in *hot dog* stand and *cowboy* hat. Thus, a speaker might say, "Brother's first little cowboy hat." The exact order of

TABLE 6.16, *continued*

Late III (MLU 2.75-3.0)	33-34 mos.	*S + aux. verb + be + X* appears. Negative *won't* appears. Aux. verbs appear in interrogatives; inverted with subject in *yes/no* type.	*But, so, or* & *if* appear.
Early IV (MLU 3.0-3.5)	35-39 mos.	Negative appears with aux. verb + *not* (*cannot, do not*). Inversion of aux. verb and subject in *Wh-* questions.	Uncontractible copula (verb *to be* as *main verb*) mastered by 90%. Pronouns *his, him, hers, us* & *they*. Noun phrase elaboration includes *Art./Dem. + Adj./Poss./Mod. + Noun.* Clausal conjoining with *and* appears. Clausal embedding as object with *think, guess, show, remember*, etc.
Late IV (MLU 3.5-3.75)	39-42 mos.	Double aux. verbs in declaratives. Add *isn't, aren't, doesn't* and *didn't*. Inversion of *be* and subj. in *yes/no* interrogatives Add *when* and *how* interrogatives.	Articles (*the, a*), regular past (*-ed*), & third person regular (*-s*) mastered by 90%. Infinitive phrases appear at end of sentence.
Stage V (MLU 3.75-4.5)	42-56 mos.	Indirect objects appear in declaratives. Add *wasn't, wouldn't, couldn't, shouldn't*. Negative appears with other forms of *be*. Some simple tag questions appear.	Pronouns *our, ours, its, their, theirs, myself* & *yourself.* Relative clauses appear attached to object. Infinitive phrases with same subj. as main verb.
Post-V (MLU 4.5+)	56+ mos.	Add indefinite negatives (*nobody, no one, nothing*), creating double negatives. *Why* appears in more than one-word interrogatives. Negative interrogatives after 60 mos.	Irregular past (*does, has*), uncontractible auxiliary *to be*, and contractible auxiliary *to be* and copula (*to be* as main verb) mastered by 90%. Remaining reflexive pronouns added. Multiple embedding; embedding + conjoining. Relative clauses attached to subj. appear.

adjectivals is more complex, requiring more explanation than space allows (see Crystal et al., 1976; Dever, 1978).

The *noun* function can be filled by subjective pronouns, such as *I, you*, and *they;* objective pronouns, such as *me, you*, and *them;* genitive pronouns, such as *mine, yours*, and *theirs;* simple singular and plural nouns, such as *boy, girls*, and *women;* and mass nouns that have no distinction between singular and plural, as in *sand, water*, and *police*. When a pronoun is used, the noun to which it refers usually has already been identified. Therefore, few noun modifiers are used, and the noun phrase is relatively simple. The noun function also may be complex or may consist of a phrase, as in *Statue of Liberty, need to succeed*, and *city of Los Angeles*, or a

TABLE 6.17
Elements of the noun phrase

Initiator	+ Determiner	+ Adjectival	+ Noun	+ Post-noun Modifier
Only, a few of, just, at least, less than, nearly, especially, partially, even, merely, almost	**Quantifier:** All, both, half, no, one-tenth, some, any, either, each, every, twice, triple **Article:** The, a, an **Possessive:** My, your, his, her, its, our, your, their **Demonstratives:** This, that, these, those **Numerical Term:** One, two, thirty, one thousand	**Possessive Nouns:** Mommy's, children's **Ordinal:** First, next, next to last, last, final, second **Adjective:** Blue, big, little, fat, old, fast, circular, challenging **Descriptor:** *Shopping* (center), *Baseball* (game), *hot dog* (stand)	**Pronoun** I, you, he, she, it, we, you, they, mine, yours, his, hers, its, ours, theirs **Noun:** Boys, dog, feet, sheep, men and women, city of New York, Port of Chicago, leap of faith, matter of conscience	**Prepositional Phrase:** On the car, in the box, in the gray flannel suit **Adjectival:** Next door, pictured by Renoir, eaten by Martians, loved by her friends **Adverb:** Here, there, (Embedded) **Clause:** Who went with you, that you saw

Examples

Nearly.........................all the one
hundred......................old college ....alumni ....attending the event
Almost all of ....her thirty ....former........................clients
Just ....half of your................brother's
                                                     old baseball.................uniforms.............in the closet

compound, as in *Tom and Bob* and *duty and responsibility*. Finally, if the noun is understood by both the speaker and the listener, it may be omitted, as in the following exchange:

"What did you and Barb do last night?"

"(We) Went to that movie at the mall."

Post-noun modifiers may take many forms, including prepositional phrases (*in the gray flannel suit*), embedded clauses (*who lives next door*), adjectivals (*next door* and *driven by my mother*), and adverbs (*here* and *there*). Post-noun modifiers may be used singly or in combination—for example, "The man *who lives in the green house on the next block* bought all of the candy that I was selling."

The development of elements of the noun phrase takes most nonimpaired children many years and continues into adolescence. As noted in Table 6.16, elaboration begins in isolation and then moves to the object position in the sentence before appearing in the subject position. This pattern is only the beginning of the development process; with increasing age, the child should use more and more noun elaborations. Adjectives and determiners appear at the two-word stage for both children with language impairment and those without (Morehead & Ingram, 1976). Initiators and post-noun modifiers appear later, with children with language impairment exhibiting a marked delay (Morehead & Ingram, 1976). For children developing normally, clausal post-noun modifiers appear in late Stage IV and V (Table 6.16).

Most 5–year–olds use no more than one modifier. Thus, most internal development of the noun phrase occurs in later childhood and adolescence. Both elaborated prenoun and postnoun modification, using relative clauses and prepositional phrases, develop during this period (Nippold, 1993; Perera, 1986a, 1986b; Scott, 1988a, 1988b). The most elaborated forms usually are produced in written language.

The speech-language pathologist is interested in the distribution of these elaborations in these positions and the average number of morphemes within noun phrases. It may be helpful for the speech-language pathologist to use a format of analysis similar to that in Table 6.18.

Children with language impairment can be expected to have simpler, less elaborated noun phrases. Pronouns offer a special problem. Children with LEP may exhibit confusion with modifier order and pronoun use.

Verb phrase.   Verb phrase elaboration consists of the verb and associated words, including noun phrases used as complements or as direct or indirect objects. The speech-language pathologist is concerned with the verbs used and those that are missing or incomplete. Other elements of the verb phrase that are present or absent are also important and reflect the maturity of the speaker's language system.

Predicates, or verb statements, show the relationship of the various sentence elements to each other. This relationship takes three forms: intransitive, in which the verb cannot take an object; transitive, in which the verb can take an object; and equative, which consists of the copula (*to be*) plus a complement of a noun, adjective, or adverb. Verb phrases can be described by the length and range of types, as demonstrated in Table 6.18.

Simple transitive (*Mommy throw*) and equative verb phrases (*Doggie big*) appear at an MLU of about 1.5 (Kamhi & Nelson, 1988). At this stage, the verbs are unmarked for tense or person, and the copula is omitted. As language becomes more complex, verbs become marked, the copula appears, and intransitive verb phrases appear. By Stage II, the progressive *-ing* marker and catenatives (*gonna, wanna, gotta, hafta*) appear. The perfective form (*have + verb-en*) and the passive voice begin to be used by Stage IV. Adverbial phrases also appear in Stage IV. Late childhood and adolescent language development is characterized by increasing verb complexity with the use of auxiliaries, modals, and perfective forms, such as *have been going*. There is also increasing use of adverbs and adverbial phrases, such as prepositional phrases of manner (*in silence*), place (*in the*

TABLE 6.18
Elements of the verb phrase

Modal Auxiliary	+ Perfective Auxiliary	+ Verb to be	+ Negative*	+ Passive	+ Verb	+ Prepositional Phrase, Noun Phrase, Noun Complement, Adverbial Phrase
May, can, shall, will, must, might, should, would, could	Have, has, had	Am, is, are, was, were, be, been	Not	Been, being	Run, walk, eat, throw, see, write	On the floor, the ball, our old friend, a doctor, on time, late

Examples:

Transitive (May have direct object)

May..................have ....wanted ....a cookie

Should...not ....throw..........the ball in the house

Intransitive (Does not take direct object)

Might.................have ....been ....walking.......to the inn

Could ....not ....talk............with you

Equative (Verb to *be* as main verb)

....is.....................not...a doctor

....was ....late

....were ....on the sofa

May ....be...ill

* When modal auxiliaries are used, the negative is placed between the modal and other auxiliary forms, for example, "Might not have been going."

city), and time (*in a week*) (Scott, 1984a). In general, children with language impairment who exhibit these more complex structures tend to use them less frequently than do children developing normally (J. Johnston & Kamhi, 1984).

Tense markers are used to describe the temporal relationships between events. For example, if the event being described is taking place while the speaker mentions it, the speaker uses the present progressive verb form (auxiliary + verb-*ing*) to indicate an ongoing activity (*walking, eating*). In contrast, the perfect form of the verb (have + verb-*en*) indicates that the action is being described in relation to the present. Thus, "I have been working here for 2 years" implies that this action is still occurring, whereas "I *have eaten* my dinner" implies that the action is now complete. Verb tense analysis can be accomplished in a form similar to that presented in Table 6.18. Table 6.16 identifies the ages at which most preschool children acquire auxiliary and modal auxiliary verbs.

Irregular past tense verbs are a special problem (Shipley, Maddox, & Driver, 1991). English contains approximately 200 irregular verbs. Many are archaic and used infrequently, but the rest, such as *went, saw, sat,* and *ate,* are among the most frequently used verbs. Development begins in the preschool years and extends into adolescence. Their irregular nature precludes rule learning and generalization, and most acquisition is by rote (Bybee & Slobin, 1982; Shipley & Banis, 1989). Some morphophonemic regularities do occur, however, and may influence the relative ease of learning (MacWhinney, 1978; Shipley et al., 1991; Slobin, 1971). The least difficult verbs to learn are those that exhibit no change from present to past, such as *cut/cut* and *hurt/hurt.* The most difficult seem to be those with a final consonant change from /d/ to /t/, as in *build/built* (Shipley et al., 1991). Other morphophonemic changes include internal vowel change (*fall/fell, come/came*), vowel change with added final consonant (*sweep/swept*), total change (*go/went*), and vowel change with a final dental consonant (*ride/rode, stand/stood*). Obviously, other factors, such as the concept expressed (semantics) and the sounds involved (phonology), also affect learning. Table 6.19 presents the ages at which 80% of children are able to use different irregular verbs in a sentence completion task.

Adverbs also mark temporal relations, in addition to manner and result. Temporal relations can be expressed between two events (*before, next, during, meanwhile*), with the continuation of an event (*for the past year, all week*), in the recent past (*recently, just a minute ago*), and with repetition (*many times, again*).

Verb aspect indicates temporal notions, such as momentary actions, duration, and repetition. Momentary actions are of short duration (*fall, break, hit*). In contrast, duration is marked by verbs of longer action with definite beginnings and ends (*sleep, build, make*). Phrases also may be used to convey a definite act

TABLE 6.19
Irregular verbs and age of acquisition

Age in Years	Irregular Verbs
3-0 to 3-5	Hit, hurt
3-6 to 3-11	Went
4-0 to 4-5	Saw
4-6 to 4-11	Ate, gave
5-0 to 5-5	Broke, fell, found, took
5-6 to 5-11	Came, made, sat, threw
6-0 to 6-5	Bit, cut, drove, fed, flew, ran, wore, wrote
6-6 to 6-11	Blew, read, rode, shot
7-0 to 7-5	Drank
7-6 to 7-11	Drew, dug, hid, rang, slept, swam
8-0 to 8-5	Caught, hung, left, slid
8-6 to 8-11	Built, sent, shook

Source: Adapted from Shipley, K., Maddox, M., & Driver, J. (1991). Children's development of irregular past tense verb forms. *Language, Speech, and Hearing Services in Schools, 22,* 115–122.

(*sing a song*), and an act without a well-defined terminal point (*sing for your own enjoyment*). Still other verbs describe repetitive actions (*tap, knock, hammer*).

The development of tense markers seems to be related to the temporal aspect of the verb. The speech-language pathologist should investigate the relationship between tenses the child uses and the verbs to which these tenses are applied. No doubt, this analysis will require a sample larger than a 50– to 100–utterance sample.

Modal auxiliary verbs, such as *can, could, will, should, shall, may, might,* and *must,* are used to express the speaker's attitude (Bliss, 1987). Syntactically, modals function in the formation of questions and negatives. They are used also in such statements as "I *will* do it tomorrow."

As with the pronoun system, modals represent a complex interaction of form, content, and use that is reflected in the slow rate of acquisition, which usually lasts from age 2 to age 8 (Fletcher, 1975; Kuczaj, 1982; Major, 1974; J. Miller, 1981). Semantic categories of modals include wish or intention (*will, would*), necessity or obligation (*must, should*), ability or permission (*can*), certainty (*will*), and probability or possibility (*may, might*) (Bliss, 1987).

Those modals associated with action, such as *can* and *will* (ability, intention, and permission request), are acquired first. During the third year, the number of modals and the categories increases. Beyond age 4, the child clarifies the different forms and their uses (Hirst & Weil, 1982).

Children with language impairment rarely use modal auxiliaries (Menyuk & Looney, 1972; Trantham & Pedersen, 1976), possibly because of the linguistic subtleties expressed. In general, children with language impairment have more difficulty with catenatives, modals, and auxiliary verbs than their language level would suggest (J. Johnston & Kamhi, 1984). The speech-language pathologist is interested in the range and frequency of modals the child exhibits.

Children with LEP and with different dialects may experience difficulty with verb tense and with auxiliary verbs. Irregular past tense verbs may exhibit substitutions. Verb endings may be omitted as a general phonological rule pattern. Verb-subject agreement is also difficult.

When analyzing a sample, the speech-language pathologist pays particular attention to the level of development, the range of semantic concepts, the variety of usage, and the types of errors (Bliss, 1987). Variety of usage is noted with different pronouns, verb tenses, negative and positive statements, and sentence types.

Sentence types.   A single event may be described by the agent that originates the action, the action or state changes, and/or the recipient or object of that action (Duchan, 1986b). The agent as a noun or a noun phrase is usually first, followed by the action word or verb, which in turn is followed by the recipient or object of that action in the form of a noun or a noun phrase ("John threw the ball" or "Mother ate the cookie").

If the agent performs the action for the benefit of some other person, that beneficiary—the indirect object—either precedes or follows the noun phrase describing the object of the action. For example, in "He painted the picture for mother," *for mother* follows the object of the sentence. Instruments used to complete the action usually are placed after the action and follow the preposition *with*, as in "He painted *with a brush*."

Sentences that differ from the predominant subject-verb-object format may be difficult for the child with language impairment to decipher and form. Often, overreliance on the S-V-O strategy is not noted until the child begins school. The child with language impairment may resist rearrangement or interruption of this form and may attach other structures only at the beginning or the end. Yes/no questions may be asked with rising intonation, rather than through transformation of the subject and verb elements. Passive sentences, which use an object-verb-subject form, may be misinterpreted.

The speech-language pathologist is interested in the range of internal sentence forms and in the different sentence types. Sentence types include positive and negative forms of the declarative, interrogative, and imperative. Declarative sentences are statements ("He likes ice cream" or "She does not want to go").

Interrogatives include three types of questions, including yes/no, *wh-* or constituent, and tag. Yes/no questions ask for confirmation or denial in the form of a yes or no response, as in "Did you fix the light?" The form of yes/no questions may vary from a statement with rising intonation ("You went to the store?") to a transformation using the copula or an auxiliary verb ("Is he happy?" or "Did she eat her pie?").

Wh- questions require more information and begin with such words as *what, where, who, why, when,* and *how.* Either the copula or auxiliary verb and the subject are transformed from their order in a statement ("What is her age?" or "Why did he go?"). A less mature form that can be used with some *wh-* questions places the *wh-* word at the end of the sentence ("She likes *what*?"). These types typically are used for clarification, however, and are discussed later.

Tag questions are statements with question tags attached ("She's lovely, isn't she?"). These questions seek only agreement.

The preschool development of questions is given in Table 6.16. Mature tag questions, because of their complex nature and infrequent use in American English, are acquired much later than are yes/no and *wh-* interrogatives. Some children do not master the mature tag form until mid-elementary school (Dennis, Sugar, & Whitaker, 1982; Reich, 1986). A less complex form using *okay* or *alright* (or the Canadian *ah*) may appear in preschool ("I do this, okay").

The range of sentence types and the maturity of form are of interest to the speech-language pathologist. These are listed in Table 6.16.

With more mature speakers, the speech-language pathologist must consider the use of emphasis, pauses, and intonation to mark different meanings for the same form. Pauses mark the end of conceptual units and direct the listener in the type of response required. For example, "Do you like football (pause) or baseball?" requires a very different response from "Do you like football or baseball?" Rising intonation is used on an entire word for unexpected or surprise events, and falling intonation for the expected. As mentioned previously, rising intonation at the end of a word or a sentence signifies a question, and falling intonation signifies a statement.

Imperatives are commands ("Eat your dinner" or "Stop that"). The subject, *you*, is understood. Speech-language pathologists must be careful not to confuse these sentence types with utterances in which the child omits the subject. The child who repeatedly omits the subject in other sentences probably should not be credited with imperative forms.

The behavior of other people may be influenced also by requests. These are discussed in Chapter 4 and in the illocutionary functions section of this chapter because of the pragmatic aspects of this form.

Negative sentences, whether declarative, interrogative, or imperative, also possess characteristic developmental forms (Table 6.16). The child's first negatives are marked by *no* and slightly later by *not*. Initially, these two forms are used interchangeably. To these are added *don't* and *can't*, also used interchangeably, followed by *won't*. Positive forms of *do, can, will*, and *would* develop later, followed by negative forms for the verb *to be* and for other auxiliaries. By school age, the child develops indefinite forms (e.g., *no one, nothing*) and indirect negative imperatives ("Watch out for the hole"). These do not require syntactic negative transformations. During the school-age years, the child masters such negative prefixes as *un-, non-*, and *ir-*.

Embedding and conjoining.   Both embedding and conjoining involve relationships between clauses. In addition, embedding involves the relationships between phrases and clauses.

A *clause* consists of a noun phrase and a verb phrase. A clause that can stand alone is an independent clause or sentence even though it contains only the noun and the verb ("John ran"). Some clauses contain both elements but are not independent. These clauses, such as "that you want," must be attached to an independent clause or sentence in a process called *embedding*. In this manner, "that you want" can be embedded in "The toy is on sale" to form "The toy *that you want* is on sale." Two or more independent clauses can be joined together in a process called *conjoining*.

Clausal embedding initially develops in the object position at the end of the sentence (Table 6.16). Called *object noun complements*, these dependent clauses take the place of the object following such words as *know, think*, and *feel* ("I know *that you can do it*"). Object noun complements using *that* (I think *that I like it*) appear at an MLU of 4.0, most frequently following the verb *think* (Tyack & Gottsleben, 1986). By an MLU of 5.0-5.9, this type of embedding accounts for only 6% of children's two-clause sentences. Object noun complements using *what* ("I know *what you did*") account for 8% of these sentences. Relative clauses attached to nouns develop next, beginning in the object position, as in "I want the dog *that I saw last night*." Finally, the relative clause moves to the center of the sentence, describing the subject, as in "The one *that you ate* was my favorite." During late childhood and adolescence, an increase occurs in relative clauses either attached to the subject or serving as the subject, as in **Whoever wishes to go** *should come to the office*. This type of clausal embedding is more common in written language than in oral (Perera, 1986a, 1986b; Scott, 1988a, 1988b).

Relative clauses appear less frequently than other forms of clausal embedding among preschoolers, although by school age, 20–30% of two-clause sentences may be of this type (Scott, 1984b). Relative clauses appear at about 48 months initially as postnoun modifiers for empty nouns, such as *one* or *thing* (Wells, 1985). The most common relative pronouns for preschoolers are *that* and *what.* During the school years, pronouns expand with the addition of *whose, whom,* and *in which.*

Phrases also may be embedded in clauses. As in clausal embedding, phrasal embedding usually develops initially at the end of the sentence. A *phrase* is a group of related words that does not contain a subject and a verb and are of several types, including prepositional, participial, infinitive, and gerund phrases. Such phrases take the place of nouns or modify nouns. Prepositional phrases also may be adverbial in nature, as in "She will arrive *in a minute.*" During late childhood and adolescence, an increase occurs in both the number and length of adverbial phrases (Scott et al., 1992).

Infinitive phrases first appear in the object position, most frequently following *want* ("I want *drink pop*"). This form with the *to* omitted emerges at a median age of 30 months (Wells, 1985). Infinitives with a different subject from the main verb ("Mommy, I want you *to eat it*") appear somewhat later.

The speech-language pathologist is interested in the number and type of embeddings. Some developmental data are included in Table 6.16. The position of these embeddings within the sentence is also important, given the developmental significance of position.

Clausal conjoining appears relatively late in preschool development, although some conjunctions appear much earlier. Conjunctions express the relationships between two entities, such as words or clauses.

Usually, *and* is the first conjunction learned; it is used to join objects in a group. Throughout the preschool period, *and* continues to be the most frequently used conjunction, being 5 to 20 times more common than *but* (Scott, 1988a). Around 30 months of age, children begin to sequence clauses, using *and* as the initial word in each sentence (Bloom et al., 1980; Lust & Mervis, 1980). As noted in Table 6.16, *and* is also the first conjunction used to join clauses. At this point, *and* is used for sequential events and is interpreted as *and then.* Even among school-age children, 50–80% of all narrative sentences begin with *and* (Scott, 1984b, 1987). With age and an increase in written communication, use of *and* decreases. Between ages 11 and 14, only 20% of spoken narrative sentences begin with *and.* In written narratives, the rate is only about 5% (Scott, 1987). Other conjunctions may express a causal relationship (*because*), simultaneity (*while*), a contrasting relationship (*but*), and exclusion (*except*). Conjunctions develop in the following order: *and, because, when, if, so, until, before, after, since, although,* and *as* (L. Lee, 1974; Loban, 1976; Scott, 1987; Tyack & Gottsleben, 1986; Wells, 1985). The most frequently used conjunctions through age 12 are *and, because,* and *when.*

Early strategies that rely on the order of mention for interpretation may persist with the child with language impairment. Thus, the child ignores the conjunctions and their intended meanings. The sentences "Go to the market before you go to the movie" and "Go to the market after you go to the movie" are interpreted as having the same meaning.

The speech-language pathologist is interested in the range and frequency of the conjunctions used and in the amount of conjoining present in the sample. This information is especially important with more mature speakers and is discussed in the following chapter on narratives.

The speech-language pathologist also should note multiple embeddings and embedding and conjoining that occur within the same sentence. Again, this usage is much more characteristic of school-age language than of preschool language. The narratives of children ages 10 to 12 years are easily distinguishable from those of preschoolers by the presence of multiple embedding and conjoining within the same sentence (Perera, 1986a, 1986b; Scott, 1988a, 1988b).

Computer-Assisted Language Analysis

Several computer-assisted language analysis (CLA) methods are available, each based on some particular model of language structure. CLAs provide the speech-language pathologist with a quick, efficient, standard analysis routine. A normative database currently is lacking but is in preparation (J. Miller et al., 1992). Thus, at present, results are criterion-referenced.

Most CLA formats have three common features (Long, 1991). First, all utterances must be coded to assist the computer in identifying structures. This time-consuming step may be shortened for the speech-language pathologist by having a trained typist make an initial transcription on a disk (J. Miller et al., 1992). The resultant disk can be corrected and readied for analysis by the speech-language pathologist. Second, the computer recognizes, analyses, and tabulates the identified structures from the transcript. Third, the program displays the results in an interpretable format. A list of available CLA syntactic and phonological software is provided in Table 6.20.

Once mastered, CLA is more efficient than analysis by hand; this efficiency increases as the complexity of analysis increases (Long & Masterson, 1993). Although CLAs may quicken the analysis phase of sampling, they cannot replace the clinical intuition of the trained speech-language pathologist. Nor can CLAs fill the deficiency caused by a poorly collected sample. In addition, only the speech-language pathologist can use the data generated to make clinical decisions.

Phonologic Analysis

A phonological analysis should describe the child's phonetic inventory; the syllable structures or word shapes produced by the child; strategies, such as avoidance of certain sounds or use of favorite sounds; and the child's phonological processes (M. Edwards, 1984). Children with SLI and other language impairments often demonstrate difficulty with the regularities of the phonological system (Leonard, Schwartz, Allen, Swanson, & Loeb, 1989). Although all of these data may not be available from one or two conversational samples, it is helpful to recall that every sound in a word provides some data.

The Computerized Assessment of Phonological Processes (Hodson, 1985), the Natural Process Analysis (Shriberg & Kwiatkowski, 1980), and a modified form of the Procedures for the Phonological Analysis of Children's Language (Ingram, 1981) seem to differ little in the amount of information they provide for the selection of intervention targets (Dyson & Robinson, 1987). Nor is there much difference in the phonological processes identified by the three analysis procedures (Paden & Moss, 1985). In addition, testing and sampling results may differ significantly (Morrison & Shriberg, 1992). Thus, a variety of processes should be sampled and, possibly, a combination of procedures used. Computer-assisted analysis software is listed in Table 6.20.

It is important for the speech-language pathologist to recognize that phonological processes are not necessarily errors. For children at certain ages, these rules or processes function as ways for them to produce sounds and sound combinations with which they have difficulty. These rules reflect "natural processes" (Oller, 1974) that act to simplify adult forms of verbal language for young children.

Just as young children simplify sentence structure, they may follow similar rules to simplify words. For example, the 2-year-old who has difficulty with long

TABLE 6.20
Computer-assisted language sample analysis software

Software	Description
Syntax/Morphology	
Automated LARSP (Bishop, 1985)	Based on Language Assessment, Remediation, and Sampling Procedure (LARSP)(Crystal, Fletcher, & Garman, 1976) Calculates MLU Uncoded transcript
Computerized Profiling (Long & Fey, 1988, 1989)	Based on Conversational Act Profile (Fey, 1986), Developmental Sentence Analysis (DSS)(L. Lee, 1974), Profile in Semantics-Lexical (PRISM-L)(Crystal, 1982), Profile of Prosody (PROP)(Crystal, 1982), Profile of Phonology (PROPH)(Crystal, 1982) Calculates MLU and type-token ratio Uncoded transcript
DSS Computer Program (Hixson, 1985)	Based on Developmental Sentence Analysis (DSS) (L. Lee, 1974) Coded transcript
Lingquest 1 (Mordecai, Palin, & Palmer, 1985)	Calculates MLU and type-token ratio Coded transcript
Parrot Easy Language Sample Analysis (PELSA) (F. Weiner, 1988)	Calculates MLU Coded transcript
Pye Analysis of Language (PAL) (Pye, 1987)	Flexible analysis categories Coded transcript
Systematic Analysis of Language Transcripts (SALT)(J. Miller & Chapman, 1985)	Based on Brown's Stages of Development Flexible analysis categories Calculates MLU, NDW, TNW Coded transcript

TABLE 6.20, *continued*

Phonology

Computerized Assessment of Phonological Processes (CAPP)(Hodson, 1985)	Based on Assessment of Phonological Processes (Hodson, 1980) using preselected set of words
Computer Managed Articulation Diagnosis (Fitch, 1985)	Analysis based on preselected set of words
Computerized Profiling (Long & Fey, 1988, 1989)	Analysis based on unrestricted words
Interactive System for Phonological Analysis (ISPA) (Masterson & Pagan, 1989)	Analysis based on unrestricted words
Lingquest 2 (Palin & Mordecai, 1985)	Analysis based on unrestricted words
Process Analysis 2.0 (F. Weiner, 1985)	Analysis based on preselected set of words
Program to Examine Phonetic and Phonologic Evaluation Records (PEPPER)(Shriberg, 1986)	Based on Natural Process Analysis (NPA)(Shriberg, 1986) Analysis based on unrestricted words
Pye Analysis of Language (PAL) (Pye, 1987)	Based on Procedures for Phonological Analysis of Children's Language (Ingram, 1981) Analysis based on unrestricted words

Source: Adapted from Long, S. H. (1991). Integrating microcomputer applications into speech and language assessment. *Topics in Language Disorders, 11*(2), 1–17.

words may adopt the strategies of dropping weak or unstressed syllables, simplifying consonant blends, and omitting final consonants. The resultant word may resemble the target only vaguely, if at all.

These processes are found in all developing children at some stage in their acquisition of verbal language. It is only when these processes do not evolve into more mature strategies that parents, teachers, and speech-language pathologists become concerned. In the following section we discuss the major phonological processes found in young children and the methods for analyzing data from a conversational sample.

Phonological Processes

With first words, children shift to greater control of articulation. Babbling requires less constrained production, but when children add meaning to sound, they need some phonological consistency to transmit their messages. After the onset of meaningful speech, there is much individual variation in the pattern and rate of vocabulary growth, the use of invented words, and the syllable structure of words acquired.

Most first words are monosyllabic CV or VC units or CVCV constructions (C. Ferguson, 1978; Ingram, 1976). Within a given word, the consonants are usually the same or noncontrasting, such as **baby** or **goggie** (doggie). It is the vowels that initially vary. Consonant contrasts usually occur in less frequent CVC constructions, such as *cup* (Waterson, 1978).

Children produce great phonological variation in their early words. The same word may be produced consistently or may vary greatly. The most noticeable phonological patterns among toddlers relate to syllable structure and include open syllables and diminutives, reduplication, and cluster reduction (Table 6.21).

As with other aspects of language, children's phonological development progresses through a long period of language decoding and hypothesis building.

TABLE 6.21
Phonological processes of young children

Processes	Examples
Syllable structure	
Deletion of final consonants	*cu* (/kʌ/) for *cup*
Deletion of unstressed syllables	*nana* for *banana*
Reduplication	*mama, dada, wawa* (water)
Reduction of clusters	/s/ + consonant (*stop*) = delete /s/ (*top*)
Assimilation	
Contiguous	
Between consonants	be*ds* (/bɛdz/), be*ts* (/bɛts/)
Regressive VC (vowel alters toward some feature of C)	nasalization of vowels: *can*
Noncontiguous	
Back assimilation	*dog* becomes *gog*
	dark becomes *gawk*
Substitution	
Obstruants (plosives, fricatives, and affricatives)	
Stopping: replace sound with a plosive	*this* becomes *dis*
Fronting: replace palatals and velars	*Kenny* becomes *Tenny*
(/k/ and /g/) with alveolars (/t/ and /d/)	*go* becomes *do*
Nasals	
Fronting (/ŋ/ becomes /n/)	*something* becomes *somethin*
Liquids: replaced by	
Plosive	*yellow* becomes *yedow*
Glide	*rabbit* becomes *wabbit*
Another liquid	*girl* becomes *gaul* (/gɔl/)
Vowels	
Neutralization: vowels reduced to /ə/ or /a/	*want to* becomes *wanna*
Mixed deletion of sounds	*balloon* becomes *ba-oon*

Source: Ingram, D. (1976). *Phonological disabilities in children.* New York: Elsevier.

During the preschool years, children not only acquire a phonetic inventory and a phonological system but also develop "the ability to determine which speech sounds are used to signal differences in meaning" (Ingram, 1976, p. 22). Some sound contrasts are very difficult for children to perceive and to produce, whereas others are relatively simple. Much of the morphological production of preschool children will depend on their ability to perceive and produce phonological units.

For this discussion, the phonological processes of children (Table 6.21) have been divided into processes relative to syllable structure, assimilation, and phoneme substitution. The greatest reduction in the use of phonological processes occurs between ages 3 and 4 (Haelsig & Madison, 1986), and most processes disappear by age 4.

Syllable structure processes.   From the moment children begin babbling, the basic unit used is the open or CV syllable, one ending in a vowel. When they begin using words, children frequently attempt to simplify production by reducing words to this form or to a CV multisyllable structure.

This basic syllable structure form affects the final consonant (Ingram, 1976; Oller, 1974). Open syllables predominate. Words with final consonants or multisyllabic words are produced frequently in a CV or CV multisyllable form (Waterson, 1978). The final consonant may be deleted, producing a CV structure for a CVC (*cup* may become /kʌ/), or may be followed by a vowel to produce a CVCV structure from a CVC (*cake* may become *cake-ah*). The diminutive, in which the child adds an /i/ to the end of a CVC word (producing *doggie* from *dog*), is another form of this process. Open syllable processes usually disappear in half of the children between ages 3 and 4.

The child also may delete unstressed syllables to simplify word production. Generally, initial unstressed syllables are deleted most frequently. This process usually disappears after age 4.

Reduplication appears to be a step in the acquisition of final consonants. Reduplication occurs when children attempt polysyllabic words (*water*) but are unable to produce the one syllable correctly (C. Ferguson, Peizer, & Weeks, 1973; Menn, 1971). They compensate by repeating another syllable (*wawa*). Usually, either the first or the stressed syllable is reproduced. This process usually disappears by age 3 but may occur occasionally with words that are difficult to produce.

Finally, consonant clusters may be reduced or simplified to one consonant, producing *top* for *stop*. These deletions are predictable and usually adhere to the following patterns:

Cluster	Deletion	Example
/s/ + plosive (/t, p, k/)	/s/	*stop* becomes *top*
plosive or fricative	liquid or glide	*bring* becomes *bing*
+ liquid or glide		*swim* becomes *sim*

Cluster reduction, which usually disappears after age 4, often is followed by a stage in which another sound is substituted for the omitted sound. Some children have continuing difficulty with consonant clusters, and we do not expect mastery until about age 7.

Assimilation processes.   Assimilation processes simplify production by enabling the child to produce different sounds in the same way. In short, one sound becomes similar to another in the same word. The process may occur on contiguous or noncontiguous sounds and may affect following or preceding sounds. For example, young children often produce *doggie* as *doddie* or *goggie,* demonstrating assimilation in either direction.

Substitution processes.   Substitution process are of several types, including stopping, fronting, and backing. Most of these processes are reduced by half between ages 3 and 4 and disappear by age 4. In stopping, plosives are substituted for other sounds. Stopping is most common in the initial position in words (Oller, 1974), as in *dat* for *that.*

In fronting, labial or alveolar sounds are substituted for palatals or velar sounds. For example, /t/ and /d/ might be substituted for /k/ and /g/, producing *tid* for *kid* and *dun* for *gun.* Within nasals, fronting might result also in /n/ being substituted for /ŋ/, producing *rinin* for *ringing.* The speech-language pathologist must be careful not to confuse dialectal variation, in which only the final sound is substituted (e.g., *walkin*), for fronting. In dialectal variation, the /ŋ/ would be modified only on the present progressive marker, producing *ringin* rather than *rinin.* Backing is the reverse of fronting, and back sounds are substituted.

Multiple processes.   To make this puzzle even more difficult for those who must unscramble these phonological patterns, children often use more than one phonological process at a time. For example, *blanket* may become /baeki/ as a result of cluster reduction and open syllabification.

Analysis Steps

Unscrambling is a good term for describing the process of phonological process analysis. Because this analysis is difficult and time-consuming, it should be attempted only when a phonological disorder is suspected from prior data. When analysis is undertaken, however, previously unrecognized patterns may reveal themselves.

The entire sample is transcribed phonetically with the addition of the applicable diacritical markers shown in Table 6.22. Target words and transcribed productions then can be transferred to an analysis sheet similar to that found in Table 6.23. Unintelligible patterns can be determined by having a familiar listener, such as a parent or a teacher, interpret the child's speech from the audiotape.

Because phonological processes are found at the syllable and/or word levels, words are analyzed individually for the presence or absence of these processes. Casual, stylistic, or everyday patterns, such as *runnin'*, *wudja get? get 'um,* and *j'eat yet?* should not be analyzed for phonological processes because they represent a very different sort of behavior.

Words, syllables, and sounds are rated for evidence of various phonological processes. The speech-language pathologist must identify processes and describe the

TABLE 6.22
Diacritical markers

Marker	Meaning	Example
/:/	Full lengthening. Place to right of phoneme to indicate increased duration of production.	Adjacent identical sounds: last time /lst:alm/ Omission of final sound results in vowel lengthening: *car* /kɔ:/
/~/	Nasalization. Place above non-nasal phoneme to indicate nasalization.	*can* /kãn/ *nine* /naɪn/
/÷/	Nasal emission. Place above phoneme to indicate audible emission through nares.	*Pete* /p̈it/
/ⁿ/	Dentalization. Place above phoneme to indicate consonant produced with tongue tip against upper teeth, as done correctly with the /d/ in *width*. Found in fronting processes and in frontal distortion or lisp.	*this* /ð̯ᴵs/ *big* /b̯ᴵg/
/^/	Lateralization. Place above phoneme to indicate a release of air around the sides of the tongue, as in a lateral distortion or lisp.	*miss* /mᴵ§̂/

consistency of each. An individual word may be affected by one or more processes. Where substitutions are suspected, further analysis is attempted at the sound level.

Most individual sound errors will be inconsistent. The data from every consonant in question is evaluated. Of interest is not only the sounds substituted but also the similarity in features of the target and the substituted sound (Fey, 1992a, 1992b). Sound contrasts may be marked by the child but incorrectly. The following procedure of analysis is suggested (M. Edwards, 1984; H. Klein, 1984; Lund & Duchan, 1988):

1. Rate all productions possible by using a form similar to Table 6.24.

2. Compute the percentage of correct production for each sound in question by dividing the number correct by the total number attempted. Note consonants that are never produced correctly.

3. Identify patterns by position in words, manner, place, and voicing of production. An arrangement such as that in Table 6.24 aids in summarizing these data. These patterns may be diagrammed to give a graphic representation of substitutions and omissions (A. Williams, 1993).

4. Sounds that experience variability of substitution patterns should be analyzed for assimilation. This task may necessitate a change in the initial portion of the analysis.

5. Note sounds that may be produced incorrectly when they occur but also may be substituted for other sounds.

TABLE 6.23
Sample phonological process analysis format

Target Word	Word Produced	No Process Evident	*Deletion of Consonants Not in Clusters			Deletion of Unstressed Syllable	Reduplication	Reduction of Consonant Clusters			*Assimilation			*Substitution		
			Init.	Med.	Fin.			Init.	Med.	Final	Init.	Med.	Final	Init.	Med.	Final

Syllable Processes

* Individual phoneme analysis (See Table 6.24) is needed.

229

TABLE 6.24
Sample analysis of phonological processes affecting individual sounds

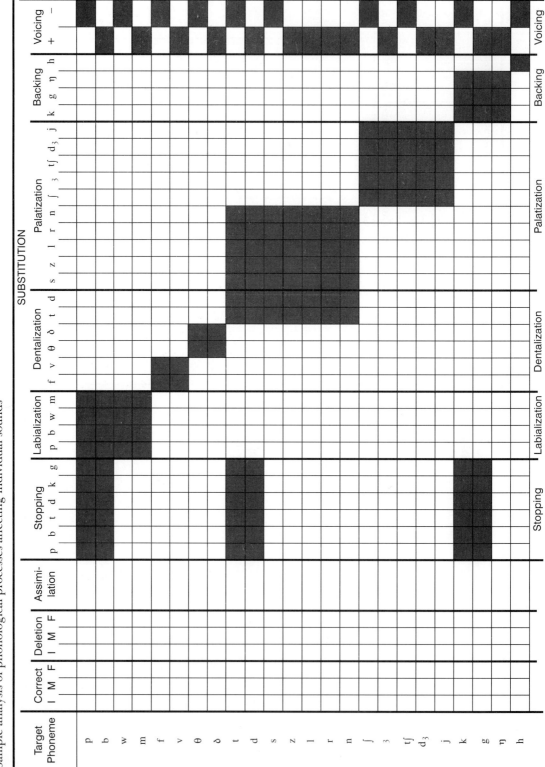

The speech-language pathologist should be cautious when using predetermined rule classification systems such as those in Table 6.24 because more than one rule system may be operating at a time (Fey, 1992b). In addition, naming a rule does not explain it. The speech-language pathologist should take pains to try to explain the process used by the child and hypothesize as to the causal factors.

Not all children with phonological disorders demonstrate the common processes noted in this section (Leonard, 1985). Occasionally, children form idiosyncratic rule systems. In this case, the speech-language pathologist should form hypotheses about the child's rule or rules and test these hypotheses through intervention (Fey & Stalker, 1986).

Although there are few criteria for decisions of impairment, there are measures of severity, such as the process density index (PDI) (M. Edwards, 1992). PDI is calculated by summing the total processes in each word and dividing by the number of words, as illustrated in Table 6.25. PDI scores are related closely to judgments of intelligibility (Wolk, 1990).

TABLE 6.25
Calculating process density index

Process Density Index (PDI) is the sum of the total processes divided by the number of words.

$$PDI = \frac{\text{Total number of processes}}{\text{Total number of words}}$$

Example:

Target	Production	Process	Number
Shoe ⟶	/pu/	sh ⟶ /p/	2 (fronting, stopping)
Stop ⟶	/tɑt/	st ⟶ /t/	1 (cluster reduction)
		p ⟶ /t/	1 (assimilation)
Go ⟶	/doU/	g ⟶ /d/	1 (fronting/dentalization)
Banana ⟶	/dænʌ/	b ⟶ /d/	1 (dentalization)
		nana ⟶ /nʌ/	1 (Syllable deletion)
		TOTAL	7

$$PDI = \frac{7}{4} = 1.75$$

Judgments of intelligibility are difficult to obtain. At present, most speech-language pathologists make gross estimates based on the severity of the phonological impairment (Gordon-Brannon, 1994). Severity can be expressed as a percentage of the words spoken. If 80 of 100 words are comprehended, then the percentage correct is 80%. Unfortunately, this value does not directly correlate to subjective judgments of intelligibility.

Scaled scores, such as 1–7 representing degrees of intelligibility, also may be assigned to a speech sample. Although accomplished more quickly, scaled scoring is not as valid as percentage correct (Kwiatkowski & Shriberg, 1992).

Selection of intervention targets can be based on different criteria suggested by a number of specialists (Dunn & Barron, 1982; Dyson & Robinson, 1987; M. Edwards, 1983; Grunwell, 1982; Hodson & Paden, 1983; Ingram, 1976, 1983; Shriberg, 1983; Shriberg & Kwiatkowski, 1980; Weiner, 1981). These criteria can be summarized as follows:

1. Select processes that occur frequently (at least 40% of the time) but are optional (less than 100% of the time).
2. Select processes that affect stimulable sounds or sounds within the child's phonetic inventory.
3. Select processes that will have the greatest effect on intelligibility.
4. Select processes that affect early developing sounds. Developmental data are included in Appendix B.

Obviously, it is impossible to meet all of the criteria at once. The knowledgeable speech-language pathologist will have to determine the most effective criteria for the clinical model.

The speech-language pathologist should describe the child's phonetic inventory—those sounds in the child's repertoire—and the child's phonemic inventory—those contrasts in the child's repertoire. It is easy to forget the child's abilities when focusing on disabilities.

Children With LEP and Different Dialects

The oral language of children who speak English as a second language or speak a nonstandard dialect will be affected to some degree by L1 or by that dialect. The speech-language pathologist must know enough about those language systems to evaluate the child's performance (Hamayan & Damico, 1991). It is best for children with LEP if the speech-language pathologist evaluates in both L1 and English. Common phonological errors of children with LEP are listed in Table 6.26.

It may be helpful for the speech-language pathologist to enlist the help of the child's language community. Teachers and aides from the child's community can be trained to rate phonological patterns in children on the basis of their own standards of severity (Bleile & Wallach, 1992). The data then can be applied to children with possible language impairments. Community standards then become the criteria for determination of disorder.

TABLE 6.26
Common phonological errors of children with LEP

Target sounds	Common errors
Vowels - American English vowel system is extremely complex.	
Back vowels	Not present in repertoire; many vowels fronted.
Long and short vowels	No duration difference.
Diphthongs	Reduced to single vowel sound.
Consonants	
Unvoiced consonants	Omitted in the final position.
Voiced consonants	Devoiced, especially in the final position.
Blends, clusters, and affricatives	Reduced to single sound.
/f,v/	Produced as labials. Some Asian languages have no labiodentals.
/d, t, n, l/	Produced as linguadentals
/Θ/	Produced as /d/
/w,u/	No lip rounding
/ʃ, ʒ, ts, dʒ/	Experience fronting
/h/	Palatalized
/r/	Distorted, trilled, or flapped. Not found in most Asian languages.

The speech-language pathologist will have to train herself to listen and transcribe carefully the child's oral language. For example, African American children delete final consonants but also mark the deletion of voiced consonants with lengthening of the preceding vowel (Moran, 1993). To note only the deletion is to do a disservice to the child. The lengthening is the child's method for marking the consonant.

CONCLUSION

The conversational sample is a rich source of data about children's language. Each utterance can be analyzed for a variety of language features within the five aspects of language. Obviously, such analysis is time–consuming. Speech-language pathologists should analyze only areas of suspected difficulty rather than attempt a blanket analysis.

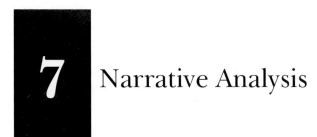

7 Narrative Analysis

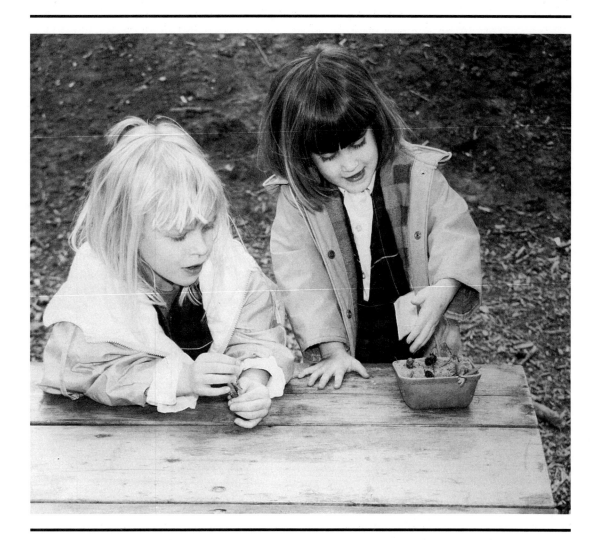

Narratives are a self-initiated, self-controlled form of discourse. As such, narratives are an important part of the language assessment of older school-age children and adolescents because they provide an uninterrupted sample of language that the child or adolescent modifies to capture and hold the listener's interest (Chappell, 1980; Crais & Chapman, 1987; Culatta, Page, & Ellis, 1983; J. Johnston, 1982b; Liles, 1985a, 1985b, 1987; Scott, 1988b).

Although narration and conversation share many qualities, they differ in very significant ways. First, narratives are extended units of text. Second, events within narratives are linked with one another temporally or causally in predictable ways. Narratives are organized in a cohesive, predictable, rule-governed manner representing temporal and causal patterns of relating information not found in conversation. Third, the speaker maintains a social monologue throughout. The speaker must produce language that is relevant to the overall narrative while remaining mindful of the information needed by the listener.

Many students incorrectly equate narratives with fictional storytelling. This misunderstanding leads to narrative evaluation consisting of the child or adolescent recounting fairy tales or formulating stories from pictures. For the purposes of language analysis, we consider *oral narration* to include the telling of self-generated stories, storytelling of familiar tales, retelling of movies or television shows, and recounting of personal experiences. Most conversations include narratives of this latter type. How often we begin conversations with, "You'll never believe what happened to me coming to work today," or, "Let me tell you what it means to get into a hassle."

Although conversation and narratives share many elements, such as a sense of purpose, relevant information, clear and orderly exchange of information, repair, and ability to assume the perspective of the listener, they are not the same thing (F. Roth, 1986). Conversations are dialogues, whereas narratives essentially are decontextualized monologues.

In decontextualized narratives, the language does not center on some ongoing activity, but usually communicates some experience not directly shared by the speaker and the listener. To share the experience, the speaker must present an explicit, topic-centered discussion that clearly states sequential and causal relationships.

The major characteristics found in narratives but not in conversation are the agentive focus and the temporal contingent structure (Longacre, 1983). Narratives are about agents—people, animals, or imaginary characters—engaged in events over time. Other differences include the narrative use of extended units of text, introduction and organizing sequences that lead to a narrative conclusion, and the relatively passive listener role that provides only minimal informational support to narratives (F. Roth, 1986).

The narrative speaker is responsible for ordering and providing all of the information in an organized whole (F. Roth & Spekman, 1985). Narratives, therefore, are found more frequently in the communication of more mature speakers and should be included in an analysis of the language of school-age children. The clinical importance of narratives can be summarized as follows:

Narrative analysis is one of the most valuable skills a language clinician can possess. People of all ages from all cultures experience stories daily . . . in representing events in their own lives and in participating in the happenings, both real and imaginary, in the lives of others. Knowledge of story structure contributes to people's understanding of how the world functions, facilitating predictions of actions and consequences, causes and effects. (Hedberg & Stoel-Gammon, 1986, p. 58)

Some studies have failed to find significant differences between the narratives of children with language impairment and those without (Hedberg & Fink, 1985; Klecan-Aker, 1985; Ripich & Griffith, 1985; F. Roth & Spekman, 1989b). In general, though, the narratives of children with language impairment such as LLD are shorter and less mature and have less mature episode and sentence structure than those of age-matched peers developing normally (Merritt & Liles, 1987, 1989; F. Roth & Spekman, 1986). Possibly because of the communication demands placed on the child in narration, the narratives of children with LLD exhibit a greater rate of communication breakdown in the form of stalls, repairs, and abandoned utterances (MacLachlan & Chapman, 1988). Although children with LLD and those without display similar patterns of cohesion, such as the use of conjunctions and unambiguous reference, children with LLD are less efficient in their use (Klecan-Aker, 1984; Liles, 1985a). In general, children with LLD use fewer conjunctions and exhibit more ambiguous reference, often failing to consider the needs of their audience (Liles, 1987). The internal story organization of children with language impairment is also less complete than that of age-matched peers (Merritt & Liles, 1987). The narratives of children with language impairment contain more statements that are not integrated into the episode structure than do those of children without impairment. Usually, such children have difficulty describing and manipulating props and activities (Sleight & Prinz, 1985).

DEVELOPMENT OF NARRATIVES

Before the appearance of first words, children have well-established notions of agents, actions, and objects and of the relationships these have to each other and to such notions as location and negation (Bates, 1979; Golinkoff, 1981; Robertson & Suci, 1980). They also have some understanding of familiar events and of the positions of some actions at the beginning, middle, and end of sequences (Bruner, 1975; DeLemos, 1981; Ninio & Bruner, 1978; Ratner & Bruner, 1978). Although children by age 2 possess basic ideas, called *scripts*, about familiar events and sequences, they are not able to describe sequences of events until about age 4 (Karmiloff-Smith, 1981; K. Nelson & Gruendel, 1979; Peterson & McCabe, 1983; Slobin, 1973).

Children speaking American English begin to tell self-generated, fictional narratives between ages 2 and 3 (Sutton-Smith, 1986). These stories may have a vague plot and usually center on certain highlights in the child's life. There is little recognition of the need to introduce, to explore with, or to orient the listener to the story, and these stories usually lack easily identifiable beginnings, middles, and ends. Disquieting events are the theme and are repeated with endless variation. Frequently children repeat phenomena that they find disruptive or extraordinary in their own lives, such as danger, violence, and deprivation (Ames, 1966).

Two-year-olds usually construct additive chains in which one sentence is added to another, as in, "This is kittie. This doggie bowl." There is no story line, no sequencing, and no cause and effect. The sentences may be moved anywhere in the text without changing the meaning of the entire text. Additive chains may describe a scene, as in, "There is kittie. Water in doggie bowl. Doggie sleep." Again, there is no temporal structure.

In these early stories is a dominance of performance and textual qualities over text (Sutton-Smith, 1986). Sound production and prosody may be used to move the story along at the expense of information (Scollon & Scollon, 1981). Between ages 3 and 7, children's narratives gradually change from prosodic poetry to prose with plots (Sutton-Smith, 1986). It is not until age 8 that children can tell narratives really well. Narration is a complex task that requires skill and practice.

Temporal event sequences emerge between ages 3 and 5. Events follow a logical sequence, for example:

> There is this kittie. He runs to door. Then he goes outside to play. He rolls in the grass and then goes to sleep in the sun.

Although there is sequencing, there is no plot and no cause and effect or causality. Temporal chains often exhibit third person pronouns, past tense verbs, and temporal conjunctions (e.g., *and, then, and then*) and have a definite beginning and ending.

Causal chains are infrequent until ages 5 to 7. Causality involves descriptions of intentions and unobservable states, such as emotions and thoughts, and the use of causal connectives. This development also can be seen among children speaking Spanish (Gutierrez-Clellan & Iglesias, 1992). Although 2- and 3-year-olds have mastered some causal expressions, they are unable to construct coherent causal narratives (Kemper & Edwards, 1986). Their stories consist predominantly of actions from which physical and mental states must be inferred. Initiations and motivations are largely absent.

Causality can be seen, however, in the use of agency, connectives, plans, scripts, and descriptions of mental states used by 2- and 3-year-olds to describe their own behavior (Kemper & Edwards, 1986). A plan is a means or series of actions intended to achieve a specified end. As an intention, a plan is a model of causality. Many of the first words of children refer to intentions and consequences, such as *all gone, there, uh-oh,* and *oh dear.* By age 2, the child has acquired the words to describe perceptions (*see, hear*), physical states (*tired, hungry*), emotions (*love, hate*), needs, thoughts (*know*), and judgments (*naughty*) (Bretherton & Beeghly, 1982).

Scripts form an individual's expectations about event sequences and, as such, are an attempt to impose order on event information (J. Johnston, 1982b). Based on actual events, scripts are not content free, as are story grammars that outline narratives. Scripts influence our interpretation and our telling and retelling of events and narratives.

Children's understanding of *agency,* the ability of humans to initiate actions and to respond with mental states, develops gradually between ages 1 and 3. By age 3, children also are able to describe chains of events within familiar activities, such as a birthday party (K. Nelson, 1981b). These familiar activity sequences or scripts (K. Nelson, 1981b) are causally and temporally ordered events within routine or high-frequency regularized activities.

"To tell a story, a child must be able to relate the chain of events in such a way as to explain what happened and why" (Kemper & Edwards, 1986, p. 14). The elements of event knowledge are seen in the narratives of 4-year-olds. Underlying every story is an event chain, a chronology of events. Events include actions, physical states (e.g., possession, attribution), and mental states (e.g., emotions, dispositions, thoughts, intentions) that are linked causally as motivations, enablements, initiations, and resultants in the chain. Causal explanations are a repetitive cycle of these events. Children gradually learn to link events serially and only later with causal connectives (Hood & Bloom, 1979). Psychological causality, such as motive, is used more frequently than physical causality or the connection between events in the narratives of 4- to 9-year olds (McCabe & Peterson, 1985). Connectives are acquired in the following order: *and, and then, when, because, so, then, if,* and *but* (Bloom et al., 1980). The fuller adult range of connectives (*therefore, as a result of, however*) is acquired gradually during the school years.

Between ages 2 and 10, the child's stories begin to contain more mental states and more initiation and motivation as causal links (Kemper & Edwards, 1986). Around age 4, children's stories begin to contain more explicit physical and mental states. Agentive actions or natural or social processes influence characters' thoughts and emotions. By age 6, children's stories describe motives for actions.

Generally, it is not until age 6 that children's narratives are causally coherent (Kemper, 1984). Narratives require the skill to manipulate content, plot, and causal structure. Although 4- and 5-year-olds have many narrative elements in their conversation, especially about common plans and scripts, they do not have the linguistic skill to weave all the elements into a coherent narrative. Between ages 5 and 7, plots emerge consisting of a problem and some resolution of that problem. Gradually, these simple plots are elaborated into a series of problems and solutions or are embellished from within.

Narratives of 7-year-olds typically involve a beginning, a problem, a plan to overcome the problem, and a resolution. Both adults and children prefer goal-directed stories, such as the overcoming of an obstacle, to non-goal-directed stories (Stein & Policastro, 1984). The plot usually centers around the past actions of a clearly fictional main character, allowing the storyteller greater flexibility. The presentation is manipulated dramatically by performance.

Causal chains may go through stages of development before they emerge as full goal-directed narratives. For example, the narrative may be truncated as in the following:

> And there was a big dragon who stole the princess and burned all the land.
> So, this little guy with a sword fixed everything up. The end.

In this example, the problem is solved, but it is unclear how this occurred. Similarly, the problem may be resolved but not because of the intervention of the principals in the story. An example of this type of story is the very complex and complicated problem that is solved when one character awakens to find that it was all a dream.

By second grade, the child may use not only beginning and ending markers (*once upon a time, lived happily ever after, the end*), but also evaluative markers, such as *that was a good one*. Story length increases, greatly aided by syntactic devices such as conjunctions (*and, then*), locatives (*in, on, under, next to, in front of*), dialogue, comparatives (*bigger than, almost as big as, littlest*), adjectives, and causal statements. Although disquieting events are still central to the theme, there has been a change from inconsistent to consistent characters and from distinct but similar episodes to a chronology (as yet there is no fully developed plot).

The sense of plot in fictional narratives is increasingly clear after age 8 (Labov, 1972; Peterson & McCabe, 1983; Sutton-Smith, 1981, 1986). Now there is definite resolution of the central problem. The child's presentation relies primarily on language, rather than on performance. The child manipulates the text and the audience to maintain attention.

In general, the narratives of older children are characterized by the following (J. Johnston, 1982b):

Fewer unresolved problems and unprepared resolutions

Less extraneous detail

More overt marking of changes in time and place

More introduction including setting and character information

Greater concern for motivation and internal reactions

More complex episode structure

Closer adherence to the story grammar model

Children learn to recognize, anticipate, respond to, tell, and read narratives within their homes and their language community. Because different sociocultural groups provide different learning situations for children, various types of narratives emerge (Heath, 1986b). Although every society allows children to hear and produce at least four basic narrative types, the distribution, frequency, and degree of elaboration of these types vary greatly. The four genres include three factual types, called *recounts, eventcasts,* and *accounts,* and fictionalized *stories* of animate beings who attempt to realize some goal (Stein, 1982).

The recount, common in school performance, brings to present attention those past experiences the child participated in, read about, or observed. Someone in authority usually asks the child to verbalize this shared experience. This form occurs infrequently outside of middle- and upper-class school-oriented families.

The eventcast is a verbal replay or explanation about some current or future event. A child often uses eventcasts to direct the actions of others in imaginative play or to try to influence others' behavior. Use of eventcasts enables the child to consider and analyze the effect of language on others.

Accounts seem to be the preferred form for children's spontaneous narratives. Within accounts, children share their experience ("You know what?"). Children initiate this narrative form, rather than report information requested by adults. Therefore, accounts are highly individualized.

In contrast, stories have a known and anticipated pattern or structure. Language is used to create the story form, and the listener plays a necessary interpretive function.

In middle- and upper-class school-oriented families, the earliest types of narratives are eventcasts that occur during nurturing activities, play, and reading with children. Caregivers share many accounts and stories, and by age 3, children are expected to appreciate and use all forms of narration. Invitations to give recounts decrease with age.

By the time most children begin school, they are usually familiar with all four forms of narration. This is not true for all children. In a white, working-class Southern community referred to as Roadville, recounts, tightly controlled by the interrogator, are the predominant form throughout the preschool years. Accounts do not begin until children attend school. Children and young adults also tell few stories, which seem to be the province of older, higher status adults (Heath, 1983).

In contrast, working–class, African American, Southern children produce mostly accounts or eventcasts and have only minimal experience with recounts because of the difficulty in gaining adult attention. As long as these children remain within their families and communities, their language helps them maintain a positive self-image. These children are at a disadvantage, however, when they encounter the expectations of educational institutions (Heath, 1986a). Likewise, Chinese American children are encouraged to give accounts within, but not beyond, their families.

Students with LLD demonstrate knowledge and use of story grammars but convey and recall less information (Weaver & Dickinson, 1982). In addition, children with LLD retrieve less information and make fewer inferences than do children who are non-LLD (Hansen, 1978; Oakhill, 1984). Although the stories of children with LLD contain all of the elements in the generally appropriate order, they are substantially shorter and contain fewer and more poorly organized complete episodes (Liles, 1990). Episodes are also less likely to be related linguistically (F. Roth & Spekman, 1985). In addition, more statements of children with language impairment are not integrated into the episode structure (Liles, 1990). This paucity of information may reflect a lack of presuppositional skills (F. Roth, 1986).

COLLECTING NARRATIVES

The quality of the narrative is influenced by the selection of appropriate stimuli and topics based on the age, verbal ability, interests, and gender of the child or adolescent (Hedberg & Stoel-Gammon, 1986). Stimuli may include objects or pictures used for original constructions and heard or read stories used for retelling. In general, the task used to elicit the narrative influences the speaker's adaptation to the listener.

As only one linguistic form used in communication, narratives should form only a portion of any child's language analysis. The results should be compared with the child's other linguistic abilities prior to making judgments on the adequacy of the child's language system.

There are many different types of stories and many different contexts within which to tell them. The story type and context affect the eventual narrative form produced (Scott, 1988b). In general, maximally naturalistic topics and contexts elicit the most representative narratives (Peterson & McCabe, 1983). Other variables that may affect the narrative form are the story genre, the child's experiential base, the task in which the narrative is told, the source of the narrative, the topic, the formal or informal atmosphere of the context, and the audiovisual support available (Scott, 1988b).

Because the unit of analysis is the entire narrative, several narratives must be collected. The wide variation in narratives that can be produced by a single child within different contexts supports this notion. Prior to collecting, the speech-language pathologist decides on the type of narratives desired and the stimuli to be used in their collection.

In general, fictionalized narratives with a vicarious experiential base may result in incomplete narratives with little emphasis on goals, characters' feelings or motivations, and endings. The pace, action orientation, and frequent commercial interruption found in television form a very different base for narratives than does experience or even traditional fables or fairy tales (W. Collins, 1983; W. Collins, Wellman, Keniston, & Westby, 1978).

The type of elicitation task will affect the child's performance (Baggett, 1979; Cook-Gumperz & Green, 1984; Gibbons, Anderson, Smith, Field, & Fischer, 1986; Griffith, Ripich, & Dastoli, 1986; Warden, 1976). Books elicit descriptive information, whereas films elicit action sequences (Gibbons et al., 1986). Films also elicit more causal sequences in retelling than do oral stories (Baggett, 1979). Pictures tend to constrain the form of the narrative and may lead to the production of additive chains. Stories in response to pictures tend to exclude character information, internal responses, or intentions (Griffith et al., 1986). Shared information may be omitted and new information treated as old even when the listener has not viewed the picture (Warden, 1976). In contrast, photographs or discussions of familiar events foster temporal chains.

Narrative retelling and recall can be used to determine the child's memory organization (Graybeal, 1981; Lovett, Dennis, & Newman, 1986; Stein, 1982). In narrative retelling, the child listens to a well-formed story and then reconstructs the story orally or in writing. Retelling of short narratives even may serve as a screening tool with young elementary school children (Culatta et al., 1983). At this age, children should be able to retell the story without deviating significantly from the original in sequence or content.

In general, children with language impairments produce longer and more complete story grammars in retold narratives than in self-generated ones (Merritt & Liles, 1989). Clause length is also greater in retold narratives. Comprehension can be assessed within retold narratives by questioning the child when the retelling is complete. In general, children with LLD perform much like younger children, recalling less of the stimulus story (Crais & Chapman, 1987).

It is important to consider the amount of structure inherent in the stimulus and its effect on retold story construction. For example, nondescript dolls or puppets or sets of vehicles provide no structure. In contrast, a sequence of related pictures provides maximal structure. In general, the more structure found in the stimuli, the less structure the child must provide. Thus, a greater degree of structure is found in the stories of children with language impairment if this structure is provided by the stimuli (Lemme, Hedberg, & Bottenberg, 1984; Merritt & Liles, 1989). Possibly, the child is better able to use the cognitive schema of story organization within the retold narrative format.

In story retelling tasks, the speech-language pathologist must consider the comprehension skills needed to understand the story, the mode of presentation (oral or written), story length, the child's past experience with the story genre (e.g., fairy tale, mystery), the child's interest in the content, and the degree of story structure (Hedberg & Stoel-Gammon, 1986). In general, more familiar, more interesting, and more structured stories result in more complete, better organized retellings.

Well-formed stories should be chosen for retelling, and these should be modified to enhance clarity and organization (Gordon & Braun, 1983, 1985). Stories should be rewritten to reduce complexity in their oral form and to summarize important sections. Subparts and transitions between parts of the narrative may need to be highlighted. Good narrative models often have repetitive elements, such as those found in myths, fables, and fairy tales (Westby, 1985).

Independent, self-generated narrative production requires the child to use her or his own organizational structure and narrative formulation. Narratives can be classified as fictional, personal-factual, or a combination of the two. Fictional or make-believe stories are good vehicles for preschoolers and may be stimulated by objects or pictures (F. Roth & Spekman, 1986; Westby, 1984, 1985). The speech-language pathologist should provide a model narrative, begin the story for the child, or ask the child to relate a story about the object or picture, beginning with, "Once upon a time. . . ." This initial structure usually results in a more literate style.

Personal-factual narratives may be collected from conversation or prompted. This type of narrative is very common in preschool and early elementary school, especially in show-and-tell activities. Preschoolers naturally create these types of narratives in conversation with each other (Preece, 1987).

The speech-language pathologist should not try to elicit these narratives with open-ended prompts, such as, "What did you do yesterday?" It may be helpful for the speech-language pathologist to establish some common experience with the child and to share a narrative about this experience as an example for the child. To get a narrative, the speech-language pathologist has to give one. Using a combination of narration and probing questions (Peterson & McCabe, 1983), the speech-language pathologist can tell a personal story related to a common event, such as going to the doctor, and prompt the child with leading questions to stir the child's memory of past events ("Have you ever been to the doctor? Have you ever hurt yourself?"). Experiential topics prompted in this fashion usually result in the longest and most complex narratives (Peterson & McCabe, 1983).

At least three story prompts should be used to elicit as many narratives from the child (McCabe & Rollins, 1994). Topics such as a new sibling or a death usually result in very truncated narratives. The child can be prompted also to relate the scariest or funniest thing that ever happened (Garnett, 1986). In addition, the child might be asked to relate a favorite movie, television show, or story, although these prompts may elicit a sequential list of events.

The speech-language pathologist should add nothing to the child's narrative other than feedback in the form of "uh-huh," "okay," "yeah," "wow," or a repetition of the child's previous utterance. These neutral but enthusiastic responses will not influence the course of the story as others might. The narrative can be resumed or the child prompted to continue by such utterances as, "And then what happened?"

Stories are enhanced also by familiarity with the physical setting and with the listener. The speech-language pathologist should decide ahead of time on strategies for terminating rambling stories and for probing to elicit longer ones. A suggested guideline is not to expect children to engage in storytelling unless their MLU is 3.0 or more (Hedberg & Stoel-Gammon, 1986).

NARRATIVE ANALYSIS

Narrative analysis is a portion of an overall language analysis. As with dialogues, narratives can be analyzed in several ways, such as narrative levels, story grammars, and cohesive devices (J. Johnston, 1982b; Lahey & Silliman, 1987; Westby, 1984). Narrative levels are concerned with the structural relationship of the narrative parts to the narrative as a whole. Events may be seemingly unorganized or organized sequentially or by causality.

Narrative levels do not have a goal-based organization, whereas story grammars (what happens in the story) do. Narrative level analysis is most appropriate for the stories of 2- to 5-year–olds (Applebee, 1978) and for school-age children with limited verbal abilities; story grammar analysis is best for those over age 5 (Glenn & Stein, 1980). The narratives of preschool children may be evaluated also by using high-point analysis to determine the type of narrative structure (McCabe & Rollins, 1994).

Story grammars describe the internal structure of a story, including its components and the rules underlying the relationships of these components (Mandler & Johnson, 1977; Rummelhart, 1975; Stein & Glenn, 1979; Thorndyke, 1977). By serving as a framework, story grammars may facilitate narrative processing (Snyder & Downey, 1983). Ideally, components of a story are told in a way that increases understanding. Story grammars may be used to remember and interpret stories (Christie & Schumacher, 1975; Mandler & Johnson, 1977; Stein & Glenn, 1979; Whaley, 1981) and to anticipate content (Baggett, 1979).

Cohesion analysis (Halliday & Hasan, 1976) describes the linguistic devices used to connect the elements of the text. In narratives, coherence, or making sense, is conveyed through cohesion. For example, appropriate use of anaphoric reference provides cohesion and indicates topical links across utterances (Newman et al., 1986). Inappropriate or inadequate use of cohesive devices results in a disjointed text that is difficult to comprehend. For example, individuals take longer to comprehend sentences in which a pronoun can refer equally to two previously mentioned nouns (Caramazza, Grober, Garvey, & Yates, 1977).

From the analysis, the speech-language pathologist should address the following questions (J. Johnston, 1982b):

- Does the narrative contain chains? If so, what type?
- Does the narrative follow the typical story grammar model? Is the story organized maturely?
- What are the guiding scripts of the narrator, and what do they reveal about the storyteller's knowledge of events and expectations?
- What linguistic means are used to create a cohesive unit?

In addition, the speech-language pathologist is interested in the sensitivity of the narrator to the perceived needs of the listener.

Narrative Levels

Children use two strategies for organizing their stories: centering and chaining (Applebee, 1978). *Centering* is the linking of attributes or objects to form a story nucleus. The links may be based on similarity or complementarity of features. Similarity links are formed by perceptually observed attributes, such as actions, characteristics, and scenes or situations. Causal links are not present, although sequential ones may be. Complementary links consist of conceptual bonds based on abstract, logical attributes, such as members of a class or events linked by cause-and-effect bonds. *Chaining* consists of a sequence of events that share attributes and leads directly from one to another.

Most stories of 2-year-olds are organized by centering. By age 3, however, nearly half of the children use both centering and chaining. This percentage increases, and by age 5, nearly three-fourths of the children use both strategies.

These organizational strategies can result in six basic developmental stages of story organization (Applebee, 1978), presented here in developmental order:

> *Heaps* are sets of unrelated statements about a central stimulus. The statements identify aspects of the stimulus or provide additional information.

The common element may be the similarity of the grammatical structure, for there is no overall organizational pattern.

> Dogs wag their tails and bark. Dogs sleep all day. A dog chased a cat.

Sequences include events linked on the basis of similar attributes or events that create a simple but meaningful focus for a story. The organization is additive, and sentences may be moved without altering the narrative.

> I *ate* a hamburger. And Johnny *too*. Mommy *ate* a chicken nuggets. Daddy *ate* a fries and coke.

Primitive temporal narratives are organized around a center with complementary events.

> I go outside and swing. Bobby push swing. I go high and try to stop. I fall. And I start to cry. Bobby pick me up.

Unfocused temporal chains lead directly from one event to another, while linking attributes, such as characters, settings, or actions, shift. This is the first level of chaining, and the links are concrete. As a result of the shifting focus, unfocused chains have no centers.

> The man got in his boat. He rowed and fished. He ate his sandwich. (Shift) The fishes swimmed and play. Fishes jump over the water. Fishes go to a big hole in the bottom. (Shift) There's a dog in the boat. He's thirsty. He jump in the water.

Focused temporal or causal chains generally center on a main character who goes through a series of perceptually linked, concrete events.

> This boy, he found a jellybean. And his mother said not to eat it. And he did. And a tree growed out of his head.

Narratives develop the center as the story progresses. Each incident complements the center, develops from the previous incident, forms a chain, and adds some new aspect to the theme. Causal relationships may be concrete or abstract and move forward toward the ending of the initial situation. There is usually a climax.

> There was a boy named Tommy. And he got lost in the woods. He ate plants and trees. And he was friends with all the animals. He builded a tent to live in. One day, he builded a fire, and the policemen found him. They took Tommy home to his mommy and daddy.

Each narrative is divided into episodes that are analyzed according to this scheme. Table 7.1 contains examples of narratives and their analysis by narrative level.

High-Point Analysis

High-point analysis is a method for identifying narrative macrostructure. The high point, or most significant point of a narrative, is revealed not in the past events recalled, but in an event's meaning to the narrator. The accompanying structure has developmental significance.

TABLE 7.1
Narrative level analysis

Example	Classification
Simple frames Granma lives on a farm. There are horsies and piggies. The cows moo. I can ride on the tire swing in a tree. And the calf licked me. That's all.	Sequence
Once there was two kids, Joey and . . . and Fred. Fred's a funny name. And they was fighting. Their mother said, "Why are you fighting?" Joey and Fred doesn't know why. They stop and be friends.	Focused chain
Complex narrative frame with episodic development The kids all went to Burger King on Halloween. Super John—that's me—got a cheeseburger. My sister got a Big Mac. Mommy and Daddy got nuggets and salad bar.	Sequence
They were eating when a big ghost came out of my milkshake. He threw milkshake on everyone and got them mad. Super John stuck the ghost with a fork. The ghost got flat. All the air came out. Daddy was so happy that he buyed ice cream cones for all the kids.	Narrative

It is best to use narratives that describe events in which the narrator is present (McCabe & Rollins, 1994). The speech-language pathologist should separate the narratives and select the longest personal event narratives for analysis. Length and complexity have been shown to be related (McCabe & Peterson, 1990). The narratives of some children with language impairment may have very poorly defined boundaries that make this demarcation difficult.

The evaluated high point is marked by children in many ways. These markings include paralinguistic features, such as emphasis, elongation, and use of environmental noises ("It went BOOM!"); and linguistic features, such as exclamations ("Wow!"), repetition, attention getters ("Here's the best part."), exaggeration, judgments or evaluative statements ("It was my favorite."), emotional statements, and explanations (McCabe & Rollins, 1994).

Once she has identified the high point of the narrative, the speech-language pathologist can analyze for narrative structure. Different types of structures are presented in Table 7.2. Next to each is the age at which these structures are most common for Caucasian, English-speaking, North American children. The speech-language pathologist can use this table to determine whether the child is using narrative structures typical of his age group.

After age 5, fewer than 10% of children produce one-event, two-event, leap-frog, and miscellaneous narratives (Peterson & McCabe, 1983). No children over age 6 produce leap-frog narratives. The chronological narrative type, common at all ages, is of little diagnostic value (McCabe & Rollins, 1994). Obviously, a small sample of a few narratives will be needed for an adequate evaluation.

TABLE 7.2
High-point narrative structure

Narrative Structure	Characteristics	Expected Age in Years
One-event narrative	Contains one event.	Below 3.5
Two-event narrative	Contains 2 past events but no logical or causal relationship in the real world or in the narrative.	3.5
Miscellaneous narrative	Contains 2 or more past events that in the real world are logically or causally related.	Very low frequency at all ages (3.5–9)
Leap-frog narrative	Contains 2 or more related past events, but the order does not mirror the real-world relationship.	4
Chronological narrative	Contains 2 or more related past events in a logical or causal sequence without a high point.	Present at all ages (3.5–9)
End-at-high-point narrative	Contains 2 or more related past events in a logical or causal sequence with a high point but no following events (resolution).	5
Classic narrative	Contains 2 or more related past events in a logical or causal sequence with both a high point and a resolution.	6+

Source: Adapted from McCabe, A., & Rollins, P. R. (1994). Assessment of preschool narrative skills. *American Journal of Speech-Language Pathology, 3*(1), 45–56.

Normal variations are to be expected within and across children. Many young children will "test the waters" by stating the high point first ("I got stung by a bee.") and, if accepted, then proceeding with the narrative. This is not an example of impaired narration and can be analyzed by using the suggested narrative structures.

Cultural differences must be considered too. African American children often tell topic-associating narratives in which events that happened at different times and places may be combined around a central theme (Michaels, 1981). The narratives of Japanese children may be succinct collections of experiences, rather than single detailed sequential events (Minami & McCabe, 1991). Children from Latino cultures often do not relate sequential events (Rodino, Gimbert, Perez, Craddock-Willis, & McCabe, 1991).

Story Grammars

Story grammars provide an organizational pattern that can aid information processing (J. Johnston, 1982b). The competent storyteller constructs the story and the flow of information in such a way as to maximize comprehension. The speech-language pathologist should note the story grammar elements present and produce a model of the child's story grammar (F. Roth, 1986).

A *story* consists of the setting plus the episode structure (story = setting + episode structure) (J. Johnston, 1982b). Each story begins with an introduction contained in the setting, as in "Once upon a time in a far-off kingdom, there lived a prince who was very sad . . ." or "On the way to work this morning, I was crossing Main Street. . . ."

An *episode* consists of an initiating event, an internal response, a plan, an attempt, a consequence, and a reaction. An episode is complete if it contains an initiating event or response to provide a purpose, an attempt, and a direct consequence (Stein & Glenn, 1979). Episodes may be linked additively, temporally, causally, or in a mixed fashion. A story may consist of one or more interrelated episodes.

The seven elements of story grammars occur in the following order (Stein & Glenn, 1979):

1. Setting statements (S) that introduce the characters and describe their habitual actions, along with the social, physical, and/or temporal context and that introduce the protagonist.

2. Initiating events (IE) that induce the character(s) to act through some natural act (e.g., an earthquake), a notion to seek something (e.g., treasure), or the action of one of the characters (e.g., arresting someone).

3. Internal responses (IR) that describe the characters' reactions, such as emotional responses, thoughts, or intentions, to the initiating events. Internal responses provide some motivation for the characters.

4. Internal plans (IP) that indicate the characters' strategies for attaining their goal(s). Children rarely include this element.

5. Attempts (A) that describe the overt actions of the characters to bring about some consequence, such as attain their goal(s).

6. Direct consequences (DC) that describe the characters' success or failure at attaining their goal(s) as a result of the attempt.

7. Reactions (R) that describe the characters' emotional responses, thoughts, or actions to the outcome or preceding chain of events.

The two very different stories in Table 7.3 present examples of story grammars.

There appears to be a sequence of stages in the development of story grammars (Glenn & Stein, 1980). Certain structural patterns appear early and persist, whereas others are rather late in developing. The apparent developmental sequence is as follows:

Descriptive sequences consist of descriptions of characters, surroundings, and habitual actions. There are no causal or temporal links. The entire story consists of setting statements.

This is a story about my rabbit. He lives in a cage. He likes to hop around my yard. He eats carrots and grass. The end.

Action sequences have a chronological order for actions but no causal relations. The story consists of a setting statement and various action attempts.

I had a birthday party. (S) We played games and won prizes.(A) I opened presents. (A) I got balloons. (A) I blowed out the candles. (A) We ate cake and ice cream. (A) We had fun. (A)

TABLE 7.3
Story grammar examples

Narrative	Story Grammar Elements
I. Single Episode	
There was this boy, and he got kidnapped by these pirates.	Setting statement (S) Initiating event (IE)
So when they were eating, he cut the ropes and got away.	Attempt (A) Direct consequence (DC)
And he lived on a island and ate parrots.	Reactions (R)
II. Multiple episode	
Once there was this big dog on a farm.	Setting statement (S)
And he got hungry 'cause there wasn't enough food.	Initiating event$_1$ (IE$_1$)
The dog . . . His name was Max . . . was sad with no food, so his owner went to find some.	Internal response$_1$ (IR$_1$) Attempt$_1$ (A$_1$)
He met a witch, but she wouldn't give him food 'til he killed a yukky toad.	Initiating event$_2$ (IE$_2$)
He was scared but he decided to build a trap.	Internal response$_2$ (IR$_2$) Internal plan$_2$ (IP$_2$)
He dug a hole and filled it with frog food.	Attempt$_2$ (A$_2$)
The frog wanted to eat the man but got caught.	Direct consequence$_2$ (DC$_2$)
The man went back to the witch and she got some hamburgers for the man and the dog.	Direct consequence$_1$ (DC$_1$)
And the man and Max ate hamburgers and were happy.	Reaction$_1$ (R$_1$)

Reaction sequences consist of a series of events in which changes cause other changes with no goal-directed behaviors. The sequence consists of a setting, an initiating event, and action attempts.

> There was a lady petting her cow. (S) And the cow kicked the light. (IE) Then the police came. (A) Then a fire truck came. (A) Then a hook-and-ladder came. (A) And that's the end. (S)

Abbreviated episodes contain an implicit or explicit goal. At this level, the story may contain either an event statement and a consequence or an internal response and a consequence. Although the characters' behavior is purposeful, it is usually not premeditated.

> There was a mommy and two kids. (S) And the kids baked a cake for the mommy's birthday. (S) They forgot to turn on . . . off the stove and burned the cake. (IE) The kids went to the store and bought a cake. (C) The end. (S)

Complete episodes contain an entire goal-oriented behavioral sequence consisting of a consequence statement and two of the following: initiating event, internal response, and attempt.

This man was a doctor. (S) He made a monster. (IE) And it chase him around his house. (IE) He run in his bedroom. (A) He push the monster in the closet. (A) And the monster go away. (C) That's all. (S)

Complex episodes are expansions of the complete episode or contain multiple episodes.

Once there was this Luke Skywalker. (S) And he had to fight Darf Invader. (S/IE) They fighted with swords. (A) And he killed him. (C) And he got in his rocket to blow up these kind of horse robots. (IE) And he shot them. (A) Then all the bad soldiers were killed. (C)

Interactive episodes contain two characters who have separate goals and actions that influence each other's behavior.

Sally never helped her mom with the dishes. (S) She got mad and said that Sally had to do it. (IE) So, Sally washed the dishes but she was mad. (IR) Then Sally dropped some dishes. (A) Then she dropped more. (A) And her mom said that she didn't have to do any more dishes. (C) And Sally watched TV every night after dinner. (S)

Specific structural properties associated with each structural pattern are listed in Table 7.4.

TABLE 7.4
Structural properties of narratives

Structural Pattern	Structural Properties	Structural Pattern	Structural Properties
Descriptive sequence	Setting statements (S)(S)(S)	Complex episode	Multiple episodes
Action sequence	Setting statement (S)		Setting statement (S)
	Attempts (A)(A)(A)		Two of the following:
Reaction sequence	Setting statement (S)		Initiating event (IE$_1$)
	Initiating event (IE)		Internal response (IR$_1$)
	Attempts (A)(A)(A)		Attempt (A$_1$)
Abbreviated episode	Setting statement (S)		Direct consequence (DC$_1$)
	Initiating event (IE) or		Two of the following:
	Internal response (IR)		Initiating event (IE$_2$)
	Direct consequence (DC)		Internal response (IR$_2$)
Complete episode	Setting statement (S)		Attempt (A$_2$)
	Two of the following:		Direct consequence (DC$_2$)
	Initiating event (IE)		Expanded complete episode
	Internal response (IR)		Setting statement (S)
	Attempt (A)		Initiating event (IE)
	Direct consequence (DC)		Internal response (IR)
			Internal plan (IP)
			Attempt (A)
			Direct consequence (DC)
			Reaction (R)
		Interactive episode	Two separate but parallel episodes that influence each other

Children with LLD produce fewer mature episodes than do their age-matched peers who are non-LLD. In addition, children with LLD make less complete setting statements and are less likely to include response, attempt, and plan statements in their narratives (F. Roth & Spekman, 1986). Interepisodic relations are also weaker in the narratives of children with LLD.

Unfortunately, there are few normative data for clinical use. In general, children developing normally produce all of the elements of story grammar by age 9. Children's narratives can be used, however, to approximate their functioning level and to determine which structural elements are present (Hedberg & Stoel-Gammon, 1986). Table 7.5 contains several narratives analyzed by story grammar structural pattern and narrative level.

Cohesive Devices

Text consists of the linguistic properties of a narrative, not the form of individual sentences (J. Johnston, 1982b). Of interest in the text are cohesive devices that linguistically connect the components. In short, any sentence element that sends the listener outside of the sentence for a referent is a cohesive device. For example, a pronoun may require referral to the previous sentence in order to determine the referent. The five types of cohesive relations are reference, substitution, ellipsis, conjunction, and lexical items (Halliday & Hasan, 1976). Of these, lexical cohesion may be the most difficult to assess reliably (Liles, 1990).

Children with language impairment and those with poor reading abilities exhibit some difficulty communicating well-organized, coherent narratives (Norris & Bruning, 1988). In general, they produce event and sentential relationships more poorly than do their age-matched peers (J. Johnston, 1982b; Liles, 1985a, 1985b, 1990; Merritt & Liles, 1985). The most common cohesive errors among children with language impairment are an *incomplete tie,* in which the child references an entity or event not introduced previously, and an *ambiguous reference,* in which the child does not identify to which of two or more referents she or he is referring (Liles, 1990).

Cohesion repairs require particular organizational strategies not found in conversation. Older children, aged 8.5 to 12.5, most often make meaning repairs in narratives and in conversation, recognizing the importance of being comprehended successfully (MacLachlan & Chapman, 1988; Purcell & Liles, 1992). Cohesion repairs of one of the five types mentioned previously also are made frequently by both children developing normally and those with language impairment, but with different levels of success (Purcell & Liles, 1992). In general, both types of children are equally successful with repairs within T-units, usually consisting of single word repair. In repairs across T-units, requiring reorganization of several sentences, however, children with language impairment are less successful. This difference may reflect underlying language skills and processes (Butler, 1986; L. Miller, 1984; Snyder-McLean & McLean, 1978; VanKleeck, 1984; Wallach & Liebergott, 1984).

Because there is little normative data on the development of these relations, descriptive analysis is the best diagnostic approach. In general, mature story gram-

TABLE 7.5
Story grammar analysis

Narrative	Story Grammar Elements	Structural Pattern	Narrative Level
I.			
We went to a farm.	(S)		Unfocused
I got to feed chickens.	(S)		temporal
Then I saw cows in the barn.	(S)	Descriptive	chain
Cows give milk.	(S)	sequence	
Cows stay in the field all day and eat grass.	(S)		
At night they come in.	(S)		
II.			
There was this boy who lived in a city.	(S)		Focused
And one day a giant bug got out of this place where they keep bugs.	(IE)	Reaction sequence	temporal chain
And the boy got in an airplane and shot it.	(A)		
III.			
Once there was two boys.	(S)		
One boy fell into a big hole	(IE$_1$)		
with rats and he was scared.	(IR$_1$)		
His brother got a ladder but	(A$_1$)	Complex	
the rats ate it.	(DC$_1$/IE$_2$)	episodes	Narrative
So, he threw his lunch in the hole.	(A$_2$)		
The rats ate it, too, and the	(DC$_2$)		
boy climbed up a rope and was safe.	(R)		

Even though the third narrative possesses advanced structural properties, it demonstrates some pronoun confusion. The relationship of the boys is not established until the third utterance.

mar develops prior to mature use of cohesive devices. It is possible, therefore, to have good episodes but poor cohesion. The two are related but not dependent. The cohesion within and between episodes becomes important as children develop complex and interactive episodes. There is a metalinguistic quality about cohesion in that the speaker must pay attention to the text apart from the story itself. Cohesive relations are discussed in Chapter 5 and are reviewed only briefly in this section.

Reference

Reference devices, which refer to something else in the text for their interpretation, consist of pronouns, definite articles, demonstratives, and comparatives. The link with the referent should be clear and unambiguous. Clarity is often a problem when the child changes the story narrator frequently, uses dialogue, or includes several characters. Pronouns and definite articles are used to refer to referents previously identified in the narrative.

In contrast, demonstratives locate referents on a continuum of proximity. Nominals, such as *this, that, these,* and *those,* refer to a person or a thing; adverbs, such as *here, there, now,* and *then,* refer to a place or a time. Use of *now* and *then* usually is restricted to referring to the time just mentioned. In addition, *now* and *then* can serve as conjunctions.

Finally, comparatives are both general, referring to similarities and differences without reference to a particular property, and specific, referring to some specific quantity or quality. General comparatives include such words as *another, same, different(ly), equal(ly), unequal, identical, similar(ly),* and *else.* Specific quantity words include *more, less, so many, as few as, second, further,* and *fewer than.* Quality words and terms consist of *worse than, as good as, equally bad, better, better than, happier than,* and *most happy/happiest.*

Substitution and Ellipsis

Substitution and ellipsis both refer to information within the narrative that supposedly is shared by the listener and the speaker. In substitution, another word is used in place of the shared information. The words *one(s)* and *same* can be substituted for nouns, as in "Make mine the *same*" or "I'll take *one,* too." Such words as *do* can be substituted for main verbs, as when we emphasize, "I *did* already." Finally, such words as *that, so,* and *not* can be substituted for whole phrases or clauses, as in, "I think *not*" or "Mother won't like *that.*"

Ellipsis differs from substitution in that shared information simply is omitted. Whole phrases and clauses may experience ellipsis. Any portion of the noun phrase may be omitted, as in the following examples:

> I have *four of her brightly wrapped red gifts.* Which is *yours*? Would you like *two*? Do you have *green*?

Verbal material also may be omitted, as in the response, "He can't," to the question, "Will John attend the concert tonight?" Clausal ellipsis may be demonstrated with the same question when the answer is "Probably."

Conjunction

The four types of conjunctive relations are additive, temporal, causal, and adversative. Whereas additive relationships usually are represented by *and,* temporal ones may be signaled with a variety of words, such as *then, next, after, before, at the same time, finally, first, secondly,* and *an hour later.* Causal conjunctive relationships may be expressed with a variety of terms, such as *because, as a result of, in that case, for,* and *so.* Finally, adversative conjunctions include *but* and others, such as *however, although, on the other hand, on the contrary, except,* and *nevertheless.*

Conjunction use may be independent of the specific clausal structure linked (Halliday & Hasan, 1976). In other words, conjunctions link the underlying semantic concepts and thus represent the relationship of these units, which many differ from the syntactic units. The way episode parts are linked may reflect the child's underlying episodic organization. We would expect, therefore, that conjunctive relationships between episodic elements would be more complex and difficult from those between sentences. This increase seems to be true for both children with language impairment and those without (Liles, 1987).

Lexical Items

Words themselves express relationships by the morphological endings used. For example, the present progressive *-ing* ending is used to express actions taking place at the present time. The following example demonstrates a clear understanding of the relationship of the process to the product:

> He *had been writing* for several months. After the book was finally *written*, he celebrated for days. He swore never *to write* another novel.

Categorical relationships can be expressed and demonstrate convergent and divergent organizational patterns. Convergent thought goes from the members to the category, as in "She had *petunias, dahlias, roses, and pansies* in her garden, but she could never have enough *flowers.*" Divergent thought goes from the category to the members, as in "She liked several kinds of *sports* but was best at *soccer, rugby, and lacrosse.*"

Finally, words can express relationships, such as opposition or part-to-whole. In a narrative, the speech-language pathologist can look for antonyms, synonyms, ordered series, and part-whole or part-part relationships. Ordered series include memorized sequences, such as the days of the week, or hierarchies, such as instructor-assistant professor-associate professor-full professor. Part-whole relationships are expressed by entities that form a portion of the whole, as in rudder-boat, pedal-bike, and January-year. Finally, part-part relations contain parts of the same whole, as in nose-chin, finger-thumb, and rudder-sail.

Reliability and Validity

Narrative analysis is not without its detractors. The reliability and validity of narrative analysis as a clinical tool has been questioned (Klecan-Aker & Carrow-Woolfolk, 1987). Naturally, reliability and validity will vary with the aspects of narratives measured.

Establishing developmental level by the number of story grammar components present appears to have very high inter- and intrajudge reliability (Klecan-Aker & Hamburg, 1991; Klecan-Aker, Swank, & Johnson, 1991). This developmental level and other quantitative measures, such as words per T-unit and words per clause, also correlate strongly with language test scores, suggesting that narrative analysis has strong construct validity.

CHILDREN WITH LEP AND DIFFERENT DIALECTS

Children entering school with good narrative abilities are better prepared to comprehend and produce the decontextualized language of reading and writing (Gee, 1989; Westby, 1984). Other children are at greater risk of academic failure (Orum, 1986; U.S. Bureau of the Census, 1990). To tell, retell, or comprehend the literate narratives found in English, a child must have a concept of story grammar and a cultural script for the story. An evaluative technique such as "Tell me a story" may be irrelevant to children not exposed to bedtime or other similar storytelling situations (Heath, 1982).

Narrative performance among various cultural, ethnic, and linguistic groups may differ greatly. These differences reflect both cultural and individual differences in storytelling. Thus, "storytelling is never context free" (Gutierrez-Clellan & Quinn, 1993, p. 2). Rather, it is the product of the contextual interaction of the narrator and the audience and of the sociocultural norms of each, which shape each's presuppositions and expectations. Even the purpose and context for narratives varies across cultures.

Telling narratives is a social event governed by cultural norms and values. Not every culture expects the narrative monologues seen in American English. Among some Latinos, Native Americans, African Americans, Jewish Americans, and Hawaiian Americans, stories are produced conversationally with audience cooperation (Erickson, 1984; Phillips, 1982; Schiefflin & Eisenberg, 1984; Scollon & Scollon, 1979, 1981; Tannen, 1982; Watson-Gego & Boggs, 1977). The story is built by the storyteller acting out the parts as the audience challenges and contradicts.

Narrative completeness will reflect also each child's experience and world knowledge (B. Ross & Berg, 1990). Pictures and topics that are used to elicit the child's narrative may be beyond the child's experiential base and result in diminished performance. It is difficult for children to tell stories with unfamiliar scripts. A child unfamiliar with a farm, for example, may use the word *truck* for *tractor* and *garage* for *barn*.

Even the temporal qualities of narratives reflect the temporal realities of different cultures. The importance to seconds, minutes, and hours in Western culture is not found in others. A good friend once told me of his grandfather, a Cherokee elder, who measured time by the slow, purposeful movement of the earth and moon.

Many of the aspects of narrative analysis discussed previously are based on American English forms and cultural expectations, such as the narrative organization and the use of linguistic devices. The analysis in this chapter assumes that all narratives are composed of an elaborated story grammar. In contrast, the narratives of Japanese children are very sparse, consisting of two-unit episodes: a complication and a consequence (Clancy, 1980).

Likewise, the narratives of African American children have less formal beginnings and endings and less chronology while containing more judgments on characters and their actions (Heath, 1983). In addition, the stories of African American and Puerto Rican children embed such evaluations within the narrative and are less likely than Caucasian children to state the point of the story explicitly at the end (Iglesias, Gutierrez-Clellan, & Marcano, 1986; Labov, 1972).

Grammatical contrasts offer further examples. In Spanish, referential cohesion is demonstrated in the introduction of and the later referral to different entities in the story. Characters, props, and places may be referenced by the nominal (*un nene/ a boy*), elliptical (*El fue a la tienda, cogio un poco de comida/ He went to the store, got some food*) (Gutierrez-Clellan & Heinrichs-Ramos, 1993, p. 560), or the demonstrative (*este/this*). In addition, characters and props may be referenced by the pronominal (*elle/she*). With increasing age, Spanish-speaking and English-speaking children use ellipsis more for place (Black, 1985; Gutierrez-Clellan & Heinrichs-Ramos, 1993). Once the setting has been introduced, it is not named again unless changed.

Whereas the use of ellipsis in English requires previous nominal reference, speakers of Spanish may omit referential information because verb endings mark this information (*tuve/I had; tuviste/you had*). A child speaking Spanish who is familiar with this practice may omit nominal reference in English too, giving the impression that he does not understand cohesion.

Still, there is much similarity in narrative development. By age 4, children speaking Spanish have a wide range of referential strategies. The nominal and elliptical forms are used for characters in the subject position, while pronominals are used for those in the object (Gutierrez-Clellan & Heinrichs-Ramos, 1993).

As children speaking Spanish get older, a greater number of props and places are introduced, and their narratives become more detailed, though not necessarily much longer (Gutierrez-Clellan & McGrath, 1991). More and more information is embedded, decreasing the number of sentences needed to express the same information. Redundant information is omitted. The number of characters changes little, however, from ages 4.5 to 8 years.

Children speaking Spanish develop causal sequences at about the same age as children speaking American English. From ages 4 to 9, there is a decrease in two-clause causal sequences and in the proportion of unrelated statements, and an increase in three-clause causal sequences (Gutierrez-Clellan & Iglesias, 1992). Action sequences predominate as a means of moving the story forward. Physical and emotional states as the cause of result of change tend to remain stable from ages 4 to 9.

Other devices, such as paralinguistics, may be used by other cultures more than in the majority American culture, which tends to rely on rising and falling intonation (Gee, 1986; Gumperz, Kaltman, & O'Connor, 1984; Michaels, 1981, 1986; Scollon & Scollon, 1979, 1981). For example, African American and Puerto Rican children use more loudness, pitch, rate, stress, rhythm, and intonation, along with exclamations and repetitions than majority children to move the story forward and to make evaluative or emotional comments (Heath, 1983; Iglesias et al., 1986; Labov, 1972). In other cultures, false starts and hesitations function as internal organizers, while slower pace through repetition, redundancy, and silence may signal the point of the story or its conclusion (Gee, 1986, 1989; Scollon & Scollon, 1979, 1981).

Narrative Collection and Analysis

The cultural variability of narratives requires the speech-language pathologist to assess narrative development in a wide variety of culturally relevant contexts approaching the natural environment of the child (Gutierrez-Clellan & Quinn, 1993). If the child does not consider the task "worthy," he may give less than his optimum or even typical performance (Iglesias et al., 1986).

The speech-language pathologist may err on the overly cautious side by assuming that all differences are cultural or that the child can only produce narratives of a familiar type in familiar contexts. A third option, discussed previously, is a dynamic assessment that evaluates the child's learning potential or teachability (Feuerstein, Rand, Jensen, Kaniel, & Tzuriel, 1987).

A dynamic assessment consists of two steps: collection/analysis and mediation (Gutierrez-Clellan & Quinn, 1993). In the first step, the speech-language pathologist collects several narratives in different contexts and analyzes each for the "rules" appropriate for that type of narration. The characteristics of each type of narration based on temporal, referential, causal, and spatial coherence are included in Table 7.6 (Gutierrez-Clellan & Quinn, 1993). The speech-language pathologist must remember that the "rules" for certain types of narration may be unfamiliar to some children and may be a difference, rather than a deficit. The types of cohesion used by the child should reveal his narrative style.

TABLE 7.6
Types of narration and cohesion

Temporal Coherence
> Is there a temporal order of events?
> Are temporal connectives necessary? If so, are they used?
> Are shifts in time marked?

Causal Coherence
> Are physical and mental states used to interconnect actions? (He was very tired, so he
>   went to sleep)
> If not, can connectives be inferred easily?
> Are causal connectives necessary? If so, are they used?

Referential Coherence

> **Participants**
> > Is adequate reference to the participants made?
> > Are new characters introduced clearly? If not, are they referred to as if introduced
> >   elsewhere in the text?
> > Are characters reintroduced in an unambiguous manner?
> > Can the referent be inferred from general world knowledge?

> **Props**
> > Is identification of specific objects necessary? If so, are props mentioned adequately?
> >   If not, are props introduced by gestures or deictics, such as "that thing"?
> > Can the identity of props be inferred from descriptions or functions?

Spatial Coherence
> Is information about location necessary? If so, are locations identified?
> Are shifts in location clearly marked?

Source: Gutierrez-Clellan, V. F., & Quinn, R. (1993). Assessing narratives of children from diverse cultural/lingual groups. *Language, Speech, and Hearing Services in Schools, 24,* 2–9.

In the second step, the different types of narratives are explained to the child by using cues, such as, "Talk like a book in school," or, "Talk like you would to a friend," and examples. Within the training, the child is given different types of narratives to produce. Feedback is used by the speech-language pathologist to seek clarification, additional information, relevant comments, and reference. After some intervention, the speech-language pathologist should attempt to determine whether the child can learn different types of narration, can transfer the types of cohesion across contexts, and can tell narratives without cuing and feedback.

Two measures that seem particularly important are the length of causal sequences and the number of unrelated statements. Among children speaking Spanish, an increase in the length of causal sequences and a decrease in the number of unrelated statements are indicators of greater causal cohesion (Gutierrez-Clellan & Iglesias, 1992).

Dynamic procedures work well with children from different sociocultural backgrounds (Feuerstein, 1979; Lidz, 1987; Pena & Iglesias, 1989; Sewell, 1987). The procedures require that the task be explained, that the reasons for certain responses be stated adequately, and that the child respond differentially to the speech-language pathologist's cues (Gutierrez-Clellan & Quinn, 1993).

CONCLUSION

In general, the more mature the narrative, the more complete the structure and the story grammar. In addition to causal chains, more mature narratives contain greater cohesion to aid the listener in interpretation. Mature narratives are structurally cohesive and proceed from one event to another in a logical fashion that demonstrates the narrator's attempt to guide the listener.

More mature narratives also include more insight into the thoughts and feelings of the central characters and greater use of devices for expressing time and place. There are fewer extraneous details and loose ends.

The speech-language pathologist should be cautious when evaluating children from cultures whose narratives do not closely follow the literary pattern described in this chapter. Children from some Spanish-speaking and some Native American cultures may have less experience with story narratives. To varying degrees, these cultures make extensive use of more descriptive narratives. The use of pictures and elicitation techniques, such as, "Tell me a story about this picture," may evoke a very different narrative from what is sought.

The near universal use of some form of narrative suggests, however, its importance in communication. As in dialogue analysis, it is important to analyze narratives simultaneously at several levels. Although there are few normative data on narrative development against which to compare a child's or adolescent's performance in any culture, the speech-language pathologist can use the model described in this chapter to analyze and describe performance.

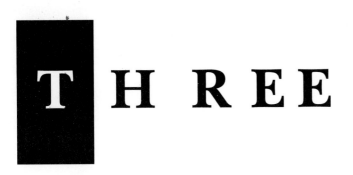

THREE

Intervention

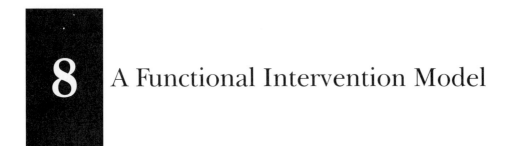

8 A Functional Intervention Model

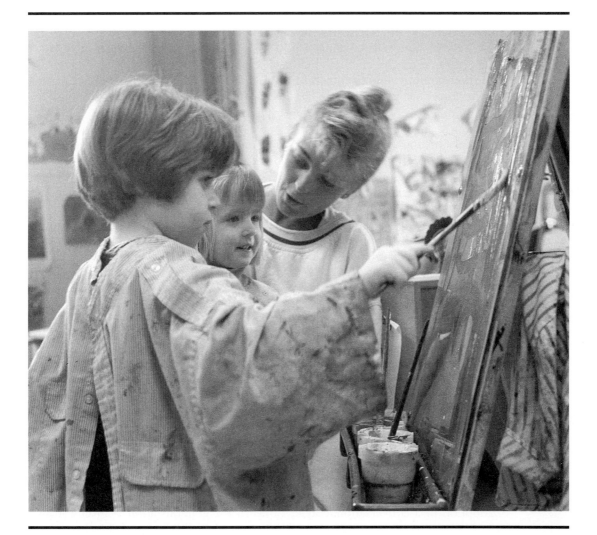

Traditional language intervention does not consider either the integrated nature of language or the context of language use. Language is viewed as a hierarchically organized set of rules, rather than as a holistic set of variable context-sensitive rules (Rice, 1986). Thus, traditional language intervention usually focuses on isolated linguistic constructs without considering the interrelationship of these units (Gullo & Gullo, 1984). Although the focus may include form, content, and use, the overall design is usually additive, rather than integrative (Craig, 1983). Often, the stated goal is to learn specific language units, not enhance communication. Language methods that emphasize very specific skills seem to have very specific, limited effects (Leonard, 1981). Although structured approaches may generalize to situations that differ in one or two respects from the teaching environment, there is little evidence that newly acquired forms will generalize to everyday conversational use (Leonard, 1981; Mulac & Tomlinson, 1977; Olswang & Bain, 1991; Stokes & Baer, 1977; Warren & Rogers-Warren, 1980; Welch, 1981; Zwitman & Sonderman, 1979).

Clinical intervention should be a well-integrated whole in which the various aspects of language combine to enhance communication (Snow et al., 1984). The purposes of intervention should be (a) to teach a generative repertoire of linguistic features that can be used to communicate in socially appropriate ways and (b) to stimulate overall language development (Russell, 1993; Warren & Kaiser, 1986a).

A functional language intervention model attempts to target language features that the child uses in the everyday context, such as the home or the classroom, and to adapt that context so that it facilitates the learning of language. Table 8.1 presents a comparison of the traditional language intervention model with a functional integrated approach.

The functional approach recognizes a need to orient language training toward the inclusion of family members and teachers as language facilitators and toward the use of everyday activities for encouraging functional communication (Mahoney & Weller, 1980). Therefore, routines within the home, school, and community are used with an array of language facilitators (Gullo & Gullo, 1984; McCormick, 1986; Rice, 1986). In this way, aspects of language can be trained as they relate to one another within the context of a meaningful experience. As a result, the intervention experience more closely approximates patterns of nonimpaired language development. Content is based on common experiences.

This functional approach, with its integrative and interactive aspects, changes the nature of the clinical interaction and the role of the speech-language pathologist (McDermott & Hood, 1982; Shultz, Florio, & Erickson, 1982). The speech-language pathologist becomes a consultant for the other language facilitators, who interact more frequently with the child, training them to modify the contexts within which language can occur and to elicit and modify the child's language. The speech-language pathologist and caregivers collaborate in the child's language intervention.

Functional language intervention, however, requires more than just the adoption of a conversational style. Concern for generalization is foremost and

TABLE 8.1
Comparison of traditional and functional intervention models

Traditional Model	Functional Model
Individual or small group setting using artificial situations.	Individual or small or large group setting within contextually appropriate setting.
Isolated linguistic constructs with little attention to the interrelationship of linguistic skills.	Relationship of aspects of communication stressed through spontaneous conversational paradigm.
Intervention stresses modeling imitation, practice, and drill.	Conversational techniques stress message transmission and communication.
Little attention to the use of language as a social tool during intervention sessions.	The use of language to communicate is optimized during intervention sessions.
Little chance or opportunity to develop linguistic constructs not targeted for intervention.	Increased opportunity to develop a wide range of language structures and communication skills through spontaneous conversation and social interaction.
Little opportunity to interact verbally with others during intervention.	Increased opportunity to develop communication skills by interacting with a wide variety of partners.

Source: Adapted from Gullo, D., & Gullo, J. (1984). An ecological language intervention approach with mentally retarded adolescents. *Language, Speech, and Hearing Services in Schools, 15,* 182–191.

governs the overall intervention approach because the goal is to train language useful in the everyday context. Planning by the speech-language pathologist, along with the language facilitators, is essential. Implementation and generalization may be hampered or impeded by any number of factors, such as the targets selected, the intervention setting, the training methods used, and caseload and scheduling considerations.

Intervention should begin with a generalization plan (Stremel-Campbell & Campbell, 1985) that identifies features of the child's communication environment relevant to generalization. All too often, generalization is the last step in the intervention planning process, rather than the overall organizing aspect.

Once the appropriate generalization variables have been identified, the speech-language pathologist can begin to design intervention strategies. The relevant features of the communication environment that have been identified can now be enlisted. Ideally, such intervention enables the speech-language pathologist to (a) develop linguistic constructs at the child's developmental functioning level, taking into account the strategies children normally use when acquiring language, (b) integrate all linguistic areas within the communication framework, and (c) provide meaningful and age-appropriate contexts (Gullo & Gullo, 1984).

In this chapter we discuss principles of intervention of the functional approach and an overall model for intervention, focusing on the variables that affect generalization.

PRINCIPLES

Use of a functional approach to language intervention requires the speech-language pathologist to change some methods and to be mindful of certain principles that aid communication with and learning for the child. It is important to engage the child in a meaningful dialogue or in some other communication event, and this event must become the vehicle for learning and generalization.

The following section includes some of the most important principles of the functional approach. Undoubtedly, some important ones have been omitted that the reader will want to include in her or his repertoire.

The Language Facilitator as Reinforcer

As communicators, we continue to interact with individuals who provide positive feedback and reinforcement. Each of us avoids communicating with certain individuals who are nonresponsive, caustic, or overly critical. Children avoid certain potential conversational partners for many of the same reasons. If speech-language pathologists want children to communicate with them, then they must be people with whom children want to communicate.

The way the speech-language pathologist approaches children is very important for future communication. By reducing the authority figure persona, demonstrating an attentiveness and a willingness to adopt the child's topics, and remaining accepting while providing evaluative feedback, the speech-language pathologist can send a message of acceptance of the child as a partner. Most children will respond in kind.

Children respond most readily to adults who convey genuine caring and respect for them. These attitudes are conveyed by the adult who tries to meet the child halfway. Adults who desire to be effective conversational partners must appreciate the world from a child's perspective. Events easily understood by an adult may be quite incomprehensible to a young child. It may help to recall that for children the world is full of wonder and delight, full of things that cannot be explained, and full of magic.

Adults demonstrate concern for children when they are willing to attend to children, to listen, and to accept their topics. As much as possible, intervention should be nonintrusive, with facilitators providing supportive, evaluative feedback to the child.

An important question in the intervention setting is, What sense is the child making of this situation? The child's sense of things will influence behavior and language within that situation (Duchan, 1986a). An activity that seems very concrete to the facilitator, such as looking at pictures, might be very abstract for the preschool child.

Few child linguistic responses are totally wrong. Even seemingly incorrect utterances demonstrate the child's understanding of the situation and of the underlying relationships. Acceptance of the child includes acceptance of these utterances. Usually, some portion of the utterance can be reinforced.

CHILD: I need ear-gloves.
SP-LANG PATH: That's right, they are like little gloves for your ears. We
                    call them ear*muffs*. Here, let me help you put on your ear-
                    muffs.

The partner has accepted the child's utterance, recognized the child's understanding of the situation, corrected the utterance, and left the child's ego intact.

The intervention setting itself should "create and sustain an atmosphere
containing fun, surprise, interest, ease, invitation, laughter, and spontaneity"
(Cochrane, 1983, p. 160). In such an atmosphere, children will be eager to participate. One of my best lessons on verbal sequencing used mime, complete with
whiteface. The children enacted familiar everyday event sequences, such as making breakfast, while other students tried to guess the name of the sequence. After
the correct guess was given, the actor stated each event in the sequence while
performing it. Finally, each actor attempted to reconstruct the sequence verbally.
The lesson was messy, fun, enjoyable, and thoroughly successful.

Children also respond favorably if the facilitator occasionally plays the
clown or buffoon. I may wear a cooking pot on my head in order to evoke a
response. On other occasions, I purposely may make incorrect verbalizations or
actions. These behaviors add to the magic of the communication situation and
encourage children to communicate in an accepting atmosphere.

Closely Approximate Natural Learning

Language intervention strategies should approximate closely the natural process
of language acquisition. The strategy should be communicative in nature and
should use language as it naturally occurs (Mahoney & Weller, 1980). Teaching
language devoid of its communicative function deprives the child of intrinsic
motivation and of one essential element of generalization.

Natural language models—parents, teachers, aides, and others—should be
the principal resources for implementation of language intervention (Broen &
Westman, 1990; Crais, 1991, 1992; Hazel, 1990; Mahoney & Weller, 1980; Whitehurst et al., 1991). These individuals serve as language models with or without
the speech-language pathologist's input. Their potential as language facilitators
can be exploited best, however, when they are guided in content selection and
trained in facilitative techniques. When using these language facilitators within
the child's everyday situations, the role of the speech-language pathologist
changes to that of collaborator (Lyngaas et al., 1983).

Follow Developmental Guidelines

The language development of children developing normally can guide the selection of training targets. As a group, these children develop language in a similar,
albeit individualistic, manner. Generally, language form is preceded by function,
with easier, less complex structures being learned first. Children use the language

they possess to accomplish language goals or uses. These uses are the framework within which new forms develop. The overall result is hierarchy that suggests steps for training language.

Of course, no speech-language pathologist would ever adopt a language intervention hierarchy without some personal adaptations. Slavish adherence to a developmental hierarchy is inappropriate for two reasons. First, the developing child's hypothesis testing of language rules occasionally results in nonproductive strategies. For example, young children learn a few irregular past tense verbs early in their language development. On learning the regular past tense -ed rule, these children apply it to the previously learned irregular verbs. This tactic results in such delightful forms as *eated* and *sitted*. No speech-language pathologist would wish to adopt these forms as training targets, although they appear in the language of children developing normally.

Second, good teaching may suggest alternative hierarchical teaching patterns (Elbert & McReynolds, 1985; Powell, 1991; Powell & Elbert, 1984). For example, children developing normally acquire the verb *to be* as both an auxiliary verb and as a main verb or copula. In intervention, therefore, these forms might be targeted separately. Our knowledge of carryover might suggest, however, that we train them together, making little distinction between the forms and aiding generalization.

Developmental hierarchies can act as guides for intervention. These hierarchies suggest several subprinciples:

1. Language evolves from nonverbal communication means.
2. Social and cognitive prerequisites are necessary for the child to use language in certain ways.
3. Simple rules are acquired before more difficult ones.
4. Development is not uniform across all aspects of language.
5. At different levels of development, children act differently.

Each subprinciple has several implications for intervention.

Because language has evolved as a sophisticated communication means from a nonverbal communication system, intervention with children who are low-functioning should begin with less sophisticated systems and progress toward symbol use (Mahoney & Weller, 1980). In addition, the speech-language pathologist needs to be mindful of the many ways in which a message may be sent by any communicator and to note development within the nonlinguistic and paralinguistic realms, as well as within the linguistic.

Although social and communicative prerequisites are important prior to the appearance of first words, these prerequisites cannot be overlooked with later development. The speech-language pathologist should be aware of the prerequisites for successful communicative behaviors at the functioning level of the child (Rieke & Lewis, 1984). The child learning plurals need not be able to count but must have a notion of one and more than one. Likewise, successful use of *why* questions and answers requires an ability to reconstruct events in reverse. These cognitive skills may need to be taught prior to attempting the linguistic manner for noting this knowledge.

Similarly, the child needs to understand the requirements and demands of different communication situations to communicate effectively within them. For example, the requirements of classroom give-and-take are very different from having a face-to-face conversation or from talking on the telephone.

As with much learning, simple rules are combined and modified or enlarged to form higher order rules. By carefully analyzing each new training target and monitoring progress, the speech-language pathologist can ensure that the child possesses the appropriate rules for new learning. It is best not to change too many aspects of the training situation at one time. For example, there may be too much new information to absorb if the child is learning new words while being taught different sentence types in which to use these words. Words used frequently by the child should be selected to train longer utterances.

Children with language impairment will not present textbook examples of language development hierarchies. They may have splinter skills or be more proficient in one aspect of language than in others. This situation is not unlike that found in children developing normally. Language development and impairment can be very individualistic and may not follow the dictates of a developmental hierarchy. Aspects of language will develop at rates influenced by perception and cognition, opportunity, needs, and training. Of more importance for intervention is the designation of training targets that help the child function more effectively within the everyday environment.

Finally, the language rules observed by most children at each level of development are valid for those children at that time. For example, young children say such things as, "Mommy eat," and, "More juice," that demonstrate adherence to simple word sequencing rules based on semantics. "Mommy eat" is not a defective form of some longer adult sentence. Children demonstrate rules appropriate to their level of linguistic competence. Requiring adult rule use negates the uniqueness of children and dismisses the importance of child rules as a step in the acquisition process.

At various levels of intervention, it is appropriate to target child rules, rather than the more difficult adult ones that will be trained later. These rules provide excellent training targets for children with language impairment who also are beginning to form two-word utterances. Likewise, the child with language impairment who is forming negatives, such as no + noun + verb, should make a logical progression to noun + no + verb, rather than to the adult rule with full auxiliary verb. To require children with language impairment to use adult sentence forms seems ridiculous, especially when we do not require such behavior from children developing normally. As adults, we sometimes think that the adult way of doing things is the only way.

Even the expectation that a child will use a new or adultlike language rule or feature following brief periods of intervention may be unrealistic (Fey, 1988). Children developing normally learn and extend or retract their language rules gradually after many encounters and trials. Over time, these rules come to resemble those of adults. Therefore, it is probably inappropriate to expect near perfect performance from children with language impairment shortly after a target is introduced. Rule learning is complicated and time-consuming. In addition, children with language impairment may form rules very different from those intended by speech-language pathologists.

As the child progresses, the language training should be modified accordingly. In other words, the speech-language pathologist *ups the ante* (MacDonald, 1985), or requires performance just above the child's current functioning level.

Follow the Child's Lead

Often, the expectation that a child will not communicate effectively becomes self-fulfilling. If facilitators expect the child to communicate and plan for it, the child will. At that time, it is essential that the facilitator give full attention to the child.

It is equally important that the facilitator attend to the content and intent of each child utterance and respond appropriately to that content and intent. "Training techniques in which teachers follow the child's lead . . . should be most effective because teaching occurs when the child is attending and because the language being taught to the child is a positive consequence" (Warren & Rogers-Warren, 1985, p. 7).

Language facilitators can either direct and maintain the child's attention or attend to what interests the child. Although the former is a trainer-oriented approach (Fey, 1986) that gives the trainer virtual control of the entire interaction, it may not be the most effective approach. For example, children with MR are less likely to follow such trainer attempts to redirect attention (Landry & Chapieski, 1990). In contrast, these children seem to learn object-vocabulary relationships more easily when trainers follow their attentional lead (P. Yoder, Kaiser, & Alpert, 1991; P. Yoder et al., 1993).

A more child-centered approach guarantees joint or shared reference, enhances semantic contingency, and reduces noncompliance by the child (McDade & Varnedoe, 1987). With semantic contingency, the adult comments on the child's topic or previous utterance, thus facilitating processing by the child. Children appear to attend most to and to be best able to comprehend speech during joint-attention activities (Tomasello & Farrar, 1986).

Responses to child actions or utterances provide contextual support. Such support may aid the processing of children with mental retardation who have memory storage and retrieval problems that complicate encoding and decoding (Bilovsky & Share, 1975; McDade & Adler, 1980; Mervis, 1990).

The child's verbal behavior should be interpreted by others in terms of intention, rather than viewed as inappropriate or incorrect. In other words, a request is still a request even though the form may be wrong, the item desired misnamed, and so on.

When the adult has an agenda different from that of the child, the interaction is diminished. Such interactions are at cross-purposes and are faulty (Duchan, 1984).

Children signal those things in which they are most interested by their actions or through verbalizations. This gauge can be used to keep child interest and motivation high in the intervention setting. Often, I will say to a child, "What toy do you want to play with?" Although the topic is open-ended, the technique is very specific—as we see later—permitting a flexible choice of topic.

When the child initiates an interaction and is responded to accordingly, the value for learning is greater than when the child's initiation is ignored or penalized (Duchan, 1984). Ignoring or penalizing the child will result in a decrease in future initiations.

While observing a lesson in a training apartment in preparation for the client's move to his own apartment, I overheard the following exchange:

SP-LANG PATH:	What are you doing?
CLIENT:	Dusting furniture. (Matter-of-factly)
SP-LANG PATH:	Good. What else are you doing?
CLIENT:	You live in apartment?
SP-LANG PATH:	You didn't answer my question. What . . .

The client obviously was interested in living arrangements and would have joined such a conversation willingly if the speech-language pathologist had followed his lead. The speech-language pathologist should follow the client's content and manipulate the conversation to encourage the desired language features. Continued use of directive responses by this speech-language pathologist will diminish the client's initiating behavior.

Actively Involve the Child

Normal language acquisition occurs with the active participation of the learner. Language learning is not a passive process (Mahoney & Weller, 1980).

In like fashion, more rapid learning occurs when the child with language impairment is participating actively in some event. In general, the more actively involved the child, the greater and more stable the generalization (Spiegel, 1983). Ideally, intervention should consist of motivating participatory activities with the potential for a variety of language use contexts (Kunze et al., 1983).

Language Is Influenced Heavily by Context

Context can be a big determiner of what is said and how it is said. Language is a socially based cultural form whose use reflects an individual's linguistic, interpersonal, and cultural competence within a given contextual situation (Rice, 1986). The individual's knowledge of the event or situation influences the way he or she uses language in that situation.

Language intervention should occur within the contexts of everyday events and within the context of conversational give-and-take or of other communication events. The language facilitator needs to create a rich context in which the child with language impairment can experience a variety of linguistic and nonlinguistic stimuli. The integration of talking and listening within conversations should be emphasized (Kunze et al., 1983).

The content for these dialogues is the common experience of the intervention setting. Ideally, this setting reflects or is a part of the child's everyday environment. The child and the facilitator talk about the focus of the activities used in training. The skillful facilitator can manipulate both the linguistic and nonlinguistic context to attain desired targets from the child.

Familiar Events Provide Scripts

A *script* is a set of expectations about routine or repeated events organized in a temporal-causal sequence (Fivush, 1984; K. Nelson, Fivush, Hudson, & Lucariello, 1983). As such, scripts contain shared event knowledge based on common experiences that aid and enhance memory and comprehension (Bower, Black, & Turner, 1979; Constable, 1986; Furman & Walden, 1989; Lucariello, Kyratzis, & Engel, 1986; K. Nelson, 1986). Scripts provide structure that describes appropriate sequences of events in particular contexts.

Routinized events for which children have scripts provide specific situations in which children can learn appropriate language (Kim & Lombardino, 1991). Familiar activities of high interest, such as making popcorn, pudding, or cake, can be used as the contexts for language intervention. The event sequences contained in scripts can be used to teach language expression and comprehension, and recall (Duchan, 1986b; Kim & Lombardino, 1991; Ross & Berg, 1990).

Naturally, scripts will differ with maturational level and, to some extent, with the individual, although even very young preschoolers remember events in an organized manner similar to adults in general structure and content (L. Light & Anderson, 1983; K. Nelson et al., 1983). As children mature, their scripts become longer, more detailed, and contain more options ("Sometimes . . ."), alternatives ("You either . . . or . . .), and conditions ("If . . ., then you . . .") (Fivush & Slackman, 1986; McCartney & Nelson, 1981; K. Nelson, 1986; K. Nelson et al., 1983; K. Nelson & Gruendel, 1981; Slackman, Hudson, & Fivush, 1986).

Individual differences may be the result of different experiences (Schank & Abelson, 1977). In general, specific event experience is more important than age alone (Chi & Ceci, 1987; Ross, 1989; Ross & Berg, 1989). The resultant personal scripts are more important for memory than a generic notion of the script (Ross & Berg, 1990). Individual experience becomes especially important when we consider intervention with children with LEP or different dialects.

Design a Generalization Plan First

Considerations of generalization are essential to treatment program design and should be identified prior to beginning training. Table 8.2 is a suggested generalization plan format. In designing such a plan, the speech-language pathologist considers the individual needs of the child and environment and the relevant variables that will affect generalization.

TABLE 8.2
Possible generalization plan format

Training targets:
Identify settings, situations, and persons in each across which training can occur.

Settings

	Situation	Situation	Situation	Situation	Situation	Situation	Situation	Situation
P								
e								
r								
s								
o								
n								
s								

Cues: _____

Consequences: _____

GENERALIZATION VARIABLES

To ensure generalization to the everyday environment of the child, the speech-language pathologist must manipulate the generalization variables most likely to result in that outcome. The variables that affect generalization can be grouped as content and context variables (Table 1.1). Content variables include the training targets and training items. Context variables include the method of training, language facilitators, cues, contingencies, and location of training. Each of these variables and considerations for intervention as they relate to a functional model is discussed in this section.

Training Targets

As mentioned previously, teaching the complex process of language use as discrete bits of language actually can retard growth (Cazden, 1972). Language intervention should be relevant to the particular needs of the child within the communication environment and should target the language use process, rather than language products or units. Therefore, intervention must answer two questions (Warren, 1985):

1. What will be the function of the forms and content we are teaching?
2. Are the forms and content being trained in the context of communication events in which the intended function can actually be accomplished?

In general, more frequently used targets are more relevant to the child's world and, therefore, are more likely to generalize. Communicative utterances observed to occur in the home, albeit incorrectly, can be introduced in therapy as natural outcomes of the context. Once introduced, they can be modified by the facilitator.

Language "is often acquired more rapidly and used more effectively if the skill called 'communicative interaction' is established first" (Rieke & Lewis, 1984, p. 44). Language targets need to be those that increase the effectiveness of the child as a communicative partner (Snow et al., 1984). The first goal of intervention should be successful communication by the child at the present level of functioning. Language goals that are too taxing may result in a lessening of successful communication and decreased initiation by the child. Through observation and language sampling, the speech-language pathologist notes communication breakdowns as a source for identifying possible training targets.

Developmental guidelines can aid target selection but should be followed cautiously. Unfortunately, "all too frequently clinicians take a 'description' of normal acquisition as a 'prescription' for the way language must be taught" (deVilliers & deVilliers, 1978, p. 270).

In 43 published language-intervention studies, those that used goals approximating a developmental sequence were more successful that those that did not (Bryen & Joyce, 1985). In general, most earlier emerging forms can be learned in fewer trials and prior to later emerging forms. In addition, earlier emerging forms seem to generalize more readily into the child's use system and at a higher level of use (Dyer, Santarcangelo, & Luce, 1987).

A functional model would suggest teaching forms useful in the natural setting while attending to the developmental order of these forms (Dyer et al., 1987). As mentioned previously, the development of children developing normally can serve as a general guideline, rather than as a curricular hierarchy. The overriding criteria for target selection should be to aid the children in communicating what is necessary in the contexts in which they most frequently communicate. This practical approach is especially important for children who experience pragmatic difficulties, such as with TBI or psychiatric disorders (Audet & Hummel, 1990; Ben-Yishay, 1985; Russell, 1993). In Chapter 10, we offer some guidelines for modifying a developmental hierarchy of intervention.

The best way to determine need is through environmental observation. If, for example, the child frequently requests items in the environment but is generally ineffective, then requesting might be chosen as a target. When there is very little opportunity for a possible training target to occur, it might be best to identify other content for training.

Infrequent opportunity for possible training targets to occur may be the result of low environmental expectations or requirements for the child to produce these forms or functions. For example, there may be few opportunities for children to ask questions when there is little expectation that they will do so. In such cases, low expectations can become self-fulfilling. The communication environment may need to be restructured to facilitate use of newly acquired communication skills. The speech-language pathologist is an invaluable expert in facilitating such language use.

The speech-language pathologist should identify both targets and everyday situations in which the target is likely to occur and in which its use will be affected by and, in turn, affect the context. For example, questions should be trained in situations in which they make sense and in which they perform their intended function of gaining information. Speech-language pathologist instructions such as, "I'm coloring a picture. Ask me what I'm doing," violate the function of questions. Usually, we do not ask questions for which we already have the answer. Similarly, the speech-language pathologist's attempt to elicit an answer with the instruction, "What am I doing?" also violates the function of questions and answers. Although we might wonder about the mental capacity of speech-language pathologists who do not know what they are doing, we can modify the situation and cue to gain this feature more appropriately. For example, the speech-language pathologist might sit behind a screen, give clues, and ask the child, "Can you guess what I'm doing?"

Training Items

The speech-language pathologist should plan to train enough examples of the feature being targeted to enable the child to generalize to untrained members

(Stremel-Campbell & Campbell, 1985). For example, it is neither desirable nor possible to train all noun-verb combinations. The goal should be to train enough examples from the noun class in combination with examples of the verb class so that the child will generalize the rule *noun + verb* to all members of these two classes. Obviously, this process is being simplified in this discussion, and more planning and thought are required. Not all nouns and verbs can be combined. For example, the combination "Desk eat" is unacceptable.

In addition, a sufficient number of items must be trained so that the child can determine both the relevant and irrelevant aspects of the communication context. For example, words or phrases such as *yesterday, last week,* and *in the past* are relevant to use of the past tense. The child forms a hypothesis that states, "In the presence of *yesterday, last week,* or *in the past,* use the past tense." Other aspects may be irrelevant, such as the specific nouns, pronouns, or verbs used. For example, the pronoun *I* is irrelevant and can be used with any tense. If the child is trained to use the form *Yesterday, I . . ., Last week, I . . .,* and *In the past, I . . .,* the resultant incorrect hypothesis might be "In the presence of *I,* use the past tense." Knowledge of both the relevant and irrelevant aspects of the context are essential for learning.

Initially, training response classes should be similar so as to limit irrelevant dimensions. For example, the child first may learn to use regular past tense with *yesterday.* Such words as *today* do not signal the tense as clearly and should be introduced later. Gradually, more irrelevant dimensions are introduced.

Not all word classes require the use of all training targets. For example, nouns do not require the past tense *-ed* marker, and *tomorrow* does not require a past tense verb. The child needs to learn those response classes in which the target is required and those in which it is not.

When a particular syntactic form or function is being targeted, it is especially important to select content words or utterances already in the child's repertoire. With the targeting and introduction of new topic words, the wise speech-language pathologist will select familiar structural frames. This principle is called "new forms-old content/old forms-new content" (MacDonald, 1985).

Processing constraints found in all human beings reflect the limited capacity of the brain to process information. When these boundaries are reached, performance sacrifices or trade-offs must occur in one area because of demands in another. For example, children omit more grammatical markers in longer, more complex sentences than in shorter, less complex ones (Nakayama, 1987). Children with language impairment are particularly susceptible to these constraints because the automatization of linguistic processing takes longer (Kamhi, Catts, & Davis, 1984). Training items that exceed the information-processing constraints of these children may result in inadequate learning and poor generalization (J. Johnston, 1988a).

Often a behavior fails to generalize because the child has not learned the rules or conditions that govern the use of the behavior. Within the typical intervention model, the child learns imitative responses, followed by elicited ones. Thus, the child internalizes this unique relationship between the communication variables.

Because the child often lacks metalinguistic awareness, rule explanation is not a viable clinical tool (deVilliers & deVilliers, 1978). The speech-language pathologist must structure the environment so that linguistic regularities are obvious.

Contrast training is one method of overcoming generalization problems (Connell, 1982). In contrast training, the child learns those structures and situations that obligate use from those that do not. For example, use of the third person -*s* marker is required with singular nouns and third person singular pronouns. The child must recognize also that plural nouns and other pronouns do not require this marker. "By contrasting sentences which obligate a target form with minimally different sentences which do not . . . the learner can recognize which parts of sentences occur regardless of the presence or absence of the target form" (Connell, 1982, p. 235).

Conversational use requires recognition of the linguistic contexts within which the training target does or does not appear. The identification of other contexts, such as events, facilitators, and settings, also should be accomplished. Using several different contexts ensures that the child does not identify the speech-language pathologist and the therapy setting as the only contexts in which to use the language being trained.

Ideally, functional training uses multiple exemplars (Stremel-Campbell & Campbell, 1985) or examples, such as the several categories of linguistic response classes or training items, several facilitators, and several settings. This feature is essential for generalization.

Method of Training

In the past, language was taught much as one would teach any other complex behavior, and intervention centered on individual discrete behaviors. The goal was to increase the frequency of these behaviors (Guess et al., 1974). Language, however, is a set of rules that allow a person to use language elements in communication contexts to express intentions (Wilbur, 1983).

A rule is an abstraction that describes similarities in behavior. Language is a rule-governed behavior. Thus, the goal of intervention should be to learn the abstract rules, rather than the behaviors that reflect these rules (Connell, 1982; Fey, 1986; J. Johnston, 1983; Leonard, 1981). Current methods of teaching language do not reflect this goal (Connell, 1987b). There is a discrepancy between the goals and the methods of teaching.

It is not practical with most children and most intervention targets simply to explain the language rule being trained. Instead, training needs to be limited to observations of the rule being applied within situations that contrast the critical conditions that apply to the rule (Connell, 1987b).

The speech-language pathologist's role is to provide organized language data to the child as an illustration of rule use (J. Johnston, 1983). Thus, the child would be presented with paired minimally different situations that do and do not invoke the rule (Connell, 1987b). For example, these situations could be sentences in which the use of a form, such as pronouns, is alternately appropriate and inappropriate.

By presenting these contrasting situations and encouraging the child to practice, the speech-language pathologist helps the child amass the data necessary to identify the critical elements of the rule. Once the child is aware of the critical elements, the speech-language pathologist has the flexibility to present these elements in any communication situation. In contrast, a behavior-teaching approach would contain none of these systematic alterations of form and function.

The strength of the rule-teaching approach is in the way it simplifies the learning task by condensing relevant input and highlighting critical conditions (Connell, 1987b). Unfortunately, not every form has a direct link to some function (Bates & MacWhinney, 1982). The passive voice, for example, does not have a clear function and may be used to answer, comment, reply, declare, and so on. Forms that do not have a clear direct function are more difficult to teach. Rules based on abstract grammatical categories are also difficult.

Theoretically, functional techniques should be effective because they incorporate behavioral principles and also use the context of naturally occurring conversations that can be modified systematically by the language facilitator. Generalization is more likely than with more structured approaches because the cues used resemble the varied ones found in communication events. In addition, the child's attention is focused on objects and events in the environment while the child is receiving linguistic input about those objects and events (Warren & Kaiser, 1986a).

A functional model provides a dynamic context for teaching language. Language training that works for the child in communication events should generalize to those events. "Language programs . . . must be based on communicative needs and must be planned with these functions in mind" (Rieke & Lewis, 1984, p. 48). Training is oriented toward communication, rather than toward discrete bits of language. The focus should not be merely the correctness of the child's language, but its communicative potential (Bauer & Sapona, 1988).

In general, functional intervention, sometimes called *incidental teaching* (Hart & Risley, 1986; Warren & Kaiser, 1986a), in combination with more structured remediation, facilitates both acquisition and generalization of language targets to usage within natural environment situations. The functional or incidental approach involves (a) selecting appropriate language targets for the child and environment, (b) arranging the environment to increase the likelihood that the child will initiate, (c) responding to the child's initiations with requests for elaboration of the target forms, and (d) reinforcing the child's attempts with attention and access to objects in which the child has expressed interest (Warren & Kaiser, 1986b). Interactions between adults and children arise naturally in unstructured situations, such as play, and can be used systematically by the adult to give the child practice in communication (Warren & Kaiser, 1986b, p. 291).

The child signals a topic by demonstrating interest or requesting assistance. Thus, the child provides the topic and the opportunity for the facilitator to teach the language form (Duchan, 1986b). The child is more likely to talk and be more interested in the content of this talk if the topic has been established by the child.

Within these communication contexts, the speech-language pathologist models the responses that fulfill the child's communication goals. Because the purpose of language already is established in the natural environment, form and content may be learned more easily (Spinelli & Terrell, 1984). In short, the child is taught a more effective way to communicate within a particular context (Audet & Hummel, 1990). The speech-language pathologist also models behaviors for the caregivers in order to facilitate training and increase the likelihood that situations will occur in which the child is successful.

When the desired interactions do not occur, the speech-language pathologist can manipulate the environment to enhance its language-training potential (J. Norris & Hoffman, 1990a). Both linguistic and nonlinguist aspects of the context can be altered to elicit the desired communication.

Activities can be planned around communication contexts that are highly likely to occur for the child. Training outside the normal environment should be as close to that environment in materials, situations, and persons as possible. Activities should include the child's usual reasons for talking and typical topics, rely on previous experiences and introduce new ones, use familiar focuses of communication, and include the child's normal communication partners (Spinelli & Terrell, 1984).

Each child's individual learning or cognitive style also must be considered by the speech-language pathologist. Children are most comfortable with new experiences and information presented in a manner consistent with that style. In part, learning styles are culturally based, a consequence of accumulated experience (Saville-Troike, 1986; B. Terrell & Hale, 1992). For example, extended families, such as those in many Asian and Hispanic cultures, may foster a less independent style of learning than more nuclear families. Studies also have demonstrated that African American children benefit from incorporation of physical activity and movement into the learning situation (Hale-Benson, 1986, 1990a, 1990b).

The speech-language pathologist must recognize that events within the child's everyday environments will differ in the amount of structure provided by the event itself (Duchan, 1986a). Some contexts are highly planned and scripted or routinized, such as bathing or eating, whereas others are relatively free and open, such as playing. The communication demands and the expectations on the child vary accordingly. Language intervention must recognize what the child brings to each context and what is demanded in return. The speech-language pathologist must attend to the child and to his understanding of the situation. New information should be organized to meet the functioning level of the child (J. Norris & Hoffman, 1990a).

Routines may provide the best vehicle for training the child who is noninteractive. The child can ease into participating through repeated exposure to a routine in which the facilitator models actions and communication. Because the event is prescribed and expectations are known, there is some security for the child. Likewise, discussions of familiar events, such as a birthday party, provide a script for communicating.

Routine event knowledge shared with a communication facilitating adult provides the scaffolding for communication. Routines provide structure and expectations, freeing cognitive processing abilities for linguistic processing (Lucariello, 1990). In such familiar situations, preschoolers are freer to discuss nonpresent topics (Eisenberg, 1985; Sachs, 1983). Overall, varied linguistic features are more likely to occur in familiar, meaningful contexts (Lucariello et al., 1986).

"Language treatment based on play and daily life experiences with an adult who provides modeling and expansion of the child's forms and meaning is similar to normal language learning processes" (Kunze et al., 1983, p. 81). For example, children at a 0-36 months functioning level learn through play and interaction with adults. Intervention with children functioning at this level should reflect this reality.

By considering why and how children use words and gestures, the speech-language pathologist increases her ability to provide the most natural and optimal situations for eliciting and teaching communication. "This combination of appropriate context as well as specifically targeted behaviors facilitates maximum carryover and generalization of language skills outside the clinical environment" (Kunze et al., 1983, p. 81).

Data from a number of studies indicate that functional intervention (a) teaches target skills effectively, (b) aids generalization to nontraining settings, times, and persons, and (c) improves both the formal and functional aspects of language (Warren & Kaiser, 1986b). Functional, conversational techniques have been used effectively to enhance vocabulary growth and grammatical complexity and to increase the frequency of language use (Hart & Risley, 1980; Rogers-Warren & Warren, 1985; Warren et al., 1984).

The technique works well with a variety of age groups and populations with language impairment and with a variety of specific language responses. Language training generalizes to classroom and home settings and to teachers and parents (Alpert & Rogers-Warren, 1984; Halle et al., 1981; McGee et al., 1983). In addition, the general effects of the technique are beneficial to the overall language learning and functioning of the child (Alpert & Rogers-Warren, 1984; Rogers-Warren & Warren, 1985).

Language Facilitators

If the goal is language use within the child's everyday context, then the lone speech-language pathologist is limited as to what she can accomplished (Snow et al., 1984). The brevity of child-speech-language pathologist contact necessitates the use of a wider variety of social contexts, including various communication partners. These partners supply a strong social base for intervention, providing a reason for language use (Paul et al., 1991). The speech-language pathologist need not question *whether* these partners should be involved, but rather *how* they should be involved (Olswang & Bain, 1991).

"Obviously, adults who are with the child throughout the day are the individuals who are most able to effect an increase in the frequency of initiated communication and lay the groundwork for the continuing emergence of language behaviors" (Rieke & Lewis, 1984, p. 47). The appropriate partners to be used in training will vary with the age and circumstance of the child. Whereas parents may be appropriate for preschool children, they may have only limited interaction with their school-age children for whom teachers and peers may be more effectual. Classroom approaches are discussed in Chapter 11. Successful use of the language taught in intervention programs depends, in part, on the expectations of these significant others in the child's environment.

Parents have been successful language facilitators with a variety of language impairment types (Broen & Westman, 1990; Fey, Cleave, Long, & Hughes, 1993; Whitehurst et al., 1991). Most success has been reported for children in early stages of language and cognitive development (Cheseldine & McConkey, 1979; Girolometto, 1988; Kysela, Hillyard, McDonald, & Ahlsten-Taylor, 1981; MacDonald, Blott, Gordon, Spiegel, & Hartmann, 1974; Manolson, 1979; McConkey, Jeffree, & Hewson, 1979; Seitz & Reidell, 1974; Tannock, Girolametto, & Seigel, 1990; Weistuch & Brown, 1987; Whitehurst et al., 1991; P. Yoder et al., 1991). Home-based training for young children is least disruptive for them and uses the everyday home environment.

The child must have the opportunity to communicate; thus, the facilitator must be attentive and responsive. The facilitator must consistently recognize the child's attempts to communicate and provide appropriate responses (Wilcox, Kouri, & Caswell, 1990).

Communication partners, such as teachers and parents, can be an effective part of an intervention team if they are trained and monitored thoroughly (Jimenez & Iseyama, 1987). The facilitator must be trained in both (a) the *how,* or the best teaching techniques, and (b) the *what,* or the goals and materials for intervention. Training of facilitators can be accomplished in a combination of ways, including direct training and modeling, in-service training, and the use of telephoned and written/illustrated instructions. Telephone systems can be used effectively to increase both parent-initiated calls and child performance, especially if the system is used to enhance intervention activities (Banch, 1989; Bittle, 1975; Fuller, Vandivers, & Kronberg, 1987; Marshall & Herbert, 1981; Minner & Prater, 1987; Schubel & Erickson, 1992).

Children with significant communication impairments accompanying such disorders as autism and mental retardation usually have serious problems with conversational interactions, primarily due to the complex nature of such interactions (Higginbotham & Yoder, 1982). In general, these individuals have difficulty organizing, coordinating, and monitoring all of the various elements that comprise these interactions, such as topic initiation and maintenance, presupposition, turn taking, conversational repair, and the like (Mirenda & Donnellan, 1986).

It is often difficult for toddlers with language impairments and their parents to establish mutually rewarding interactional patterns (Cunningham, Reuler, Blackwell, & Deck, 1981; Eheart, 1982; Jones, 1978; Rieke & Lewis, 1984; Terdal,

Jackson, & Garner, 1976). Such children are less likely to succeed in a preschool setting. Their experience level and their success in communicative interaction are often minimal, and they may exhibit poor listening skills. Children who are not successful in communication often become resistant or negative and develop attention-getting behaviors.

According to the interactional view, the difficulties experienced by these children reflect their everyday contexts more than their so-called disorder. If this is so, then conversational partners must assume some of the responsibility for the communication failures of these children. For example, the quality and quantity of spontaneous conversational behavior of children with language impairment are inversely related to the number of verbal initiations and directives by their adult conversational partners (Prizant & Rentschler, 1983; Semmel, Peck, Haring, & Theimer, 1984).

Partially in response to these children's language deficits, adults modify their own language to include more imitations, semantic expansions, directives, and questions (Goldberg, 1977; Marshall, Hegrenes, & Goldstein, 1973; Nakamura & Newhoff, 1982; Scherer & Owings, 1982). The frequency of parental self-imitations is negatively correlated with the rate of language growth. Mothers of children with language impairment repeat more than do mothers of children developing normally. Most of these maternal repetitions are imperatives (demands) or directives (commands), which also correlate negatively. "A highly directive interaction style is certain to provide the child with minimal opportunity for immediate comparisons between his or her own utterances and those of the caretaker since there is no necessary connection between the use of a directive and any utterance of the child" (Lieven, 1984, p. 16). In turn, the children's contributions are determined by the complex contribution of social, environmental, and cultural factors (Mishler, 1979).

Adult verbal control of interactions seems to affect adversely the verbal output of children with language impairment. For example, although the question-answer style of adult communication may aid children functioning around age 2 to maintain a conversational topic, it can discourage children from commenting outside the topics initiated by the adults (Bloom et al., 1976; Mirenda & Donnellan, 1986; Moerk, 1977). As children with disabilities and those without move beyond this developmental level, the use of a question-answer strategy is counterproductive to the goal of spontaneous conversational behavior.

The use of an adult facilitative style of conversation can increase the use of topic initiations, questions, and topic comments by children with language impairment (Mirenda & Donnellan, 1986). An adult facilitative style (a) allows the child to control and initiate conversational topics, (b) follows the child's conversational lead, and (c) encourages the child to participate in various ways.

In contrast, an adult directive style includes verbal conversational behaviors that (a) control and initiate conversational topics, (b) lead the conversation, and (c) structure the nature of the child's contribution (Mirenda & Donnellan, 1986). These behaviors ensure a cohesive and fluent conversation at the expense of the child's spontaneous initiations.

The facilitative adult is less interested in conversational flow than in providing an opportunity for the child to participate and to assume control of the conversation. Specific behaviors that define each style are given in Table 8.3 (Duchan, 1983a; McDonald & Pien, 1982; Olsen-Fulero, 1982).

Several conversationally based parent-training programs have demonstrated an increase in parent responsiveness and a decrease in directiveness toward their preschool children with language impairment (Broen & Westman, 1990; Cheseldine & McConkey, 1979; Mahoney & Powell, 1986; McConkey & O'Connor, 1982; Price, 1984; Seitz, 1975; Weistuch & Lewis, 1986). Other changes include increased willingness to follow their child's lead, more equality in turn balancing, shorter parental MLU, and fewer questions.

Mothers who receive facilitative training are more responsive to and less directive of the children's behavior than are untrained mothers (Girolometto, 1988; Tiegerman & Siperstein, 1984). These changes in parental behavior are related causally to such child language changes as increased MLU, increased number of utterances, increased lexicon, and improved standardized test scores. Children whose parents receive training initiate more topics, are more responsive, use more verbal turns, and have a more diverse vocabulary. These results suggest that the effect of parental conversational strategies may be greater on semantics and pragmatics than on linguistic form.

An increase in the percentage of semantically related or contingent utterances can, in turn, provide greater opportunity for topic maintenance and turn taking (Tiegerman & Siperstein, 1984). With more opportunity to participate, the child gains more control over both the adult's behavior and the exchange process.

TABLE 8.3
Characteristics of the directive and facilitative styles

Directive	Facilitative
Initiate at least half of the topics of conversation.	Initiate fewer than half of the topics of conversation.
Use direct questions to initiate most topics.	Use indirect questions or embedded imperatives to initiate most topics.
Use primarily direct questions and occasional imitations or expansions to maintain topics.	Use primarily direct statements, encouragements, imitations, expansions, or expansion questions and occasional direct questions to maintain topics.
Do not ask for clarification directly, relying instead on encouragement, imitation, and expansion strategies.	Use direct clarification questions or statements when necessary and appropriate.
Do not allow lapses in turn taking to occur, but use direct questions to require the child to respond.	Allow lapses between turns to occur and after a short wait, initiate topics as noted above.

There is an ongoing debate, however, on the form of language to be addressed to children with language impairment. Parents of language learners developing normally use child-directed language patterns. These differ in syntactic completeness from the language employed in many teaching programs. Language directed at children developing normally in natural settings consists of reduced, syntactically complete utterances (deVilliers & deVilliers, 1978). In contrast, language used in teaching programs is often syntactically incomplete (Page & Horn, 1987).

Children with language impairment differ in comprehension of different language styles according to their linguistic stage (Page & Horn, 1987). Children in early Stage I (R. Brown, 1973) use a semantically based comprehension strategy, especially agent + action and action + object, rather than one based on syntax (J. Miller & Yoder, 1974). In addition, these reduced adult forms facilitate the production of two-word semantic relations for some children with language impairment (Nestheide & Culatta, 1980). The use of either adult forms or reduced forms does not seem to affect the comprehension or production of children in Stage II with language impairment (Page & Horn, 1987).

Children's spontaneous verbalizations can be enhanced also when adult facilitators provide a high level of verbal feedback coupled with little verbal directing (Broen & Westman, 1990; Woods, 1984). Examples are given in Table 8.4. Data from several studies suggest that children's conversational abilities can be increased by adult behaviors that are highly responsive to the children's spontaneous communicative behaviors.

One effective technique that can be used to increase verbalizations is a time delay procedure (Halle et al., 1981; Halle, Marshall, & Spradlin, 1979; McLean & Snyder-McLean, 1988b; Snell & Gast, 1981). First, the child is trained to pro-

TABLE 8.4
Examples of minimally directive verbal feedback to children

CHILD:	I went to the zoo, yesterday.
PARTNER:	Oh, that's one of my favorite spots. I love the monkeys best.
CHILD:	I have a birthday party, tomorrow.
PARTNER:	Oh, that should be fun. What do you want for your birthday?
CHILD:	We went whale watching on vacation.
PARTNER:	I've always wanted to do that. Bet it was exciting. Tell me about it.
CHILD:	My picture is a cowboy.
PARTNER:	A big cowboy on a spotted horse.
CHILD:	I'm gonna be a ghost for Halloween.
PARTNER:	Don't come to my house; I'm afraid of ghosts. I think I'll be a witch and scare your ghost.

In each of these five exchanges, the adult followed the child's lead by commenting on the child's topic and then cueing the child to provide more information or waiting for a reply.

duce verbal requests for a desired reinforcer in response to a direct verbal cue, such as, "What do you want?" Later, the facilitator withholds the cue while waiting for the child to vocalize or verbalize spontaneously. Gradually, the child learns to respond to the naturally occurring stimulus, rather than to the adult verbalization. Other techniques are discussed in following sections.

Language facilitators plan their role in the communication event and their communication turns to maximize the learning opportunity for the child. Within each turn, the facilitator responds to the child while troubleshooting the child's previous utterance, maintains the conversation by taking a meaningful turn, and provides an opportunity for the child to respond (see Table 8.4) (Craig, 1983).

The use of parents, teachers, and others as language facilitators does not diminish the role of the speech-language pathologist. It is essential that she remain very involved in the intervention and also become a facilitator. Whereas parents sometimes find it difficult to adapt their behavior to a more facilitative style, speech-language pathologists can more readily provide this input on a consistent and uniform basis (Fey et al., 1993). Best results seem to occur when other facilitators receive frequent, regular, structured training, including role playing and critiques.

There is a distinct difference between parental involvement and family-centered or family-focused services in which all family members participate (Crais, 1991; Turnbull, Summers, & Brotherson, 1983). Public law 99-457, regarding education of special needs populations, focuses on the family as integral to intervention, recognizing the characteristics of the family that transcend any single individual. In a family-centered model, families are treated as valued, equal partners and are encouraged to participate at all stages of decision making. Families are recognized as a constant in the child's life, while special services are recognized as more transient by nature. In such an arrangement, the speech-language pathologist-family relationship becomes a collaborative one. The aspects of this collaborative model are presented in Table 8.5.

Although each family is individualistic, culture is one of the most important influences on it, affecting such aspects as structure, interaction, function, and life cycle. Family *structure* includes the number of individuals and types of relationships, but more importantly, the cultural values and beliefs about family structure. Members of Asian American families that a majority culture speech-language pathologist might consider to be distant relatives may be very important in decision making involving the child with language impairment.

Family *interaction* is the way family members relate and the roles they play within the family. The relative importance of certain roles will vary with the culture. For example, a child who is an unmarried adult will be treated very differently, depending on the family background. Interactions are governed by the cohesion of the family, its adaptability or ability to change, and patterns of communication (Summers, Brotherson, & Turnbull, 1988). Japanese American forms of communication may seem extremely formal to a speech-language pathologist from the majority American culture.

Family *functions* are the responsibilities that families are expected to assume for their members. Again, this aspect of families varies widely across cultures.

TABLE 8.5
Guidelines for implementing a family-centered collaborative model

Define your role and explain your approach to intervention.
Convey respect by

1. Providing real choices for the family and encourage them to make decisions
2. Providing requested information and services immediately
3. Ensuring confidentiality
4. Recognizing cultural/ethnic values, traditions, and beliefs
5. Explaining the purposes of procedures and methods
6. Providing a rationale for procedures and methods
7. Ensuring a role for the family in both assessment and intervention
8. Meeting at times and locations convenient for the family
9. Attending to family concerns before professional concerns

Ensure that the family attends all discussions and decision-making meetings.
Use language that can be comprehended easily by the family.
Speak to family members forthrightly, completely, honestly, and in an unbiased manner.
Design intervention plans to fit the family's routine.
Be flexible in intervention planning.

Source: Adapted from Crais (1992); Johnson, McGonigel, & Kaufmann (1989); McWilliams & Winton (1990); Winton & Bailey (in press)

Some cultures may value overprotection of children more than the speech-language pathologist's goal of increased independence.

Finally, family *life cycle* describes the changes in families over the course of their development. Nuclear families may have periods of isolation after children have grown or in old age, whereas extended families may not experience this phenomenon.

Cultural identity is not a stereotype. Families within the same culture will differ. Recognition of cultural contributions by the speech-language pathologist, however, will increase the likelihood of appropriate and effective intervention. Table 8.6 presents guidelines for speech-language pathologists to follow when interacting with culturally diverse families.

Speech-language pathologists should be mindful of the differing expectations and perceptions of various ethnic and racial minorities. The role of parents, the expectations for children, and the attitudes toward disability, medicine, healing, self-help, and professional intervention within a minority population should be understood thoroughly prior to intervention. Children and professional intervention services are viewed quite differently across Asian, Hispanic, and African American cultures. Likewise, the speech-language pathologist's conversational style may have a great effect on future involvement with members of that community (Matsuda, 1989). Successful speech-language pathologist-family collaboration should be characterized by mutual respect, trust, and open communication

(Wayman, Lynch, & Hanson, 1990). These characteristics only evolve when the speech-language pathologist is sensitive to the cultural background of the families with whom she interacts.

The model of intervention proposed in this text is based on North American psycholinguistic research of white, middle-class families and, therefore, contains an implicit cultural bias (van Kleeck, 1994). Other cultures may not value either child talking or child conversational initiation or feel especially predisposed to accommodate the needs of young children. In addition, the two-party conversational interactions proposed may not be appropriate for the childrearing practices of other cultures. Indeed, the very foundation of child and parent as equal conversational partners may be anathema to some clients' beliefs and practices.

The parent-as-caregiver model found in white, middle-class, North American homes is less characteristic of African American, Latino, Native American, and Hawaiian communities in which siblings take a greater responsibility (Werner, 1984). Samoan and Mexican American children also participate in more multiparty and fewer two-party interactions (Briggs, 1984; Eisenberg, 1982; Ochs, 1982).

Family-centered training must be culturally congruent with each individual family structure and belief system (van Kleeck, 1994). The model proposed in this text will need to be adapted to best serve families with various cultural backgrounds.

Training Cues

If one accepts the premise that pragmatics is the governing aspect of language, then the speech-language pathologist must be concerned with the context within

TABLE 8.6
Guidelines for interacting with culturally diverse families

Do not make assumptions based on cultural stereotypes.

Cultural rules govern each encounter for both the family/child and the speech-language pathologist. Be aware that responses to stimuli, such as a clinic room, may be very different across cultures.

Learn about the cultures of the families and the children you serve.

Use cultural mediators or interpreters when necessary.

Learn to use words, phrases, and greetings from the culture of the family/child.

Be patient; allow more time for interactions. Use as few written instructions as possible, unless a family member has good English reading comprehension. Allow time for questions.

Recognize that the family may not be prepared for the amount of professional-family collaboration found in functional approaches.

Encourage family input without embarrassing family members. Involve the family to the extent that they wish to be involved.

Ensure that goals and objectives of the professionals and the family match.

Involve the cultural community when possible.

Source: Adapted from Lynch & Hanson (1992); Taylor (in press); Wayman, Lynch, & Hanson (1990)

which training occurs. Certain linguistic and nonlinguistic contexts require or provide an expectation of certain linguistic units.

In part, the problem of lack of success in generalization is due to *response programs* "in which children are taught specific responses to specific, often carefully worded, directions or questions" (Rieke & Lewis, 1984, p. 49). The child's everyday world lacks this careful control. The everyday context contains many irrelevant stimuli that do not and cannot elicit trained communication behaviors.

At the same time, parents and teachers may be presenting cues and prompts in such a diverse manner as to inhibit learning. They can be trained to focus their attention and to manipulate the environment to elicit the behaviors desired (Lucariello, 1990).

Relevant, common stimuli within the everyday communication context can serve, however, to elicit the child's new language targets if these stimuli are included in the training (Stremel-Campbell & Campbell, 1985). Targets can be trained across several behaviors, facilitators, and settings to ensure generalization. For example, the child's toys or everyday items and daily routines are used in the training.

The systematic introduction of increasingly more irrelevant stimuli from the communication environment into the training context has been termed "loose" training (Stremel-Campbell & Campbell, 1985). The overall goals are for the newly trained behavior to be emitted in response to a variety of stimuli and for a single stimuli to result in a variety of responses. These goals can be achieved by using concurrent behaviors, response variations, and linguistic and nonlinguistic cue variations. In concurrent behavior training, relevant and irrelevant stimuli are presented together so that the child learns which ones affect the newly learned behavior.

Response variation teaches the child that several responses can be used to achieve the same communication goal. For example, a drink can be attained by saying, "Want drink," "Drink please," "May I have a drink?" "I'm thirsty," and, "Are you as thirsty as I am?"

Verbal and nonverbal cues can be varied to ensure that the child does not become dependent on one stereotypic stimulus. Too often, the traditional approach has relied on very narrow and somewhat stilted cues unlike those found in conversation. The use of these traditional cues, such as, "Tell me the whole thing," may result in training characterized as apragmatic pseudoconversational drills (Cochran, 1983). Pragmatically, the cues do not make sense—for example, asking a question to which the speaker already knows the answer. As a result, the conversations within which training occurs are little more than drill with a conversational veneer.

Use of a functional conversational approach requires the speech-language pathologist to assess thoroughly the effects of certain cues and to explore the possibilities of eliciting language with a variety of linguistic and nonlinguistic cues (Constable, 1983). Those speech-language pathologists who rely on traditional cues are unaware of the rich variety of cues available for creating contexts in which language targets can occur.

Contingencies

Once the language facilitator has elicited language from the child in a conversational manner or the child has initiated language, the facilitator can begin to modify that language if necessary. In short, the child's utterance is the stimulus to which the facilitator responds. These responses or contingencies help form the context for the child's utterance.

Children learn language within the context of several different and individualistic interactional contexts. Nonetheless, several particular aspects of parent-child communication affect the rate of language acquisition. Overall, the amount of parental speech is correlated positively with language growth. Mothers of children with language impairment communicate less with their children and in a much less intelligible fashion than do mothers of children developing normally (Grimm, 1982; Schodorf, 1982).

Natural maintaining consequences should be identified prior to beginning training. As much as possible, these consequences should be related directly to the response. Such consequences as "Very good" and "Good talking" should be avoided (Stremel-Campbell & Campbell, 1985). When the child message ("I saw monkeys") and the consequence ("Good talking") are unrelated, the child's language fails to retain its communicative value. Instead, communication behaviors can be maintained by conversational responses ("Oh, I think monkeys are funny. What did they do?"). Often, simply attending to the child is sufficient to maintain the child's participation.

As much as possible, conversational consequences should be semantically and pragmatically contingent and should serve to acknowledge the child's utterance. *Semantic contingency,* the relatedness of a parent's or facilitator's response to the content or topic of a child's previous utterance, has a positive effect on the rate of language development (Barnes et al., 1983; Cross, 1978, 1981; R. Ellis & Wells, 1980; K. Nelson, 1981c; K. Nelson & Denninger, 1977; Newport, Gleitman, & Gleitman, 1977).

Adult speech that is semantically contingent on the child's immediate utterances decreases the amount of processing the child has to do to understand and analyze the structure and meaning of the adult's utterances (Shatz, 1978). The sharing of a conversational topic and common vocabulary decreases the child's memory load for processing and increases the ease of immediate language production. The facilitator's utterance provides a prop or scaffolding (Scollon, 1979) for the child's own analysis and production. In contrast, frequent topic changing or refocusing of the child's attention by the adult impedes the child's language acquisition (Snow et al., 1984).

It is not enough, however, just to comment on the child's topic. In the following example, the facilitator's response is semantically contingent but lacks *pragmatic contingency.*

> CHILD: I want cookie, please.
> FACILITATOR: Johnny wants a cookie.

The facilitator's response should make sense within the conversational framework. In this example, more appropriate responses would be, "What kind of cookie do you want?" "Okay, but just one," "Help yourself," and, "No cookies until after lunch." This example shows that such contingencies as "Good talking" violate pragmatic contingency and do not help continue the interchange. The child's language is reinforced more naturally when its purpose and intention are met (Arwood, 1983; McCormick & Goldman, 1984; Spradlin & Siegel, 1982).

In brief, parental behaviors that attempt to increase the child's participation in the interaction, that is, a child-centered interactional style, enhance the child's language skills (Lieven, 1984; McDonald & Pien, 1982). By relinquishing some control and adopting the child's topics, language facilitators can ensure more child participation and interest. This interactive, child-centered style can be the therapeutic model for children with language impairment (Lieven, 1984; Wood, 1983).

As a group, parents of children with language impairment are less positive and accepting of their children's utterances than are the parents of age-matched or language-level-matched peers. In other words, parents of children with language impairment acknowledge their children's utterances less frequently (R. Ellis & Wells, 1980; Furrow, Nelson, & Benedict, 1979).

It is possible that we have a cycle in which the child responds to the adult's language infrequently, causing the adult to interact less. This, in turn, provides less reinforcement for the child, so the child communicates less and the process begins again. We have no idea which participant begins the cycle, but it probably evolves as an interactional pattern for each dyad over a lengthy period of time.

Overall, in the clinical setting, it is important that facilitators accept a child's utterance as representative of the child's understanding of the world and of the requirements being asked. Answers considered wrong by the adult may, in fact, represent the child's somewhat different perspective. The child's response meaning can be negotiated by the facilitator and the child as the conversation continues. This degree of acceptance translates into indirect acceptance of the child.

Location

Location of training includes both the physical location in which training occurs and the conversational context formed by the child and the facilitator. In many ways, the conversational context is more important for generalization because it does not depend on physical setting and transcends the clinic, classroom, and home (J. Johnston, 1988a). In the light of the flexibility of these natural communication sequences, training is more a matter of *how* than *where* (Craig, 1983).

Physical Location

When possible, training should occur wherever the child is likely to use the newly trained language skill. Most communication takes place within familiar events that influence the way the participants communicate. For example, storytelling, conversation, and classroom participation have different rules for participation that affect the language used. Therefore, language intervention should take place within these types of discourse events as they occur in the child's everyday physical locations. The everyday environment provides natural and familiar stimuli for intervention and for generalization facilitation (Caro & Snell, 1989). Children with lingering pragmatic deficits, such as those with TBI, are particularly in need of environmentally based intervention (Russell, 1993).

Obviously, parents and teachers will need to be trained for their new roles as language facilitators. Parents may come to the clinic or the school to be trained. If this is not possible, evening group sessions or written guidelines can be used. Even if the parents only modify their expectations for the child, this will help with the generalization of language training.

Conversational Context

Behavior must be evaluated and trained within some dynamic context in order to make sense. Language and communication are influenced heavily by the context of what precedes and follows (linguistically and nonlinguistically) and by the expectations for participation with that specific context. For example, the expectations for storytelling are different from those for conversation. Ordering at a fast-food restaurant presents different expectations from chatting with a friend on the phone. Each event follows certain scripts.

Sentences trained out of context are, therefore, more difficult for the child to learn. The speech-language pathologist is not training static forms but a generative, versatile system. The contextual expectations and scripts must be examined prior to beginning intervention within each context.

Conversations provide a dynamic context in which language serves a purpose or function. Although these conversational sequences may mirror natural sequences, the speech-language pathologist and other language facilitators are mindful of the teaching situation and the facilitator-child model (Craig, 1983). Communication strategies can be provided to the child as needed (Spinelli & Terrell, 1984). Teaching approaches used previously can be adapted to this setting to approximate more closely conversational exchange.

CONCLUSION

By carefully considering the variables that affect generalization, the speech-language pathologist can modify training to maximize this effect. Targets and design decisions can be made on the basis of the likely effect on generalization and on ultimate use within the events and situations of the child's everyday environment. Language can be elicited and modified by using techniques that mirror the conversational style used by the child's usual partners within these contexts. Motivation is provided by the child's desire to participate in enjoyable activities with responsive and attentive adults.

Facilitators should adhere to the following guidelines:

1. Expect the child to communicate.
2. Respond to the child's topics and initiations.

3. Respond conversationally and build the child's utterances into longer, more acceptable ones.

4. Facilitate communication within the everyday activities of the child.

5. Cue the child in a conversational manner to elicit the language desired.

All of these principles are discussed in Chapter 9.

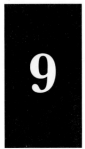

9 Manipulating Context

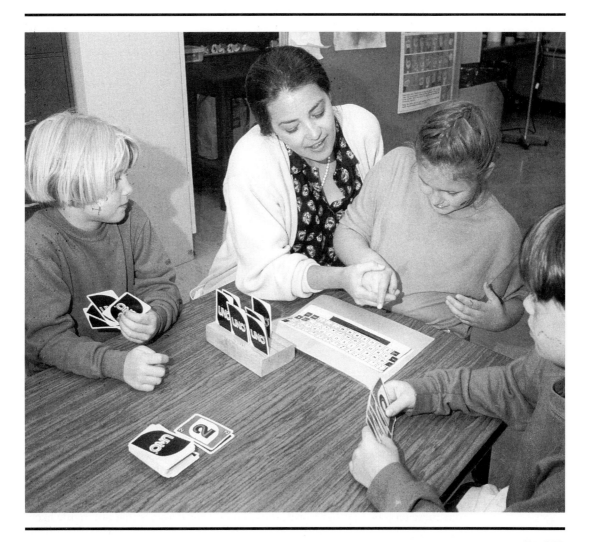

Language is pragmatically based in that the demands of the nonlinguistic and linguistic context give rise to both the form and content of the language expressed (Bates, 1976a, 1976b; P. Cole, 1982; Gallagher & Prutting, 1983; Prutting, 1982). Therefore, a primary goal of language intervention should be for the child to learn the appropriate language skills to function effectively within everyday communication contexts or environments.

Within each activity, the facilitator strives to provide an active experience with language use. It seems appropriate, then, that the speech-language pathologist and other language facilitators learn to manipulate these contexts to provide the child the maximum learning possible. The facilitator's role is "to accept the child's spontaneously occurring verbal or nonverbal behavior as meaningful communication, interpret it in a manner that is contextually appropriate, and become a collaborator with the child in communicating the message more effectively" (J. Norris & Hoffman, 1990b, p. 78).

When language can be used to achieve goals within everyday communication contexts, the chances of generalization to these contexts increases. Language acquires a purpose or function. The training becomes functional in nature.

In this chapter we explore various strategies that can be used to manipulate the nonlinguistic and linguistic contexts in which language occurs. These strategies can be used within the everyday activities of the child and, thus, can become a part of that natural environment. As much as possible, natural and conversational strategies are recommended. But the reader should be forewarned that there may be even better, more interactional ways to train children than are presented here.

NONLINGUISTIC CONTEXTS

Speech-language pathology is so oriented toward linguistic forms of communication that it is easy to overlook the nonlinguistic aspects. Yet, the nonlinguistic context—what happens in the environment—offers a rich source for eliciting language. The speech-language pathologist can manipulate the nonlinguistic contextual cues to elicit desired language and to ensure that the child initiates language. All too often, the training paradigm of the child with language impairment allows the child little control. Therefore, the child assumes a passive, responsive role to the speech-language pathologist's linguistic cues.

Certain nonlinguistic contexts naturally elicit more language than do others. For most adults, cocktail parties are more likely to elicit language than are theater engagements. Inherent in the theater experience is the necessity to remain silent during the performance.

Some situations also dictate the type of language used. Most adults do not question and challenge sermons—at least not while the sermon is being delivered. In contrast, learning situations, such as in a classroom, are supposed to encourage questioning. Fast-food establishments are likely to elicit demands or requests.

If targets have been selected to help the child communicate better, then the speech-language pathologist already has identified the contexts in which the child attempts these targets. In other words, the nonlinguistic contexts that are highly likely to elicit the target are known. Although the child is expected to perform, the speech-language pathologist believes that the performance will be in error because the target was chosen from aspects of language with which the child has experienced difficulty.

Likewise, the speech-language pathologist has some control of the topics the child will discuss. The facilitator's role "is not to change the topic, once the child has chosen it, but to determine through environmental arrangement what topics the child will choose" (Hart, 1985, p. 80).

Ideally, the nonlinguistic context serves to elicit the target language behavior; the speech-language pathologist then can help the child modify the target into a correct form for that situation. In theory, the child who makes a meaningful response in context will be interested in that response and motivated to change it in the desired manner. This corrected response should generalize more easily to everyday use because it is being trained within the context of everyday events and conversations.

Table 9.1 contains a sample of nonlinguistic contexts and the type of language each may elicit. Small group projects or tasks usually elicit lots of language

TABLE 9.1
Nonlinguistic contexts and language elicitation

Turn taking and requesting objects:
Provide only one plastic knife for children to share as they make a fruit salad.
Provide one highly desirable outfit in the dress-up corner of the class.
Provide only enough art supplies for half of the children and request that children share equipment.

Following directions and directing others:
While working in a group, re-create the teacher's construction paper collage. The teacher should be careful not to supply precut paper or to help children with the color tints. The goal is to get the children to ask for help and to direct others and themselves.
In groups of two, duplicate a cake decoration previously completed by the teacher.
As a group, plant seeds in cups as the teacher has done previously. A more involved project might involve planting a garden, keeping the different crops straight, and making signs.
Bake while following a written or pictured recipe.
Put together a model by following written or oral directions.
Play dumb. By making lots of mistakes, the teacher can have children direct or correct the behavior.
Have a child explain how to do something known by only that child.
Have children direct each other through activities blindfolded.
Have the child be the teacher.

Requesting information:
Give only partial directions for completing a task.
Put objects that the children need for a task in an unusual location so that they will need to ask for the location.
Introduce visually interesting items but do not name them or explain their function to the children.

Giving information:
Have children explain class projects to children from another class.
Have children explain class projects to parents at a special event or Parents' Night.
Have children tell about events they experienced: for example, summer vacation, a weekend trip, a birthday party. This task and explaining how something is accomplished are excellent vehicles for sequencing.
Have children request information from children who need to improve their ability to give information.
Have children tell make-believe stories.

TABLE 9.1, *continued*

Reasoning:

Have children try to float or submerge objects in water. Include objects that float and those that do not so that the children must find various combinations.

Build a suspension bridge from straws, string, toothpicks, and tongue depressors.

Design a city with transportation, schools, recreation facilities, and residential, industrial, and business areas.

Play initiative games in which groups of children must solve a common problem.

Make large projects in connection with class projects. For example, children might design the "perfect" world, make montages that demonstrate male and female roles, or design a board game, such as On the Way to Your Birthday, that illustrates stages of fetal development.

Requesting help:

Pose problems that children cannot solve themselves.

Sabotage activities, such as holes in paper cups, dried markers and paints, glue bottles glued shut, not enough chairs, missing gloves and hats, and so on. The list is endless.

Imagining and projecting:

Set up a drama or dress-up center. Set up a puppet stage with a variety of characters.

Set up simulated shops and stores or a housekeeping center.

Role-play. (Role play can elicit a variety of intentions.)

Protesting:

Play dumb, as in forgetting to give children peanut butter and jelly with which to make sandwiches.

Miss a child's turn or withhold needed objects.

Violate a routine or an object function by using objects in novel or nonsensical ways.

Give a child too much of something or more than is needed.

Put away objects before the child is finished using them.

Ask a child to do something that is not physically possible (but safe).

Initiations:

Pose problems and *wait* for children to initiate communication.

Ask children to talk to lonely animals for you.

Source: Author's experience, Constable (1983); Kunze, Lockhart, Didow, & Caterson (1983); Staab (1983)

from children. For younger children, role play and dress-up are good contexts for language. Routines also can be established within the home or the classroom for asking for desired objects or privileges.

Within these nonlinguistic contexts, language may be elicited through the use of delays, introduction of novel elements, oversight, and sabotage (McLean & Snyder-McLean, 1988b). Delaying or waiting for the child to initiate communication is often a very effective strategy, especially after the child has mastered a desired behavior (Hart, 1985). Too frequently, adults do not expect the child to communicate, and this expectation becomes self-fulfilling when the adult communicates for the child.

The language facilitator waits for the child to initiate the interaction. The facilitator may sit near the child and look questioningly or display some interesting item while looking at the child (Hart, 1985). When the child looks at the adult, the adult does not speak for a specified period of time unless the child does. If the child does not verbalize, the adult models or prompts the desired verbalization. Upon successful completion, the child is given the desired item.

If the item is edible, it should be small and quickly consumed. In a camp situation, I was able to maintain communication initiations of a small child with autism over 8 days with two large sugar cookies crumbled into very small pieces. Nonedible items may be used for specific, limited tasks, such as gluing one piece of colored paper to another, and then returned to the facilitator.

Novel or unexpected events can be introduced into the situation to evoke communication. Most individuals will notice and remark on such events. For example, a kitten, guinea pig, or bright toy might be found in an unexpected spot. Even children functioning at the single-word level will comment on elements in the situation that are novel, different, or changing.

Oversight or forgetting by the facilitator will elicit language from the child eager to become the teacher. I often play dumb, forgetting object locations or children's turns. Needed objects, such as glue or scissors, can be omitted or used in unusual ways.

Finally, sabotage of activities or routines involves taking actions or introducing elements that will not permit the activity to continue or to be completed (Constable, 1983; Lucas, 1980). My favorite example is the classroom teacher and aide who would buckle the children's boots together and turn their coats inside out sometime during the day. One can imagine the chaos at the end of the day and all of the language elicited as children requested assistance.

LINGUISTIC CONTEXTS

The goal of language use within a conversational context necessitates a thorough evaluation of the linguistic cues used with children in the training situation. Cues such as, "What do we say?" and, "Now, tell me the whole thing," are examples of pseudoconversational cues mentioned previously.

Eliciting language through constant prodding or interrogation can be unpleasant and result in less talking by the child. Such communication is one-sided, with the child assuming the role of receiver or occasional reluctant speaker (McDade & Varnedoe, 1987).

Linguistic contexts can be divided into those that model language with or without a child's response, those that directly and indirectly cue certain behaviors, and those that do not cue these behaviors. A particular utterance will cue one type of behavior but not others and, thus, can be used in contrast training to teach contextual discrimination.

Modeling

In comparative studies, the efficacy of the modeling approach has been demonstrated repeatedly (Courtright & Courtright, 1976, 1979; Prelock & Panagos, 1980; M. Wilcox & Leonard, 1978). *Modeling* is a procedure in which the speech-language pathologist produces a rule-governed utterance at appropriate junctures in conversation or activities but does not ask the child to imitate. The technique compares favorably with more active techniques, such as question-answer, that require responses by the child (Weismer & Murray-Branch, 1989).

Modeling can be used in any of the following ways:

1. As a high-frequency response in very structured situations (Connell, Gardner-Gletty, Dejewski, & Parks-Reinick, 1981; Courtright & Courtright, 1976, 1979; Culatta & Horn, 1982; Leonard, 1975; Leonard et al., 1982; Schwartz et al., 1985; M. Wilcox & Leonard, 1978)

2. As general language stimulation containing a number of language targets simultaneously (J. Cooper, Moodley, & Reynell, 1978, 1979; Evesham, 1977; L. Lee, Koenigsknecht, & Mulhern, 1975)

3. As an element in comprehension training in which the child points to pictures that illustrate the utterance modeled (Paluszek & Feintuch, 1979; Ruder, Smith, & Hermann, 1974; Winitz, 1973)

In general, modeling closely approximates the language-learning environment of children developing normally and is an effective language-learning strategy for the child with language impairment (Lucas, 1980).

It is expected that the child will acquire some aspect of the language behavior of the facilitator and use it in a similar context later. Unlike direct instruction techniques, interactive modeling considers the child to be an active learner who abstracts the rules used in forming utterances and associates these utterances with events and stimuli in the environment (Leonard, 1981).

It is best to model the training target for the child prior to attempting to elicit the target. Within such *focused stimulation*, the speech-language pathologist produces a high density of the targets in meaningful contexts without requiring the child to respond. Two varieties of this stimulation are *self-talk* and *parallel talk*. In self-talk, the speech-language pathologist talks about what she is doing, whereas in parallel talk, discussion centers on the child's actions. Obviously, activities must be chosen carefully to provide sufficient opportunities for the target to occur.

Focused stimulation should be semantically and pragmatically appropriate (Fey et al., 1993). The target feature is presented frequently while little pressure is placed on the child. Such frequent modeling plus recasts of the child's utterances has been effective in facilitating use of certain language structures (Camarata & Nelson, in press; Camarata et al., 1991; Culatta & Horn, 1982; Leonard et al., 1982; Orazi & Wilcox, 1982; Watkins & Pemberton, 1987; M. Wilcox, 1984; Willbrand, 1977).

Once a target has been modeled thoroughly, the speech-language pathologist asks the child to respond in a manner similar to the model. Children who are young, low-functioning, or delayed may need imitation training, with a complete model presented immediately before their response. *Imitation* is a procedure in which the child repeats the language behavior of a facilitator, with the expectation that the child will acquire some aspect of the facilitator's language.

Imitation can be used as a first step in programs to teach specific language targets (Connell, 1987a, 1987b; Courtright & Courtright, 1976; Friedman & Friedman, 1980; Gottesleben, Tyack, & Buschini, 1974; Hegde, 1980; Hegde,

Noll, & Pecora, 1979; Zwitman & Sonderman, 1979) or as a correction procedure when the child fails to respond or responds incorrectly (Hester & Hendrickson, 1977; L. Lee et al., 1975; Warren et al., 1984). The procedure has been used successfully with several types of language impairment. By monitoring the child's progress, the speech-language pathologist can provide varied cues, including partial models and/or delayed imitation.

The child may respond also to questions for which the speech-language pathologist has modeled the answers. Initially, the modeled answer may follow the question, but this format can be altered so that the answer precedes the question, is given partially, or precedes the question by increasingly longer periods of time.

Although the modeling procedure seems stilted in writing, it can be applied very flexibly and works well with groups of children. In small groups, children who have acquired a certain target can serve as models for those who have not. By varying turns, the speech-language pathologist ensures that sufficient models are provided for different children with different targets. In a reversal of roles, the speech-language pathologist can serve as a model for the child, while the child cues the speech-language pathologist.

Some studies have found modeling to be less effective than other, more structured methods (K. Cole & Dale, 1986; Connell, 1987a; Connell et al., 1981; Friedman & Friedman, 1980). Whereas modeling is effective in changing the behavior of children developing normally, it is less effective than imitation with children with language impairment (Connell, 1987a). More structured approaches include imitation, elicitation in the form of fill-ins, stimulation, and comprehension training.

Direct Linguistic Cues

Linguistic cues for certain targets can be direct or indirect. Direct elicitation techniques might include the following target questions:

To elicit. . .	*Use. . .*
Verbs	"What is he doing (are you doing)?" Use any tense. A benefit is that the question contains the target tense.
Noun subjects	"Who/what is verbing?" Again, the tense can be altered for the situation.
Noun objects	"What is he/she verbing?" Tense can be altered for the situation. Obviously verbs that do not take objects should not be used.
Adverbs or adverbial phrases	"When/where/how is he/she verbing?" Tense can be altered. "How" questions can be used also to elicit process answers, as in "How did you make the airplane?"
Adjectives or adjectival phrases	"Which one . . .?" Tense can be altered. There should be an obvious contrast between choices for the response, such as *big* and *little*. These differences might be noted prior to questioning.

Responses of a particular type can be modeled, as
in, "Which one ate the cookie, the littlest bear, the
middle-size bear, or the biggest bear?" To keep the
child from responding, "That one," the speech-language pathologist may want to cover her eyes or
use some barrier.

Specific words   Completion sentences, as in, "She is playing in the
___." Rising intonation after the last spoken word
will signal the child to respond. If the speech-language pathologist plays dumb or acts forgetful, the
child's behavior makes more sense conversationally.

Substitution requests also can be used. For example, pronouns can be substituted for old information. The facilitator might make a statement, such as giving
one descriptor ("The dog is little"), and then ask the child to make a comment
("What can you tell me about the dog?"). This procedure can take the form of a
guessing game, as in, "Is the dog little? Well, if the dog isn't little, what can we
say?"

Although these linguistic cues are conversational in nature, they will seem
very nonconversational if used in nonlinguistic contexts in which they make no
sense pragmatically. Questions should be used when the facilitator really desires
the answer and when the child is interested in the topic of discussion.

The speech-language pathologist can model a response prior to asking the
child a question, for example, "I think I want the yellow one. What about you?"
This type of cue is more likely to elicit a longer utterance and is more conversational in tone.

One variation of the direct linguistic cue is a *mand model* (Hart, 1985; Hart
& Rogers-Warren, 1978; Rogers-Warren & Warren, 1985; Warren et al., 1984;
Warren & Kaiser, 1986a, 1986b). This technique has been used effectively with
preschoolers and with children with SLI (Olswang & Bain, 1991). This procedure
follows a routine that is established prior to beginning any activity. The routine
serves as a chain in which one stimulus cues the next. The mand-model approach
usually is used for teaching new language features.

Access to desired items is through the teacher, who determines the criterion
for acceptability. In this way, the teacher, not the object, becomes the stimulus for
talking. According to this procedure, "it is likely to be not so much what the
teachers do—the forms of language they model—as the interactional context in
which the adults' models occur that facilitates children's progress in language
learning" (Hart, 1985, p. 81).

In the four-step training sequence, the teacher first attracts the child's
attention by providing a variety of attractive materials. This inducement may not
be necessary if the child already displays an interest. Thus, the teacher establishes
joint attention with the child. In the second step, after the child has expressed
interest, the teacher (de)mands, "Tell me about this," or, "Tell me what you
want," requesting a behavior trained previously. If there is no response, the

teacher moves to step three and prompts a response or provides a model to be imitated. In step four, the teacher praises the child for an appropriate response and gives the child the desired item.

Preschool peers can be trained to use the mand-model technique effectively (Venn et al., 1993). Production may generalize to unprompted productions.

Indirect Linguistic Cues

Indirect linguistic cues are more conversational and situational in nature. For example, when attempting to elicit questions, the speech-language pathologist might use unfamiliar objects hidden in boxes to set the nonlinguistic context. Beginning with, "Boy, is this neat," the facilitator peeks into the box. An exchange might continue as follows:

CHILD:	What's in there?
FACILITATOR:	This. (Takes the object out. Waits.)
CHILD:	What is it?
FACILITATOR:	A flibbity-jibbit. It does everything.
CHILD:	What it do?

It is easy to see the interplay of nonlinguistic and linguistic cuing.

Another indirect linguistic technique requires the language facilitator to make purposefully wrong statements. A child's clothing can serve as the focus of this conversation, a technique I have dubbed "the emperor's new clothes."

FACILITATOR:	(Touching child's red sweater) What a nice blue blouse.
CHILD:	This no blue blouse.

In both examples, the child has given a response that may be something less than what is desired. The speech-language pathologist now can respond and begin to shape the child's previous utterance into an acceptable form.

These examples are only a very few of many indirect techniques. Others are listed in Appendix H.

Contingencies

Conversational consequences can be divided roughly into those that do not require a child's response and those that do. Each type provides some feedback to the child, and each differs with the functioning level and degree of learning exhibited by the child.

Contingencies Requiring No Response

Contingencies that require no response from the child are nonevaluative or accepting in nature and can be used to increase correct production or highlight incorrect production for self-correction. When the child initiates or responds to some cue, the facilitator focuses full attention on the child, creating joint focus on the child's topic. Because the child has established the topic, it now acts as a reinforcer for the child and can be used to modify the child's language. Techniques used to modify the child's response include *fulfilling the intention, use of a continuant, imitation, expansion, extension* and *expiation, breakdowns* and *buildups,* and *recast sentences.*

By *fulfilling the intention* of the child's utterance, such as handing the child a requested item, the facilitator signals the child that the message was acceptable as received. No verbal response is required.

A *continuant* is a signal that a message has been received and acknowledged. These signals usually consist of head nods or verbalizations, such as "uh-huh" and "okay." Continuants fill the speaker's turn by agreeing with the previous utterance.

In *imitation,* the facilitator repeats the child's utterance in whole or in part but makes no evaluative remarks. Rising intonation, signifying a question, is not present. Again, this behavior acknowledges the child's previous utterance. Imitation is especially helpful to the child when correctly produced features of interest are emphasized ("She *is* riding the bike"). Imitations might be preceded also by phrases such as *That's right* ("That's right, she *is* riding the bike").

In contrast to imitation, *expansion* or recast/expansion is a more mature or more correct version of the child's utterance that maintains the child's word order, for example:

CHILD: It got stolen by the crook.
FACILITATOR: Uh-huh, it *was* stolen by the crook.

The use of expansion as a teaching tool is very limited for children functioning above about 30 months of age. In a variation of expansion, the speech-language pathologist can prompt the child to imitate the expansion, although such requests disrupt the flow of conversation. A more appropriate variety of expansion for older children is a reformulation in which two or more child utterances are combined into one utterance that includes the concepts of each, as in the following:

CHILD: The dog bit the man. The man ran away.
FACILITATOR: Oh, the dog bit the man, who then ran away.

For older children, extension is a more appropriate response. *Extension* is a reply to the content of the child's utterance that provides additional information on the topic, as in the following:

CHILD: It got stolen by the crook.
FACILITATOR: Oh, I wonder if the crook stole anything else.

Much of our behavior in conversations consists of replies to the content of the other speaker, and these comments can be used effectively regardless of the age or functioning level of the child. Extensions signal the child that the facilitator is attentive and interested.

Breakdowns and buildups consist of dividing the child's utterances into shorter units and then combining them and expanding on the child's original utterance. I use this strategy as my hearing-impaired and senile great-great-uncle used to do to aid the processing of information, mulling it over before commenting.

CHILD:	It got stolen by the crook.
FACILITATOR:	(Emotional, disbelieving) It was. (Hmmm) It was stolen. Stolen by the crook. (Disgusted) By the crook. (Finally) It was stolen by the crook.

This strategy works well, especially if the speech-language pathologist plays dumb or uses a silly puppet who just does not seem to get things right. The child may shake his head or say, "Uh-huh," in agreement between the facilitator's utterances.

Finally, *recast sentences* are a changed form of the child's utterance that maintains the same relations as the original, as in the following.

CHILD:	It got stolen by the crook.
FACILITATOR:	Was it stolen by the crook?
	OR
	It was stolen by the crook, wasn't it?
	OR
	The crook stole it.
	OR
	Did the crook steal it?

These sentences can be recast in whatever form the speech-language pathologist has targeted, although comments are easier than question forms.

If the child says little, the speech-language pathologist can recast her own utterances. If the child will not stop talking, the speech-language pathologist can interrupt with "yeah" or "uh-huh" and insert a recast sentence.

Contingencies Requiring a Response

Contingencies that require a response are used when the child is able to produce the target reliably but has failed to do so or has produced the target inaccurately in conversation. A skilled use of both nonlinguistic and linguistic contextual cues should set the stage for production of the target in a situation in which it makes good pragmatic sense. As a fully participating conversational partner, the child has an interest in the conversation and in his own utterance. Thus, the child is motivated to modify production in order to maintain the conversation and receive the adult's attention.

Most of these contingencies note the child's error, or require the child to find the error, and request that the child produce the target more correctly. A second contingency type requests repetition or a correct or expanded utterance to strengthen correct production. A hierarchy of both types, ranging from contingencies used in initial training to those used when the target is learned, would be *correction model/request, incomplete correction model/request, reduced error repetition/request, error repetition/request, self-correction request, contingent query, repetition request, expansion request,* and *turnabouts* (Duchan & Weitzner-Lin, 1987; L. Lee et al., 1975; Muma, 1978).

In a *correction model/request,* the facilitator repeats the child's entire utterance, adding or correcting the target that was omitted or produced incorrectly, for example:

CHILD:	I *builded* a big tower out of blocks.
FACILITATOR:	I *built* a big tower out of blocks. Now you say it.

The child is requested gently to repeat the facilitator's model.

Initially, the target may be emphasized to aid the child in locating the corrected unit. Later training, except that involving person markers on the verb, might restate the child's utterance as a question, as in, "You *built* a big tower out of blocks?"

Because the entire utterance is desired in the child's response, the facilitator should act confused to maintain the conversational nature of the interaction.

FACILITATOR:	You *built* a tower out of big blocks? No, you *built* a big tower out of blocks? Oh, I'm confused, tell me again.

In a correction model/request, the child is provided with a complete or only slightly altered model of the correct utterance.

The facilitator should require the child to produce correctly only those units that are currently in the child's repertoire. It is difficult for facilitators to reinforce utterances even when they contain errors, as in the following example:

CHILD:	I *builted* the most biggest tower out of blocks.
FACILITATOR:	You *built* the biggest tower out of blocks?
CHILD:	Yeah, I *built* the most biggest tower out of blocks.
FACILITATOR:	Uh-huh, how big was it?
	OR
	What kind of blocks did you use?
	OR
	Where is the tower now?

A conversational approach requires the language facilitator to remain focused on the target and on the hierarchy of teaching strategies being used.

In contrast to a correction model/request, an *incomplete correction model/request* provides only the corrected target. The child must provide the rest of the utterance, as follows:

CHILD:	I *builded* a big tower with blocks.
FACILITATOR:	*Built.*
CHILD:	I *built* a big tower with blocks.

Initially, the child will need a cue to repeat the utterance with the corrected target.

Once the child has learned the target reliably within more structured situations, the language facilitator can use other techniques that require the child to supply the missing or correct target. With *reduced error repetition/request,* the facilitator repeats only the incorrect structure with rising intonation, thus forming a question. This contingency informs the child that the language unit in question is incorrect and must be corrected, for example:

CHILD:	I *builded* a big tower with blocks.
FACILITATOR:	*Builded?*
CHILD:	*Built.*

The facilitator's question is more conversational than the cue found in correction model/requests and is less disruptive to the flow of conversation. If the child fails to recognize the error, the facilitator can provide a corrected model by using an incomplete correction model/request.

With *error repetition/request,* the facilitator repeats the entire utterance with rising intonation. The child must locate the error or omission and correct it, as in the following:

CHILD:	I *builded* a big tower with blocks.
FACILITATOR:	I *builded* a big tower with blocks?

The emphasis on the error can be increased or decreased as needed. For example, increased emphasis might be used to aid the child in finding the error. If this technique is unsuccessful, the facilitator might provide a reduced error repetition/request.

Once the child's target knowledge is reasonably stable, the facilitator can use the error repetition/request even when the child is correct. This procedure helps children scan their productions spontaneously and to self-correct.

A *self-correction request* does not provide the child with a repetition of the previous utterance. Instead, the facilitator asks the child to consider the correctness of that utterance from memory, for example, "Is/was that right/correct?" and, "Did you say that correctly?" If the child is unsure, the facilitator can provide an error repetition/request.

In contrast to the somewhat stilted tone of the self-correction request, the *contingent query* is very conversational. It is concerned more with comprehension of the message being sent than with specific targets. Nonetheless, this technique can be used effectively to signal the child that something may be amiss with the production. The child is left to scan recent memory to determine where communication breakdown occurred.

Use of contingent queries should be limited because they can disrupt communication and frustrate the speaker who is continually asked to repeat. Young school-age children dislike having to repeat more than once or twice.

Contingent queries may be specific or general, depending on the abilities of the child. In response to the sentence "I *builded* a big tower with blocks," the facilitator might respond, "What did you do with blocks?" "What did you do?" or simply, "What?" If the child falsely assumes that his production was correct and merely repeats the error or omission, the facilitator might use a self-correction request.

Correct productions of the target can be reinforced by asking the child to repeat. With a *repetition request,* the facilitator simply says, "Tell me that again," or, "Could you say that again?" This technique also can be used conversationally, implying that the listener missed some portion of the transmission, not that the transmission was in error.

If the child produces the target correctly but in a smaller unit than desired, such as a one-word response following a reduced error repetition/request, the facilitator can use an *expansion request.* The typical cue "Tell me the whole thing" is not conversational in tone. It is better for the facilitator to fake confusion and ask for a total restatement, as in the following example:

FACILITATOR: *Built?* What was *built?* Who *built* it? I get so confused. You better tell me again.

The advantages of using this routine to elicit language from children were discussed previously.

Turnabouts may be more effective than repetition requests and are more conversational in nature. In a *turnabout,* the facilitator acknowledges the child's utterance or comments and then asks for more, as in, "Uh-huh, and then what did you do?" or, "Wow, what will you do next?" or, "That sounds like fun; what happened then?"

The turnabout technique has been taught to high school peers and parents and has been used effectively in conversation with children with language impairment (Hunt, Alwell, & Goetz, 1988, 1991). This partner-as-facilitator strategy reportedly can improve conversation skills significantly.

The *wh-* questions used in turnabouts should be of a topic-continuing nature and thus support the child's efforts to maintain the topic (P. Yoder, Davies, Bishop, & Munson, 1994). This style of responding is especially helpful to preschool children and children with language impairment.

Several relational terms also may be used in open-ended utterances to aid the child in providing more information of a specific nature. For example, the facilitator might repeat the child's utterance with the addition of *but* to elicit contrary or adversative information, or *and* to elicit complimentary information.

CHILD: We played games at the party.
FACILITATOR: What fun. You played games at the party *and* . . .
CHILD: And we had cake and ice cream.

Other types of relationships and terms are as follows (J. Norris & Hoffman, 1990b, pp. 78-79):

TABLE 9.2
Hierarchy of conversational contingencies

For the examples, the child's utterance is, "I sawed two puppies." The facilitator should use the contingency farthest down on the list that ensures the child's success with minimal input.

Conversational Contingency	Example
Correction model/Request	I *saw* two puppies. Can you tell me again? (The cue to say it again is optional, unless the child does not repeat spontaneously.)
Incomplete correction model/Request	*Saw.* Can you tell me again? (Again the cue is optional.)
Reduced error repetition/Request	*Sawed?*
Error repetition/Request	I *sawed* two puppies?
Self-correction Request	Was that right?
Contingent query	I didn't understand you. Say it again, please. (Other options include *Huh?* and *What?* or in this example *What did you do?*)
Expansion request	Tell me the whole thing again.
*Repetition request	Tell me again.
*Turnabout	You did; I love puppies. What did they look like?

Example of hierarchy in use:

CHILD: I sawed two puppies.
PARTNER: Was that right? (Self-correction request)
CHILD: Uh-huh.
PARTNER: I sawed two puppies? (Error repetition/request)
CHILD: Yeah.
PARTNER: Sawed? (Reduced error repetition request)
CHILD: Saw. I saw two puppies.
PARTNER: Uh-huh, tell me again. (Repetition request)
CHILD: I saw two puppies.
PARTNER: I think I love puppies more than kittens. Where did you see them? (Turnabout)

* Used with complete, correct responses.

Temporal	*and then, first, next, before, after, when, while*
Causal	*because, so, so that, in order to*
Adversative	*but, except, however, except that*
Conditional	*if, unless, or, in case*
Spatial	*in, on, next to, between,* etc.

These contingencies can be arranged in a hierarchy similar to that in Table 9.2. This arrangement will differ with the language unit being targeted. The facilitator who is familiar with this hierarchy can respond to the child's utterances in a manner that enhances language stimulation and facilitates language learning.

CONCLUSION

Both the nonlinguistic and linguistic contexts can be manipulated by the speech-language pathologist and other language facilitators to teach language to the child and to encourage use of structures recently acquired. By using the various techniques described in this chapter, facilitators can maximize interactions with the child with language impairment. Although it would be ideal if facilitators used the full range of techniques, even the adaptation of some would help make learning more conversational in nature.

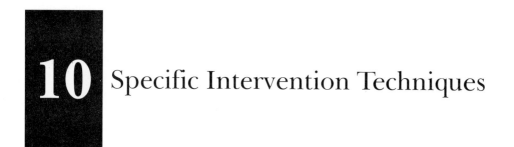

10 Specific Intervention Techniques

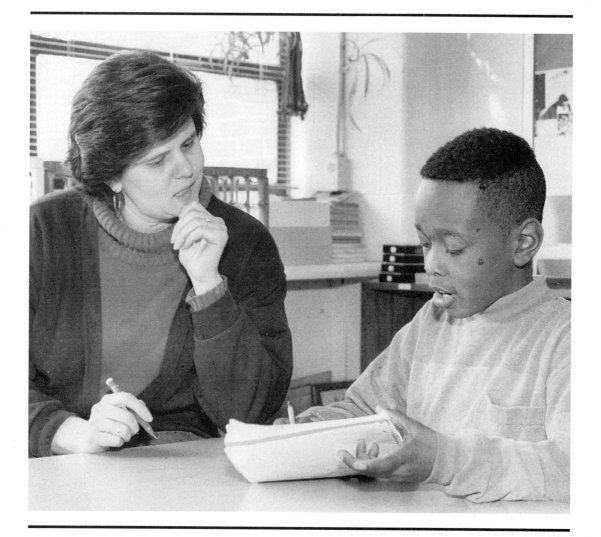

A number of training approaches effectively teach the use of linguistic features to children with language impairments. The success of intervention varies with the particular linguistic feature trained, the manner and duration of the training, and the characteristics of the individual child (Leonard, 1981).

Prior to beginning intervention, the speech-language pathologist should examine all deficit areas for a given child and apply a "What's the point?" criterion (Lilius, 1993). In short, the speech-language pathologist is concerned with the importance of individual deficits on the child's overall communication. Each deficit should be evaluated to the extent that it contributes to the child's communicative functioning. Deficits that greatly affect functioning should be targeted first for intervention. Those that do not affect overall communication fail the "What's the point?" test.

It is important that the speech-language pathologist consider generalization at the beginning of intervention and make crucial training decisions on the basis of generalization to the use environment. Even in a direct teaching approach, at least a portion of each lesson should involve the conversational context. Intervention that focuses solely on linguistic form can result in limited progress and lack of generalization (Goetz & Sailor, 1988; Halle, 1988). Preferable are specific situations in which language form skills are necessary, such as ordering in a fast-food restaurant and using the telephone (Mire & Chisholm, 1990).

In general, in this chapter we discuss a developmental hierarchy of intervention, modified where appropriate by sound teaching principles. It is important to remember that development is a gradual process with much overlap between structures. A child will reach performance levels gradually, and it is unrealistic to expect 90-100% correct performance for many language features when they are initially targeted. It may be more practical to expect a lower performance level followed by a plateau and then further change. During these plateaus, other features can be targeted.

Development is also not "domain-specific" (Kamhi & Nelson, 1988). Rather, changes in one area of language can affect other areas, just as overall developmental changes can affect language.

When possible, I apply the functional approach explained throughout this text. At all levels of instruction, some elements of the functional intervention model can be used.

Intervention should be fun and challenging, using real conversational exchanges between the child and partners wherever possible. Thus, both partners are involved actively in the process. "The child must be an active speaker who engages in communicative behavior that is effective at changing the attitudes, beliefs, or behavior of the hearer" (Lucas, 1980, p. 31).

In this chapter we explore some proven and some promising techniques for language intervention. For clarity, I have divided the chapter into the five aspects of language: pragmatics, semantics, syntax, morphology, and phonology. We discuss hierarchies for training and techniques that lend themselves well to each area. The final portions of the chapter deal with the special needs of children who are bilingual and bidialectal and the clinical application of computers.

The best intervention presents language holistically so that the child can experience newly acquired language as it is used in communication. Some speech-language pathologists accomplish this goal by targeting skills in more than one area of language or by using a stage approach in which a few training targets from a stage of development are targeted simultaneously (Prutting, 1979). The holistic aspect of intervention is discussed at the end of the next section, and suggested activities are presented in Appendix I.

PRAGMATICS

As children mature, they gain increasingly more complex categorizational or word-associational strategies and increasingly more complex organizational word and structure systems. The most appropriate and effective way of expressing oneself depends on a number of variables that are stylistic, socioemotional, personal, and contextual. In other words, linguistic variation is the result of skills in pragmatics or language use.

Many children do not use language as an effective tool for learning about their environment. They do not ask questions or request materials. Making mistakes and being corrected is easier for them than asking questions. They wait for the environment to act in some way, and then they respond. Often, adults in the child's world lose their expectation that the child will initiate communication.

The constituation of effective communication varies with the communication situation and with the age of the child. For example, with young adolescents the speech-language pathologist may need to target academic and personal-social success. As the youth nears adulthood, academic concerns yield to vocational (Larson & McKinley, 1993). The communication skills required for success in these contexts varies considerably. Intervention might begin at the point of communication breakdown (Nippold, 1993). In general, conflicts with peers are easier to modify than those with adults, and personal difficulties are easier than vocational (Selman et al., 1986).

Traditional language intervention goals, however, are usually product rather than process oriented (Wilkinson & Milosky, 1987). In other words, language forms are targeted, whereas language use is ignored. Although a theoretical shift has occurred toward pragmatic models of language, many treatment programs continue to emphasize syntax and semantics (Connell, 1982; Fujiki & Brinton, 1984; Goldstein, 1984; Tyack, 1981). In general, communicative context is used only to create fun or as an afterthought relative to generalization (Culatta & Horn, 1982).

Children can acquire very complex forms without totally comprehending them. It is essential, however, that they understand the functional qualities or use of the form (Snow & Goldfield, 1983). Thus, the effect of communicative need overrides the effect of syntactic complexity. We might do better to identify and train pragmatic behaviors and to teach the appropriate contexts in which to use these behaviors. When targeting pragmatics, form errors should be ignored unless they interfere with the intended purpose of the child's utterance.

When appropriate, however, forms can and should be targeted within a functional context. For example, the speech-language pathologist might teach requesting as a function of the goal of gaining information, action, or materials. She can help children identify the goal first and then the form that goes with each goal. Subsequently, she may teach alternative forms for such requests.

Through role playing and the use of videotaped interactions, the speech-language pathologist can teach the child to identify situations in which the desired information, action, or material was requested inadequately, inaccurately, or inappropriately (Lloyd, Baker, & Dunn, 1984). She also can train either repairs or reattempts or requests for clarification. Likewise, she can help the child to identify the requested goal of another speaker and to respond appropriately.

The speech-language pathologist may target a number of pragmatic skills within a single lesson and should use many everyday events and play activities to teach a single pragmatic skill (A. Johnson, Johnston, & Weinrich, 1981). For example, telephone conversations teach acknowledgment of the interaction, conversational opening and closing, topic maintenance, and referential communication. The use of situational cards and different voices on the other end of the phone can help the child adapt to differing situations. Pretending that she is lost or cannot see, the speech-language pathologist can teach requesting and giving assistance and information, roles, and following directions.

Construction toys, such as Legos, clay, and Play-Doh, or construction paper, used to copy a model, can teach requesting assistance, referential communication, giving and following directions, and topic maintenance. More difficult tasks will require more assistance.

Several children's stories can be enacted to help the child learn roles. Recitation of stories or nursery rhymes to different audiences will aid growth of register. The use of different puppets or dolls or different costumes will aid the learning of role taking.

Finally, the speech-language pathologist can use any number of activities for referential communication. Children can describe objects seen in Viewmasters or through periscopes, felt in paper bags, or hidden. Such activities as I Spy and Twenty Questions also aid referential communication growth and foster requesting and giving information.

If we "provide the child with the tools and an opportunity to be a successful communicator . . . the child has been given a purpose to maintain linguistic communication" (Lucas, 1980, p. 201). These tools might take the form of speech acts or conversational abilities.

Speech Acts

Children select and acquire utterances that are communicatively most useful (Snow et al., 1984). This fact explains why request forms and words that mark the initiation of favorite activities are acquired before labels and descriptive terms (K.

Nelson, 1981a). In training, however, the speech-language pathologist is concerned with the breadth of illocutionary functions that the child is able to express.

The following section addresses the training of several illocutionary functions (Bedrosian, 1985, 1988; Constable, 1983). In Chapter 11, some methods to be used in the classroom are discussed. Appendix H also provides several indirect linguistic cues useful for eliciting different functions.

Calling for Attention

Calling for someone's attention requires the presence of a person whose attention the child seeks or who is essential to completion of a task. In general, children seek attention from adults who provide it. Adults or facilitators might give the child an object within a situation and ask him to take it to an adult who, for the purpose of training, initially ignores the child. The child also might be asked to relay a message to someone else.

Adults or facilitators should attend to the child as soon as the child requests attention. If the child continually demands attention or uses inappropriate behavior to get attention, the facilitator will have to set some limits, such as only responding in certain situations and never responding to inappropriate behavior.

The form is usually the child calling the facilitator by name or gaining attention by some other means, such as tapping the listener's shoulder, moving into the visual field of the listener, leaning in the direction of the listener, or using eye contact. The child also may specify how the facilitator should respond.

Requests for Action

Requests for action can be trained at mealtime, within small group projects, or during almost any physically challenging task. Again, the child assumes that the facilitator can provide what is requested.

The facilitator will need to design situations in which children require assistance to complete the task. To encourage requesting, she can use initiative games in which children must solve problems. Tasks also may be sabotaged (see Table 9.1). As in requests for objects, attention is gained first, and the form of the utterance is interrogative or imperative.

Requests for Information

Children with language impairment often do not see other persons as sources of information and may produce few such requests. Although the environment can be manipulated to encourage requests for objects and actions, it is not as easy to encourage or increase the child's need and desire to seek information.

Requests for information require that the facilitator omit essential information for some novel or unfamiliar task, such as an art project, a new game, or some challenging academic task. Objects unknown to the child may be introduced without being named or their purpose explained. The child can be prodded gently to ask questions if asking does not occur spontaneously.

The child must recognize both the need for this information and that another person possesses the knowledge. Recognition of need is often the most difficult aspect of this training. Confrontational naming tasks, with objects known and unknown to the child, may encourage initial requesting for information. The form of requests for information is either a *wh-* or *yes/no* interrogative with rising intonation.

The facilitator also might encourage the child to ask questions by questioning him about other people's feelings or actions of which he has little knowledge. The child then can be cued with, "Why don't you ask (name)."

The child should be expected to ask questions that reflect the form the child is capable of producing. The facilitator's verbal responses discussed in Chapter 9 can be used to help the child modify incorrect, inappropriate, or immature responses.

Requests for Objects

The facilitator can easily train requests for objects within art tasks, group projects, snacktime, job training, or daily living skills training, such as dressing and hygiene. It is essential that the child desire the object requested and that the facilitator can provide it.

The facilitator can change the environment to increase both the opportunities for requesting and the caregiver behaviors that direct the child's attention to these opportunities (Olswang, Kriegsmann, & Mastergeorge, 1982). Many situations, especially those with groups of children, provide an opportunity for overlooking a child's turn, thus encouraging requesting. Of particular importance is a coordinated program designed to teach requesting for the everyday environment by approximating that environment and training those within it to model and elicit requests. Table 10.1 includes general guidelines for caregiver elicitation techniques.

The speech act usually begins with eye contact or some attention-getting behavior, such as using a name. The form, usually accompanied by a reaching gesture, is interrogative or imperative and specifies the desired object. Form training can occur within the actual need situation.

Responding to Requests

Responses may take the form of an answer to a question or a reply to a remark. These forms are very different and require different skills.

In responding to questions, children must recognize that they possess the answer and that they are required to reply. Initial training should disregard the correctness of the answer in favor of reinforcing answering in general. At this stage, teaching *wh-* question responses should reflect the *appropriateness-before-accuracy* pattern found in early question development (Parnell et al., 1986). In a situation in which the facilitator asks about objects known to the child, it is fairly certain that the child will give the appropriate answer, although it might be inaccurate. The information requested can expand gradually to conform to the child's ability to respond.

Replying is more difficult to teach because a response is expected but not required. The child's response may be in the form of nonlinguistic compliance or

TABLE 10.1
Guidelines for caregiver elicitation of requests

Make statements throughout the day about objects that the child might prefer. Wait for a response.

Use elicitation behaviors to accompany high-interest activities and play. These behaviors include the following:

Modeling with an imitative prompt. Facilitator provides a model of a request and asks the child to imitate.

Direct questioning. Facilitator asks, "What do you want?" or, "What do you need?"

Indirect modeling. Facilitator provides a partial model followed by an indirect elicitation request, such as, "If you want more X, let me know (or, "ask me for it") or, "Would you like to X or Y?"

Obstacle presentation. Facilitator requests that the child accomplish some task but provides an obstacle to accomplishment.

"Please get me the chalk over there." (There is no chalk.)

"Pour everyone some juice." (The container is empty.)

General statement. Facilitator makes a verbal comment about some activity or object that the child might want to request. The facilitator entices the child.

"We could play Candyland if you want to."

"I have some Play-Doh on that high shelf."

Set up specific situations to elicit requesting.

Provide direct and indirect models as often as possible without requiring the child to imitate.

Provide a model at appropriate times when the child appears to need assistance or is looking quizzical.

Have the child attempt difficult tasks in which help is occasionally needed.

Respond *immediately* and *naturally* to any verbal request.

Source: Adapted from Olswang, L., Kriegsmann, E., & Mastergeorge, A. (1982). Facilitating functional requesting in pragmatically impaired children. *Language, Speech, and Hearing Services in Schools, 13,* 202–222.

a linguistic response. Children's comprehension of different requests will vary with age (Ervin-Tripp, 1977). Table 4.4 contains the ages at which different types of requests are understood.

The child's ability to reply may be hindered by an inability to determine the topic or to formulate a response. The facilitator may enhance linguistic processing by having the child repeat the request. Over time, she can modify this procedure to whispered imitation, mouthing, and silent repetition until the process is internalized. She can help children in identifying important information in requests and in formulating responses.

The speech-language pathologist can elicit denials by giving the child something other than what he requested or by giving the child something undesirable. The child can reject either an action or proposal. The speaker uses emphatic stress, and the utterance is in a negative form.

Statements

Show-and-tell, discussions, and current event activities help children state information. During discussions of high-interest topics, such as dating, holidays, pets, or competitive games, the facilitator can encourage children to offer their opinions. She also can use mock radio and television broadcasts. With a little cutting and some paint, she can convert a large appliance box into a console television from within which children can deliver daily newscasts of information.

The facilitator may either know the information the child is sharing or not. In the first instance, the child is recalling a shared event; in the latter, the child is presenting new information and can assume that the facilitator has very limited information. Each situation has different informational needs and requires some presuppositional skill to determine the necessary amount of information to convey.

The form is declarative. Initially, the child must secure the listener's attention and state the discussion topic. Statements can be expanded into narratives whose purpose is also to convey information.

Conversational Abilities

More than other areas of language intervention, the training of conversational abilities requires the use of actual conversational situations. Ritualized communication that interferes with interpersonal communication, such as echolalia, can be modified gradually into acceptable and conventional routines, such as greetings, conversational initiations, and requests for repair (Lord, 1988; Lord & Magill, 1988; Magill, 1986). Social routines can be memorized and practiced in different situations that help the child become more flexible in their use. Variations can be taught through different facilitators and situations. For example, one does not offer to shake hands when the potential partner has her or his arms full (Lord, 1988). If nothing else is accomplished in training, the child learns appropriate entry into conversations (Prizant & Wetherby, 1985).

Several clinical programs are commercially available that teach conversational skills in actual or role-played situations (Blank & Marquis, 1987; Carson, 1987; Hoskins, 1987; Larson & McKinley, 1987; L. Schwartz & McKinley, 1984; Weinrich, Glaser, & Johnston, 1987; Wiig, 1982a). In the following section I present methods for training selected conversational abilities.

Presupposition

The speaker's semantic decisions are based on her or his knowledge of the referents and the situation and on *presuppositions,* or social knowledge of the listener's needs. The speaker needs to provide information that is as unambiguous as possible. In other words, the speaker and the listener need to share the same linguistic context.

Often, children with language impairments are unaware of their audience's needs (Bliss, 1992). With maturity, children developing normally are increasingly able to perspective-take, the greatest growth occurring in middle childhood (Livesley & Bromley, 1973; Selman & Bryne, 1976). In contrast, children with language impairment seem to improve little with age. Breakdown could occur in social-cognitive processes and/or linguistic production (Bliss, 1992). Significant improvement can occur, however, from training speakers to be aware of listener needs (Shantz & Wilson, 1972).

The two aspects of this training are (a) what information to relay and (b) how much. The first can be trained with descriptive or directive tasks in which the child is the speaker. The listener tries to guess or draw the described object or to follow the directions. The facilitator can use barrier games, in which she places an opaque barrier between the speaker and the listener, for teaching speakers to be aware of their listeners' needs (Muma, 1978; Wallach, 1980). Some clinical materials are available commercially (McKinley & Schwartz, 1987). Because the speaker and the listener do not share the same nonlinguistic context, the bulk of the information must be carried by the linguistic element in an unambiguous manner if the listener is to comprehend.

When the child is the listener, the speech-language pathologist can send ambiguous or incomplete messages or directions to give the child an opportunity to identify the missing semantic elements. Obstacle courses are also a good vehicle through which the child can be directed or direct others.

Training the correct amount of information to transmit may be more difficult. Of course, giving insufficient information in the tasks mentioned in the last paragraph would make the directions difficult to follow. The speech-language pathologist can train children to give more, as well as more accurate, information. For the child who gives too much information, these tasks may be trained initially one descriptor or one step at a time. These tasks then can be grouped into multidescriptor or command steps so that the child experiences offering more information. The relating of very discrete or limited events, such as drawing a picture or washing your face, also can control the amount of information to be relayed.

The speech-language pathologist can help the child monitor his own production to know when redundancy occurs. She can gently remind the child that certain information was relayed previously. In subsequent training, she can quiz the child about the novelty of information presented.

Referential Skills

Referential skills include identifying novel content and describing this content for the listener. Children with LLD have been trained successfully to use referential skills through the use of barrier games (Bunce, 1989). The description of physical attributes is somewhat easier to teach than are relational terms, such as location.

It may be best to pair a child with LLD with another child, rather than with an adult, because the child may assume that the adult partner intuitively knows the object or is pretending not to know. Thus, the child may provide less information to an adult partner.

Topic

Topic performance is an important intervention target for the following reasons (Bedrosian & Willis, 1987):

1. Its use is one means of coordinating conversations and actions, thereby fostering development of interpersonal relations.

2. It regulates the sequence of a conversation.

3. It involves the initiation of conversation.

4. It requires listening and comprehension to maintain the flow of conversation.

5. It provides a framework for making relevant contributions (Grice, 1975).

In short, topic offers an encompassing framework for considering other language skills.

Unlike greetings, which vary only slightly across situations, topics and methods of topic introduction and identification are context-dependent (Lord, 1988). Topic identification is a complex process that develops gradually through school-age and adolescence (Dorval & Eckerman, 1984). A successful strategy is to engage in whatever everyone else in the conversation is doing (Dodge, Coie, & Brakke, 1982).

Topic initiation.   *Initiation* is the verbal introduction of a topic not currently being discussed. Children often do not understand the purpose of conversations or are reluctant to introduce topics for discussion. Topic initiation, a form of conversational manipulation, implies an active conversational strategy. The child with language impairment may not be adept at introducing topics clearly or may have very limited topics (Dollaghan & Miller, 1986). Children with autism may introduce unusual or inappropriate topics (Baltaxe, 1977; Rumsey, Rapoport, & Sceery, 1985).

Adolescents with moderate-to-severe mental retardation have been taught to initiate a topic through the use of facilitator waiting and through training in the purpose of conversation (Downing, 1987). In the first step of training, the facilitator maintains eye contact for 10 seconds but does not speak. Planned delay can be an effective strategy for prompting clients to initiate conversation (Halle et al., 1981).

If the child does not initiate the conversation during this wait, the facilitator can explain the purpose of conversation and the enjoyment that can result (Downing, 1987). She also can describe the roles of speaker and listener. Then the facilitator returns to the waiting strategy. If the child still does not respond, the facilitator can suggest that the child find something of interest to discuss by looking through a magazine. The facilitator then returns to the waiting strategy. If the child fails to initiate again, the facilitator can model a topic initiation.

Some children fail to initiate conversations and topics because of a history of failure. It is important that the facilitator focus fully on the child when he initiates and follow his lead. The facilitator should try not to interrupt the child (DeMaio, 1984).

She might first teach the child to gain the listener's attention. When the child inadequately introduces a topic, the facilitator can request further information to identify the topic. Focused activities, such as describing pictures or a shared event or following directions, will show the child the need to share the referent with the listener.

The facilitator initially can tolerate inappropriate topics to give the child some success. Gradually, she can discuss the inappropriateness of these topics and gently steer the conversation to more appropriate ground. She can suggest topics ("Maybe you'll tell me about . . .") and leave it for the child to initiate. She also can train the child to ask other people about their likes and dislikes, favorite foods, sports, TV shows, or exciting trips or vacations in order to include other-oriented topics in the child's repertoire.

Traditional therapy often centers on the immediate context and may inhibit generalization by failing to incorporate displacement or nonimmediate contexts (Spradlin & Siegel, 1982). In part, the discussion of the immediate context is related to the stimulus items used with children. To increase the frequency of memory-related topics, the facilitator can encourage the child to talk about feelings or activities engaged in prior to the conversation (Bedrosian & Willis, 1987). Elicitation can be direct ("What did you do yesterday?") or indirect ("I wonder what you did yesterday"). She can encourage the child to ask the same information of the language facilitator. In addition, she can engage the child in activities and then ask him to discuss what was done. The speech-language pathologist can provide feedback in the form of expansions of the child's utterances. Future-related topic initiations are similar, such as discussing what the child will do next. The use of such conversationally based strategies can increase nonimmediate topic initiations, as well as the general level of syntactic performance (Bedrosian & Willis, 1987).

Topic maintenance.   The speech-language pathologist can continue the conversation by commenting on the topic the child initiated and by cuing the child to respond (Downing, 1987). She can use turnabouts—usually a comment followed by a cue for the child to respond, such as a question—to keep the conversation flowing and on-topic. Questions should make pragmatic sense; that is, the facilitator should not know the answer prior to asking. Table 10.2 is a list of various turnabouts.

Off-topic responding may indicate that the child is inattentive or cannot identify the referent or topic presented. Children who are inattentive may be distracted easily and need help determining the focus of their attention. Children with autism may make off-topic comments because of a lack of assumed background information and experience or a lack of realization that such background is available (Lord, 1984; Lord & Magill, 1988; Rutter, 1985; Tager-Flusberg, 1981b).

The facilitator can help the child who cannot sort through the information to identify the referent or topic through the use of questions and prompts that highlight those semantic cues of importance to the child (Mesibov, 1984; T. Williams, 1989). Practice conversations with various partners and topics can provide an opportunity to learn and generalize (McGee, Krantz, & McClannahan,

TABLE 10.2
Variety of turnabouts

Type	Example
Tag	Child: Baby's panties. Mother: It's the baby's diaper, *isn't it?*
Clarification (contingent query)	*Huh?* *What?*
Specific request	*What's that?*
Confirmation	*Horse?* *Is that a hippopotamus?* (Hand object to partner and give quizzical glance)
Expansions	
Suggestions	*I want one.*
Corrections	*No, it's a zebra!* (Expectant tone)
Behavior comment	*You can't sit on that.*
Expansive question for sustaining conversation	*What would the police officer do then?*

Source: Drawn from Kay, K., & Charney, R. (1981). Conversational asymmetry between mothers and children. *Journal of Child Language, 8,* 35–49.

1984). The facilitator can keep the child on-topic with such cues as, "Anything else you can tell me about (topic)?" or, "Tell me more about (topic)." Later, she can use contingent queries to keep the child on-topic.

Specific words may confuse the child. The speech-language pathologist must be careful to limit the use of words, such as *what,* that can be used to obtain specific nominative information ("What is this?") and explanations ("What happened at the zoo?").

When the facilitator and the child have shared the same experience, the facilitator can act as a guide to keep the child on-topic. The facilitator also can help the child sequence events through the use of questions ("Then what happened?") or probes ("Are you sure that happened next?").

The facilitator should avoid dead-end conversational bids. Dead-end bids result in a short response that ends the interaction. A common dead-end bid is the overused, "What did you do today?" to which every child knows the answer: "Nothing."

Duration of topic.   The facilitator may help the incessant talker by using very limited topics with definite boundaries, such as, "What animals did you see at the zoo?" If the child strays beyond the topic, the facilitator should interrupt. She then can remind the child of the topic and gently bring him back to it.

The facilitator also should alert the child when he has provided enough information or is redundant. Such phrases as, "You've already told me about *X*" or, "I'll only answer that question one more time," help the child establish boundaries.

Children who provide too little information can be encouraged to provide more with, "Tell me more." The speech-language pathologist also can play dumb with such utterances as, "Well, I guess it was pretty boring if that's all that happened." In general, children remain on-topic longer when they are enacting scenarios, describing, or problem solving (Schober-Peterson & Johnson, 1989).

Turn Taking

It is important not to initiate turn-taking training while also attempting to train topic maintenance. Too many new training targets may confuse the child. The facilitator may have to tolerate off-topic comments initially to correct inappropriate turn taking.

Turn taking can begin at a nonverbal, physical level. The facilitator and the child can pass items back and forth as they use them. The item then can become the symbol for talking. Many structured games also require turn taking. The facilitator also can provide a turn-taking model by imitating the child. She can use verbal games and motion songs with groups of children. Later, she can use turnabouts or a question-answer technique to help the child take verbal turns. Nonlinguistic cues, such as eye contact and nodding, can signal the child to take a turn. She can decrease questioning gradually in favor of these nonlinguistic cues and wait for the child to take a turn. She can teach the child attention-getting devices, such as increased speaking volume, to gain a turn. She can change conversational partners for those with whom the child is more assertive and initiates more frequently. Games in which the child directs other people are highly motivating.

Turn taking is appropriate if it does not interrupt others. The child who is overly assertive and who continually interrupts may need to be reminded not to do so. The facilitator might focus instruction on identifying when speakers have completed their turns. She also should explain appropriate interruptions, as in emergencies. Structured exchanges through use of an intercom or CB radio may help children understand the importance of turn allocation. Structured games, such as Twenty Questions, also foster turn-allocation learning.

Conversational Repair

Through monitoring, each conversational partner detects and reacts to conversational breakdowns by other people when she or he is speaking and alone when a partner is speaking (Markman, 1981). Children with language impairment often seem unaware of the distinction between understanding and failure to understand and rarely act even when they do not comprehend.

The speech-language pathologist may modify comprehension monitoring through the use of audiotaped language samples in the following training sequence (Dollaghan & Kaston, 1986):

1. Identification, labeling, and demonstration of active listening
2. Detection of and reaction to inadequate signals
3. Detection of and reaction to inadequate content
4. Identification of and reaction to comprehension breakdown

Although this sequence can be trained easily in an audiotaped mode with first graders, generalization to actual conversational use should not be neglected. The introduction of puppets, dolls, or role playing at each step can facilitate this generalization. Written scripts may be used with older children.

Comprehension monitoring can be facilitated when the child takes an active role in the process. The child is taught first to identify, label, and demonstrate active orientation to listening behaviors, such as sitting, looking at the speaker, and thinking about what the speaker says (Dollaghan & Kaston, 1986). After learning to distinguish successful and unsuccessful performance of the three active listening behaviors, the child labels and demonstrates each. The child also might repeat the previous speaker's utterance or reply to such questions as, "What did (name) just say?"

Next, the child is taught to detect and react to *signal inadequacies,* such as insufficient loudness, excessive rate, or competing noise. These concrete obstructions that prevent representation of the message are relatively easy to identify and enable the child to learn the difference between understanding and not understanding (Dollaghan & Kaston, 1986).

Within everyday activities, the facilitator can encourage contingent queries from the child by mumbling or talking too fast. This technique works especially well when giving directions needed to complete some fun task. The facilitator occasionally can ask the child, "What did I say? How can we find out?"

Once able to identify signal inadequacies, the child can be taught a variety of responses for requesting clarification. Requests may include general appeals, such as, "Pardon?" (or "What?"), "I can't hear you," and, "Wait . . . Now say it again" (or "Again please"), or more specific requests, such as, "Talk louder please" (or, "Louder"), "Could you talk more slowly?" (or, "Slow down"), and, "Did you say *X*?" It is best to begin with more general requests and then move to more specific ones. The request form should reflect the child's overall syntactic level.

Next, the child can be taught to detect and react to *content inadequacies,* such as inexplicit, ambiguous, and physically impossible commands. For example, because inadequate content may not always be obvious, the speech-language pathologist can ask the child to repeat the message to himself and/or to the speaker and to attempt the task demanded (Dollaghan & Kaston, 1986). Again, the child is taught various methods for requesting clarification of inadequate content. Requests may include, "What do you mean?" "Which one?" "Where?" "I can't do that" (or, "I can't"), "Do you mean *X*?" and, "That doesn't make sense."

This part of the training can be great fun, with the facilitator making outrageous statements and ridiculous demands of the child. She can insert intentional content inadequacies into any number of daily activities.

Finally, she can teach the child to identify and react to messages that exceed his comprehension capacity by the presence of unfamiliar lexical items, excessive length, and excessive syntactic complexity. This level of comprehension breakdown may be the most difficult to detect because of the often abstract nature of the breakdown.

The child can practice identification and reaction in the form of clarification requests in real-life situations in which these difficulties are likely to occur.

Most novel activities include unusual jargon that the facilitator can use to confuse the message. For example, cooking offers such words as *ladle, simmer,* and *skillet.*

Requests for clarification might include, "Say those one at a time" (or, "One at a time"), "That was too long for me," "I don't know that word" (or, "I don't know"), "Can you tell me a different way?" "What does X mean?" (or, "What do you mean?"), and, "Can you show me?" (or, "Show me"). As training progresses, the child should identify the point of actual breakdown for the speaker.

Narration

Language intervention with narratives may focus on the organization of the narrative, cohesion, or comprehension. Specific targets will vary with the maturity of the child.

Narrative Structure

Young children use a script-based knowledge organization system (McCartney & Nelson, 1981; Wimmer, 1979). Although older children and adults retain this system, they also use taxonomic or categoric knowledge for processing (Lange, 1978; Mistry & Lange, 1985).

Scripts are sequences of events that form unified wholes. When this event sequence is placed in linguistic form, it is called a *text,* the basis of narratives. Narratives generally are organized by a story grammar consisting of an initiating event, a reaction by the main characters to the event, an attempt to respond to the event, a consequence or outcome to the event, and an ending (J. Johnston, 1982b; Stein & Glenn, 1979).

Knowledge of episode structure forms a framework within which the child can interpret complex events and unfamiliar content. The speech-language pathologist can facilitate development of internalized narrative schemes or story grammars through the following (Hewitt, 1992; N. Nelson, 1986b):

1. Involve children in organized activities, such as daily routines, to help them organize their own real-life scripts.

2. Use scripted play in which children enact everyday activities that gradually become more variable and less contextualized.

3. Read and tell real-life stories with clear scripts.

4. Help children transfer from activities to linguistic organization by telling them narratives with clearly structured story grammars and then having them dramatize the stories (Moeller & McConkey, 1984).

These exercises also may be written.

Scripted play is especially useful with preschool and early school-age children. Initially, it is very important that the scripts describe familiar motivating events, such as going to the market or getting ready for school. The script should be introduced and discussed prior to play, with expectations stated.

Today, we're going to play "shopping at the market." How many of you have gone shopping with someone? Good. Whom did you go with, Tiera? Okay, and whom did you go with, Andre? Good. What do we buy at the market? Uh-huh. Yes. Good. I have some things right here. What's this, Jewell? Good. What's this, T. J.? Right. Do we buy this at the market? That's right, we don't buy this at the market. What's this, Rochelle? Good. Do we buy this at the market? Good, that's right, we do. What is the first thing that happens when you get to the market? (And so on.)

The script is played and discussed afterward.

With each replaying, the children change roles, modify the events, and use less concrete objects. As children become more adept at recounting the script, the speech-language pathologist encourages telling of the narrative without an enactment. Again, familiar roles and situations are used. These procedures work especially well with groups of children and will be discussed in more detail in the following chapter on classroom intervention.

The speech-language pathologist can facilitate production of event descriptions by having children describe familiar events as they occur or as recalled from slides, pictures, or videotapes (Duchan, 1986b; Lewis, Duchan, & Lubinski, 1985). Children can role-play and describe familiar events as they occur. One of my favorite language lessons included mime and the acting out of familiar situations. Later, these events were described without role playing.

Pictures of familiar events as the child draws them can be used for sequencing. The facilitator can help the child identify the setting and characters by asking him to describe the picture; for example:

FACILITATOR:	Well, what do we have here?
CHILD:	This is me in the kitchen, and I'm making breakfast.
FACILITATOR:	So, we might say, "This morning, I was in the kitchen making breakfast." What did you do first? (Or, Then what happened? or, What's this next picture?)

After completing a step-by-step description, the child can be encouraged to tell the entire narrative.

Children then can progress to fairy tales or their own stories. The facilitator can use questions to move children to more sophisticated ways of organizing and expressing concepts and relationships. Chapter 11 includes a discussion of replica play and narratives in the classroom.

Narrative discourse is the next logical step. Children should have the opportunity to practice forms of narration within a variety of role-playing situations (Heath, 1986b). Narratives can be cued by statements such as, "Tell me what you did at . . ." or, "Tell me how you did . . ."

It is unclear whether cohesion can be taught directly. Increased organization may reflect maturation of children's cognitive-social-linguistic knowledge system (K. Nelson, 1985; Rice, 1984). Contextualized training can provide the structure needed to foster the development of cohesion in children's communication.

Cohesion

It is best to teach story grammar structure prior to cohesion (Liles, 1990). Although the two are related, it is possible for a narrative to have a good story grammar and poor cohesion. Cohesion requires some metalinguistic skill because the narrator must pay attention to the text apart from the sequence of events being presented.

Cohesion is of three types: conjunctive, referential, and lexical. (Lexical cohesion, using terms such as *yesterday, in the future, prior to,* and *ate/will eat,* is difficult to measure reliably and is very individualized. It will not be discussed here.) *Conjunctive* reference is the easiest form of cohesion to teach. Children's oral narratives can be collected and transcribed into a "book." Use of conjunctions and the relationships expressed can be analyzed. Simple stories containing various clausal relationships also can be read to children. In a retelling, a child usually will not express relationships and conjunctions that he does not use.

Once the child's narrative relationships and conjunctions have been analyzed, the speech-language pathologist can begin to introduce other conjunctions. A developmental order of introduction may be helpful, although the first priority should be conjunctions omitted or used incorrectly in the relationships expressed. For example, in " . . . stoled all his money. He robbed a bank. He was starving . . .," cause and effect are suggested but without the use of *because.*

The speech-language pathologist can introduce narrative relationships with or without a conjunction and then, using a question-answer technique, prompt the child to produce the desired conjunction. If the child responds incorrectly, the speech-language pathologist can reread or retell the relevant portion of the narrative, model a response including the conjunction, discuss the meaning, and prompt the child to respond again. The important aspect of the training is an understanding of the relationship expressed, not a regurgitation of the correct conjunction. The final stages of training would include original narratives produced by the child.

Referential cohesion uses nouns, pronouns, and articles to designate old and new information in the narrative. Again, questions and answers can be used to direct the child as a narrative is told. Retellings by the speech-language pathologist might use a *cloze* technique, in which the child fills in the appropriate word. Gradually, less narrative-structured and more expository materials can be introduced. It is more difficult to comprehend and produce cohesion without the narrative frame.

Comprehension

Narrative comprehension can be improved by beginning with predictable narratives concerning everyday events or routines familiar to the child. The child's internalized event script aids both comprehension and recall. As in scripted play, variations in the narrative are introduced gradually, and the text moves to more unfamiliar and fictionalized events and stories. Comprehension and recall can be facilitated by having children draw or write event sequences.

Some data suggest that the use of subjectivity or the character's thoughts and feelings can enhance comprehension of fictional narratives (Hewitt, 1992). Children can be taught to focus on a character's thoughts and feelings as a way of making sense of the events in the narrative. Thus, the child focuses more on the reasons for and outcomes or results of events within the narrative. There are no right or wrong answers; rather, the child's responses explain events in a manner comprehendible to the child.

SEMANTICS

Semantic intervention consists of several different but related levels of intervention. Word meanings form relationships with other words that help categorize and organize not only the language system but also cognitive processes, particularly for older children. For this reason, semantic intervention involves a variety of interrelated intervention strategies much more complex than simply training vocabulary words.

At its core, word meaning consists of concepts or knowledge of the world. Words do not name things, but rather refer to these concepts (Olson, 1970). These conceptual complexes are formed from many experiences with the actual referents.

The process of forming and organizing concepts may reflect general cognitive organization and, in turn, influence that organization (N. Nelson, 1986b). Semantic training must recognize the importance of these underlying concepts and include cognitive aspects of concept formation. Several commercial resources are available for training cognitive skills essential for conceptualization (Cimorell, 1983).

Inadequate Vocabulary

Reference or *meaning* is the relationship of the sign or word to the underlying concept. Different strategies are used by different children and by the same child at different developmental times to construct meanings.

Children with language disorders often use one strategy exclusively or predominantly. For example, the meanings of children with autism seem to be unanalyzed, experience-based chunks that are very situationally related (Fay & Schuler, 1980; Prizant, 1983b). Children with mental retardation are often deficient in their ability to form complex concepts. Other children may have conventional concepts but experience difficulty relating these underlying concepts to linguistic symbols or words.

The speech-language pathologist may assist with the building and extending of individual reference systems by providing situations in which children encounter the physical and social world. Dynamic events seem to encourage early concept development better than do static ones (N. Nelson, 1986b). Therefore, feature learning can be enhanced by focus on movement, contrast, and change. The most successful strategy is to (a) build on an experiential or prior knowledge base and establish links to new words, (b) teach in meaningful contexts, and (c) provide multiple exposures (Nagy & Herman, 1987). The experiential base is important, especially for the child below age 7. The child should have the opportunity to have meaningful, real experiences.

World knowledge, or what the child knows about her or his world, is very important for vocabulary growth. Early word meanings are acquired within event-related experiences, especially predictable, everyday routines and their accompanying scripts (Bruner, 1978b; K. Nelson & Brown, 1978; K. Nelson & Gruendel, 1979; N. Nelson, 1986b; Peters, 1984; Snow, 1977b; Snow & Goldfield, 1983). Gradually, meanings generalize and decontextualize. Between ages 5 and 9, the child developing normally reorganizes her or his vocabulary from event-based processing to more linguistic, semantic-based processing (K. Nelson, 1977; Petrey, 1977).

Groups of children on a field trip can experience the world by touching, smelling, and even tasting an old log and describing the sensation. Language facilitators can encode features of events and entities to which children attend (N. Nelson, 1986b). Older elementary school children can learn from the experiences of others, much as adults do (Lucas, 1980).

Vocabulary is acquired in a two-phase process. First, words are *fast-mapped*—a small portion of the meaning is acquired on the first exposure (Carey, 1978). The child's world and word knowledge affect which features of the definition she or he acquires. The second phase is a later, more gradual one in which repeated exposure results in a more complete map of the word's meaning (Carey & Bartlett, 1978).

Children and adolescents with language impairment need to learn how to use the context to establish word meaning (McKeown & Curtis, 1987; Nippold, 1991; R. Sternberg, 1987). Contexts provide a number of cues that can be classified as temporal (time), spatial (location), value (relative worth), stative descriptive (physical description), functional descriptive (use), causal (cause and effect), class membership (type), and equivalence (similarity/difference) (R. Sternberg & Powell, 1983). Class membership and functional descriptive are the easiest for children, whereas stative descriptive seems to be the most difficult (R. Sternberg, 1987). Context should be established for the child prior to introducing the word numerous times. The child will need help in determining what he knows from the context and repeated exposures. Narratives also may provide a context for introducing a novel word (Crais, 1987).

No one likes to give verbatim definitions. Learning benefits if the child and the facilitator can use the word to discuss a relevant topic in context. It is important to remember that the child may not need a full adult definition when the word is first introduced. A less full definition may suffice (Kameenui, Dixon, & Carnine, 1987).

The facilitator should not expect dictionary definitions from children below age 12. By that age, however, the child should be able to define words, draw conclusions, and make inferences.

Child and adult definitions, especially categorical ones, seem to be organized around a prototype or best exemplar. Examples given to the child should be of the prototype or best exemplar variety, as these will enhance learning of salient features (Lucas, 1980). In addition, the facilitator should expose children to multiple examples of events and things in familiar contexts in order to perceive these features of events and entities. Language facilitators can act as mediators framing, focusing, and providing salient features of experiences for the child (N. Nelson, 1986b).

Within activities, children can be encouraged to describe features. Descriptors then can be used to determine similarities and differences and to label the world. Instead of naming unfamiliar entities, such as types of leaves, children can be encouraged to stretch their existing language and give descriptive names, such as *five-pointed leaf tree.*

Facilitators also can target words used frequently at home and school in everyday activities and events. In general, it is easier to learn words for known concepts than to learn both words and concepts (Crais, 1990). The choice of which words to teach should be based on the likely frequency of use, normal development, need within the classroom and use in textbooks, and likelihood of the child learning the word from context alone (E. Dale & O'Rourke, 1981; Graves, 1987). Even slang expressions might be taught to aid socialization, especially among adolescents (D. Cooper & Anderson-Inman, 1988).

Training should include words along with others that mean the same (synonyms), sound the same (homonyms), or are opposites (antonyms). This training will help the child organize language for easy storage and retrieval of information. Prefixes and suffixes are also important, as is syllabication. The child's existing meanings can be consolidated by building on the child's current vocabulary while correcting errors and misconceptions of meaning (Elshout-Mohr & van Daalen-Kapteijns, 1987).

Understanding and training should progress from these general meanings to more specific ones. It is important for the child with language impairment to expand meanings beyond the often obvious best exemplars. Training also should proceed from more contextual meanings, as in "hit the ball," to less contextual, more figurative meanings, such as "hit the roof," and multiple meanings, such as, "a hit musical." Abstract terms, such as *except, instead,* and *until,* should be targeted last.

The semantic features of words can be analyzed to expand the characteristics associated with words and to aid categorization (Crais, 1990). Words can be classified according to their semantic features, as in Figure 10.1. Sorting tasks perform a similar function, and children can be encouraged to make their own associations.

Multiple meanings should be related to specific academic subject areas or contexts. The facilitator should help the child understand that meaning varies with context (Graves, 1987).

A root-word strategy can be used with school-age children to help them discover meanings and their modifications (Crais, 1990). Suffixes are easier to learn than prefixes and should be introduced first (see morphology section of this chapter). Prefix training should begin with concrete, easy-to-define prefixes, such as *un-,* and proceed to more abstract ones. The most frequently used prefixes in American English are *un-, in-, dis-,* and *non-.*

	Transportation	Four-wheel	Two-wheel	Engine-powered	Peddle-powered	Runs on rails
Motorcycle	X		X	X		
Bicycle	X		X		X	
Car	X	X		X		
Bus	X	X		X		
Train	X			X		X

	Animals	Bird	On farm	Wild or zoo animal	Gives milk	Four-legged
Chicken	X	X	X			
Duck	X	X	X			
Cow	X		X		X	X
Elephant	X			X	X	X
Goat	X		X		X	X

FIGURE 10.1
Analyzing semantic feature similarities

Materials should provide for adequate semantic development. Pictures are too abstract for some children; single examples too limited. "Materials that isolate word meanings from the total concept are too abstract" (Lucas, 1980, p. 21). Referents should be presented in a variety of ways to build a total concept. Varying contexts provide for maximum usage and exposure. Storytelling in which a novel word must be used is also a good strategy and uses context to facilitate use.

Many commercially available games can be used as is or modified for vocabulary training, including Boggle, Pictionary, and Scrabble (Beck, McKeown, & Omanson, 1987; Graves, 1987). Semantic organizers, such as spidergrams, can be used to build associations. Children can use semantic organizers to "brainstorm" or to tell all they know about a word (C. Nelson, 1991). Figure 10.2 is a typical spidergram.

Children also enjoy creating words such as "sniglets"—words that do not exist in the dictionary but should. Such original words can be used along with real words to try to encourage children to make educated guesses about the meaning (Atkinson & Longman, 1985; Hall, 1984). Table 10.3 contains several sniglets.

Semantic Categories and Relational Words

Meaning extends beyond the word level. As children develop beyond the single-word level, they are able to encode meaning in the form of the utterances produced. Words with the same referent can fulfill different semantic roles or cases

FIGURE 10.2
Spidergram of word meanings and associations

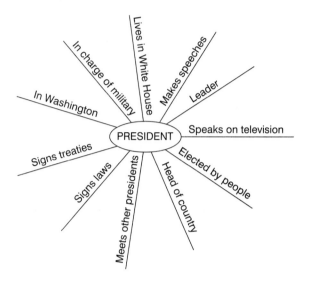

that specify the relationships among those referents. Table 6.7 presents the most common cases or semantic classes. Thus, the child forming a sentence must keep in mind both the referent and the semantic role.

Words and phrases also modify the meaning of basic syntactic elements by indicating qualities, such as perceptual attributes, manner, and temporal aspects, and relationships between larger sentential units, such as additive (*and*) or causal (*because*). As a listener, the child can only comprehend other people to the extent that she or he understands the various relationships underlying their utterances (Creaghead & Donnelly, 1982).

TABLE 10.3
Examples of "sniglets"

Sniglet	Definition
Bathquake	n. The violent quake that rattles the entire house when the water faucet is turned to a certain point.
Lotshock	n. The act of parking your car, walking away, and then watching it roll past you.
Maggit	n. Any of the hundreds of subscription cards that fall from the pages of a magazine.
Petrool	n. The slow, seemingly endless strand of motor oil at the end of the can.
Shoefly	n. The aeronautical terminology for a football player who misses the punt and launches his shoe instead.

Source: Hall, R. (1984). *Sniglets (Snig'lit): Any word that doesn't appear in the dictionary, but should.* New York: Macmillan.

Semantic Classes

The speech-language pathologist can teach words to children and place the words in different semantic classes. A portion of word definition is the semantic class into which a word can be placed. She also can teach other word types that relate to that class. Children with language impairment may find it difficult to identify and use semantic classes of words.

The agent function found in the subject position of a sentence offers a unique example for semantic category training (Connell, 1986b). English is a subject-prominent language in which a large number of morphosyntactic and transformational elements are associated with the subject of the sentence (P. Cole, Harbert, Herman, & Sridhar, 1980; Keenan, 1976; Li & Thompson, 1976). These elements include subject-verb agreement, as with the verb *to be* and the third person singular, present tense marker; pronouns; and auxiliary verb inversions in questions. These elements are not critical to the content of a sentence, and they can be omitted without greatly affecting the understanding of the sentence.

The speech-language pathologist may facilitate teaching these elements by teaching the concept of *subjecthood* (Connell, 1986b). She can accomplish this by using a functional approach in which she teaches the child the purpose of a subject.

The function of a sentence's subject, represented by a noun or a noun phrase, is to designate the perspective used in the sentence (Dik, 1980). In contrast, the topic designates the focus of discourse. If the sentence contains action, the agent designates the actor. In the sentence "John ate the salami" (Connell, 1986b, p. 482), all three elements are the same. In "*John* was arrested by the police" (ibid.), *John* is the topic and the subject, but *police* is the agent.

Subjects can be identified by the pronouns used with them. Subjects take nominative case pronouns, whereas topics and agents may take different types. Subjects also agree with predicates, whereas topics and agents need not.

The speech-language pathologist can train children to identify the topic and the subject by using the following forms (Connell, 1986b):

1. Objecive   nominative   verb/
   case   +   case   +   *be*   +   adjective/
   pronoun   pronoun   adverb/noun
   (*Him*,   *he*   *is*   *running*)

2. Nominative case prononun + *be* + verb/adjective/adverb/noun
   (*He*   *is*   *running*)

The first is taught in response to a "Which one is . . .?" type of question, and the second in response to a "What is the man doing?" or "Who is . . .?" type of question. Children can induce the function of the subject and its separateness from the topic by the varying sentential contexts in which they are used.

Children can learn each sentence form by imitation and then in response to questions within ongoing activities. Training should begin with the second sentence type because it is included within the first. Once children have learned the formats, the questions can be alternated. Later, the habitual or simple present form of the verb, such as *eat* or *drink,* can be introduced to teach children subject-verb agreement within the same subject-highlighted format.

Other semantic classes may be taught in a similar manner. Table 10.4 presents suggestions for training.

Relational Words

Relational words fulfill many functions in language. Relationships may be based on quantity or quality and may be general or specific. Other relational words are used to mark location and time. Conjunctions are relational words that relate one clause to another. Each type of relational word requires specific considerations.

In general, relational terms can be acquired through descriptive tasks, in which the child must differentiate between one entity and another, or through narrative tasks, in which the child must aid the listener to differentiate characters. The speech-language pathologist can help the child initially by keeping the task context-bound and by controlling the number of items or characters. By playing dumb or acting confused, the facilitator can help the child provide additional or essential information. Narratives are also effective vehicles for acquiring

TABLE 10.4
Suggestions for training semantic classes

Instrument
Initially, this class can be trained in the final position of the sentence preceded by the word *by,* as in "The wood was split *by his axe.*" Position and the preposition *by* act as signals for this class. This class can also be signaled by the verb *use,* as in "John *used the rake* to gather the leaves." This sentence type can be prompted by questions such as "How did . . .?" and "What did John use to . . .?"

Patient/Object
This class may be taught initially by using the final position in the sentence as a direct object to transitive verbs. Question prompts such as "What did Carol throw?" may be used to elicit this class.

It is somewhat more difficult to teach this class in the subject position because that position is usually occupied by an agent. If agents are taught in response to a *who*-type of question, patients might use *what,* as in "What grew in the park?"

Dative
The dative class is most frequently and obviously used as an indirect object. This function can be clearly signaled initially by use of the prepositions *to* and *for.* Question prompts can include these cues and the word *whom,* as in "For whom did Mary buy the flowers?"

Temporal, Locative, and Manner
These classes are relatively easy to teach because each has specific questions that prompt usage. Prepositions, such as *in, on,* and *at,* are used with these functions, as are *to, with,* and *by,* which are used to mark other semantic class use.

Accompaniment
The final position in the sentence and the use of the preposition *with* should be used in training to signal this class. *With whom* question prompts can be used to elicit response.

---

conjunctions, especially when the facilitator synthesizes larger, more conceptually complex sentences based on those of the child.

Quantitative terms.   A child does not need to be able to count to learn quantitative terms. Initial training can begin with the concepts of *one* and *more than one*. The second concept can be marked variously by *many, much, some,* and *more.* Such terms as *these* and *those* should be introduced with some caution because of deixis or interpretation from the perspective of the speaker. Deixis is mentioned in the pragmatics portion of this chapter and is covered briefly in the following section.

The distinction between *many* and *much* is complex and should be ignored with children functioning at a preschool level. In general, *many* is used with regular and irregular plural nouns, such as *cats, shoes,* and *women.* In contrast, *much* is used with mass nouns—nouns that refer to homogeneous, nonindividual substances, such as *water, sand,* and *sugar.* It is not surprising that children have difficulty with the two terms *much* and *many.*

Before going beyond the quantity words mentioned, the child must learn to count and have a concept of the relative values of different numbers. In other words, the child must know that four is greater than two, not that four merely follows in a sequence.

Later quantifiers can include words such as *few* and *couple.* These can be followed by other quantifiers, such as *nearly, almost as much as,* and *half.* Table 10.5 presents common quantitative words. The ordering of these words in the noun phrase is very important and is discussed in the syntax section of this chapter.

Qualitative terms.   Qualitative terms include such words as *bigger* and *tallest,* which use the *-er* and *-est* morphological markers, and such phrases as *as big as,*

TABLE 10.5
Common quantitative and qualitative terms

Quantitative	Qualitative
One, two, three, four . . .	Big, little, long, short
Many, much, lots of	Large, small, fat, thin
Some, few, couple	Soft, hard, heavy, light
More, another	Same, different, alike
Nearly, almost all	Old, young, pretty, ugly
As much/little as	Blue, green, red, . . .
Plenty	Hot, cold, warm, chilly
Half, one-fourth, two-fifths	Wide, narrow
10%, 75%	Sweet, sour
Units of measure: Inch, foot, mile, cup,	Nice, mean, funny, sad
pint, quart, gallon, centimeter, meter,	Fast, slow
kilometer, liter, ounce, pound, gram,	Smooth, rough
kilogram, acre	Angry, afraid
Clean, dirty	Comparative and superlative relationships:
Empty, full	*-er, -est,* as *x* as, *x-er* than

not as wet as, smaller than, and the like. Table 10.5 also presents common qualitative terms. In general, children learn to use the comparative *-er* before the superlative *-est,* and training should follow that pattern. It is best to begin with the regular use of these two markers before introducing exceptions, such as *better* and *best.* Words can be expanded into phrases, for example, *bigger* to *bigger than.*

Children seem to acquire concepts one semantic feature at a time (E. Clark, 1973). A corollary to this hypothesis is that broad, nonspecific concepts (e.g., *big*) are learned before more specific concepts (e.g., *long*). In this example, *big* refers to overall size, whereas *long* refers to size only in the horizontal plane. Several studies have confirmed this acquisition order (Richards, 1979).

The speech-language pathologist should introduce terms and relationships in the order in which comparative terms develop. Table 10.6 includes common pairs of comparative terms and the approximate age at which most children can use them correctly.

In general, conceptual word-pairs are acquired asymmetrically, one prior to the other, on the basis of their polarity. Children ages 3 to 7 appear to learn the positive-pole member of conceptual pairs, the one that represents more of the dimension characterized by the conceptual pair, prior to learning the negative member (Bracken, 1988; Greenberg, 1966). For example, *big* and *little* are opposite poles of the dimension *size. Big* represents more size and is, therefore, the positive member. These data suggest that positive members should be taught first to children with language impairment. In addition, positive-type comparisons

TABLE 10.6
Common comparative word-pairs

Positive-Negative (age)	Positive-Negative (age)	Positive-Negative (age)
same-different (36–60 months)	open-close	on-off (24–36 months)
in front of-behind (48–54 months)	inside-outside	up-down (36–60 months)
into-out of	over-under (42–48 months)	high-low (42–60 months)
top-bottom (48–54 months)	front-back (48–52 months)	forward-backward
rising-falling	above-below (66–72 months)	happy-sad
healthy-sick	right-wrong	old-young
big-little (30–48 months)	heavy-light (30–48 months)	large-small (78–84 months)
deep-shallow	tall-short (30–84 months)	long-short (horizontal) (54–60 months)
thick-thin	loud-quiet	hot-cold
hard-soft (30–42 months)	sharp-dull	dark-light
smooth-rough	solid-liquid	tight-loose
more-less (42–72 months)	full-empty (36–48 months)	a lot-little
all-none	with-without (48–54 months)	fast-slow
old-new	arriving-leaving	early-late
before-after (66–72 months)	first-last (60–66 months)	always-never

(The overall order does not reflect the order for teaching conceptual pairs.)

Source: Bracken (1988); Edmonston & Thane (1990); Wiig & Semel (1984)

should be taught before negative ones. In other words, *bigger than* should be introduced before *smaller than* and *not as big as.* Positive comparisons seem to be easier for children to process.

Spatial and temporal terms.   Several words are used to mark both space or location and time and, thus, are potentially confusing. Among the most commonly used words in English are prepositions, such as *in, on, at,* and *by.* Each of these small, seemingly insignificant words has several definitions. In the syntax section of this chapter I discuss prepositional training. In addition, other words, such as *first* and *last,* also note place and time.

Spatial concepts are best taught first in relation to the child; then with "featured" or fronted objects, such as a television, chair, or person; and finally with nonfeatured objects, such as a wastebasket or a ball (Edmonston & Thane, 1990). The latter is more difficult to learn because it involves deixis. In general, vertical dimensions are learned before horizontal. Horizontal front and back terms, such as *in front of* and *behind,* are learned before horizontal side-to-side terms, such as *beside* and *next to.*

The order of temporal term learning reflects the underlying concepts of order, simultaneity, and duration (Edmonston & Thane, 1990). Terms that denote order, such as *before, after, first,* and *last,* usually are learned before terms for simultaneity, such as *at the same time* and *when.* Duration terms, such as *a long time,* generally are acquired last.

Children with psychological disorders have difficulty with the concept of time and with event boundaries. Thus, changing activities is often difficult. Intervention needs to begin with awareness (Audet & Hummel, 1990). The use of timers or other reminders can help these children monitor and regulate their behavior. Concrete event boundaries, such as the completion of a project, can aid transitions. Schedules and/or pictures of sequential events also may increase awareness.

In general, it is better to begin with concrete definitions and progress to more abstract ones. For example, with *first, last, before,* and *after,* training can begin with objects in a line. The facilitator can have the child touch individual objects, then a short sequence of objects, and finally a reverse sequence. Objects should be used first before terms for events and the concept of time sequencing.

One context is not enough for teaching concepts of space and time. The greater the number of contexts, the more learning and generalization that will occur. Language can be used to help the child organize the environment by marking experiences of space and time. Table 10.7 includes common spatial and temporal terms.

The speech-language pathologist can use direction following and activities to train children about space and time. It might be best to begin with routines that the child knows, such as those that occur at home or in the classroom, and then move into less familiar activities, such as using a pay telephone or changing a tire, in which the child must rely more on linguistic input.

Later, the speech-language pathologist can use sequenced pictures or storytelling in the training. Pictures may seem very abstract to some children, espe-

TABLE 10.7
Common spatial and tempo-
ral terms

Spatial	Temporal
Next to	Next
Before	Before
After	After
On, on top	Into
In, into	Soon
In between	Later
Between	Now
Middle	Above
Above	Yesterday
Under	Today
Over	Tomorrow
Below	Calendar dates
Corner	Months
Bottom	Seasons
Inside	Numerals for years
Outside	Morning
Side	Afternoon
End	Evening
In front of	Days
Behind	Weeks
Beside	Hours
Right	Minutes
Left	Through
Through	Away from
High, tall	Toward
Upside down	Sometimes
Together	

cially school-age children with mental retardation and preschoolers, and should
be used with caution.

Deixis and the use of deictic terms are very difficult concepts to teach. The
facilitator who takes the role of speaker and prompter for the child violates the
roles in a conversation. The simple example of *here* and *there* is illustrative.

The request, "Put the ball *here*," is said from the speaker's perspective. To
the listener, the speaker's *here* is most likely *there*. If the speaker then shifts to the
listener or the child's perspective and says, "Yes, put it *there*," it may confuse the
child further.

When training the child about deictic terms, it is best to sit next to the child so
that you can share a perspective. From this shared perspective, some deictic terms,
at least those for location, would be similar. Another facilitator, puppet, or prere-
corded tape may act as the other conversational partner. The teaching of deixis is
discussed also under the topic of pronouns in the syntax section of this chapter.

Conjunctions.   The facilitator should teach conjunctions in the order in which
they develop by noting for the child the relationships expressed in each (Klecan-

Aker, 1985). For example, *because* represents cause and effect and may not be fully acquired until about age 12 by children both with LLD and without (Tyack, 1981; Wiig & Semel, 1984). Table 10.8 presents the general order of conjunction acquisition. The conjunction *and* can first be taught to combine entities, as in "cats *and* dogs." In a cooking activity, the facilitator might say, "Which two types of cookies do you like best?" or, "Tell me your two favorite types of cookies." In similar fashion, *but* can be used for like/dislike distinctions ("I like cookies, *but not beets*").

Wiig & Semel (1984) suggest using a *main clause + conjunction + subordinate clause* format initially to help the child acquire the underlying relationship. For example, sentences might be presented as follows:

> We wear a coat *because* it is cold.
>
> We wear a coat *if* it is cold.
>
> We wear a coat *when* it is cold.

Once the child understands these relationships, the order of the clauses can be reversed, as in, "Because it is cold, we wear a coat."

Next, the speech-language pathologist can present new clauses for the child to complete. She also may use a breakdown and buildup technique, as described in Chapter 9, in which the child identifies clauses and conjunctions and then reconstructs the sentence (Klecan-Aker, 1985).

Word Retrieval and Categorization

Word-retrieval difficulties can result from two possible sources (Kail et al., 1984; Kail & Leonard, 1986). The first is lack of elaboration or lack of a well-established, thorough representation of the word within the child's lexicon. Word knowledge is related to storage ability in that growth in word knowledge results in a larger storage capacity. An increased lexicon requires greater semantic networks in which to group words. In general, children who exhibit difficulties often have less extensive vocabularies and poor word knowledge (Kail & Leonard, 1986; C. Smith, 1991).

TABLE 10.8

Acquisition order for English conjunctions

Source: Based on Bloom, Lahey, Hood, Lifter, & Fless (1980); Clark & Clark (1977); Corrigan (1975); Hood & Bloom (1979); Kuhn & Phelps (1976); L. Lee (1974); Wiig & Semel (1984)

And
And then
But, or
Because
So, if, when
Until, before-after
Although, while, as
Unless
Therefore, however

Data from studies are very variable, and this list is only a rough guide.

The second source of problems is in retrieval. In general, children with this problem are less efficient in retrieving words from storage. Whereas elaboration difficulties may occur alone, retrieval problems usually do not and may be an additional difficulty found in some children with elaborative problems (Kail & Leonard, 1986).

A number of activities have been suggested that facilitate word-finding skills (McGregor & Leonard, 1989; Wiig & Semel, 1984; Wing, 1990). Children appear to benefit from both elaboration and retrieval activities (McGregor & Leonard, 1989). Word-finding activities can be incorporated easily into a number of everyday activities and conversations about these activities.

Prior to beginning intervention, it is important to determine the source of the word-retrieval problem (German, 1992). In short, children with poorly established word meanings have a semantic storage problem. In contrast, those with word-retrieval problems on words that they understand have poor retrieval skills. Finally, some children have problems in both areas. These last children should receive intervention services that combine the goals of the other two.

Children with storage problems have difficulty understanding and retrieving words that are not stable in their memory. Inadequate storage is the result of shallow meanings, reference-shifting problems, and poor analytical and synthesizing skills (German, 1992). The goal of intervention is to improve word knowledge and storage (Wiig & Semel, 1984).

Those with retrieval-only problems have difficulty with search and recovery. Somewhere in the process of discriminating the desired word from among competing words and constructing the phonological specifications for production, the process breaks down (Bjork & Bjork, 1992). The goal of intervention is to improve access.

Memory storage seems to be affected by the depth or level of processing (Craik & Lockhart, 1972). In general, recall is best for words processed at the deepest levels, which are elaborative by nature (Lockhart & Craik, 1990). Theoretically, acoustic processing, such as rhyming, is surface processing; categorical is mid-level; and semantic/syntactic is deep.

Words are remembered in relation to other words and form meaning networks. Such relationships might be morphological (Mackay, 1978; Nagy et al., 1989). When one member of the family is accessed, it activates others. These relationships are based on meaning, not just linear sound or letter strings. In other words, *ride* does not elicit *stride,* nor does *cad* elicit **cadet**.

Semantic similarity and, to a lesser degree, phonetic similarity do affect judgments of relatedness, especially for literate adults (Derwing, 1976; Derwing & Baker, 1979). Networks of semantic-related morphemes are part of each individual's memory system. Thus, *stain, stained glass,* and *stainless steel* are perceived to be related.

Elaboration training focuses on organization of the child's lexicon and generalization of word meanings to everyday use (Kail, 1984; Kail & Leonard, 1986). In children developing normally, increased word knowledge results in increased storage strength. In short, a larger vocabulary means a more extensive database.

In elaboration training, the speech-language pathologist can use semantic focus strategies, such as nonidentical exemplars and word comparison tasks. She presents nonidentical exemplars, or examples of the word in several linguistic contexts, to enrich the child's definition and word associations. Nonidentical exemplars for *house* might include *dollhouse, house fly,* and *greenhouse.* In comparative tasks, she expects the child to identify similarities and differences between two words with related meanings, such as *house* and *hotel.*

A mnemonic or "key word" strategy (J. Levin et al., 1984) also might be used to aid elaboration and recall of new vocabulary. New words are linked with acoustically or visually similar words with which the child is familiar. For example, *dogged* might be linked with *dog.* This initial linkage is modified to a semantic one with deeper processing.

In the mnemonic method, pictures and written descriptions are used to link two words. A known word is used to aid learning and storage of an unknown one. In the above example, a *dog* would be portrayed being stubborn or determined (dogged). Under the picture, it might read *The **dog** was **dogged** and would not give up.* Other examples are given in Figure 10.3. The key word now becomes the retrieval cue.

Children using this approach reportedly are able to recall 50% more definitions than those taught vocabulary by a more traditional method (J. Levin et al.,

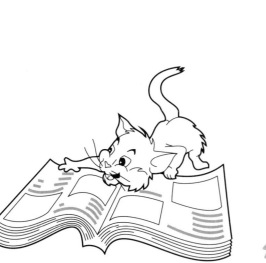

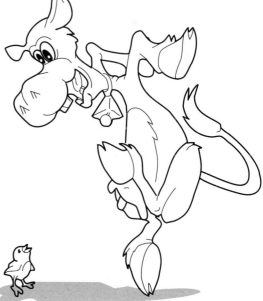

The **cat** is ordering from the **catalog.**   The **cow** is a scared **coward.**

FIGURE 10.3
Examples of mnemonic strategies

1984). In addition, the combined picture and sentence format appears to be more effective than either used separately (Condus, Marshall, & Miller, 1986).

Children seem naturally to enjoy word games and word play, and these teaching strategies can be incorporated into many types of activities. As a communication partner, I like to get very "confused" and use words in silly ways. Children laugh and freely correct their somewhat slow-witted communication partner. Retrieval training may include categorization tasks, such as naming members of a category or identifying the category when given the members. Categories include animals, clothing, grocery items, and the like. Categories also may be formed by the initial sounds of words and by rhyming.

As a group, children with language impairment are less likely than children developing normally to discover semantic organization strategies on their own and usually require more examples to determine a basis for organization and for generalization of organizational skill. Word-retrieval errors should demonstrate the predominant organizational framework of the child and alert the speech-language pathologist to the patterns that need strengthening.

Categorization tasks, especially such familiar ones as Saturday morning cartoon shows, in which the child names members of the category, facilitate recall by building associational and categorical linkages between words. The child usually recalls a word by first accessing the category to which it belongs. The possibility still exists that he will access the right category but retrieve the wrong member (Wolf, 1982, 1984).

Categorization tasks can be elaborative in nature when members of more than one category are presented together. For example, the items *chair, bed,* and *table* can be classified as furniture; *chair, swing,* and *bicycle* are things on which you sit; and *bicycle, car,* and *bus* are vehicles. The facilitator could present these items together and ask the child to classify them in as many ways as possible.

Training might begin with actual objects and children making piles of objects that go together (M. Cole & Cole, 1981). As a child, I sorted my comic books by main character and my baseball cards by team. Similar tasks are found in several everyday activities. Children can make collages in school of things that go together. Items might be classified by description (e.g., cold) or by function (e.g., things that you ride on). The facilitator should encourage the child to use as many different sensory descriptions as possible to describe objects.

Verbal training should begin with common words for everyday concrete objects (Nippold, 1992). Familiar everyday objects and events should be used. This notion is sometimes difficult for adults to understand, especially if they are attempting to bring interest and variety into the training. I am reminded of a teacher who tried to teach zoo and farm animal categories but found the children very unresponsive. Both categories were outside their realm of experience. When one child suggested the category of animals seen "squashed" on the highway, every child became a participant. Although the example is somewhat gruesome, the lesson for speech-language pathologists is very practical. Everyday natural environments provide specific cues that aid memory (Nippold, 1992).

Word-finding difficulties can be helped by (a) naming/descriptive tasks ("It's a bicycle; you ride on it by peddling"), (b) associational activities ("Red, white, and ___"), and (c) sentential elaboration tasks based on syntactic characteristics of two words drawn at random ("The *trailer* was parked near the *restaurant* while the driver ate") and open-ended fill-ins and completions ("We eat with a ___") that involve deeper levels of processing (Casaby, 1992). Word-sorting tasks can aid in the development of categorization and recall skills (Bjorkland, Ornstein, & Haig, 1975). Taxonomy charts, especially for newly introduced classroom content, also can help children develop categorization strategies.

Categorical identification by the facilitator seems to be the best cue for recall (Wiig & Semel, 1984). By naming the category, the facilitator can help the child locate the desired word. Partial word cues also may help the child and are less confusing than synonyms. Sentence completion and nonverbal, gestural cues are also aids.

Although semantic strategies appear to work well, they are not the only ones. In preliminary studies with limited numbers of subjects, a combination of phonological and perceptual strategies is reported to be even more effective than semantic elaborative methods alone (Wing, 1990), although semantic elaboration and retrieval activities produce better results than phonological strategies alone (McGregor & Leonard, 1989). In phonological training, the child participates in segmentation exercises such as rhyming, initial sound matching, and counting syllables and phonemes. The rationale for this method is that, in part, break-down is the result of poor phonological representation of the word.

Perceptual training involves imagery activities, such as simultaneous picture and auditory exposure, visualization with eyes closed, and silent name repetition. This procedure progresses to matching pictures to a "memorized" sample of names.

The facilitator can help a child note perceptual and functional features and attributes that determine how members are categorized. The child with a language learning disability will have particular difficulty abstracting salient features and, therefore, will have difficulty forming categories based on these features.

It is important that children note a similar attribute on more than one object. Otherwise, children may begin to associate certain attributes with specific items. For example, several very different objects may be described as *wet*. This kind of task naturally leads to categorization. Attributes should appear also in many different linguistic forms.

Speed and accuracy of retrieval are important. In general, retrieval improves with increased speed and accuracy (Cirrin, 1983; German, 1986/89, 1990; Guilford & Nawojczyk, 1988; Wiegel-Crump & Dennis, 1986). In children developing normally, all three improve with maturity. Retrieval using picture cues is easier than naming to a description. Naming to a rhyme is the most difficult (Wiegel-Crump & Dennis, 1986). Several retrieval strategies are listed in Table 10.9. Retrieval units should move from single words to discourse.

As mentioned previously, it is important to keep in mind the "What's the point?" criterion. The relationship of responses to naming exercises and word finding in conversation is unknown. Overall, responses to pictures may be of relatively little value. At a minimum, it is essential that training include a strong conversational element to ensure generalization of word-finding skills (Dennis, 1992).

TABLE 10.9
Word-retrieval strategies

Retrieval strategies		Descriptions
Attribute cuing	Phonemic cuing	The initial sound, vowel nucleus, digraph, or syllable is used to cue the target word.
	Semantic cuing	The category name or function is used to cue the target word.
	Graphemic cuing	The graphic schema is used to cue the target word.
	Imagery cuing	A revisualization of the referent is used to cue the target word.
	Gesture cuing	The motor schema of the target word action is used to cue the target word.
Associate cuing (*story* for *book*)		An intermediate word is used to cue the target word.
Semantic alternates	Synonym/category substitutions	Semantic components (synonym or category words) are substituted for the target word.
	Multiword substitutions	Semantic components (functions or descriptions) are substituted for the target word.
Reflective Pausing		Constructive use of pausing is used to reduce inaccurate competitive responses.

Remedial techniques		Descriptions
Stabilization of phonological specifications	Rehearsal	Students practice saying or writing the target words five times alone and then in five different sentences.
	Rhythm + rehearsal	Each syllable is marked with a tap during the above rehearsal of the target word.
	Segmenting + rehearsal	A line is drawn between each syllable during the above rehearsal of the target word.
Rapid naming		Students rapidly say names of and phrases with target words until their response time is reduced.

Source: German, D. J. (1992). Word-finding intervention for children and adolescents. *Topics in Language Disorders, 13*(1), 33-50. Reprinted with permission.

It may be helpful to teach the child strategies for circumventing blocks (German, 1992). Synonyms, category names, and multiword descriptions may enable the child to continue the conversation and to work through the word-retrieval difficulty. Compensatory programming, such as modifying classroom tasks, also may aid the child with word-retrieval difficulties (Table 10.10). It is essential that those in the child's home and classroom modify expectations and cue the child in the most advantageous manner.

Comprehension

Very young children, lacking good word definitions, use their knowledge of familiar event sequences to structure their responses (Paul, 1990). Familiar events provide scripts that aid comprehension. Even later, when children and adults rely on lexical and syntactic cues, it is still easier to comprehend information in familiar events and contexts (Haviland & Clark, 1974; Kieras, 1985).

In early preschool, the child matures from reliance on the immediate context to reliance on stored experience for interpretation. This stored experience is called *world knowledge*. The child uses world knowledge to structure a "probable event" strategy of interpretation. Only gradually does the child gain the ability to rely on word order (Golinkoff, Hirsh-Pasek, Cauley, & Gordon, 1987; Roberts, 1983).

By late preschool, ages 3½ to 5, word order is used more consistently for interpretation (Tager-Flusberg, 1989). Linguistic knowledge becomes the preferred comprehension strategy, although no clearly dominant strategy is evident (Bridges, 1980). Preschoolers still rely more readily on contextual knowledge.

It is not until ages 5 or 6 that children use syntactic and lexical interpretation more consistently (Keller-Cohen, 1987). They still make errors, of course, usually by ignoring clausal boundaries and interruptions in the flow (Wallach & Miller, 1988). By ages 7 to 9, children are more sensitive to boundaries, embedding, and temporal connectives (Fluck, 1979).

Humor in the form of jokes, a school-age development, requires extensive use of linguistic interpretation. The linguistic incongruity in the punch line must be understood in order for the joke to be funny.

Children with a range of language impairments perform similarly on language comprehension tasks (Bishop, 1982). They exhibit poorer comprehension than their peers developing normally (D. Bernstein, 1986; Nippold, 1985; Spec-

TABLE 10.10

Classroom oral questioning modifications for word-retrieval problems

Word-finding profile	Content areas	Classroom activity	Recommended modifications for teacher	New materials
Difficulty retrieving specific words: inaccurate namer	All	Oral questioning	1. Use multiple-choice frames 2. Accept volunteer participation only 3. Provide target word cues (e.g., initial sound, syllable) 4. Use questions that require yes/no or true/false response	Advance organizer
Difficulty retrieving specific words: slow namer	All	Oral questioning	1. Prime student for questioning 2. Give student additional time to answer 3. Use multiple-choice frames 4. Use questions that require yes/no or true/false response	List of possible questions

Source: German, D. J. (1992). Word-finding intervention for children and adolescents. *Topics in Language Disorders, 13*(1), 33–50. Reprinted with permission.

tor, 1990). In general, there is a greater tendency among school-age children with language impairment to rely on word-order strategy and to retain this strategy longer than do children developing normally (F. Roth & Spekman, 1989a).

Among preschool children with language impairment is an earlier overuse of word-order strategies and less use of world knowledge (Lord, 1985; Paul, Fisher, & Cohen, 1988; Tager-Flusberg, 1981c, 1985). In other words, the comprehension strategy is less flexible; there are fewer alternative strategies than in children developing normally (Paul, 1989a, 1989b). It is not surprising that higher interpretative skills, such as those used to comprehend humor, are often not observed in children with severe language impairment.

Even mature language users rely on world knowledge to some extent (Milosky, 1990). *Comprehension* consists of both decoding the syntactic and semantic information and interpreting that information based on the linguistic and nonlinguistic context and world knowledge (Clark, 1983; Garrod & Sanford, 1983; Marslen-Wilson & Tyler, 1980; Waltz & Pollack, 1985).

The goal of intervention is to teach the child to retrieve relevant word and world knowledge as a comprehension aid and to help the child decide how and what to remember from what he hears or reads (Trabasso & Van Den Broek, 1985). Comprehension and memory are aided by familiar, meaningful contexts; thus, intervention should occur within familiar routines and locations (Milosky, 1990). The degree and type of experience the child has with events strongly shapes his expectations and, thus, his comprehension. Meaningful activities are more comprehensible; they make more sense.

The level of involvement also affects memory and comprehension (Lehnert & Vine, 1987; Miall, 1989). The more involved the child, the more he comprehends and recalls. Songs, nursery rhymes, and finger play can be used to help the child make active associations between words and the nonlinguistic context (Paul, 1990). The repetitive nature and limited focus of such activities help shape expectations and aid comprehension and memory. In "Where Is Thumbkin?" the structure is *where . . . here* with the phrases repeated several times. Similarly, "Farmer-in-the-Dell" uses an *agent* + *action* + *object* format in each verse (*The farmer picks a wife . . .*) (Paul, 1990).

Finally, comprehension intervention should be pleasurable. Fun activities keep children engaged, a necessity for comprehension and comprehension training (Pellegrini & Galda, 1982). Involvement is fostered by the type of facilitator feedback. A pleasing manner encourages responding and making use of such feedback (Paul, 1990).

Initial comprehension training may need to be very concrete and highly contextual. Preschool children benefit more from direct labeling instruction than from less direct use of narratives (Kouri, 1994). The use of gestures and a slower rate of talking by the language facilitator also enhances comprehension by young children (Weismer & Hesketh, 1993). As children approach school age, training should become more decontextualized, similar to many of the literate activities found in school.

Comprehension training might begin with recall from pictures or objects and progress to literal recall of one or more details from verbal sources (M. Cole & Cole, 1981). Gradually, the speech-language pathologist can require the child to recall more details. Later, the child can detail these in sequence, possibly using sequential pictures, photographs of past events, or comic books as aids. Daily events can provide a script to aid comprehension. Next, she can require the child to relate cause and effect from familiar or recently read narratives. Once able to reconstruct these relationships, the child can begin to make inferences, to draw conclusions, and to predict outcomes from stories, riddles, and jokes. Finally, the child can learn to synthesize information and create subjective summaries of the meanings of narratives, TV shows, or movies.

To assist comprehension, the speech-language pathologist can shape question-response strategies by manipulating the semantic content, complexity, context, and function (Parnell & Amerman, 1983). The therapy process moves from simple, context-embedded questions to the use of questions in more abstract contexts, while controlling the length of the questions to highlight semantic content (Moeller et al., 1986). In the first stage, the facilitator attempts to build awareness and enhance emerging skills by using topics of high interest as the question contexts. She concentrates on establishing repeatable responses to yes/no questions by using a second adult as a model, multiple-choice alternatives ("Did the ball roll under the sofa? Yes or no?"), visual cues to signal that a response is desired, and the child's natural, everyday contexts.

In stage two, early developing *wh-* question forms become the targets, and yes/no questions are used to highlight the semantic content desired. Take, for example, the question, "What is the girl wearing on her head?" A nonresponse, an inappropriate response, or an inaccurate response might be followed by, "Is she wearing a shoe on her head?" If the child responds negatively, the prompt would be, "That's right, what is she wearing on her head?" Print, pictures, or signs can be used to highlight the *wh-* words and, thus, emphasize the information desired. These prompts can be faded gradually. In the third stage, new *wh-* forms are added systematically. In the final stage, stimulus content is shifted gradually from concrete, predictable, factually based academic topics to more abstract, less predictable conversational ones.

School-age children might manipulate objects or pictures and match them with the sentences heard (Wallach & Miller, 1988). For example, the child might be told to place a small red ball on top of a large yellow box. Similarly, the child might select a picture described by the facilitator from among a set of pictures. Written cues also could be used.

The child also might match sentences with similar meaning. Synonyms can be introduced. Metalinguistic skills can be enhanced by tasks in which the child judges similarity and difference among sentences (van Kleeck, 1984).

Idioms are a form of figurative language that are particularly troublesome to comprehend for children with language impairment and for children with LEP and different dialects (Donahue & Bryan, 1984; Lutzer, 1988; Nippold & Fey, 1983; Seidenberg & Bernstein, 1986). The most common error is literal interpretation. Although idioms are a concise, colorful, and intriguing way to express complex meanings, they are very diverse and, thus, difficult to learn as a group (Bromley, 1984). Idioms vary along several continuums, including single words-to-clauses, colloquial-to-formal, and concrete-to-abstract.

Difficulty with idioms can affect classroom comprehension because of their frequent occurrence (Nippold, 1991). Approximately 11.5% of teacher utterances contain at least one idiom, with a range from 4.7% in kindergarten to 20.3% in eighth grade (Lazar et al., 1989). Similarly, 6.7% of the sentences in textbooks contain idioms, with a range from 6% in third grade to 9.7% in eighth (Nippold, 1990).

The meanings of idioms are inferred gradually from repeated exposure in context. Children with language impairment may lack a strategy for determining meaning. Some common idioms are listed in Table 10.11.

Intervention should begin with comprehension of transparent or easily decipherable idioms. Narratives may be the best teaching milieu because of the contextual support (Nippold, 1991). The child can be instructed prior to the narrative that it will contain a certain idiom and that he will be able to figure out the meaning from the story. Questions can be used throughout the narrative to help the child attend to important information. Answers can be redirected to ensure that the child is attending to salient points. After repeated exposure and the child's correct interpretation, he can be encouraged to invent his own narratives that illustrate use of the idiom. Finally, conversationally appropriate use can be discussed and role-played.

Microcomputers can be used to teach figurative language comprehension. Computers have special advantages, including inherent motivation, active involvement, nonjudgmental feedback, and an independent, self-paced mode of operation (Fitch, 1986; Lasky, 1984; Sanders, 1986; Shearer, 1984).

Unfortunately, commercially available software does not reflect current developmental knowledge, does not offer a clear rationale for instructional methods, and does not offer comprehensive instruction (Nippold, Schwarz, & Lewis, 1992). In addition, these programs provide for little or no customizing and offer only minimal use of animation, graphics, synthesized speech, or sound effects that might aid children with reading problems. At best, current computer software can complement intervention by the speech-language pathologist (Nippold, Schwarz, & Lewis, 1992). Each speech-language pathologist should analyze software carefully to determine the best way to use it. In addition to concerns for content and instructional methodology, the speech-language pathologist should consider the compatibility of computer-based intervention and her teaching style.

SYNTAX AND MORPHOLOGY

Although language use improves syntax, the reverse is not true (Lucas, 1980; Mundell & Lucas, 1978). It is important, therefore, that syntactic training be as conversational as possible.

When language forms or constructions are taught outside a communication context, the forms may be mastered without the knowledge of how to express ideas within and across these forms (J. Norris & Bruning, 1988). In addition, utterances produced in context strengthen cohesion and relationships across linguistic units.

TABLE 10.11

Common American English idioms

Source: Compiled from Boatner, Gates, & Makkai (1975); Clark (1990); Gibbs (1987); Gulland & Hinds-Howell (1986); Kirkpatrick & Schwarz (1982); Palmatier & Ray (1989)

Topics

Animals
- A bull in a china shop
- As stubborn as a mule
- Going to the dogs
- Playing possum
- A fly in the ointment
- Clinging like a leech
- Grinning like a Cheshire cat

Body Parts
- On the tip of my tongue
- Raise eyebrows
- Turn the other cheek
- Put your best foot forward
- Turn heads

Clothing
- Dressed to kill
- Hot under the collar
- Wear the pants in the family
- Fit like a glove
- Strait laced

Colors
- Grey area
- Once in a blue moon
- Tickled pink
- Has a yellow streak
- Red letter day
- True blue

Foods
- Eat crow
- Humble pie
- That takes the cake
- A finger in every pie
- In a jam

Games and Sports
- Ace up my sleeve
- Cards are stacked against me
- Got lost in the shuffle
- Keep your head above water
- Paddle your own canoe
- Ballpark figure
- Get to first base
- Keep the ball rolling
- On the rebound

Plants
- Heard it through the grapevine
- Resting on his laurels
- Shrinking violet
- No bed of roses
- Shaking like a leaf
- Withered on the vine

Vehicles
- Fix your wagon
- Like ships passing in the night
- On the wagon
- Don't rock the boat
- Missed the boat
- Take a back seat

Tools and Work
- Bury the hatchet
- Has an axe to grind
- Hit the nail on the head
- Jockey for position
- Throw a monkey wrench into it
- Doctor the books
- Has a screw loose
- Hit the roof
- Nursing his wounds
- Sober as a judge

Weather
- Calm before the storm
- Haven't the foggiest
- Steal her thunder
- Come rain or shine
- Right as rain
- Throw caution to the wind

The linguistic techniques discussed in Chapter 9 are particularly applicable to syntactic and morphologic training. Methods requiring an imitative or spontaneous response by the child are reported to be superior to those presenting only a model (Connell & Stone, 1992). Feedback is also very important.

During training, it is important that the facilitator control for vocabulary and/or sentence length, especially when teaching new structures. If the facilitator changes too many variables at one time, it may confuse the child or make the task too complex for successful completion.

The facilitator should be careful not to require metalinguistic skills beyond the child's abilities. Although recognition and comprehension usually precede production, judgments of correct usage do not. Judging a sentence to be grammatically correct is a metalinguistic skill that develops in the middle elementary school years. Asking children to form sentences with selected words also requires metalinguistic skill. In short, any task that requires the child to manipulate language abstractly takes some degree of metalinguistic skill.

The development of syntactic and morphologic forms is well documented and provides a guide for intervention. In the following section, hierarchies for intervention with several different forms are discussed. The purpose is to offer general guidelines for the ordering of structures to be taught.

Just as development is a gradual process, especially for older children and adolescents, so too is intervention. It may be unrealistic to expect error-free production following teaching (Nippold, 1993). Some low-frequency forms are difficult even for adults.

Morphology

Inflectional suffixes develop early and lend themselves well to teaching within a conversational milieu. Other morphemes may best be taught in a more explicit manner first, beginning with derivational suffixes, followed by prefixes (Rubin, 1988). Common bound morphemes are listed in Appendix G. Because derivational relationships are complex and irregular, memorization is of little value as a learning tool (Adams, 1990). It is essential that the child understand the changes in meaning that are occurring.

Although data for school-age morphological development are scarce, some suggestions for the order of teaching can be suggested. These are presented in Table 10.12. Training should begin with the most transparent and most common morphemes and proceed toward those that are more complex and cause phonological and orthographic or spelling changes.

The school-age child should be taught to analyze from derived words to word stems and to synthesize from word stems to derived words (Moats & Smith, 1992). Meaning relationships should be emphasized. The metalinguistic skill of awareness of word structure is essential to the analysis of complex structures. These skills should be taught and used at all levels from word imitation to conversational use.

Young school-age children who read and have some metalinguistic skills can be taught to differentiate word structures (Rubin, 1988; Rubin et al., 1991).

TABLE 10.12

Suggested order for teaching morphemes

1. Establish awareness of syllables and sounds. Practice counting both.

2. Identify roots and affixes. Practice pronouncing and defining roots and affixes in contrasting words that are similar in sound or appearance, such as *happy-sunny*, and *include-conclude*.

3. Generate a formal definition in the form "A/An *X* is a (superordinate category) that (restrictive attributes)."

4. Discuss relationships with other words.

5. Use words in meaningful contexts and in analogies and cloze activities.

6. Use words in reading activities if appropriate.

7. Introduce spelling and spelling rules if appropriate.

Source: Adapted from Moats & Smith (1993)

Words can be contrasted on the basis of structure and rhyming, as in *money-funny, wise-pies,* and *pinned-wind,* or on small structural changes that affect meaning, as in *winner-winter.*

Mid-school-age children can be taught complex derivational morphology (Moats & Smith, 1992). Training can occur in both the oral and written modes. Training for mid-school-age children also should include Latin and Greek roots because of the frequency of these in science, math, and social studies (Henry, 1990).

Verb Tensing

Verbs are very difficult for children with language impairment, partly because of the many ways they are treated syntactically and morphologically. Although the typical 2-year-old developing normally has a notion of action words, the child does not understand the many forms these verbs can take; nor does the child comprehend other verbs that express notions such as state. Verb learning takes several years, with the rules being mastered slowly.

The teaching of verb tensing can be adapted easily to everyday activities in which children discuss what they are doing at present, did previously, or will do in the future. Art projects and building toys are especially useful. Appendix I offers a number of activities for targeting verb tensing.

Training should begin with *protoverbs,* such as *up, in, off, down, no, there, bye-bye,* and *night-night.* These verblike words usually are used in relation to some familiar action sequence (Barrett, 1983). General purpose verbs, such as *do,* might be targeted next.

More specific action verbs should be introduced in their uninflected or unmarked form. The facilitator can cue by asking what a child is doing or by directing the child, "Tell *X* to verb." To facilitate learning, action word meanings might be taught with specific actions or objects. Children first describe their own actions, not those of others (Barrett, 1983; Huttenlocker, Smiley, & Charney, 1983; K. Nelson & Lucariello, 1983). While playing, the facilitator can hide her eyes or turn away from the child and ask, "What are you doing?" Although the cue requires an -*ing* ending on the verb in the response ("Eating"), this form is not required at this level of training.

Familiar event sequences, such as play or routines, facilitate action verb usage because of the mental representations of these sequences that children possess (K. Chapman & Terrell, 1988). These event sequences enable the child to focus on the communication, rather than on the extralinguistic elements of the event (Constable, 1986).

Once the child is able to form simple two- and three-word utterances with an action word, as in "Doggie eat meat," the present progressive verb form can be introduced without the auxiliary verb. The language facilitator can model this form through self-talk and parallel talk. She can cue the child to use this form with, "What's doggie doing?" or, "What's he doing?" Pronouns, such as *he*, must be used with caution at this level.

At this level of training, the child only needs to deal with the immediate context. A sense of time beyond the present, however, is essential for further verb training.

The facilitator can use a few high-usage irregular past tense verbs, such as *ate, drank, ran, fell, sat, came,* and *went,* to introduce the past rather quickly and to forestall overgeneralization of the regular past *-ed,* the next target form. With both past tense forms, storytelling, show-and-tell, and recounting past events are good vehicles for training and use. Initially, the facilitator can ask the child such questions as, "What did you eat (or other action verb)?" to teach the child the form. When the child responds with, "Cookie," or another entity, the facilitator can reply, "What did you do with cookie?" Later, the sequence can begin with the question, "What did you do?" The child responds, "Ate cookie," or, "I ate a cookie." It is important that question cues not violate pragmatic contingency, which requires that questions make sense. Facilitators should not ask questions to which they know the answers. This strategy is achieved easily by asking about unobserved actions or having a puppet ask questions.

Before training additional verb forms, the facilitator should introduce singular and plural nouns and subjective pronouns because the child will need these for the third person singular present tense *-s* marker and for present tense forms of the verb *to be.*

The facilitator can introduce the third person marker with singular and plural nouns. Subjective pronouns can be introduced gradually. She can elicit the third person marker with such cues as, "What does he do every day (all of the time)?" or such fill-ins as, "Every day, the girls (verb)," or, "All of the time, he (verbs)."

She should not target the phonological variations of the *-ed* marker (/d/, /t/, and /Id/) and those of the third person *-s* (/s/, /z/, and /Iz/) in initial training. When the marker is first being emphasized in training, the facilitator should use one form exclusively, such as the /d/ or the /s/. As the emphasis on the marker becomes more natural or lessens, its cognate can be introduced.

Facilitators should not expect the child to understand the phonological rules relative to ending sounds and added markers. Usually de-emphasis of the marker's sound will allow the child to produce naturally either two voiced or two unvoiced sounds at the end of each word. The /Id/ and /Iz/ markers should be avoided until much later. Children developing normally usually employ the cognates by late preschool. It takes them a few more years to acquire the /Id/ and /Iz/ forms.

Use of pronouns enables the child to begin training on the verb *to be* both as an auxiliary verb and as the copula or main verb. Because the form is noun (or pronoun) + *be* + X, in which the X can be a noun, adjective, adverb, or verb, these two forms can be trained together, thus facilitating carryover. The distinction between auxiliaries and main verbs is too complex to try to explain here. As a rule, the uncontractible form is taught first, the uncontracted contractible next, and the contracted contractible form last.

The verb *to be* is a "regularist's" nightmare, with different forms for various persons and tenses. Therefore, different forms should be introduced slowly. Children developing normally generally learn the *is* form first. Other auxiliary verbs, such as *do*, also can be introduced to facilitate the development of more mature negatives and interrogatives. The negative form of *do* can be elicited with, "Tell X (some person) not to *verb.*" *Do, can,* and *will/would* appear first in the negative form in the language development of children developing normally. In other words, *can't, don't,* and *won't* appear before *can, do,* and *will/would.*

Using the present progressive form *be* + *going,* the child can begin to form early future tense forms. Facilitators should be willing to accept this form because it marks the concept (Bliss, 1987). The more mature *will* form can be trained later.

Training should begin with *going to noun,* as in "going to the zoo," before *going to verb,* as in "going to eat." The former is more concrete and does not require use of an infinitive phrase, such as *to eat.* The more mature *will* form of the future tense can be introduced later.

Guidelines for training *can, do,* and *will/would* include the following (Bliss, 1987):

1. Allow some delay between mastery of one form and introduction of another in order to avoid confusion.
2. Use self-reference in the form of either first person pronouns or the child's name initially because this is the first referent associated with these forms (Fletcher, 1979).
3. Link these forms with actions because this is the first association of children developing normally (Fletcher, 1979).
4. Initially, use short utterances with the word at the end in order to increase saliency ("Can you jump?" "Yes, I *can.*")

5. Provide meaningful situations in which the concepts and forms serve some purpose.

With the addition of the future tense, the child now can discuss the past, present (progressive), and future, somewhat like the preacher whose lengthy sermons "Tell 'em what I'm gonna tell 'em, tell 'em, and tell 'em what I told 'em." Language activities can include planning, execution, and review.

After teaching other auxiliary verbs, the facilitator can introduce *modal auxiliaries*. These are helping verbs that express mood or feeling, such as *could, would, should, might,* and *may.* The shades of meaning across the various modal auxiliaries are often very subtle, and the facilitator should not expect mature usage for some time. Most adults have difficulty with the distinction between *may* and *might.*

Finally, the facilitator may wish to target verb particles, multiword units, such as *pick up* and *come over,* that function as verbs. Although verb particles emerge in early preschool years, they are not fully acquired and differentiated from prepositions until age 5 (R. Brown, 1973; E. Clark, 1978; Goodluck, 1986; K. Nelson, 1973; Tomasello, 1987; Wagner & Rice, 1988).

The particle—*up, down, in, on, off*—may either precede or follow a noun phrase, as in *kick **over** the pumpkin* or *kick the pumpkin **over,*** or follow pronominal noun phrases, as in *kick it **over.*** Prepositions, in contrast, always precede noun phrases, even the pronominal variety, as in *over the box* or *over it.* The acquisition of verb particles is especially difficult for children with language impairment, possibly because they are unstressed units and may appear in either position vis-à-vis the noun phrase (Watkins & Rice, 1991).

Particles should be introduced with a limited set of verbs used regularly by the child. It might be helpful to use position cues to teach the distinction between particles and prepositions. Particles could be taught following the noun phrase and prepositions preceding. Particles preceding the noun phrase could be introduced later.

Procedures for teaching verb tensing should make sense both semantically and pragmatically (Bliss, 1987). Examples are, "I bet you can/can't . . .," "Mother, may I?," asking the child to perform various tasks ("Will you please . . .?"), problem solving ("What will happen if . . .?" "What might happen if . . .?"), and role playing ("What should we do if . . .?"). Many children's books—discussed in the next chapter—lend themselves to predicting tasks.

Pronouns

Pronouns are extremely difficult to learn because the user must have syntactic, semantic, and pragmatic knowledge. In general, the facilitator should teach the underlying concept first and should model appropriate use for the child. Use of pronouns requires an understanding of the semantic distinctions of number, person, and case. The noun in the sentence generally determines use, but the conversational context is also a determinant.

Several parent and teacher practices that make language easier for the child to process may, however, confuse pronoun learning and use. Overuse of nouns or of the royal *we* (e.g., "*We* are tired" to mean that the speaker is tired) model inappropriate use.

Children often avoid making an overt pronominal error by overusing nouns. This mistake can be avoided somewhat in training by limiting the number of referents. For example, if the speech-language pathologist uses too many characters in a story format, the child may overuse nouns in an attempt to remember who is being discussed. Using nouns can help children use their memory, which is somewhat more limited than that of adults.

In general, the first person *I* should be trained before the second person *you*, followed by the third person *he/she*. This developmental order reflects increasing complexity with shifting reference and the number of possible referents.

Deictic terms, such as *I* and *you*, are difficult to teach, as noted in the semantics portion of this chapter. A second speech-language pathologist, facilitator, or child can serve as a model to avoid confusing the child's frame of reference.

Development by children who are nonimpaired would suggest that facilitators target subjective pronouns (*I, you, he, she, it, we, you, they*) before objective pronouns (*me, you, him, her, it, us, you, them*). Possessive pronouns would follow (*my, your, his, her, its, our, your, their*), and, finally, reflexive pronouns (*myself, yourself, himself, herself, itself, ourselves, yourselves, themselves*). Although there are exceptions to this hierarchy, it approximates normal development (Haas & Owens, 1985).

This hierarchy and the error patterns of young children suggest that reflexives might be trained initially as possessives (*my self*). The exceptions (*himself* and *themselves*) can be introduced later.

One exception to the training hierarchy might be third person singular pronouns. It appears easier for children to learn *her-hers-herself* than *him-his-himself*, probably because of the consistency in the feminine gender (Haas & Owens, 1985). The three feminine pronouns might be trained before the masculine.

Conversational training with so many varied forms can be very confusing. Initially, the facilitator must target carefully the desired pronouns and practice cues to elicit these forms.

Plurals

To learn plurals, the child must have the concepts of *one* and *more than one*. Numbers or words such as *many* and *more* may serve as initial aids.

As with the past tense *-ed* and third person *-s* markers, the facilitator should not expect mastery of the phonological rules until later. Again, training should begin with either the /s/ or the /z/, gradually introduce the other, and wait some time before introducing /Iz/.

The facilitator may wish to introduce a few common irregular plurals to forestall overgeneralization. As mentioned in the semantics section of this chapter, words such as *water* and *sand* are not irregular plurals and present a special case, especially with the modifiers *any* and *much*.

Articles

Articles are extremely difficult for children to learn because of the two different operations they perform. Articles may mark definite (*the*) and indefinite (*a*) reference and also new (*a*) and old (*the*) information. When in doubt, preschool and early elementary school children tend to overuse *the*.

The facilitator can use objects and pictures and instruct the child to describe what is seen ("A puppy"). Next, she and the child can describe each object or picture, as in the following exchange:

FACILITATOR:	Tell me what you see.
CHILD:	A duck.
FACILITATOR:	A duck? Let's see. I can tell you that *the duck is yellow. What can you tell me?*
CHILD:	The duck is swimming.

The *an* should not be introduced until the child is functioning at the early elementary school level.

Once pronouns have been introduced, the facilitator can switch back and forth between pronouns and articles, as in the following:

FACILITATOR:	Here's *a* puppy. What can you tell me about *him?*
CHILD:	*He* has a cold nose.
FACILITATOR:	Who does?
CHILD:	*The* puppy.

The possibilities are endless within a conversational paradigm.

Prepositions

Although nine prepositions (*at, by, for, from, in, of, on, to,* and *with*) account for 90% of preposition use, these nine have a combined total of approximately 250 meanings. No wonder some children with language impairment have difficulty with this class of words. Prepositions are discussed briefly in the semantics section under relational terms.

Development of prepositions suggests the following hierarchy of training (J. Johnston, 1984; J. Johnston & Slobin, 1979; Washington & Naremore, 1978):

in, on, inside out of

under, next to

between, around, beside, in front of

in back of, behind

Such terms as *in front of* and *behind* should be trained initially by using fronted objects, for example, a television. Nonfronted objects can be introduced later.

In general, children will learn more easily when real objects are used in training. Actual manipulation of these objects, however, may interfere with learning (Harris & Folch, 1985). Such experience may be better at the level of conceptual rather than linguistic training. Spatial and directional aspects should be trained with a number of objects and/or examples so that the child understands the concept separately from any specific referent. Variety may preclude the child's focusing on the objects and referents in favor of the relationship. Large muscle activities also can be used as children go *in* and *out* of boxes or closets, *on* and *off* tables and chairs, and the like. Thus, the child's body becomes a referent (Messick, 1988). Spatial terms may be taught in a naturalistic context of play with puppets, dolls, action figures, or the child's body. In one lesson, I played the tiger who pursued a preschool child *in* the cage, *out* of the cage, and so on.

Word Order and Sentence Types

Word order and different sentence types are best trained within conversational give-and-take, although school-age children and adolescents also may benefit from both oral and written training (Nippold, 1993). Devices such as the *Fokes Sentence Builder* (Fokes, 1976) have been used effectively and efficiently to train sentence structure, but they can become very repetitive. Such devices can be used creatively to allow the child to form his own sentences, even nonsensical ones.

Miniature linguistic systems have been used to teach word combinations (Bunce, Ruder, & Ruder, 1985). In these systems, a matrix is developed with one class of words on the ordinate and another on the abscissa. The child need not learn all possible combinations to acquire the rule. Good generalization to untrained combinations has been reported. Figure 10.4 presents some sample matrices and the teaching models that have been effective.

Noun phrases initially can be expanded in isolation. A question-answer paradigm will enable the facilitator to target specific aspects of the noun phrase. Once placed within a sentence, the noun phrase can be expanded in the object position, followed by the subject position. The order of noun modifiers is discussed in Chapter 6 under analysis of the noun phrase (Table 6.17).

Adjectives can be taught in contrastive situations in which the child must distinguish between two objects that differ along one parameter, as in *big ball* and *little ball* (Kamhi & Nelson, 1988). Incorrect or inadequate adjective use in conversation would result in misunderstanding and the misinterpretation of the child's message. In a similar fashion, post-noun modifiers can be used with objects in different locations, as in *the ball in the box* and *the ball on the table*.

Verb phrases and accompanying clause types should be chosen carefully. Specific verbs that clearly illustrate transitive and intransitive clauses might be chosen. Equitive verb phrases and the use of *be* can be trained in elliptical answers to questions, as in *He is* and *We are* responses to questions such as, "Who is at the

	Cookie	Cake	Pudding	Pie	Bread
Eat	X	X	X	X	X
Bake	X				
Mix	X				
Want	X				
Give	X				

	Pet	Dog	Cat	Horse	Ferret
Feed	X	X			
Bathe		X	X		
Groom			X	X	
Walk				X	X
Brush	X				X

Verbs on one axis are combined with nouns on the other to form short phrases. Each combination taught is marked with an *X*. Rule learning will generalize to the untrained combinations.

FIGURE 10.4
Miniature linguistic systems

zoo?" The uncontractable form of the verb is very salient in this format. A similar method of teaching transitive and intransitive verbs can be used to teach auxiliary verbs, as in, "Who is eating?" and, "Who can jump?" (Kamhi & Nelson, 1988).

Using both oral and written techniques, the facilitator can aid later-school-age children and adolescents to form longer sentences and more concise sentences and to use more low-frequency structures and intersentential cohesion (Nippold, 1993). Compound and complex sentences can be formed from the youth's own simpler sentences. Subordinate clauses, such as *who is driving the red car*, can be transformed later into more concise phrases, such as *The girl **driving the red car** is from Iowa*. Low-frequency structures, such as apposition (*Mary **my sister**...* or *John **the psychologist** will...*), complex noun phrases (*the large red dog with the bushy tail* or *teachers such as Ms. Meeker or Ms. Lilius*), perfect aspect (*has been verbing*), and passive voice (*The cat was chased by the dog*). Finally, intersentential cohesion can be attempted by using adverbial conjuncts such as *therefore* and *however.* Acquisition is often very gradual. Less common types, such as *conversely* and *moreover,* should be introduced to mature language users.

Several strategies discussed in Chapter 9 can be used very effectively to strengthen word order. For example, expansion can provide a more mature model than the child's utterance, and buildup/breakdown strategies help the child analyze relationships.

Table 6.16 presents some guidelines on the acquisitional order of certain sentence types. By the time most children developing normally begin school, they are using adultlike declaratives, imperatives, and *wh-* and yes/no interrogatives in both the positive and negative forms. Later developing forms include clausal and multiple embedding and conjoining, passive voice, and tag questions.

PHONOLOGY

Not every child with speech sound errors is a candidate for a phonological approach. A child who has limited articulation errors, such as a *k/t* substitution or a distortion of */s/*, would benefit more from traditional articulation training. In general, children use immature phonological processes to make the phonology of word production simpler and more manageable. The processes are applied across sound classes and syllable sequences. The child whose errors are not limited to specific sounds, but rather reflect such patterns as producing all error sounds as plosives, is more suited to a phonological approach.

Although consonants may be correct when they occur in stressed syllables, especially in the initial position, the same sounds may be omitted or substituted with a more easily produced sound when they occur at word ends, in consonant clusters, or in unstressed syllables. Naturally, these simplification processes will affect speech intelligibility (Hodson & Paden, 1981).

A phonological rather than a phonetically based phoneme-by-phoneme approach is a more effective and efficient way of remediation because the former focuses on the reduction or elimination of general processes affecting many sounds (Weiner, 1981). Thus, "remediation should focus on phonological patterns to be acquired rather than on isolated phonemes" (Hodson & Paden, 1983, p. 44). Such a procedure also recognizes the interdependence of syllable structure and phonemes (R. Schwartz, 1992). The goal of such intervention is not just better speech but also a cognitive reorganization of the child's phonological system (Fey, 1992b). Problems exist in the child's conceptual organization, not in his production abilities (Catts, 1991; Kamhi, 1992).

The best targets for training occur frequently in the child's daily living, such as those that affect his name. Intervention is likely to result in improved overall intelligibility. The more powerful the child's utterance in achieving his conversational needs, the better target it is for intervention.

Several other criteria exist for target selection (Edwards, 1984; Hodson, 1992; Louko & Edwards, 1990). For example, the speech pathologist might target position-specific or optional processes because they occur intermittently. She also might target both processes that affect stimulative sounds or those that occur early in development. Better results might be achieved by processes that are emerging—produced correctly about 40% of the time—rather than those rarely produced correctly or those well on the road to mastery (Hodson, 1992). The speech-language pathologist must select the process or processes and the affected sounds to target.

As with other aspects of language training, the speech-language pathologist can train phonological rule use within conversational activities (P. Hoffman, 1992; Hoffman, Norris, & Monjure, 1990; Low, Newman, & Ravsten, 1989; J. Norris &

Hoffman, 1990b). Often, she accomplishes this training working with children in a group setting. She uses appropriate, real-life or role-played situations that provide opportunities to use language and that result in natural consequences.

Children with phonological impairments are aware of the effect of their errors on listener comprehension and will make adjustments to enhance vital comprehension (Campbell & Shriberg, 1982; Paul & Shriberg, 1982). These adjustments can be incorporated into training at a conversational level with emphasis on communicative success (Hoffman et al., 1990).

Phonological production is linked to other aspects of production. In short, as the demand to be understood increases, so does phonological correctness (Campbell & Shriberg, 1982). Unfortunately, as children move between isolated word production and connected speech and the return, correctness varies, decreasing with complexity (Andrews & Fey, 1986). As with other aspects of languages, complexity affects performance (Panagos & Prelock, 1982).

Knowledge is transmitted between humans via language. In the oral medium, speech and speech sounds are the link that transmits meaning or knowledge (Hoffman, Schuckers, & Daniloff, 1989). It seems logical, therefore, to use a conversational intervention method in which comprehension is based on meaning-sound contrasts.

Within a conversational milieu, the facilitator can scaffold the child's turn to maximize appropriate feedback relative to the efficacy of the child's messages (J. Norris & Hoffman, 1990b). In intervention, the facilitator uses familiar, predictable events and helps the child organize the event, the incoming information, and the child's turn. Books, predictable narratives, such as story retelling, replica play, and a cloze procedure provide adequate structure for the child (P. Hoffman, 1992).

Facilitator conversational feedback demonstrates the reinforcing value of listener comprehension. This feedback becomes part of the child's reorganized phonological system. Feedback might include expansion and specific requests for repair. Both techniques are effective in modifying children's productions (Shelton, Spier, & Lewis, 1984; Warren & Bambara, 1989). Requests such as, "Did you say ___ or ___?" are particularly effective in changing phonological processes, possibly because a model of the correct response is included in the request (F. Weiner & Ostrowski, 1979).

In short, the functional or conversational method is based on successful communication of a message to the listener (Grunwell, 1985; Weiner, 1981). If a phonological error is present, the result is miscommunication. Correcting the errors, either alone or with help, repairs the breakdown.

Changes made at the higher levels of communication simultaneously affect lower sound production levels. Compared with children using a minimal pairs strategy, discussed later in this chapter, children using a functional conversational approach make greater improvements in overall expressive language, as well as similar changes in improved phonological performance (Hoffman et al., 1990).

A reason for this difference might be found in a metaphonological explanation. *Metaphonology* is the ability to judge the correctness of phonological productions. It is possible that the child has a model or underlying representation of the message to be sent and communication breaks down when there is a mismatch between the model and the actual message produced by the child (Mele-McCarthy, 1990). Intervention can target either the underlying representation, as a conversational approach attempts to do, or phonological production.

Metaphonological processes may be targeted directly via a method called *metaphonological awareness* or *metaphon*. Metaphonology is knowledge about sounds and syllables and the ability to manipulate these sounds out of context. Young school-age children might learn metaphonological awareness through rhyming activities, rhythmic syllable games, and "silly word" creation (Hodson, 1992). Children's books and action songs offer a good source of materials.

Training might begin with the child being instructed to tell a narrative. A puppet might serve as the listener, while the speech-language pathologist acts as prompter for the child. After each child turn, the puppet can make requests for clarification, for added information, or for increased sentence complexity by using the strategies discussed in Chapter 9. Requests for clarification that require phonological adjustments by the child should be emphasized. For example, the puppet might respond as follows:

> "You said '*tenny,*' that's an old sneaker, and your brother's name is '*Kenny.*' Well, I've never been to a party for a sneaker. I don't understand. Did you have a good time?

This strategy can be very effective when used with the minimal pairs strategy discussed later in this chapter.

The speech-language pathologist can aid the child to clarify or to increase the length and complexity of the narrative. This format emphasizes the importance of communication clarity and offers numerous opportunities for modeling, feedback, and revision.

Phonological Approaches

Many nonconversational language-based intervention approaches incorporate both word meaning and sound contrast aspects of language (Blache, Parsons, & Humphreys, 1981; Ferrier & Davis, 1973; Monahan, 1984; Weiner, 1981; E. Young, 1983). This method attempts to use the child's semantic and conceptual abilities and to stress the important linguistic function of sounds. Words that differ by one sound, called *minimal word pairs,* are used to teach the sound contrasts necessary to convey meaning (Blache & Parsons, 1980). This instruction may be accomplished in a minimal pairs approach or in a metalinguistic approach called *metaphon.* In the final portions of the phonology section, these language-based procedures are discussed in detail. They can be incorporated into intervention for deletion of final consonants, consonant cluster reduction, and deletion of weak syllables. A modified procedure also can be used with sound substitutions.

Minimal Word Pairs

Although minimal word pairs approaches are not strictly conversational in nature, they do incorporate different aspects of language into intervention. Sound-meaning contrast training is most appropriate for children with severe phonological impairments, although training also should include conversational approaches similar to those mentioned previously.

One variant of this method, called *perception-production/minimal pairs*, consists of five levels of training: one sound perception level in isolation and in word pairs, and four production levels (Tyler, Edwards, & Saxman, 1987). Perceptual training is accompanied by pictures illustrating each member of the pair, such as *sew/toe*. Production levels include word imitation, independent naming, minimal pairs, and sentences. At the minimal pairs level, the child is required to produce the correct word of the pair in situations in which incorrect production would cause semantic confusion. The CVC type of words are used, and no other error sounds are included.

Each member of the minimal word pair may be pictured as a *rebus* symbol, rather than as a printed word or actual picture (E. Young, 1987). A *rebus* is a picture or symbol that conveys meaning. For the training of phonological rules, the association is sound referenced. In sound-referenced rebus symbols, the symbol for *their*, *there*, and *they're* would be the same because these words sound alike. The rebus does not relate to the meaning of the word, but merely sounds like part of the word. For example, the rebus *shoe* might be used to facilitate production of *tissue*.

Training also might include auditory bombardment at the beginning and end of each session (Hodson, 1980; Hodson & Paden, 1983; Monahan, 1986), during which the speech-language pathologist repeats a list of minimal word pairs emphasizing the process(es) being targeted. Auditory bombardment is designed to heighten the child's awareness of target sounds.

Metaphon Approach

One promising technique mentioned previously is called *metaphon* (Howell & Dean, 1991), which stands for metaphonological approach. *Metalinguistics* is knowledge about language and the ability to manipulate language out of context. Similarly, *metaphonology* is knowledge about the sound system, word segmentation, and communication of speech sounds and their effect on others. Metaphonological skills include rhyming, alliteration, and the like. It is believed that many metalinguistic skills do not develop until school age, but preschool children can gain some metalinguistic awareness through simplified tasks.

Metaphon techniques are based on the premise that phonological disorders represent immature rule systems and that intervention should occur at this level. *Change occurs in the mind of the child, not in the mouth* (Dean, Howell, & Waters, 1993).

As with much that has been discussed in this text, intervention occurs in play situations involving real communication. The child is engaged actively in the play and learning situations. Familiar routines are used as much as possible to free the child's cognitive energy for concentration on speech sounds.

In the Phase 1, the goal is for the child to develop a metalinguistic awareness, to become familiar with limited metalinguistic knowledge, and to reach the realization that communication breakdown can occur from phonological errors.

Training begins at the concept level. The child is introduced to a new vocabulary that describes the phonological processes affected. For example, the child who is fronting sounds might be introduced to the concepts of *front* and *back* in nonlinguistic play situations. The child might place decorations on the front and back of a Christmas tree or wash the front and back of a doll. In similar fashion, the contrast between plosives and fricatives might become *short* and *long,* plosives being of relative short duration and fricatives being sustainable. The child might sort short and long toys or doll clothes or draw short and long tails on animal pictures. No phonological sounds are used in this phase.

Training then moves to the sound level and on to phonemes. At these levels the child learns to classify sounds according to the parameters established at the concept level—front/back, long/short. With speech sounds, the child is shown how the classification system can be used with many sounds, not just those in error. Pictures such as *Ms./Mr. Front* and *Ms./Mr. Back* or *Cat-with-long-tail* and *with-short* are used to strengthen the concept and to enhance learning. The child might place either *Ms. Front* or *Ms. Long* in the car when he hears a short or long sound.

For children with syllable simplification processes, the sound and phoneme levels of training are replaced with a syllable level. Open syllables (CV) might be *short* and closed (CVC) *long.*

In the final level of awareness training, the child classifies words according to the contrasts learned. Minimal word pairs are used, and the importance of comprehension is stressed. Using meaning and meaning comprehension, the speech-language pathologist demonstrates how important it is for others to understand a speaker, as in, "Do we want to 'call a *cop*' or 'order *pop*'?" Again, pictures such as *Ms. Short* are used for visual reference. Sorting and matching games can be used (Dean, Howell, Hill, & Waters, 1990).

Phase 2 includes phoneme production to encourage the child to transfer learning from Phase 1, and to develop self-monitoring and self-repair. The child begins with words and then sentences. Games and the visual reference begun in Phase 1 are continued. This phase may be unnecessary for some children because of the success demonstrated by receptive awareness training alone (Dean et al., 1993).

Deletion of Final Consonants

Deletion of final consonants is a carryover from the child's early word-making strategy of linking open syllables in a string. *Open syllables* are formed by a consonant and a vowel, as in *ma,* and are strung to form such words as *mama.* Many early words follow this same CVCV syllable form, for example, *baby* and *cookie.*

The facilitator can teach the use of final consonants by using two complementary methods—a key word and minimal word pairs approach and a chaining approach. Although the methodology differs, the two apparently do not conflict or confuse children (H. Johnson & Hood, 1988). In both methods, intervention should begin with sounds already present in the child's repertoire because the introduction of new sounds might frustrate the child by requiring too much learning.

Key Words and Minimal Pairs

In this method, the speech-language pathologist uses groups of two or three words that contain a key word, differ in meaning on the basis of the final sound, and are easy to illustrate in pictures. For example, the key word *bee* could be used with words that begin with these sounds but that differ in their final consonants, such as *bean, bead, beat,* and *beak*. Other examples include the following (E. Young, 1983):

four	paired with *fork, force,* and *fort*
pea	paired with *peek, peel,* and *piece*
bow	paired with *both, bone,* and *boat*
see	paired with *seed, seat,* and *seal*
tea	paired with *team, teach,* and *tease*
die	paired with *dice, dime, dive,* and *dine*

The key word can be contrasted with the others, all of which are homonyms without the final consonant. Short periods of auditory bombardment may help reinforce the learning of contrasts (Monahan, 1986). Ending markers, such as plural *-s* and past tense *-ed*, also can be incorporated into this approach. The intervention steps are as follows (E. Young, 1983):

1. Teach the meaning contrasts between the words, beginning with a single pair, by having the child point to a picture when given a clue or asked a question, for example, "Which one lives in a hive?"

2. Have the child point to pictures when named randomly, as in, "Which one is *beat?*"

3. Have the child produce the target words correctly using the following seven substeps. Errors can be managed by returning to contrasting meaning, such as, "You said 'bee,' but the picture of the 'bee' is way over here. What do we call a bird's mouth? Yes, a bird's mouth is called a 'beak'." Final consonant substitutions consistent with the child's level of maturity should be accepted. Immature substitution errors can be corrected through traditional articulation therapy. The seven substeps are (E. Young, 1983):

    a. Imitate the word model correctly.
    b. Name the word correctly without a model.
    c. Use the word correctly in the carrier phrase, such as, "This is a ___."
    d. Imitate the word correctly in a sentence that illustrates the word's meaning, such as, "I eat bean soup."
    e. Generate spontaneous sentences with each word.
    f. Use ending consonants consistently in monitored speech in the therapy setting. Nontrained words also should be monitored.
    g. Use ending consonants outside the therapy setting.

Chaining

Chaining can be used along with minimal pairs training (H. Johnson & Hood, 1988). Emphasizing transitions between sounds, this method targets the ending position of the first word in a two-word phrase, such as "Jum*p* up" and "Pu*sh* in." Training occurs within daily play activities. Other combinations include the following:

jump/take/push/pitch/make—up/out/in/it

A number of consonant sounds from the child's repertoire are used for the target sound at the end of the first word. A variety of consonant sounds are used because this method teaches chaining as a coarticulation rule (H. Johnson & Hood, 1988).

Initially, correct production of this sound and of the ending or arresting consonant of the second word is not required. Any consonant used in the target position is accepted. Phrases are taught in the CV form that the child already uses. Thus, "Make it" is taught as "May kit" (CVCV(c)) to facilitate production of the final /k/ on *make*.

Production criteria and syllable boundaries are tightened gradually. Despite a lack of research data, it is reported that most children learn to generalize their new learning to closed syllables.

Cluster Reduction

Cluster reduction is one of the most common and longest lasting phonological processes (Haelsig & Madison, 1986; Ingram, 1976). Children use it to simplify complex articulatory demands, and the types of simplification used are often predictable among children. In English, consonant clusters tend to be associated with word beginnings.

An intervention approach that uses a shift in stress and a visual cue in the form of a rebus symbol can be effective with consonant cluster reduction and deletion of unstressed syllables (E. Young, 1983, 1987; E. Young & Sacks, 1982). Backward chaining can help simplify consonant cluster production. The procedure for cluster reduction follows (E. Young, 1987):

1. Each rebus symbol is introduced and named by the speech-language pathologist and the child. The speech-language pathologist slowly produces the target word for the child, demonstrating that the initial sound of that word and the rebus symbol will sound close to the production of the word. For example, the child is introduced to the rebus symbol for *tool* and repeats the word with the symbol. Then, the child is introduced to *stool* and is shown that *s* + rebus = target word. The child repeats the target word slowly as two distinct segments (sound + rebus).

2. Using the visual rebus symbol as a cue, the child repeats the facilitator's production of the word with no separation of sound and rebus.

3. The child repeats the speech-language pathologist's production with the rebus obscured.

4. The child produces the target word without a model.

5. The child uses the word in phrases, sentences, and conversation.

The correction procedure at each step is to return to the previous step.

Cluster reductions with the /s/ phoneme are the most predictable and are common among children. The minimal word pair technique using words that differ on the basis of deletion or nondeletion of the /s/ can be applied. Examples are as follows (E. Young, 1983):

/sk/	cool/school, care/scare, cold/scold, key/ski, core/score
/sp/	pool/spool, pin/spin, pie/spy, pot/spot, pill/spill
/st/	team/steam, top/stop, tool/stool

Unstressed Syllables

In English multisyllabic words, the initial syllable usually is emphasized. Children more easily perceive and more consistently produce these primary or maximum stress syllables (Ervin-Tripp, 1966; Martin, 1972). They may delete, reduce, or replace unstressed syllables by a substituted sound or syllable in a simplification purpose similar to deletion of final consonants and cluster reduction (Ingram, 1976; Klein, 1981). Substitutions may be related to reduplication, in which a stressed syllable is repeated; to assimilation, in which the unstressed syllable is modified toward the sounds in the stressed syllable; or to replacement by an overused speech sound. Disyllabic words can be used in intervention by changing them in two ways: (a) stressing the weak syllable so that both syllables have the same stress, and (b) associating meaning with the unstressed syllable by means of a visual rebus symbol (E. Young, 1987). These cues focus attention on the difficult portion of the word, the weak syllable.

To emphasize the unstressed syllable, the speech-language pathologist can use a backward chaining technique in which she teaches the final portion of the word and then incorporates it into the word. For unstressed sounds that approximate words but are omitted or substituted, the unstressed syllable can be pictured in a rebus. For example, the second syllable in *cookie, monkey, turkey,* and *donkey* sounds like *key.* The association is sound based, not meaning based. The picture of a *donkey* and a rebus of a *key* can be paired to reinforce the association. Training should begin with sounds that the child uses in the initial position in words but omits in unstressed syllables. Otherwise, *key* can be taught first and then incorporated into *monkey* (E. Young, 1983, 1987).

The training procedure for weak syllable reduction consists of the following steps (E. Young, 1987):

1. The speech-language pathologist presents and names the rebus symbol for the child. The child repeats the correct production of the symbol

name. The speech-language pathologist then slowly produces the target words with *equal stress on both syllables and use of the rebus symbol* with production of the unstressed syllable. For example, if the target words are *apple, people, purple,* and *chapel* and the key word is *pull,* the child can hear *a-pull* while noting the *apple* picture followed by the rebus *pull.* The child repeats each facilitator production. Both syllables should receive equal stress.

2. The facilitator again presents the disyllabic words and pictures with the rebus symbol, but this time using the natural stress pattern. The child repeats each word.

3. The facilitator presents the rebus symbol, but obscures the card in some manner. The child imitates her production with natural stress.

4. The child correctly produces each word without use of a verbal model or rebus cue.

5. The child uses the words in phrases, sentences, and conversation.

Incorrect production results in the child's receiving the extra cues of the preceding training step. Other possible word pairs are (E. Young, 1983):

pea	paired with *happy, sleepy, puppy, snoopy*
bull	paired with *table, label, marble*
knee	paired with *tiny, funny, honey, pony*
sir	paired with *mixer, answer, dancer, boxer*
kit	paired with *rocket, jacket, locket, pocket*

The present progressive can be taught with pictures depicting *sing, ring,* and *king* to be used as follows:

sing	paired with *dancing, chasing, kissing, bouncing*
ring	paired with *cheering, pouring, tearing*
king	paired with *knocking, picking, licking*

Assimilation

Key words and facilitating contexts can be used together to modify assimilation processes (Weiner, 1979). The intervention approach is very similar to the paired stimuli methodology. A word like *dog,* which might be pronounced "/gɔg/," is paired with a word in which assimilation does not occur with this child, such as *dime.* Through repeated exposure, the child recognizes that both words begin with the same sound. Do not choose a word like *dead* for the paired word because the child might modify /gɔg/ to /dɔd/ to better approximate *dead.* Conversely, when the child initially produces /dɔd/, the word might be paired with *frog* or *hog* to help the child recognize the final /g/ sound.

A *facilitative context* is one in which the nearby sound fosters production of the correct consonant. For example, /i/ facilitates /I/ because both are high front sounds. Consonants placed together, as in *mad dog,* also facilitate production of targeted sounds.

Sound Substitutions

To simplify production, the child follows production rules relative to unknown sounds. For example, unknown sounds may be produced in the front of the mouth or as plosives, two processes called *fronting* and *stopping,* respectively. To promote generalization and prevent overgeneralization, it may be best to work on more than one process at a time (M. Edwards, 1984). Learning a few new sounds or a new process may affect the entire phonological system (Elbert, Dinnsen, Swartzlander, & Chin, 1990). Emphasis should be on communication, rather than on individual sounds. The goal of functional use of speech is realized in a truly phonological approach (Fey, 1992a).

Although developmental guidelines can aid target process selection, it is best for generalization to select targets that will have the greatest effect on overall communication (Elbert & Gierut, 1986; Gierut, 1989). The easiest processes, those that develop early and/or are inconsistent or stimulable, might improve without intervention (Gierut, Elbert, & Dinnsen, 1987; Powell, 1991; Powell, Elbert, & Dinnsen, (in press). Intervention targeting sounds not likely to self-correct may have the greatest overall effect (Powell, 1991). In fact, correcting of the most severely disordered phonemes may generalize more because of the child's motivation to be understood (Elbert et al., 1990).

Substitution processes may be addressed by an approach that incorporates (a) auditory bombardment with several sounds within the pattern, (b) conceptualization training using perceptual sorting tasks and lexical production, and (c) phonemic contrast that enables the child to perceive semantic differences in minimal-contrast word pairs (Elbert, Rockman, & Saltzman, 1980; Monahan, 1986; Montgomery & Bonderman, 1989). The type of problem will determine which processes are best (Elbert, 1992). In general, omission of sounds is a phonetic problem requiring both perceptual and production training. Sound substitutions or phonemic errors may not require as much emphasis on production (Dean et al., 1993).

The training procedure mentioned above for sound substitutions has the following steps:

1. Auditory bombardment can occur with and without amplification. Two groups of children can work independently, one concentrating on and receiving target words amplified through headphones, and the other completing some project with the words being heard in the background. Rather than concentrating on individual sounds, auditory bombardment can concentrate on enough phonemes within a sound pattern to affect pattern generalization to the child's repertoire (Hodson & Paden, 1983).

2. During the perceptual portion of conceptualization training, individual phonological targets are highlighted. The child is trained to perceive the

phoneme contrasts and semantic differences in minimal word pairs or words that differ only in the correct and substituted sounds, as in *toad-code*. The contrasting sounds differ only along a single feature or dimension. Using lexically unique words, the child learns that different sounds signal different meanings. While presenting a picture that illustrates the word, the speech-language pathologist says each word in the pair, emphasizing the contrasting sounds (*debt-get*), and follows each production with an explanation ("That had a *front* sound," "That had a *back* sound"). She then asks the child to sort the pictures into two stacks of front and back sounds. Rebus symbols can be used to emphasize the contrast between the presence or absence of the sounds and the difference in the target words.

3. In the production portion of conceptualization training, the child participates in practice by using the pictures and a facilitator's verbal model. The facilitator reinforces the child for each response that does not contain the error process. For example, when producing a word with a back sound, she reinforces the child for producing *any back sound, not just the correct target sound* (Fey, 1992a). This procedure more closely reflects natural phonological process acquisition (Weiner, 1981). In other words, correct production occurs through a gradual process of modification. The following activities can be used (Monahan, 1986):

   a. Find a card. A specific card is sought from a display of several cards arranged face down. The name of the card is repeated frequently by both participants in sentences, such as, "Find the ___," and, "I found the ___." The players take turns being the finder.

   b. Playing teacher. The child as teacher holds up each card and says, "This is ___." The actual teacher supplies the missing word. The child as teacher corrects or confirms the teacher's production (often purposely incorrect).

   c. Silly sentences. The facilitator and the child take turns making sentences containing both words in the contrast pair ("I *get* in *debt* if I shop too much").

   d. The facilitator also can use art activities, music, drama, and circle games with conversation centering on the activity carefully chosen to elicit the specific phonological targets in question (Montgomery & Bonderman, 1989).

4. Using a picture cue, the child repeats the facilitator's productions. Only correct productions are reinforced.

5. The child repeats the productions correctly with the picture obscured.

6. The child produces the word correctly without any model.

7. The child uses the word in phrases, sentences, and conversation.

The minimal-contrast approach is not the only effective methodology. The modified cycles procedure, unlike the minimal-pairs method, targets several processes within a short period of time (Hodson, 1992; Hodson & Paden, 1991; Tyler et al., 1987). In this approach, auditory bombardment is used heavily. Although the cycles methodology focuses on correct production of a target sound and its sound substitution, it automatically shifts to another contrast every 2–6 weeks unless correct production falls below 20%. The target change prior to error-free production is because phonological learning is a gradual process. Mastery is not one phoneme at a time. In this manner, several processes can be targeted nearly simultaneously.

A third approach, maximal opposition, contrasts sounds that differ along several parameters (Elbert & Gierut, 1986; Gierut, 1989, 1992). Presumably, children are free to choose and attend to those specific features of the sounds they identify as relevant. This approach is based on the initial maximal perceptual distinctions of children in which they concentrate on the wide extremes of sound contrasts. In addition, maximal opposition treats children as active participants who form their own hypotheses from examples of language and then generalize these hypotheses to actual use. The overall procedures are similar to those for minimal pairs.

Whichever method of intervention chosen, the speech-language pathologist can measure overall change by using a percentage of consonants correct (PCC) in connected speech (Elbert et al., 1990). PCC is computed as follows:

$$\text{PCC} \quad = \quad \frac{\textit{Number of consonants correct}}{\text{Total number of consonants produced}} \quad \times \quad 100$$

A value could be computed also for individual consonants or groups of similar consonants.

Phonology and Reading

Beginning reading is a match between children's oral language and the written language of their books. It is built on the assumption that children are aware of words and phoneme sequences. This sound pattern awareness begins to emerge and mature within rhymes, action songs, finger plays, chants, and repetitive stories of the preschool years.

The ability to recognize syllable and word boundaries is fundamental to reading readiness (Bradley & Bryant, 1985; Liberman & Shankweiler, 1985; Mattingly, 1972; Rees, 1974; Sawyer, 1981; Wagner & Torgeson, 1987). This phonological awareness is related to phonological production (Swank, 1994). Children with reading deficits often exhibit phonological problems (Frith, 1981; Liberman, 1983; Torgeson, 1985). Teaching phonological awareness and the relationship of sounds to written symbols can have a positive effect on both reading and spelling.

Children with poor phonological awareness may have difficulty with oral rhythmic or repetitive language activities, sound-symbol associations, such as Stop or Restroom signs, and syllable or word counting. Many of the activities presented in this section can increase phonological awareness. Written words with target sounds highlighted can accompany pictures. Alliteration and rhyming tasks and repetitive songs and stories also can be used (Jenkins & Bowen, 1994). Explanation and discussion within these activites enhances instructional quality.

Summary

Although the speech-language pathologist cannot always use all elements of the functional model simultaneously, she usually can use several elements within any given teaching situation. Her target selection certainly should reflect the child's overall communication needs. Facilitators within the environment, everyday activities, and conversational give-and-take usually can be adapted to the individual child and language target(s). Some training, such as phonological intervention, may necessitate the initial use of structured approaches. Generalization to conversational use, however, will require incorporating these settings into the training. Appendix I contains activities that are adaptable for intervention and the multiple training targets within each. The speech-language pathologist can select several targets for a single child or can work on different individual targets with several children within the same activity.

CHILDREN WITH LEP AND DIFFERENT DIALECTS

Schools are among the most multicultural institutions in American society. It is estimated that in New York State more than 130 languages are spoken by children in the public schools. Children newly immigrant are increasingly poor and older than in the recent past. These children are less successful in school than their monolingual classmates speaking English and are more likely to become dropouts. In general, these children are overrepresented in programs for those with special educational needs and underrepresented in programs for the gifted.

Although it is preached that having limited English proficiency is not a disorder, practice is quite different. Children who may lack a foundation in L_1—a deficit that affects learning of English—or L_2 are placed in English-only classes as soon as possible. Instead, these children should remain in L_1 programs until they have a sufficient basc.

In addition, most children remain in bilingual programs for only 2 or 3 years before being thrust into regular English-only classrooms. Although they may have gained some conversational proficiency with English, most do not possess sufficient English for classroom learning. It is estimated that it takes approximately 5-7 years to attain such proficiency. These children often are referred for special education services on the basis of their classroom performance.

In short, the cognitive/academic language proficiency (CALP) acquired in L_1 can be transferred to CALP in L_2. A unitary system of language provides a foundation for both languages. Enhancing either language enhances the entire system, although its effect on a specific language will vary. The child able to manipulate L_1 in decontextualized situations has resultant facilitated learning in L_2 (Cummins, 1979b, 1981).

Our present well-intentioned educational model is based on the belief that immersion in English is the best way to learn English. Children with a deficient base in L$_1$ nearly always are placed in English-only programs despite the wishes of the child, family, or community. Quantity of input alone, however, is not the answer. Quality time spent conversing with an adult in English could be much more beneficial at initial stages of language learning.

Language in the typical English-only classroom is treated as one of many academic subjects. The bottom-up approach that begins with grammar and builds toward communication requires good metalinguistic skills that may be lacking in the child with an inadequate base in either language.

The solution to this problem can be found, in part, in the model of intervention that we have discussed throughout this book. The child should remain in an L$_1$ program until she or he has a sufficient language base. Later English-only training should be functional, reflect its ultimate use, and contain a top-down or communication-through-conversation focus.

An individual must develop to a certain level in one language to benefit fully from instruction in a second one (Cummins, 1979b, 1981). Children with LEP and children who are bilingual taught linguistic concepts such as prepositions and pronouns in L$_1$ and then instructed in L$_2$ learn these concepts twice as fast as those taught only in L$_2$ (Perozzi & Chavez Sanchez, 1992). Instruction in L$_1$ facilitates acquisition in L$_2$ (Garcia, 1983; Kiernan & Swisher, 1990; Legarretta, 1979; Perozzi, 1985; Sandoval-Martinez, 1982; Rosier & Farella, 1976; Vorih & Rosier, 1978). In short, L$_1$ provides input for comprehending L$_2$ (Krashen, 1981, 1983).

It is not true, however, that instruction in either language improves the other. Teaching vocabulary in L$_2$ has little effect on L$_1$ when the words are unknown in both (Perozzi, 1985).

In an English-only classroom, the environment should stimulate use and facilitate production and comprehension of English (Krashen, 1981, 1982, 1983; Terrell & Terrell, 1983). The teacher should act as facilitator and encourage group work that fosters language use.

Language is meaningful and used for real communication. New vocabulary is introduced in context, bound to experiences, and associated to other words in the child's lexicon. Language is integrated into other subject areas.

Teachers facilitate language acquisition by surrounding children with visual examples of English (Krashen, 1981, 1983). The whole language approach discussed in the next chapter lends itself particularly well to an environment of language.

The teacher's speech is modified for vocabulary complexity and use of idioms. She speaks more slowly, uses simple sentences, and emphasizes and repeats key words to enhance comprehension. Although the teacher expects children to communicate and raises these expectations as they progress, she attempts to keep anxiety low and the motivation for language use high by employing the conversational feedback techniques discussed in Chapter 9.

In the first stage, the teacher will want to focus on preproduction or comprehension in which the child develops the ability to extract meaning from utterances directed to him (Terrell & Terrell, 1983). In this stage, the child listens and follows simple instructions, responding with gestures, body movements, names, and one-word answers. One type of extended listening experience is called *total physical response* (TPR), in which the child participates in active singing, rhythming, and movement activities that include language. Language is pairing with nonlinguistic elements of learning that happen to be a lot of fun. Suggested TPR materials are listed in Table 10.13. In the next chapter, we shall explore the use of children's literature and music.

In the second stage, after 6 months or more of comprehension training with only minimal English production, focus is shifted to simple production with a strong receptive element (Heberle, 1992). The goal is limited English production with continued vocabulary growth. The facilitator uses *yes/no* and *either . . . or* questions with content that the child has used repeatedly in comprehension training. All production attempts are encouraged, and the child is not penalized for mispronunciation or errors of form. Production is usually at the one-word or phrase level. This stage of English training may last for approximately 1 year.

In the third stage, the child is required to use a more extensive production vocabulary and to begin to use grammar more correctly. Again, communication, not syntactic learning, is the goal. The facilitator uses repetition and expansion, respectively, to reinforce and correct the child's productions.

Finally, the child progresses to the final stage, conversational fluency. The facilitator still will have to modify the linguistic context to aid the child's production and comprehension.

Children with different dialects offer a similar challenge. Although dialects are rule-governed forms of the theoretical standard language, which in our case is Standard American English (SAE), some dialects are closer to the standard than others. Dialects that vary greatly from the standard are called *nonstandard*.

Nonstandard dialects are neither crude approximations of the standard nor haphazard, unpatterned forms. Nor do they reflect disordered language or disor-

---

TABLE 10.13
Suggested total physical response materials

Before the Bell Rings, Prentice-Hall/Alemany
Brown Bear, Brown Bear, What Do You See? Holt, Rinehart & Winston
Chicken Soup With Rice, Harper Trophy
The Children's Response, Prentice-Hall/Alemany
Here Comes the Cat, Scholastic
Jazz Chants for Children, Oxford
Look Who's Talking, Prentice-Hall/Alemany
The Magic of Music, Movement, and Make-Believe, DLM
Mary Wore Her Red Dress, Clarion
More Songs for Language Learning, Communication Skill Builders
Movement Plus Music, DLM
Oxford Picture Dictionary, Oxford
Purple Cows and Potato Chips, Prentice-Hall/Alemany
Songs for Language Learning, Communication Skill Builders
Where Is Thumbkin?, Gryphon House

ganized thinking on the user's part. These dialects are valid forms of the standard language within themselves, and this validity should be reflected in the intervention planning of public schools. Notions of dialectal superiority reflect prejudicial thinking and have led to educational approaches aimed at eradicating nonstandard dialects. The American Speech-Language-Hearing Association (1983) has labeled this approach "inappropriate." Targeting dialectal differences for eradication questions the minority groups that speak these dialects.

Bidialectal education should be fostered instead. This approach recognizes the validity of dialects and also the educational and employment needs of the individual. Smitherman (1985) found that only those speakers of Black English (BE) who master code switching, the successful use of both BE and a second dialect closer to the standard, achieve educational success.

As discussed previously, the speech-language pathologist must not regard dialectal differences as language disorders. Language is impaired when the child demonstrates inappropriate, incorrect, or immature use within his dialectal community. This position suggests, therefore, that intervention should teach both nonstandard and standard equivalents for disordered structures (Adler, 1988, 1990). For example, if the child with language impairment speaks Black English, use of the verb *to be* should be taught in both BE and the standard. Only this approach truly serves the child, who must function within both a dialectal community and the larger society.

In effect, the linguistic standard (SAE) is taught as a second dialect or D_2 (L. Campbell, 1993). D_2, the dialect of education, is taught while maintaining the dialect spoken at home and/or in the community. The goal is not eradication of D_1, but proficiency in an alternate dialect (O. Taylor, 1990). Using the child's knowledge of D_1, the speech-language pathologist can teach the contrasting features of D_2. Role play can be used effectively to increase the child's knowledge of both dialects and their use environments (Gee, 1989; O. Taylor, 1986b).

USE OF MICROCOMPUTERS

Microcomputers can enhance language instruction when well integrated into an overall language program in a cohesive manner (O'Connor & Schery, 1989; Steiner & Larson, 1991). Primarily a drill and practice tool at present, the computer can complement—but should never replace—face-to-face learning situations.

Children enjoy using computers. Preschoolers prefer computer-based training to traditional therapy drills and desktop activities (Shriberg, Kwiatkowski, & Snyder, 1989). Most training programs are user friendly, possessing a "forgiving quality" that lowers the threat to children with language impairment (Rosegrant, 1985).

The goals of intervention and the methodology should be established prior to determining the role of the microcomputer and integrating it into the overall plan. It is all too easy to fall into the trap of allowing the computer program to determine intervention goals.

Children with language impairment are best served by microcomputers when both the child and the speech-language pathologist actively participate, when their use is individualized, and when software specific to the intervention goal is used. The most effective integration of the microcomputer occurs when the speech-language pathologist or other facilitator and the child interact around the program being used, commenting and discussing choices offered and the child's selections. In this way, computer programs can be tuned more to the

TABLE 10.14
Integrating computer activities into language therapy

Sample language objectives	Word processing activity	Pre-/postcomputer activity	Extended project
Giving directions Taking another's point of view Sequencing events	Copy a recipe Explain special terms or translate for younger children to use	Make the recipe Tell others how it was done Take photograph of finished dish	Collect recipes into a notebook "Publish" the recipe book and display with photographs
Summarizing information Taking another's point of view Using verb tenses	Write daily entry in "speech journal" (5 minutes at end of each session)	Discuss the therapy session Plan what to write	Make a success report for mom, dad, teacher
Initiating topic Using correct question syntax Maintaining topic Changing topic Closing conversation	Write interview plan Write a "dialog" of the interview (focus on content, not punctuation) Based on the dialog, write a biography or story	Watch videotape of interview on TV Interview someone familiar (cook, bus driver, music teacher) Role-play being the interviewer or interviewee	Make "This is Your Life" display Start a school newsletter
Carryover any new syntactic or phonologic skill Sequencing events Explaining what will happen Explaining what did happen	Write a project plan Write a letter asking for permission to have contest Make signs and invitations Write a letter inviting a newspaper or yearbook photographer to the contest After the contest, write an announcement of the winners to be read over the school PA system	Plan a contest Discuss what will be needed Discuss what contestants must do Discuss what makes "news"	Hold a contest (bubble blowing, poster making, ball throwing, Twister)

Source: Cochran, P. S., & Bull, G. L. (1991). Integrating word processing into language instruction. *Topics in Language Disorders, 11*(2), 31–49. Reprinted with permission.

needs of each child. Similarly, software designed to address specific language problems (Ertmer, 1986; Meyers & Fogel, 1985; Wilson & Fox, 1983) is better than generic, mass market software.

Microcomputers seem especially useful for writing training. A four-step approach of prewriting, writing, revision, and publication can be used effectively to teach both writing and organizational skills (Cochran & Bull, 1991). Writing software includes Kidwriter, Explore-A-Story, and Explore-A-Classic for younger school-age children, and Logowriter. Speech synthesizers that can "read" the story heighten the child's awareness of the audience and can have a positive effect on writing (Borgh & Dickson, 1986; Espin & Sindelar, 1988; Kurth, 1988; Kurth & Kurth, 1987; Macarthur, 1988; Meyer & Rose, 1987; Rosegrant, 1985; Rosegrant & Cooper, 1987). Possible intervention activites are presented in Table 10.14.

CONCLUSION

We have discussed only a few of the intervention techniques for specific disorders. Limited space necessitates a rather cursory examination of the procedures. Speech-language pathologists should seek further information in source materials or in published clinical materials. They should conceive their own creative and innovative methods for intervening in language impairments. It is hoped that these methods can be adapted to fit the conversational model presented in Chapters 8 and 9.

Not all specific language problems are treated easily with a functional approach, but the entire model does not have to be discarded. Caregivers, for example, are a valuable resource and can be used in various ways, whatever the specific language problem being targeted. In Chapters 11, 12, and 13, we explore the adaptation of functional intervention to the classroom and with children who are pre- and minimally symbolic.

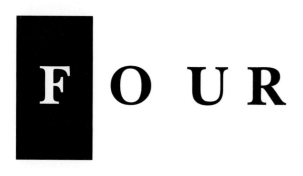

F O U R

Application to Special Locations and Populations

11 Classroom Functional Intervention

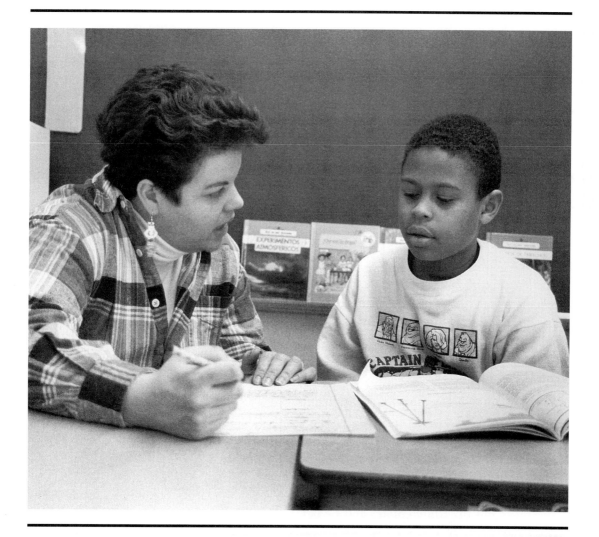

anguage and communication play many vital roles in school success and in the development of reading (N. Nelson, 1988a; Silliman, 1984; Simner, 1983; Wallach & Liebergott, 1984; Wallach & Miller, 1988; Westby, 1984). Five effective warning signs of potential school failure are (a) in-class attention span, distractibility, or memory span, (b) in-class verbal fluency or the use of precise words to convey or describe, (c) in-class interest and participation, (d) the ability to recognize numbers and letters, and (e) the number and types of printing errors made when copying (Simner, 1983). School-age children with language impairment experience difficulties not only with language but also with academic performance (Catts & Kamhi, 1986; Cooper & Flowers, 1987; Hasenstab & Laughton, 1982; Simon, 1985; Wallach & Butler, 1984; Westby, 1985; Wiig & Semel, 1984). The child with language impairment cannot interpret or express ideas at an adequate level to achieve academic success.

In school, children encounter the language of instruction, which presents discourse experiences that are very different from the child's previous conversational interactions (Cook-Gumperz, 1977; N. Nelson, 1984, 1985; Ripich & Spinelli, 1985). Language is treated in the abstract as children learn to talk about it and to manipulate it to learn about other things. Metalinguistic skills are very important. The child with inadequate language skills or inadequate strategies for making sense of different situations is apt to become lost (N. Nelson, 1989).

More than communicating with other people, "in school, language must also be used to regulate thinking, to plan, reflect, evaluate, and to acquire knowledge about things that are not directly experienced" (J. Norris, 1989, p. 206). On an oral-to-literate continuum (Westby, 1985), school tasks are at the extreme literate end, requiring the child to understand and express information displaced from her or his own experiential base. Language itself creates the context in which information is conveyed to other people so that they can comprehend it and understand an event without having shared in the experience (Jorm, 1983; Spekman, 1983).

The functional model discussed throughout this text can be adapted to these differing classroom needs. In fact, some of the recent trends in education, such as inclusion, collaborative teaching, and whole language, espouse some of the same principles we have been discussing. In this chapter, we will examine these trends and propose some models of classroom intervention. Following that, we will describe the new role of the public school speech-language pathologist and elements of a classroom intervention model, including specific intervention targets for preschool and school-age children. Finally, we will discuss implementation of classroom intervention.

BACKGROUND AND RATIONALE: RECENT EDUCATIONAL TRENDS

Language training within the school classroom offers a special challenge for the speech-language pathologist and the classroom teacher. School systems throughout the United States and Canada are adopting and modifying many models of intervention to provide more appropriate and effective intervention. These new models reflect recent educational trends of inclusion, collaborative teaching, and whole language.

Inclusion

Educational legislation in the 1960s and 1970s in the United States resulted in increased educational benefits for children with disabling conditions. One outcome of this legislation, intended or not, was two parallel educational systems: one for children developing normally and another for children with disabilities. Special education includes separate placement, separate teachers, and a separate curriculum. Special services such as speech-language pathology usually are accomplished by removing the child from the classroom.

As a result, the *pull-out* or *isolated therapy model* of intervention now prevails in public education (Marvin, 1987). The pull-out model tends to fragment the child's intervention, especially if the child needs more than one pull-out service. Such patchwork schedules are extremely difficult for children with few strategies for making sense of the world. Increased need results in increased fragmentation until there is little continuity, and the child's progress suffers as a result (Bashir, 1987).

Usually, there is little generalization with the pull-out model, and the content of such intervention may be irrelevant to the child's classroom needs (Anderson & Nelson, 1988). Children may resist leaving class because poorer performance results from the classroom absence.

Larger criticisms—just or otherwise—of the overall separate special education model include the inherent segregation, the focus on labeling and categorization of children, the "slow it down, water it down" educational approach, and a general frustration with a "once in, never out" treadmill. Beginning in the 1980s and continuing today, a movement has developed to raise education standards for all children and to share decision making through more local control and more teacher-parent shared involvement.

These changes have led to inclusive schooling and to the Regular Education Initiative (REI). **Inclusive schooling** is an educational philosophy that proposes one integrated educational system based on each classroom becoming a supportive environment for all of its members—children and teachers (Stainback & Stainback, 1990; Stainback & Stainback, 1992). The notion is not one of mainstreaming children with special needs because mainstreaming presupposed a second system of education for such children. Nor does inclusive schooling envision an end to special education. These services still will be essential for children with special needs.

Instead of separate systems of education, inclusive schooling proposes a unitary system of education flexible enough to meet individual children's needs in a flexible manner. The result is (a) a shift in focus from the deficits to the abilities of children with special needs, (b) collaborative learning, (c) curriculum-based intervention, and (d) placement of all children in regular education classrooms with special services as needed (Silliman, 1993).

REI is the movement toward a regular education continuum (L. Hoffman, 1993). This continuum extends from regular education classrooms with regular educational expectations for most children to regular education classrooms with extensive withdrawal to adaptive environments for compelling educational reasons for a small majority of the children most severely involved. At this end of the continuum, children will require services from trained professionals and curriculum-based intervention services to enhance their classroom participation.

Ideally, children developing normally will serve as models for children with language impairment, although integration alone may be insufficient to ensure interaction (Snyder, Apolloni, & Cooke, 1977). In such classrooms, preschool children with language impairments will spend a considerable amount of time talking with adults (Erickson & Omark, 1980; Weiss & Nakamura, 1992). Models of children developing normally need to be chosen carefully and trained in simple techniques (Weiss & Nakamura, 1992). Children in self-contained special education classrooms often do not form friendships with children developing normally and thus often do not have typical peer models (Roller, Rodriquez, Warner, & Lindahl, 1992).

The result is not an end to special education, but rather a change in emphasis and a new way of educating children. Some administrators and school boards see these changes as a way to scrap costly special education programs for inclusion with few services. This is not the intent of inclusive teaching; rather, it is increased educational opportunity for all children.

Collaborative Teaching

Language intervention should reflect more closely what we know about language development and use (N. Nelson, 1986a, 1988a; Wallach & Butler, 1984; Wallach & Miller, 1988). Functional intervention theories describe language as it occurs throughout the child's many experiences. Assessment and intervention theories that flow from this model stress language processing within a variety of relevant contexts, such as the classroom (L. Miller, 1989). Thus, the model is process, not product oriented (Moses & Maffei, 1989).

A functional approach to intervention shifts the focus from the child as the source and solution of the language problem to a holistic view that includes the child and the child's language uses and learning strategies, the contextual demands, the expectations and beliefs of other people within that context, and the child's interaction, the context, and the child's communication partners (L. Miller, 1989). Thus, the focuses of intervention become the contexts that surround the child with language impairment and the manipulation of these contexts.

The classroom's cognitive activities are an excellent context for stimulating language growth (Moses & Maffei, 1989). Within the classroom's constructive activities, children create, change, relate, and compare entities, set goals, encounter and try to overcome problems, make errors, reflect on success or failure, and note problem-solving procedures.

The negative effects of pull-out are not found in classroom intervention. The ongoing classroom activities can serve as the basis for intervention, with content coming from the child's assignments and projects and the interactions of the classroom (Wallach & Miller, 1988). Thus, intervention is relevant for the environment in which it is being used. In addition, the child can benefit from the social dynamics of the classroom (N. Nelson, 1988b).

The variety of formats for classroom intervention includes the following (Blank & Marquis, 1987; Catts & Kamhi, 1987; DeSpain & Simon, 1987; Dudley-Marling, 1987; L. Miller, 1989; Simon, 1985):

1. Speech-language pathologist teaches a self-contained classroom, usually at the elementary level, for students needing a focus on language and language processing (Buttrill, Niizawa, Biemer, Takahashi, & Hearn, 1989).

2. Speech-language pathologist team-teaches with the regular classroom teacher and other specialists, usually the resource room teacher (J. Norris, 1989; Roller et al., 1992). This teaching may include both specialists teaching small groups simultaneously, or one specialist, such as the teacher, working with the larger class, while the other, such as the speech-language pathologist, works with a smaller group. Goals and objectives, individualized educational plans (IEPs), and the monitoring and reviewing of individual programs are the team's joint responsibilities.

3. Speech-language pathologist provides one-on-one classroom-based intervention with selected students in the classroom by using course materials (N. Nelson, 1989). The intervention usually centers on language strategies for classroom use.

4. Speech-language pathologist acts as a consultant for the classroom teacher and other specialists. As such, she advises (not supervises) personnel, assisting primary caregivers with intervention strategies. Consultative models of intervention usually involve joint goals and objectives that the classroom teacher implements.

    This collaborative consultation model is the one most frequently suggested in the professional literature (Marvin, 1987). This model is very flexible and may include elements of several other formats. Because this model has obvious advantages for generalization (Damico, 1987), it is the basis for discussion in this chapter.

5. Speech-language pathologist provides staff training and curriculum development to the school or district.

The model for discussion incorporates some elements of each of these formats, although primary emphasis is on the collaborative format.

Collaborative teaching is a combination of consultation, team teaching, direct individual intervention where needed, and side-by-side teaching in which the teacher and the speech-language pathologist share the same goals for individual children (Lyngaas et al., 1983; Montgomery, 1992a). In partnership, the speech-language pathologist and the classroom teacher combine their efforts to serve children with language impairment. Parents are used when possible. The collaborative-consultative model stresses interaction and integration of the knowledge and expertise of the individuals involved (Confal, 1993). The approach is a problem-solving one in which all participants share the responsibilities of decision making, planning, and implementation. All aspects of speech and language services are built around the skills a specific child needs to function better in the classroom environment.

Collaborative teaching also involves active choices by children. Within limits, children can select the focus of learning just as they can select the topic of conversation. In this way, children have a stake in what is being learned. They are actively involved.

This model includes, but is not limited to, the following elements:

1. The speech-language pathologist provides in-service training for staff and parent training.

2. The classroom teacher helps identify potential children with language impairment through observation of classroom behavior. The speech-language pathologist evaluates the speech and language skills of these children and others who fail speech and language screenings. Such evaluations are an ongoing and integral part of the intervention process.

3. The speech-language pathologist, classroom teacher, and aide provide individual and small and large group intervention services within the classroom and the curriculum. In addition, the speech-language pathologist continues to provide individual or small group therapy outside the classroom to children in need.

4. The classroom teacher, aide, and parents interact daily with the children in ways that facilitate the development of language skills.

The speech-language pathologist is not a paraprofessional aide for the classroom teacher.

To use the context of the natural environment, the speech-language pathologist should be in that environment and use communication situations occurring in that context (Spinelli & Terrell, 1984). Thus, the speech-language pathologist increasingly provides individual and group intervention within the classroom and conducts small group activities in which newly acquired language skills are used.

Classroom training has been shown to be effective in increasing both elicited and spontaneous language production (Dyer et al., 1991; Haring, Neetz, Lovinger, Peck, & Semmel, 1988; Koegel, Dyer, & Bell, 1987; Koegel & Johnson, 1989). With very young children, a classroom intervention model for teaching an initial lexicon is superior to individual intervention methods in generalization of learned words (Wilcox, Kouri, & Caswell, 1991). This model can be used also to train phonology within everyday classroom activities (Masterson, 1993a). In short, the collaborative classroom model is both effective and cost-efficient (Langenfield & Coltrane, 1991; Montgomery & Bonderman, 1989).

These results reflect the more numerous natural opportunities for communication available in the typical situations and contexts of the classroom and the many potential language facilitators in the classroom (L. Miller, 1989). Ideally, the classroom provides an interactive model in which a high density of language features are modeled and used in a conversational format embedded in familiar, ongoing activities (K. Cole & Dale, 1986; Leonard et al., 1982; N. Nelson, 1989; Snyder-McLean & McLean, 1987). For collaboration to be successful, "each member of the team must be comfortable with his or her teaching style and must be willing to take risks" (Roller et al., 1992, p. 366).

Real conversations and meaningful activities provide motivation and experiences that are usually not available in isolated individual intervention targeting discrete bits of language (Bricker, 1986). Activities are meaningful and experience-based. Communication is child-initiated and controlled. The speech-language pathologist, teacher, and other children respond to the child's naturally occurring communication (Blank, Rose, & Berlin, 1978; Bricker, 1986; Fey, 1986). In this way, naturalistic classroom intervention is consistent with the principles of whole language.

Whole Language

Most remedial programs for children with language impairment are reductionist (Smith-Burke, Deegan, & Jaggar, 1991). Language features are taught as isolated skills or discrete bits (Allington, 1983). Tasks are reduced by the trainer to subsets of skills based on the child's learning deficit. Thus, learning is initiated and controlled by someone other than the child.

Whole language is a very different philosophical or theoretical approach to teaching language (Altwerger, Edelsky, & Flores, 1987; D. King & Goodman, 1990). It is not a set of techniques. In most classrooms, whole language becomes language-based, meaning-driven reading and writing instruction, but it can be much more (Sawyer, 1991).

Basic Tenets

The assumptions of whole language are as follows (Cambourne, 1988; Cambourne & Turbill, 1987; Cummins, 1983; K. Goodman, 1986a, 1986b; Jaggar, 1985; D. King & Goodman 1990; Newman, 1985; Smith-Burke et al., 1991):

1. Language is an integrated, component-complex system, not a sum of its fragmented parts (Cummins, 1983; Oller, 1979; Shuy, 1981a). All components are simultaneously present and interacting at any given time (K. Goodman, 1986a, 1986b; Rumelhart, McClelland, & PDP Research Group, 1986; F. Smith, 1982a, 1982b).

2. Learning proceeds from whole to part. Language is learned through use. Learners are not aware of increasing knowledge of subsystems

because all aspects are present and integrated in natural communication. Teaching in isolation reduces meaning and makes language learning more difficult (Rhodes & Dudley-Marling, 1988; F. Smith, 1973).

> More traditional approaches to reading instruction are summarized by Amy, age 6: "I used to think reading was making sense of a story but now I know it is just letters" (Michel, 1990, p. 43). Children naturally use background knowledge and pictures—their present level of knowledge—to extract meaning from language or the written story. This global strategy gives way to written cues when more information is needed (Mooney, 1988). In other words, children's strategies are naturally whole-to-part. Similarly, whole language approaches emphasize the integrity of language.

3. Children acquire language through immersion in a language-rich environment, not bit by bit. All subsystems of language are present simultaneously. Most children learn oral language easily, incidentally, and without direct instruction. Written language can be learned in the same way—by using it (Altwerger et al., 1987).

4. Language learning should be life-related, functional, and integrative. Motivation and learning occur when the learner is trying to accomplish something within a social context (J. Norris, 1992).

> "Language comes to life only when functioning in some environment" (Halliday, 1978, p. 28). Thus, use occurs in some context that is critical to the meaning of the language being used. Children expect language to be meaningful in the context of social interaction.

5. Language and literacy learning are constructive, self-generated, creative, sense-making processes (Y. Goodman, 1985; Jaggar, 1985; D. King & Goodman, 1990). Whatever its mode, language is a set of signals that serve intra- and intercommunication needs. Learning comes from making sense or meaning from each experience.

> The learning process involves investigation, experimentation, hypothesis testing, approximation, and discovery (Cambourne, 1988; Cambourne & Turbill, 1987; Jaggar, 1985). The complex cognitive processing necessary for language learning is not guaranteed by direct instruction (Weaver, 1991).

6. Language learning is social and collaborative, a transactional process. Interaction is essential to forming one's own meanings. It is not a solitary act. Parents and other supportive adults assist language learning by providing models, listening carefully, and responding appropriately to children's communication attempts. The child refines her or his language with each input and output.

7. Language learning is individualistic and idiosyncratic, not measured against others or some mythical norm. Children direct their own learn-

ing to accomplish personal communication goals. To learn, a child must be interested and personally involved. Language learning is an active process.

8. Language varies with the cultural and social background of the user. Culture defines what is true, logical, reasonable, and appropriate. These are reflected in language. For example, most Native American cultures lack a notion of imposing one's will on another except by physical force. Thus, most Native American languages have no words for *oblige, make, compel, order, command,* or *ought to* (D. King & Goodman, 1990).

9. Spoken language and written language are directly compatible (Shapiro, 1992). Systematic, explicit, and isolated focus on the structure of words, as in reading and writing instruction, is unnecessary and detrimental (K. Goodman, 1986a).

10. Skilled readers rarely attend to print. Print is used to confirm their predictions of the language to come. Reading is a combination of visual and contextual information.

In short, all elements of language are necessary for language to be meaningful, usable, and learnable.

Classroom Application

If language is not whole, it does not exist (D. King & Goodman, 1990). Wholeness makes language easy to learn (Table 11.1). Language teaching should be holistic or top-down, a whole-to-parts model. The language trained should be meaningful and real, not artificial. Thus, pragmatics and semantics assume new prominence.

There is no whole language curriculum per se. In the whole language classroom, however, children learn language and reading and writing by doing it. They are surrounded by interesting and meaningful language (Chaney, 1990).

TABLE 11.1
Ease of learning language
Source: Goodman, K. S. (1986a).
What's whole in whole language?
Portsmouth, NH: Heinemann, p. 8.

Language is easy to learn when . . .
  It's real and natural.
  It's whole.
  It's sensible.
  It's interesting.
  It's relevant.
  It belongs to the learner.
  It's part of a real event.
  It has social utility.
  It has purpose for the learner.
  The learner chose to learn it.
  It's accessible to the learner.
  The learner has power to use it.

Goodman, 1986, p. 8

Subskills are taught as needed. The approach is similar to that espoused throughout this book. Our concern is with communication and the child's success.

All aspects of the curriculum are interrelated. Language is a part of every classroom activity, not a separate area of training. Literacy is integrated into every aspect of the curriculum.

Language is multidimensional, so language teaching targets several language goals at once. Multiple formats and activities usually are based on a theme so that recurring ideas and common events are experienced over again and again (K. Goodman, 1986a; Newman, 1985).

In the light of these assumptions, the role of the teacher and the speech-language pathologist change (Smith-Burke et al., 1991). They become collaborators with each student. Rather than directly instruct, teachers create an atmosphere of language learning. Teachers and other adults provide opportunities for the child to participate and scaffold with cues and prompts to facilitate the child's language (Feuerstein, 1980; Langer & Applebee, 1986; J. Norris & Hoffman, 1990b). The manipulating contexts aspects discussed in Chapter 9 are applicable.

Training is individualistic—proceeding from each child's abilities—social, and meaningful. The curriculum is made to fit the learner, not the reverse. Interactions are at an appropriate developmental level for the child.

Each learner's perspective should be valued. The individual child's experience is her or his basis for using and interpreting language. Thus, differing cultural perspectives are to be esteemed.

> A first grader should understand that his or her culture is not a rational invention; that there are thousands of other cultures and they all work pretty well; that all cultures function on faith rather than truth; that there are lots of alternatives to our own society. Cultural relativity is defensible and attractive. It's also a source of hope. It means we don't have to continue this way if we don't like it. (Vonnegut, 1974, p. 139)

Without this recognition by the teacher, perspectives by minority students are not respected and are treated as inferior. The result is one of "cultural discontinuity" in which the experiences at school are not compatible with those in the child's culture. As a result, classroom teaching becomes less meaningful, less relevant to that child.

Dynamic interactic strategies replace one-way demonstrations and explanations (Stone & Wertsch, 1984). Direct teaching occurs where needed but in the context of real activities that involve transmitting and comprehending meanings (Sawyer, 1991).

Emphasis is on natural language use rather than artificial activities such as drill. "If an activity or procedure is not one that occurs naturally outside of schooling, then its value as a schooling activity is questionable" (D. King & Goodman, 1990, p. 223).

Language learning, especially reading and writing, is assumed to be social (Berthoff, 1981; Bloome, 1985; Heath, 1983; Levine, 1986; Street, 1984). Learning is not a solitary act, but occurs within a supportive environment. The child's response to written material reflects an integration of the text and the child's knowledge. Social aspects of reading and writing include the writer-reader relationship, shared definitions, shared and group reading, guided reading and conferencing, problem-solving, and small group work (Bloome, Harris, & Ludlum, 1991; Holdaway, 1979). Of course, there is also independent reading and writing. Rote practice and memorization are de-emphasized. Redundancy may be necessary for learning, but rote drill is not.

Contextual knowledge is important for learning as understanding moves from general concept to specific knowledge (K. Nelson, 1985; Piaget & Inhelder, 1969). Learning occurs best in the most familiar contexts or within the most familiar concepts, and thus repeatable contexts provide the best environment for learning language.

Whole language stresses contextual information that children use to predict written meanings (K. Goodman, 1969; F. Smith, 1988). Visual or printed information confirms these predictions. Training in print deciphering is de-emphasized (Rhodes & Dudley-Marling, 1988).

The most meaningful and enduring learning is that in which the learner is engaged voluntarily. Thus, within limits, the child chooses what to learn and how. This choice facilitates a sense of ownership of the learning and engages the learner in the task (Cambourne, 1988).

Efficacy

Several studies demonstrate the benefits of a whole language approach. The lack of a single curriculum, however, makes comparisons difficult. In general, children in whole language classrooms have better vocabularies and better reading skills than those in traditional skills-based, bottom-up classrooms (Gunderson & Shapiro, 1987; Ribowsky, 1986). Even readers who are at risk and children with LLD seem to benefit (Stice & Bertrand, 1989, 1990).

Despite its successes, whole language is not without its detractors (Kamhi & Catts, 1989; Liberman & Liberman, 1990). Whole language is, after all, a language arts program, not a remedial one. Written language requires oral language awareness and skills, especially in phonology. Early literacy activities, such as rhyming, chanting, word games, and exposure to print, do not result in phonological awareness for all children, especially for those with language impairment (Chaney, 1990; Stanovich, 1991). Poor readers may reflect basic difficulties with language processing, rather than deficits in reading ability alone (Alvermann, 1983; Chall, Jacobs, & Baldwin, 1990; Kamhi & Catts, 1989; Turner, 1989; Vellutino, 1977). Direct intervention by a speech-language pathologist is necessary with these children. Even here, however, we need not return to the traditional methods of irrelevant drill, drill, drill.

Summary

Several educational trends—inclusive schooling, collaborative teaching, and whole language—have combined to change the teaching and remediation of language. A result of whole language theory may be recognition by the speech-language pathologist that children conceptualize their physical and social environment, function as active participants therein, and integrate language within their existing knowledge of this environment (P. Cole, 1982; McLean & Snyder-McLean, 1978; Muma, 1978). Thus, in many schools, the speech-language pathologist is working with children and their language impairments within a naturalistic language curriculum in regular education classrooms.

"Speech-language pathology . . . is moving away from the behaviorism of the past 60 years and its fragmented view of language. . . . moving toward a more dynamic and integrated construct of language proficiency" (J. Norris & Damico, 1990, p. 219). The principles we have been discussing are a near perfect match to the demands of this intervention situation.

ROLE OF THE SPEECH-LANGUAGE PATHOLOGIST

Any classroom intervention model raises questions about the speech-language pathologist's role and about others' expectations of the intervention team. These questions include the following:

What is my new role? Who am I?

Are there special language needs within the routines of the classroom situation?

How do I address individual needs within a classroom?

How do I justify my new role to an administration that gauges my work in individual contact hours?

What is the relationship of language arts and language remediation?

How do I educate teachers?

The classroom model is still evolving, and there are no quick answers. Our discussion of the elements of the classroom model addresses some of these questions.

The speech-language pathologist is a problem solver who, with the guidance of a few principles, applies and adapts a variety of methods in seeking solutions. Whole language emphasizes the holistic, integrated nature of language; the individual and variable forms; the importance of social, cognitive, and perceptual abilities in language learning; and the prevailing role of culture (K. Goodman, 1986a; D. King & Goodman, 1990; Reutzel & Hollingworth, 1988; Teale & Sulzby, 1986; Winitz, 1983). In the final analysis, the model of intervention that evolves is a blend of the child's needs and the desires of the school, the individual teacher, and the speech-language pathologist. The speech-language pathologist will assume the roles of co-teacher, consultant, and direct service provider and will be integrated fully into the classroom (Farber, Denenberg, Klyman, & Lachman, 1992).

The speech-language pathologist is the school's language expert. As such, she advises administrators, teachers, and special needs committees about children and language impairment. She is also responsible for speech and language assessment, for the planning and implementation of all speech and language programming, for record keeping, and for training personnel who will work with the children with language impairment.

Relating to Others

Environmental intervention such as that in the classroom necessitates coordination of intervention goals and schedules. This coordination requires that the speech-language pathologist interact daily with a variety of individuals.

Classroom Teachers

The speech-language pathologist is uniquely qualified to assist the classroom teacher is assessing each child's level of functioning, analyzing the language requirements of various activities and materials, and developing intervention strategies in conjunction with the classroom teacher. She helps the teacher identify children with language impairments and suggests techniques to facilitate development. This is an ongoing process, accomplished through in-service training and individual consultation and training, as well as co-teaching within the classroom.

The speech-language pathologist and the classroom teacher have unique skills that they can use to help each other and the child with language impairment. The speech-language pathologist understands language development and the remediation of speech and language impairments. The classroom teacher knows each child and understands the use of large and small group interactions for teaching.

Difficulties usually arise over turf or territory. The classroom teacher may feel threatened by the presence of another "teacher" in the classroom and may resent being shown how to talk to students to maximize each child's language learning. The speech-language pathologist may feel like a classroom aide, undervalued for her expertise. These differences and potential problems should be discussed openly prior to beginning intervention. Each professional's role should be delineated and clearly understood. The speech-language pathologist and the classroom teacher should exchange clear and valuable information. This ongoing exchange is especially important at the beginning of intervention.

The speech-language pathologist and the classroom teacher are part of the intervention team and should contribute in that fashion. Each has special expertise to impart. Neither one is there to spy on the other, and their personal opinions of each other have no place in the classroom.

Parents

Not all parents can or wish to participate in their children's speech-language intervention. Parents tend to fall into three identifiable groups, the largest being those who desire participation. Next are those who desire no participation, and the smallest group is composed of parents who only want more information (Andrews, Andrews, & Shearer, 1989). The first group of parents can be involved in planning and implementation of intervention, and parents who want information can be served through parent meetings and in-service training.

School Administrators

The speech-language pathologist's new role may require some education of the administration. Traditional patterns of instruction change slowly, and administrators may not understand generalization and the need to provide language remediation within the classroom. Caseload dictates and contact hour requirements may have to be modified to accommodate the classroom model.

Administrators will need to be impressed with the increased efficiency gained through the co-teaching of the speech-language pathologist and the classroom teacher. Discussion should center on how best to serve the children and how to use professional time commitments most efficiently.

Finally, the speech-language pathologist's new role should be viewed within the perspective of a comprehensive school or districtwide program that includes early childhood intervention, bilingual and bidialectal services, and the training of English as a second language (Koenig & Biel, 1989). Public law is dictating an extension of speech-language and educational services to these children.

Language Intervention and Language Arts

Classroom teachers and administrators are sometimes confused about the difference between language arts and language remediation. Unless this distinction is clear, the speech-language pathologist's role also may be misunderstood, especially as it relates to classroom intervention. *Language arts* accomplishes several things:

1. Provides children with labels for the language units they have been using in their speech

2. Requires children to stretch their language abilities into new areas, such as fictional and expository writing

3. Enables children to have language growth experiences, such as performances

4. Helps children reason and problem-solve by using linguistic units

All of these valuable accomplishments presuppose that each child has a well-formed language system.

Language remediation cannot make this supposition. In *language remediation,* the child is taught language units or behaviors that are not present or are in error in the primary mode of communication—that is, in language transmitted via speech. Secondary modes, such as reading and writing, are a concern when problems with oral language affect them. Through training, teachers and administrators become aware of this distinction and of the valuable contribution of each to the child's education.

ELEMENTS OF A CLASSROOM MODEL

The model consists of identification (assessment), intervention, and facilitation. In each phase, the classroom teacher and the speech-language pathologist, although a team, have individual inputs that affect the delivery of quality services for the child.

Identification of Children at Risk

Teachers play a vital role in identifying children with speech and language impairments. Most teachers are not trained in language development or impairment, and the speech-language pathologist must alert them to the behaviors that signal a possible impairment.

Teacher training can be accomplished in in-service sessions. Teachers also can be given aids to use in identifying a potential speech and language problem. Table 11.2 presents a list of some signs for recognizing children having difficulties in the classroom. Appendix J contains an analysis format for classroom interactions that can guide teachers in determining the locus of breakdown in communication interactions in the classroom (Vetter, 1982). Table 11.3 or its adaptation might be used by teachers for referral to the speech-language pathologist.

Teachers should be trained to observe and describe classroom behaviors as precisely as possible. The speech-language pathologist's complaint that teachers refer children who have rather nonspecific vocabulary problems or are inattentive reflects poorly on the speech-language pathologist's training of teachers in language impairment and its manifestations. Teachers are a valuable source of raw data on classroom performance when they know what to observe and measure.

TABLE 11.2
Recognizing children with language impairment in the classroom

---

The child may have some or all of the following:
- Seems to fail to understand and follow instructions.
- Is unable to use language to meet daily living needs.
- Violates rules of social interaction, including politeness.
- Lacks ability to read signs or other symbols and to perform written tasks.
- Has problems using speech to communicate effectively.
- Demonstrates a lack of appropriate organization and sequence in verbal and written efforts.
- Does not remember significant information presented orally and/or in written form.
- May not recognize humor or indirect comments.
- Seems unable to interpret the emotions or predict the intentions of others.
- Responds inappropriately for the situation.

Source: Adapted from Nelson, N. W. (1992). Targets of curriculum-based language assessment. *Best Practices in School Speech-Language Pathology, 2,* 73–86.

TABLE 11.3
Teacher referral of children with possible language impairment

---

The following behaviors may indicate that a child in your classroom has a language impairment that is in need of clinical intervention. Please check the appropriate items.

____ Child mispronounces sounds and words.
____ Child omits word endings, such as plural -*s* and past tense -*ed.*
____ Child omits small unemphasized words, such as auxiliary verbs or prepositions.
____ Child uses an immature vocabulary, overuses empty words, such as *one* and *thing,* or seems to have difficulty recalling or finding the right word.
____ Child has difficulty comprehending new words and concepts.
____ Child's sentence structure seems immature or overreliant on forms, such as subject-verb-object. It's unoriginal, dull.
____ Child's question and/or negative sentence style is immature.
____ Child has difficulty with one of the following:

____ Verb tensing	____ Articles	____ Auxiliary verbs
____ Pronouns	____ Irreg. verbs	____ Prepositions
____ Word order	____ Irreg. plurals	____ Conjunctions

____ Child has difficulty relating sequential events.
____ Child has difficulty following directions.
____ Child's questions often inaccurate or vague.
____ Child's questions often poorly formed.
____ Child has difficulty answering questions.
____ Child's comments often off topic or inappropriate for the conversation.
____ There are long pauses between a remark and the child's reply or between successive remarks by the child. It's as if the child is searching for a response or is confused.
____ Child appears to be attending to communication but remembers little of what is said.
____ Child has difficulty using language socially for the following purposes:

____ Request needs	____ Pretend/imagine	____ Protest
____ Greet	____ Request information	____ Gain attention
____ Respond/reply	____ Share ideas, feelings	____ Clarify
____ Relate events	____ Entertain	____ Reason

____ Child has difficulty interpreting the following:

____ Figurative language	____ Humor	____ Gestures
	____ Emotions	____ Body language

____ Child does not alter production for different audiences and locations.
____ Child does not seem to consider the effect of language on the listener.
____ Child often has verbal misunderstandings with others.
____ Child has difficulty with reading and writing.
____ Child's language skills seem to be much lower than other areas, such as mechanical, artistic, or social skills.

In addition, the speech-language pathologist and the classroom teacher can identify the individual classroom or grade level's special communication requirements as a gauge against which each child can be measured to assess achievement. Called *curriculum-based assessment,* this method uses the child's progress within the school curriculum as a measure of her or his educational success (Tucker, 1985). Children are assessed against the curriculum within which they are expected to perform. Thus, intervention focuses on changes in the child's behavior that are relevant to the educational setting.

From preschool through high school, the curriculum not only becomes more difficult but also changes in the types of demands made on the student. Wiig and Semel (1984) outline these changes as follows:

> Preschool: Learning focuses on sensorimotor, language, and socioemotional growth with materials that are manipulative, three dimensional, and concrete.
>
> Early grades (K-2): Learning focuses on perceptual-cognitive strategies with materials that are one dimensional, abstract, and symbolic.
>
> Middle grades (3-4): Learning places higher demands on linguistic and symbolic skills with less direct instruction. The child is expected to make inferences, analyze data, and synthesize information.
>
> Upper grades (5-6): Learning focuses on content areas, with the child expected to recall past learning and display fluency with basic academic skills.
>
> Middle and high school: Learning emphasizes lectures in content areas, with students expected to reorganize material as they listen and to gain the main or important points. From 75% to 90% of the day may be spent receiving information.

By identifying the overall requirements for the class, the teacher has provided a list of potential skills with which the child with language impairment may experience difficulty. Some school districts have identified skills that children need to succeed in each grade. Table 11.4 presents some of the skills needed in the first three grades.

In addition to the school's official curriculum, which is an outline of the material to be learned in each grade, children encounter several other curricula (N. Nelson, 1989). These include the *de facto curriculum* that is actually taught and the cultural and school curricula needed to succeed within each context. The expectations of the latter are often very confusing for the child with language-processing problems. The implicit expectations of individual teachers and other children form a fourth curriculum.

The speech-language pathologist first must become familiar with the curricula that affect the individual child with language impairment. She can assess the child through a combination of interview and observation of the child's ability to meet the language demands of the curricula. The interview phase can provide information on the curricular expectations, and observation can focus on the specific linguistic demands made of the child.

An analysis of the linguistic demands must consider all aspects of language and the many reception and production modes. Such an analysis should note metalinguistic skills demanded in these various aspects and modes (N. Nelson, 1989).

TABLE 11.4
Some possible language skills needed in the first three grades

First Grade. The child will be able to:
Recognize correct word order auditorily.
Identify singular and plural common nouns and proper nouns.
Identify regular and irregular past and present verbs.
Identify descriptive and comparative adjectives.
Use nouns and pronouns, adjectives, and verbs correctly in sentences, including verb-noun agreement.
Give and write full sentences.
Categorize words by opposites, by sequence, by category, and as real/nonreal.
Retell a story.
Identify the main idea in a paragraph.
Classify narrative and descriptive writing.
Rhyme words and identify words that begin with the same sound.
Identify declarative and interrogative sentences and use correct ending punctuation for each.
Capitalize the first word in a sentence, days, months, people's names, and the pronoun *I*.
Alphabetize.
Give directions and explanations and follow two-step directions.
Read aloud.
Listen attentively and courteously to others.

Second Grade. In addition to the skills needed for first grade, the child will be able to:
Use correct word order.
Identify incomplete sentences.
Recognize singular and compound subjects of a sentence.
Identify possessive and plural nouns, contracted verbs, and superlative adjectives and use correctly.
Capitalize holidays, titles of people, books, stories, and places.
Identify correct comma use.
Use an apostrophe in contractions.
Identify the topic sentence and sentences that do not relate in a paragraph.
Write an explanation or set of directions.
Address an envelope.

An educational language assessment should focus on the child's oral and written abilities and capacity to learn, rather than on his deficits (Silliman, 1993). Data should be gathered by direct testing and real-life observation within the classroom. The level of support necessary for learning should be determined, including evaluation of the effectiveness of various instructional and intervention strategies. Most standardized tests are too global, and more specific measures should be used to measure the child. The parents and the teacher, as well as the child and the speech-language pathologist, should participate.

The speech-language pathologist must follow up these reports and collect her own data within the classroom setting. These data can be corroborated by further testing and sampling.

Write rhyming words to complete a poem.

Identify figurative language and synonyms.

Recognize characters, plot, setting, and the major divisions in a story or play, and the difference between fiction and nonfiction.

Tell and write a clear, original story.

Use the title page and table of contents in a book.

Use the dictionary for spelling and meaning.

Read critically for sequence, main idea, and supporting details.

Use tables and graphs as sources of information.

Recognize types of poetry.

Listen discriminately for rhyming, sequences, and details.

Third Grade. In addition to the skills needed for first and second grade, the child will be able to:

Identify imperative and exclamatory sentences, simple and compound sentences, and run-on sentences.

Recognize compound predicates in a sentence.

Recognize articles and conjunctions in sentences.

Use an exclamation point.

Use an apostrophe in possessive nouns.

Define a paragraph and identify the main idea and supporting sentences.

Write a paragraph, a book report, and a letter with correct capitalization and punctuation.

Write a clear, original story with title, beginning, middle, and end.

Recognize the difference between biography and autobiography.

Use a dictionary for pronunciation.

Use an encyclopedia, telephone book, newspapers, and magazines as references.

Identify compound words, homophones, and homographs.

Use prefixes and suffixes.

Read critically for sequence, main idea, and supporting details.

Organize information by category and sequence.

Recognize real and make-believe, relevant and irrelevant, and factual and opinionated statements.

Identify characteristics of different types of narratives.

Teachers should be informed about the results of such testing and sampling and advised on the best methods of intervention. Classroom teachers can be apprised periodically of the child's progress and involved intimately in the intervention process.

Assessment With Preschool Children

The speech-language pathologist is interested in pragmatic abilities at both the utterance, cross-utterance and cross-partner, and event levels; semantics, especially the child's lexicon, and language structure; and narrative form and story grammar rudiments. Additional areas of importance for literacy education include role play and representational play, decontextualization, literacy, and adaptations for non-oral responding (Culatta, 1992; Culatta, Horn, Theadore, & Sutherland, 1993; Westby, 1988).

Play is particularly important for preschool children, especially as a context within which to experiment with language (Westby, 1988). Of particular importance are the level of decontextualization, thematic content, organization, and self/other relations (Culatta, 1992; Culatta et al., 1993; Westby, 1988). Play can be very context-bound, using only real objects, or relatively decontextualized, using imaginary or symbolic objects. The familiar versus unfamiliar themes of play are also important for later intervention. The organization of play can demonstrate cohesion, logical connections with the theme, and planning. Finally, the roles the child takes and assigns may be important for later training and may tell the speech-language pathologist something about the child's ability to take the perspective of others and to code switch.

Decontextualization of the child's language is important for later reading and is demonstrated by reference to nonpresent entities and to past and future tense. Reading is very decontextualized because all meaning comes from print and little from the physical context.

Even though the child cannot read, literacy skills are important for further development. The speech-language pathologist is interested in the child's comprehension of text, knowledge and awareness of print, and sound-symbol associations and decoding abilities.

Finally, non-oral methods of communicating are important. These include gestures, facial expression, and body posture, but also drawing and "writing."

Assessment With School-Age Children and Adolescents

In addition to considering the language features mentioned in Chapters 4-7, the speech-language pathologist is interested in the child's language as it relates to the specific requirements of the classroom. An authentic or real assessment should be a *train-test-train* procedure, with both the speech-language pathologist and the classroom teacher acting as "participant observers," determining the best instructional strategies for individual children (Silliman, 1993). Such an evaluation consists of systematic observation of real teaching and learning in the classroom that yields meaningful information on student progress on an ongoing basis.

Systematic observation might include rating scales and checklists, narrative records, and descriptive tools by the teacher, speech-language pathologist, and student (Silliman, Wilkinson, & Hoffman, 1993). Possible rating scales for use with school-age children and adolescents are listed in Table 11.5. Teacher logs, notes, journal entries, and student assignments and self-evaluations should be gathered to ascertain the child's oral and written language skills. Of interest is the amount of scaffolding or structure and assistance needed by the child for success.

Interviews with the student are also helpful (N. Nelson, 1992). Students can be asked to describe their most difficult and easiest subjects and their strengths and weaknesses, to relate recent classroom events that made them feel bad, and to prioritize changes they would like to make in themselves and in the classroom and manner of instruction.

TABLE 11.5
Tools for assessment of classroom skills

Observation/Interviews

Clinical Discourse Analysis (Damico, 1985a)

Environmental Communication Profile (Calvert & Murray, 1985)

An Interview for Assessing Students' Perceptions of Classroom Reading Tasks (Wixson, Bosky, Yochum, & Alvermann, 1984)

Pragmatic Protocol (Prutting & Kirchner, 1983, 1987)

Self-Attribution of Students (SAS) (Marsh, Cairns, Relich, Barnes, & Debus, 1984)

Social Interactive Coding System (SICS) (Rice, Sell, & Hadley, 1990)

Spanish Language Assessment Procedures: A Communication Skills Inventory (Mattes & Omark, 1984)

Spotting Language Problems (Damico & Oller, 1985)

Systematic Observation of Communication Interaction (SOCI) (Damico, 1985b)

Testing

Classroom Communication Screening Procedure for Early Adolescence (CCSPEA) (Simon, 1987)

Curriculum Analysis Form (Larson & McKinley, 1987)

Interactive Reading Assessment (Calfee & Calfee, 1981)

Lindamood Auditory Conceptualization Test (Lindamood & Lindamood, 1979)

Test of Awareness of Language Segments (Sawyer, 1987)

The speech-language pathologist may gain additional information by informally sampling the child's performance. For example, Larson and McKinley (1987) recommend a procedure for comparing a secondary school child's notes with those of a higher performing student in the same class. Audiotapes of classroom instructions can be analyzed to determine the level of complexity that each child must be able to process. The speech-language pathologist might collect samples of the child's oral reading or help the child complete assignments, noting the child's language-related work skills.

Within a whole language curriculum, the speech-language pathologist would want to investigate several specific language features in addition to those mentioned in chapters 4-7 (Westby, 1990). Whole language is used in naturalistic contexts for real communication purposes. Therefore, the speech-language pathologist is interested in a variety of pragmatic functions and skills. Within the classroom, children use language for self-monitoring, directing, reporting, reasoning, predicting, imagining, and projecting thoughts and feelings (Tough, 1977). Of interest is the breadth of functions demonstrated in conversation and narration.

School semantic development includes the addition of abstract terms, refinement and decontextualization of word meanings, the ability to define words, multiple word meanings and figurative language, organization of a semantic network, and use of metalinguistic and metacognitive terms (N. Nelson, 1985; Pease, Gleason, & Pan, 1989). Many of these features of language have been discussed previously in this text.

TABLE 11.6
Common metacognitive and metalinguistic terms

afraid	assert	assume	believe	concede	conclude
confirm	disgusted	doubt	embarrass	feel	forget
guess	happy	hypothesize	imply	infer	interpret
know	mad	predict	propose	proud	remember
sad	surprised	talk	think	understand	

Semantic networking or relating ideas to a theme is a popular whole language activity; thus, this is an important skill for children to acquire (Heimlich & Pittelman, 1986). Those with better-formed, more extensive networks are better able to comprehend and follow a topic or theme (Westby, 1990). Networks can be evaluated by having the child name everything he can related to a given topic or category or place pictures and words into categories. Matching and categorization tasks can be used. Picture tasks can be made more challenging by the use of pictures with differing perspectives.

Success in the classroom requires that the child be able to explain decision making, to discuss mental processes, and to reflect on mental processes of others and himself (Bretherton & Beeghly, 1982; Lewis & Michalson, 1983; Olson, 1984; Wellman, 1985). Metalinguistic and metacognitive terms are listed in Table 11.6. Some terms appear prior to school age, but many are not mastered until adolescence.

Syntax and morphology gradually change throughout the school years. Initially, structure is more complex in oral language rather than in written, but this reverses. Therefore, the speech-language pathologist is interested in the structure of both. Analysis would include clause and t-unit length and elements of the noun phrase and verb phrase. Cohesive elements such as pronouns and conjunctions are especially important (Beilin, 1975; L. Chapman, 1983; French & Nelson, 1985; Karmiloff-Smith, 1983; Nippold, 1988a).

Poor readers and writers often have poor cohesive skills and are unable to go beyond a single sentence or bit of information (Irwin, 1988). Linguistic cohesion relies on a set of semantic and syntactic relationships or ties, such as reference, substitution, ellipsis, conjunction, and lexical. These are described in Chapters 5 and 7.

In short, the more cohesive ties in a text and the more explicit they are, the more readable the text (Irwin, 1980a, 1980b; Irwin & Pulver, 1984; Kintsch & Vipond, 1977; Marshall & Glock, 1978). Inferring connections requires the use of prior knowledge, which can be very difficult for poor readers (Irwin, 1986; Webber, 1978). Cultural background can affect the ability to infer connections (Steffensen, 1986). As might be expected, younger children and poor readers have the most difficulty inferring cohesion (Bridge, Tierney, & Cera, 1977; Chai, 1967; L. Chapman, 1981, 1983; Irwin & Pulver, 1984; Moberly, 1978; Monson, 1982; Paris & Upton, 1976).

Narrative and expository writing and speaking also should be analyzed. Difficulty at these levels may signal underlying problems. Narrative analysis is discussed in Chapter 7.

Expository texts are different from narrative ones. Some are descriptive and with no overall structure, requiring the child to rely on memory for comprehension. Some are sequential or procedurally organized and are easier than descriptive, especially with familiar content. A typical sequential text explains how something is accomplished. Finally, cause-effect and problem solving are more difficult for children because they refer back to previous events (Britton & Black, 1985; Meyer, 1987; Richgels, McGee, Lomax, & Sheard, 1987).

Expository texts can be elicited as prescribed in Table 11.7. It is important to pose familiar and unfamiliar themes. Key words, such as *describe, compare, contrast, cause,* and *solve,* can cue the child for the type desired. Grammatic, semantic, and cohesive analysis suggested for narratives would be important for expository texts.

It is not until sixth grade that children go beyond simple one-way connectives related to a single topic (McCutchen, 1982; McCutchen & Perfetti, 1982). The most difficult type of cohesion is intersentential. Cohesive factors relate to both reading and writing ability (Chall & Jacobs, 1984; Gundlach, 1981; Haslett, 1983; Rentel & King, 1983; Shuy, 1981a, 1981b).

Pictures can be used in an assessment to elicit both oral and written samples. Cohesive analysis of writing can identify some problems. Of interest are the clarity of cohesion and the types employed (Irwin & Moe, 1986). Questions based on the student's reading can be used to evaluate comprehension of text cohesion.

Reading and writing errors can be analyzed to determine the strategies used by the child. Semantic and syntactic acceptability are especially important. Even though a word is incorrect, it may be semantically or syntactically acceptable. For example, in the following sentences incorrect words may or may not make semantic or syntactic sense.

TABLE 11.7
Eliciting expository text

Sequential/Procedural
   "Tell me how to make (something simple)."
      Tell me how to make cookies.
      Tell me how to use a pay phone.
Cause-effect
   "Tell me what would happen if (something familiar wasn't so)."
      Tell me what would happen if children didn't go to school.
      Tell me what would happen if you missed the school bus.
Problem-solution
   "How would you. . . ." or "What would you do if. . . ."
      How would you save the children in the story?
      How would you find a police officer?
      What would you do if it was raining very hard and you didn't want to get wet going home?

Target:	He went into the *house*.	
	He went into the *home*.	Semantically and syntactically acceptable
	He went into the *hotel*.	Syntactically acceptable but semantically unacceptable
	He went into the *heavy*.	Semantically and syntactically unacceptable

The types of substitutions made may highlight the type of processing—auditory or visual—being used by the child.

Word substitutions may signal word-retrieval problems. A curriculum-based assessment should attempt to identify the discrepancy between the child's knowledge of classroom content and his ability to retrieve it (German, 1992). The speech-language pathologist should note the presence of word-finding strategies discussed in Chapters 3 and 6.

Auditory discrimination and articulation skills are important for spelling and should be assessed. Phonemic awareness is important for writing and reading.

Some poor readers give up in despair and failure (Abramson, Garber, & Seligman, 1980). They perceive the events of the classroom as out of their control with outcomes independent of their own behavior. They have learned to be helpless (Seligman, 1975). Each failure confirms their condition further.

Good learners and readers guide and control their own learning (Baker & Brown, 1984; A. Brown, 1978; A. Brown & Palincsar, 1982; Flavell & Wellman, 1977). They read purposefully and flexibly with intention, effort, and selectivity (R. Anderson, Hiebert, Scott, & Wilkenson, 1985).

The poor reader's lack of such strategies reflects his misconceptions about the task and his acceptance of failure (Diener & Dweck, 1978; P. Johnston & Winograd, 1985; Torgesen, 1980). The child becomes passive, lacking persistence and accepting low self-esteem, and displays apathy and resignation as a result of his perceived lack in his own abilities (Butkowsky & Willows, 1980; Thomas, 1979). These affective problems interfere with subsequent development (Winograd & Niquette, 1988).

Learned helplessness cannot be assessed readily on standardized tests (P. Johnston, 1987; Lipson & Wixson, 1986). Instead, information can be better obtained by interviews and observation. Interviews should focus on the child's perceptions and attributions regarding reading. Questions should include the child's perceptions of the reason reading is important, different types of reading and associated difficulties, and self-perception and its bases (Wixson, Bosky, Yochum, & Alvermann, 1984). Scaled responses, such as a 0-5 disagree-agree scale, also can be used with statements such as "Reading is difficult for me" or "My teacher doesn't help me learn how to read better" (Paris & Oka, 1986).

Observation can confirm the child's responses. Behavioral changes related to learned helplessness are nervousness, withdrawal, aggression, and chronic worry. Lack of task persistence can be noted in the amount of time or the number of attempts made to decode a word (P. Johnston & Winograd, 1985). A very high or very low number of requests for teacher assistance also can be a good indicator. In addition, self-verbalizations blaming himself ("I'm so dumb") or others ("This story is stupid" or "Why didn't you tell me I was next") rather than stating alternate strategies for success also may signal helplessness.

Curriculum-Based Intervention Within the Classroom

Within the classroom, the speech-language pathologist can work with individuals or small groups of children. Group projects can provide the context for intervention by using the techniques discussed in Chapter 9. Other children can serve as models. The teacher can work with the rest of the class at this time. If they are working on similar projects, the teacher can observe the speech-language pathologist and use some of her techniques. Small group instruction is efficient and effective and increases generalization and interaction (Shelton, Gast, Wolery, & Winterling, 1991).

An axiom of the classroom is "Busy little hands are productive ones" (Pearson, 1988). Group activities may center on art or construction projects using modeling clay or Play-Doh, pegboards, beads, puzzles, construction paper and glue, and the like.

Children's individual needs can be addressed if the speech-language pathologist or teacher carefully interacts with each child in ways that foster the targeted aspects of language. Signs posted conspicuously will remind the teacher or aide how to interact with each child. With planning, this training can be accomplished individually even in groups of children.

The goals of classroom intervention are for the child to learn new ways of communicating and to have ample opportunity to practice newly acquired skills (McCormick, 1986). The environment should be responsive so that the child learns that language can have some effect on that environment. "Communication intervention should focus on increasing the frequency of communicative behaviors, shaping production of increasingly more sophisticated language functions, and encouraging expression of familiar functions with more advanced language forms" (McCormick, 1986, p. 125). The language of effective classroom communicators is characterized by fluency of word-finding skill, coherence or content organization, and effectiveness and control (National Council of Teachers of English, 1976).

The child's learning within the classroom is a function of individual learning style and the environment (Samuels, 1983; Schumaker & Deshler, 1984). Both must be considered when assessing or attempting to intervene with learning. The language of the child's classroom and materials can provide the context and content for intervention. A number of sources provide intervention materials for use within the classroom curriculum (Cosaro, 1989; Hoskins, 1987; Larson & McKinley, 1987; N. Nelson, 1988a; Pidek, 1987; Simon, 1985; Wallach & Miller, 1988).

School-Age and Adolescent

With advancing grades, the emphasis shifts increasingly to independent work and to listening and note-taking abilities. Each of these tasks is extremely complex.

Intervention helps students learn strategies for analyzing various tasks and for determining the steps to take to accomplish them. The speech-language pathologist might teach language-impaired students time management skills, study skills, critical thinking, and language use (Buttrill et al., 1989). She might develop a book of listening activities for teacher use within the classroom (Cosaro, 1989).

Study skills training might include text analysis, study strategies, note taking, test-taking strategies, and reference skills. Through text analysis, the child can be helped to understand the organization of texts and their more efficient use.

Study strategies might include active processes for reading (Greene & Jones-Bamman, 1985), such as identifying the main ideas and reviewing periodically to organize the material. Children also can learn associative and other memory strategies.

Critical thinking is the collection, manipulation, and application of information to problem solving (Alley & Deshler, 1979). Language is an integral part of this process (Narrol & Giblon, 1984). Therefore, the child with language impairment may experience difficulties with organizing information and with decision making. Likewise, sophisticated metalinguistic judgments also would be difficult. Critical thinking training might target the three components of general thinking, problem solving, and higher level thinking (Buttrill et al., 1989).

General thinking includes observation and description, development of concepts, comparisons and contrasts, hypotheses, generalization, prediction of outcomes, explanations, and alternatives. *Problem-solving skills* include analyzing the problem into smaller parts, developing options, predicting outcomes, and critiquing the decision (Alley & Deshler, 1979; Schwartz & McKinley, 1984). *Higher level thinking* includes deductive and inductive reasoning, solving analogies, and understanding relationships. These tasks are increasingly more abstract and require greater reliance on linguistic input.

With increased emphasis on lectures at the secondary level, listening skills become even more important. In general, good listening skills are highly correlated with good overall language performance (National Council of Teachers of English, 1976). Students can be taught to tune in to what they hear and to listen actively (Kail & Marshall, 1978). Subsequent training can focus on recognition and understanding of lecture material. The child's semantic, syntactic, and morphological repertoire can be expanded as a base for comparison with new information from lectures. Such training might include word meanings, relationships and categories, sentence transformations, active and passive voice, embedding and conjoining, and segmentation (Buttrill et al., 1989). Through critical listening training, the child learns to supply missing information, complete stories, find important information, and recognize absurdities in spoken information.

In oral language production, the child can express the language repertoire trained receptively. In addition, the child can sharpen word-retrieval and figurative language skills. The speech-language pathologist can teach children to verbalize important critical reasoning skills, such as questioning, comparing, and analyzing, and to discuss a task or topic and to give examples.

She can enhance written language training by using computers and topics of interest to the child. Computer intervention can have a positive effect on language, especially vocabulary, and even can improve social-interactive skills (Schery & O'Connor, 1992). Organizational skills gained in critical thinking training can be used in expressive writing training.

Finally, she can enhance conversational skills by role playing and practice (Schwartz & McKinley, 1984). The child with language impairment can be helped to identify different communication contexts and their requirements.

Written information can be used to train oral language skills. Within a conversational or small group framework, this written information can be used for practice in communicating between speaker and listener (J. Norris, 1989). Written material can be controlled systematically to ensure that it is well organized and cohesive and that it offers a variety of topics, roles, and situations.

Prewritten textual information allows the speech-language pathologist to teach language holistically, using all aspects of language, rather than fragments (Laughton & Hasenstab, 1986). The use of social interactions enables the child to learn language as an integrated social-cognitive-linguistic experience.

Adolescents can offer a special challenge if they are not treated with respect and included in intervention decisions. Pull-out services are not practical because the student will miss required classes. In addition, exiting and entering a class calls attention to the teen in a manner perceived as negative (Holzhauser-Peters & Andrin-Husemann, 1990).

It is the very structure of the adolescent's day that highlights the need for some stability in the teen's language input. Many adolescents plateau at grade levels well below assigned grade (Schumaker & Deshler, 1988). These students need more time than short classes allow. In addition, each teacher's contact with individual students is limited to class periods. No one is responsible for the teen's overall language functioning and success (Larson, McKinley, & Boley, 1993). Some school districts have designed program prototypes that attempt to meet some of the needs of adolescents (Larson & McKinley, 1987; Larson et al., 1993; Work, Cline, Ehren, Keiser, & Wujek, 1993).

Essential to any successful adolescent program is destigmatization and the awarding of credit. Rooms selected for language group classes should be mixed with other classes. Classes should have names similar to other classes, such as "oral communication skills," rather than "speech therapy." The giving of credit aids motivation and gives the speech-language therapist clout and credibility (Larson et al., 1993).

A program such as Contextualized Adolescent Language Learning (CALL) Curriculum (Ehren & Mullins, 1988) may serve as a model. It consists of two strands, academic and functional. The academic portion targets items in the regular curriculum, while the functional emphasizes immediate daily living demands. Academic targets can be emphasized by the speech-language pathologist during classroom teaching.

The overall intervention model might incorporate elements of two instructional approaches called *strategy-based* and *systems* models. The **strategy-based**

model of intervention assumes that learning problem-solving strategies is more powerful than learning factual content and will generalize more readily (Deshler, Alley, Warner, & Schumaker, 1981; McKinley & Lord-Larson, 1985; Schwartz & McKinley, 1984; Wong & Jones, 1982). Teaching includes strategies for verbal mediation and for the organization and retrieval of linguistic information (Buttrill et al., 1989; J. Norris, 1989; Tattershall, 1987; Wallach & Miller, 1988; Wiig & Semel, 1984). This model is highly appealing because of its potential for generalization outside the intervention setting.

In contrast, a **systems model** assumes that the source of the language impairment lies in the interactions of the child, the primary caregivers, and the content to be learned. Thus, learning is a function of this complex system (N. Nelson, 1986a). Intervention strategies should reflect the child's varying learning needs across several learning contexts (N. Nelson, 1989; Wallach & Miller, 1988).

Throughout this text, we discuss the benefits of teaching rules or strategies, rather than discrete bits of language. The model presented assumes that this teaching would occur within the interactions of the child and significant others.

Although classroom intervention may suffice for some children with mild language problems, others too will need individual services. This service can be accomplished in the classroom or through the more traditional pull-out model. The functional conversational model is still very appropriate, as noted in Chapter 8. Children also may work individually within the classroom, using computer-aided instruction (Schetz, 1989).

The speech-language pathologist can demonstrate individualized targets and techniques for the teacher with the child or discuss them in meetings with the child's teachers, aides, and parents. Parents who cannot receive instruction in individualized training techniques are better used as general facilitators, rather than direct trainers.

Language facilitator education can be accomplished in in-service workshops and at parent meetings. The speech-language pathologists should not try to impart all of her knowledge to teachers, aides, and parents at these meetings. A general outline of language development and an introduction to principles of instruction will suffice.

Linguistic Awareness Intervention Within the Classroom

In addition to providing individual or group services within the classroom setting, the speech-language pathologist can increase linguistic awareness itself for all children. Within such activities, she can be especially mindful of the needs of those children with language impairment. Each child should be encouraged to participate at her or his ability level.

Preschool

Whole class, preschool, preliterate activities may include replica and role play, narrative development, and the use of children's books. Each contributes to the general notion of narration and narrative form.

Replica and role play.   Play and narrative development are very similar (Stein & Glenn, 1979; Westby, 1988). For children developing normally, the language of social make-believe play and the language of literacy have similar functions (Pellegrini & Galda, 1990). Language must be modified for the audience or participants, meaning must be conveyed, language is elaborated, and there are cohesive ties and integrated themes.

The imaginative function of the language of play is acquired during preschool (Pellegrini, 1983). Typically not performed during solitary play, imaginative language is more characteristic of social interactional play (Martlew, Connolly, & McLeod, 1976). The language is also very explicit in order to convey meaning crucial to directing such play ("You be the baby now"). Language is used to refer to objects within the situation ("*This* is my horse") and to negotiate and compromise ("Okay, you can talk like that if you're the baby"). Integrated themes are evident in the beginnings and ends of play episodes, in the temporal organization, and in the enactment of everyday events or previously heard or seen narratives (Galda, 1984; Pellegrini, 1985).

Imaginative language is heavily influenced by context. Preschool children prefer same-gender paired play with no adults present (Hartup, 1983; Pellegrini & Perlmutter, 1989). Both boys and girls prefer replica toys, such as dolls, a simulated store, a dress-up, and boys also prefer blocks. Toys generally are used as props for their intended purposes. Older preschoolers and kindergartners are more willing to use ambiguous props and to assign meaning (Pellegrini & Perlmutter, 1989).

Preschoolers use language forms in their play that later are used in school literacy events. Linguistic verbs used in play are a good predictor of reading ability later. School success is also dependent, in part, on a child's ability to comprehend and use these linguistic verbs (Torrance & Olson, 1984). Finally, reading is often in the temporal sequential mode similar to the narratives found in play.

Play has been used effectively to increase language skills of preschool children developing normally. Children can make significant gains in play-related conversation, vocabulary, and sentence lengthening (Lovinger, 1974; Smilansky, 1968). Other cognitive and social benefits also occur.

Unfortunately, many children with disabling conditions do not play like children developing normally (Westby, 1988). Sometimes, they do not have the experiential base for replica and role play. Thus, their event representations may be dissimilar. All children are more likely to engage in interactive communication when they share a social script (K. Nelson & Gruendel, 1979). In addition, children with language impairment often are isolated in the regular preschool class, engaging in solitary play. Given the importance of play for later narrative development, it is essential that these children have normalizing play interactions.

As mentioned previously, play would be assessed within the framework of an overall communication assessment. In addition to concern for language features and narrative skill for story retelling and generation, the speech-language pathologist is interested in play analysis relative to decontextualization of props and language, thematic content of the scripts presented, organization, and the roles assigned by the child to himself and others (Culatta et al., 1993; Westby, 1988). Also of interest are emerging literacy skills (Culatta et al. 1993; Edmaiston, 1988; Sulzby, 1982). These skills include recognition of situationally dependent print, such as a stop sign; independent interactions with a book; book handling skills; book knowledge, such as retelling, asking questions, and pointing to a page and its parts; and letter and sound recognition.

Prior to beginning play training, the speech-language pathologist must plan the event carefully (Culatta et al., 1993; Sonnenmeier, 1992). First, she must create a play script. Theme selection should be based on the child's familiarity with the theme or script and the child's level of play. It is best to begin with everyday events. Table 11.8 presents events based on familiarity. For a child unfamiliar with replica play, the speech-language pathologist might select getting ready for school or going to the market. By providing a supportive context, familiar routines are natural events within which language occurs. Our goal throughout this text has been for the child to have language that works in everyday situations.

Some events emphasize roles; others emphasize sequences. For example, riding on the school bus is more role-dependent, while making a cake is sequential. Different types of events should be chosen over time to aid generalization.

A note of caution is in order. Event representations vary with cultures. A child in a preschool classroom from a different culture may not readily adapt to the event chosen. Even within the "American culture" experience, levels are very different on the basis of race and ethnicity, family income and education levels, and geographic location.

Next, the speech-language pathologist determines each child's involvement in planning and develops the script. Children unfamiliar with play should be very involved in planning so that the play can be explained and have some contextual reference. The script should begin with one sequence and progress to multi-

TABLE 11.8
Themes for training replica play

Every day	Once in a while	Very seldom	Fantasy[*]
Getting ready for school	Baking a cake	Going to the zoo	Being the teacher (police, grocer, mommy, etc.)
Getting dressed	Having a birthday party	Going to the circus	
Eating lunch	Going to a birthday party	Seeing a parade	Being a dinosaur
Riding on the school bus	Getting a haircut	Going on a boat ride	Going to Mars
Going in the car	Going to the doctor	Going on an airplane	Piloting a plane
Getting a bath	Going to the market	Visiting _____	Being a caveman hunting game
	Celebrating (holiday)	Going to an amusement park	Painting a picture
	Going to temple	Going to a show/concert	Flying with wings
	Eating at McDonald's		

[*] To preschool children

TABLE 11.9
Sequence of sociodramatic script training

Step 1: Present script.

Step 2: Model roles including spoken parts.

Step 3: Have children re-present event and script. If needed, teacher prompts children for turn changes and for what to say and do. Prompting decreases over time.
    Prompts for motor-gestural response.
        Tell child what to do and give full physical prompt.
            Gradually decrease the prompt to a partial one and then to a physical assist.
        Tell child what to do and gesture or point.
        Tell child what to do.
        Point or gesture.
        Ask child, "What do you do next?'
    Prompts for verbal response.
        Ask child to imitate and present child with model ("You say, 'I want a hamburger.'").
        Ask child to imitate and present a partial model ("You say, 'I want. . . .'")
        Tell child it's his/her turn and gesture or point.
        Point or gesture.
        Repeat prior child's behavior and ask, "What do you say?"
        Ask, "What do you say to X (other child's role)?"

Step 4: When children are familiar with roles, reassign.
    Offer fewer prompts.

Step 5: Modify roles and script.

Source: Adapted from Culatta, Horn, Theadore, & Sutherland (1993); Goldstein, Wickstrom et al. (1988); Sonnenmeier (1992)

scheme events. More detail should be added gradually, along with more story grammar components.

Once children have progressed through this type of replica play, they can reenact selected texts from children's books. Appendix K includes a list of children's books for reading and enactment. The use of literature is discussed in following sections.

Decisions will need to be made about roles, props, repetitive elements in the narrative, and elaboration. In general, children with disabling conditions should be assigned initially to familiar roles. Props should be real objects. Gradually, roles can be modified and reassigned, and prop use can become more decontextualized and symbolic.

Table 11.9 presents a possible format for the training of play. The script is presented first in such a way as to provide a context for play. General play and the specific theme of this particular play are discussed. Then the adult models the appropriate roles. Children then re-create the event. This step is replayed many times with varying roles and elaboration of the basic theme.

At each juncture, children are encouraged to describe and discuss the event enacted. The language of group discussion and decision making is important for school success and helps stabilize learning more firmly.

Narrative development.   Training for narrative development and production is similar in many ways to that for play and may occur at the same time or following more advanced forms of replica play. Children enact familiar event sequences with increasing elaboration. Gradually, the events become more decontextualized through the use of puppets or cutouts and imaginary or substituted objects. Children can take turns narrating the story as it continues.

After decontextualized enactment, the narrative is related to the group and retold. With retelling, sequences can become even more elaborated so that a familiar event such as getting ready for school is modified with late arising, no clean socks, burnt toast, no toothpaste, a flat tire, and so on. Preschoolers must be cautioned to stay within the story frame. You do not get attacked by giants at the market nor rescued by the Ninja Turtles on the school bus.

Gradually, the speech-language pathologist can introduce stories with familiar event sequences that have not been enacted by the children. These, too, can be retold and modified by the children. Finally, children's literature can be used and these narratives retold by the children.

Children's literature.   Sharing children's literature with preschoolers is not just reading to them. Prereading, reading, and postreading activities can enhance the experience and make it more meaningful while bonding the class together (Montgomery, 1992a). Appendix K presents a list of children's books with suggested uses within a preschool classroom.

Children's literature must be presented to children within a framework or context that makes sense. Books should be introduced by their title and related to world knowledge that children already possess. The following is an introduction to *Brown Bear, Brown Bear, What Do You See?*:

> I'm going to read a book today called *Brown Bear, Brown Bear, What Do You See?* This is the cover. First, can anyone tell me what a bear is? That's right, Angel. Angel said a bear is like a big dog. Where does he live? Does he live in your house? No, he **doesn't** live in your house. Does he live in your neighborhood? Good, Antonio shook his head "No." He doesn't live in your neighborhood. Does he live in the woods? Yes, he lives in the woods. And in the zoo, good, Shawna.
>
> Now, this bear is brown; he has brown hair. Who has brown hair? John, point to someone with brown hair. That's your hair, John. Point to . . . yes, Billie Sue has brown hair. Put up your hand if you have brown hair. Good, Maria . . . and Katie . . . and Michel. What color hair do I have? That's right, Angel, black hair just like you.
>
> Well, our bear has brown hair. Here's a tough one: Do bears have any other color hair? . . .

As is obvious, the children can bring a lot of information to the task. When the story is read, each child can use her or his personal knowledge to interpret the story.

Notice that some children were allowed to respond by pointing. The speech-language pathologist can ensure that every child has an opportunity to participate. She facilitates their success by structuring their participation.

Often, children with language impairment do not understand books, temporal and causal sequences, story grammars, or logical consequences. The speech-language pathologist can guide them.

Within the classroom, books might be used for chanting, rhyming, or predicting activities or for specific language targets. Art activities, sequential memory, and consequential language (if . . . then) can follow reading. These activities and several resource books are listed in Appendix K.

School-Age and Adolescent

Whole language programs attempt to establish a language environment wherein books are centrally located and prominent within a hands-on activity center. Language is learned through thematic topics. Activities are organized around these themes to help children develop semantic networks and facilitate expansion of schema knowledge. Words and concepts are presented within the context of known words and concepts, not in isolation. Children are exposed to communication in print and are expected to communicate in print.

Adults model appropriate language for children within the classroom and orient children to various language functions. Not all children can benefit from this nondirective approach (Westby & Costlow, 1991).

Even schools that do not provide a whole language model require extensive language skills from their students. Reading and writing are an essential part of the educational system. Speech-language pathologists can encourage language use and aid development for those experiencing difficulties by actively engaging in classroom intervention. Skills targeted in therapy sessions can be enhanced in classroom application. Classroom linguistic awareness activities might include structuring classroom activities for success, semantic networking, and cohesion training.

Structuring classroom activities.   As mentioned, some children find school too frustrating, success too elusive. They give up. Different learning contexts within the classroom can reduce feelings of failure (P. Johnston & Winograd, 1985; Nicholls, 1979). For example, a noncompetitive environment can keep students task-involved, rather than ego-involved. Motivation is the key. Motivated students are more persistent and more likely to expend the energy necessary to access, monitor, and evaluate their language activities (Butkowsky & Willows, 1980).

The speech-language pathologist can make all students aware of the metacognitive and metalinguistic aspects of learning and employ strategies that enhance their application. She can explicitly teach learning strategies and provide guided practice and feedback. Each student can be guided and encouraged to participate at his functioning level.

Students can be aided in recognizing the features that influence comprehension and recall and the processing and retrieval demands of a task (A. Brown, Campione, & Day, 1981). General comprehension strategies to be taught include self-monitoring, drawing inferences, and resolving ambiguities. Study strategies that might be targeted include paraphrasing, summarizing, and note taking (Seidenberg, 1988). In general, metacognitive strategies have been effective in enhancing memory, comprehension, and spelling (A. Brown & Palincsar, 1982; Gelzheiser, 1984; Gerber, 1983, 1986; Palincsar & Brown, 1984, 1986; Pflaum & Pascarella, 1980; Schumaker, Deshler, Alley, Warner, & Denton, 1984; Wong, 1986; Wong & Jones, 1982).

Identifying the main idea.   Children often cannot find the main idea or organizing frame even in simple texts (Baumann, 1983). This task is fundamental to success in comprehension and academic success. The overall organizational abilities of some children may account for reading and writing problems (L. Baker, 1982; Freston & Drew, 1974). Incoming information needs to be organized for comprehension.

Structure of narrative and expository texts differs greatly and affects comprehension and memory. Readers or listeners go through a process of deleting, generalizing, and integrating the propositions of a text until they reach a macrostructure that summarizes the propositions presented (Kintsch & van Dijk, 1978). This process is dependent on underlying cognitive classification skills and world knowledge (J. Williams, 1984). Text often is evaluated for its "goodness-of-fit" to the reader's expectations (Rumelhart, 1984). World or prior knowledge also provides organizational strategies for writing (F. Smith, 1982b; Squire, 1983). Children vary in their ability to make use of prior knowledge (Pehrsson, 1982; Pehrsson & Denner, 1985).

Informational understanding develops as the readers progressively revise their expectations until they approximate the meaning of the author (Collins, Brown, & Larkin, 1980). Organizational clues supplied by the author enable the reader to interpret the passage and determine the main ideas (Tierney & Pearson, 1983).

Several textual features signal important information, including graphic features, such as italics, boldface, and type size; syntactic features, such as word order; semantic features, such as summaries and introductions; and schematic features, such as text structure (van Dijk, 1979). Of course, it is easiest to determine the overall organization if the topic is stated explicitly in the first sentence (Flood, 1978; Kieras, 1981; J. Williams, Taylor, & Granger, 1981).

Good readers are sensitive to the text organization. They "discover" the organizing structure (Mandler & Johnson, 1977; Meyer, 1975).

In general, poor readers are less sensitive to important information (Bridge, Belmore, Moskow, Cohen, & Matthews, 1984; B. Taylor, 1980; M. Taylor & Williams, 1983; Winograd, 1984; Wong, 1979). Many children with language impairment have difficulty comprehending and producing narratives because they fail to realize the internal organization of the text (Graybeal, 1981; Hansen, 1978; Weaver & Dickenson, 1979; Yoshinaga-Itano & Snyder, 1985). In general, these children fail to integrate new information with prior knowledge or fail to use the author's clues (Pehrsson & Denner, 1988). Poor readers use a fragmented organization or impose an unrelated structure. Even though third and fourth graders are able to recall important information, they have difficulty deciding what information is important in a text (A. Brown & Smiley, 1977).

Intervention might include comprehension strategies, such as predicting, questioning, clarifying, and summarizing; semantic networking; generative tasks in which the child generates a summary sentence; and familiarization with different text structures (Armbuster, Anderson, & Ostertag, 1987; Bridge et al., 1984; Dee-Lucas & DiVesta, 1980; Englert & Hiebert, 1984; Palincsar & Brown, 1983; Richgels et al., 1987; J. Williams, 1988).

In general, by second grade, children are aware of strategies for summarizing text. Strategies used by older children include deletion of unimportant information, deletion of redundant information, substitution of category names for various category members, and selection of or creation of a topic sentence (A. Brown & Day, 1983). Direct instruction in these strategies results in the best performance (Baumann, 1984; Englert & Lichter, 1982; Rinehart, Stahl, & Erickson, 1986; J. Williams, 1986).

Semantic networking or organizing is a method of teaching organization (Hanf, 1971; Heimlich & Pittelman, 1986; D. Johnson & Pearson, 1984; Pehrsson & Denner, 1988; Pehrsson & Robinson, 1985; Wiig, 1984; J. Williams, 1988). Helping children organize and reorganize structure during and after reading improves reading comprehension, writing cohesion, retention, and recall (Denner & Pehrsson, 1987; Pehrsson & Mook, 1983; Reutzel, 1985; Rumelhart & Ortony, 1977; Schultz, 1986; B. Taylor, 1980).

Ideas are displayed in semantic networks as clusters resembling spiders. Major ideas are circles or other shapes. Lines form related ideas or connect major ideas. Semantic clusters can be taught with a guided study approach that helps the child develop generalizable strategies (A. Brown, 1982). Slowly, students adapt and internalize the methods of the speech-language pathologist.

Organizational patterns are of two types: cluster and episodic (Figure 11.1). Cluster patterns are for superordination and subordination. In Figure 11.1, the topic or superordinate aspect is in the center. Related ideas radiate outward. Episodic organizers representing change move from event to event as in narration. These also can be used for problem-solution and cause-effect diagrams.

Children can begin to use semantic organizers in kindergarten or first grade, drawing pictures for the sequence of events in a narrative. Older children can write events in each cluster, either to aid recall or to structure narratives for telling or retelling. Variations, such as the story map, can help children develop story grammars (Figure 11.1). Similar diagrams, such as the mind map, can be adapted to various purposes, such as a book report, newspaper article, or argument (Montgomery, 1992a). Likewise, classroom brainstorming can help children realize their prior knowledge by examining all they know about a given topic (Dodge & Mallard, 1992).

As speech-language pathologists, we are interested in language and in helping children make sense of the language they receive and produce. Semantic networking is just one method of doing this.

Cohesion training.   Cohesion can be taught directly by explaining, modeling, and guided practice (Baumann & Stevenson, 1986; Irwin, 1986). Building on the

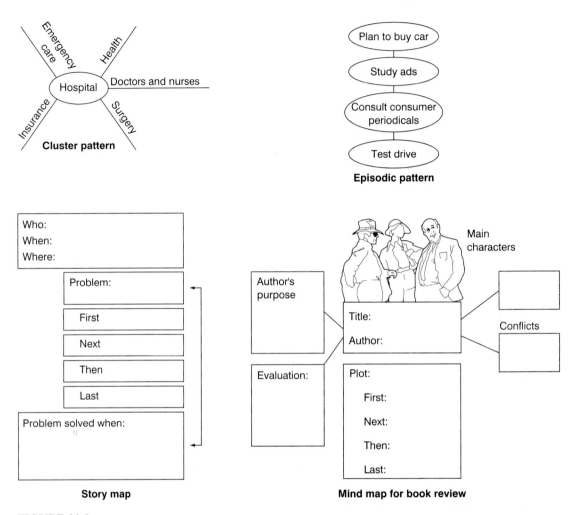

FIGURE 11.1
Examples of semantic networking
Source: Adapted from Montgomery (1992a); Pehrsson & Denner (1988)

children's prior knowledge, the speech-language pathologist can review a topic prior to reading and then help children seek meaning (C. Clark, 1986). Other exercises include phrase, clause, and sentence combining (Mackie, 1982; McAfee, 1980). These can be modified to include rewriting sentences, substituting pronouns for nouns, and filling in cohesive words, first using a cloze procedure, then in more open-ended tasks.

Summary

The speech-language pathologist can provide classroom language instruction that addresses the needs of the entire class while enabling every child to participate. She can provide the linguistic scaffolding that teachers often fail to provide, helping children become meaning makers, be successful. In addition, she can provide preteaching for the child with language impairment, helping that child be successful.

Language Facilitation

Language facilitation includes (a) identifying the needs of certain contexts and giving children the opportunity to experience this context successfully and (b) talking to children in ways that facilitate growth and highlight production. The classroom is a special context with its own demands. Facilitative techniques can be used there and in conversational interactions between children and their teachers, parents, and peers.

Classroom Language Requirements

Much of the classroom training should focus on the interactional patterns of the caregiver/facilitator and the child with language impairment. Most teacher-child classroom interactions consist of providing the right information. The child is taught to provide the correct answer and then be quiet. This behavior does not encourage an interactive conversational pattern (Rieke & Lewis, 1984).

Whereas conversations are relatively egalitarian and observe the rules of turn taking, classroom interactions usually are controlled by the teacher, who allocates turns. In contrast, conversational partners evaluate the acceptability of each utterance, but they are not expected to guess the correct utterance the other desires, as children must do in classroom responding. Finally, conversational turns may be expected but only rarely required. In the classroom, the teacher asks questions that require responses. The abstraction level of certain question forms is difficult for some children. Some question forms demand statement of fact, whereas others expect the child to reason and explain processes that may require inductive or deductive reasoning.

Often, the type of language used in the classroom is very different from what the child experiences at home. For example, the teacher's language consists of many indirect requests and statements. Questions or statements, such as, "Can you show us where the answer is written?" or, "I can't hear Lori because others are being impolite," contain requests or demands.

There is still plenty of room for conversational give-and-take in nondidactic exchanges, however, and these contexts also must be considered. The children have classroom time to participate in social conversation. Classroom programs and materials can be manipulated to maximize the opportunity for interaction. Language functions found in a typical classroom are enhanced through such manipulation.

Often the work occurs in small groups working on some common project. Children working alone have little opportunity to interact with others. Groups should reflect the classroom's composition, with opportunities for children who are high- and low-functioning to interact.

The skill of knowing how to get things done in the classroom is not usually taught to children, but rather is taken for granted by teachers (Wilkinson &

Milosky, 1987). The lack of such knowledge can be problematic for the child with language impairment asked to work with others to accomplish some task. The usual instructions are to help each other.

The child must be able to request and give information, action, and materials and to make judgments on the correct language and communication behaviors in and out of context. Each child is expected to be able to identify the information needed by all involved to complete a task and also to judge the appropriateness of information that is given.

Classroom language functions include (a) relating socially to others while stating personal needs, (b) directing others and self, (c) requesting and giving information, (d) reasoning, judging, and predicting, and (e) imagining and projecting into nonclassroom situations (Tough, 1973, 1979). Relating socially to others while stating one's own needs contains a number of behavior categories, such as referring to psychological or physical needs ("I want to leave now" or, "I'm hungry"), protecting one's self and self-interest ("That's mine"), agreeing or disagreeing ("You're wrong"), and expressing an opinion ("I hated that dessert") (Staab, 1983). This function can be elicited through activities organized around a highly desirable object that is not available to all participants, such as one bean-bag for a toss game involving three children.

The "directing self and others" function includes the categories of directing one's own actions, directing the actions of others, collaborating in the actions of others ("You be the mommy, and I'll be the daddy"), and requesting direction ("How do you do this?"). This function can be elicited by requiring children to accomplish some task they cannot do without help (Staab, 1983). There will also be a need to direct others and to follow others' directions.

The "giving information" function includes labeling ("That's a pinata"), referring to events ("Yesterday, we got a kitty"), referring to detail ("That kitty is black and white"), sequencing ("We went to the party, and then we went to the movies"), making comparisons ("Yours is bigger"), and extracting the general point ("We're making Hanukkah presents"). To elicit this function, the child shares an experience with someone who did not originally share it, as in show-and-tell (Staab, 1983).

Often, classroom discussions involve activities in which the entire class has participated, and children do not feel the need for their information to be as precise or detailed. They presuppose that their classmates share much of the information. This presumption cannot be made when classmates do not share the information.

Requests for information vary with the type of information sought. For example, adults and children tend to use more direct requests when there are few, if any, obstacles to receiving the answer, as in checking short answers to problems (Francik & Clark, 1985; Milosky & Wilkinson, 1984). In this situation, the request is very direct: "What's the answer to number 4?"

As children mature, they learn to identify the type of information needed to help a requester. In general, children become more aware of the importance of information specificity. Children are also more likely with maturity to provide information on the process of solving a certain problem, rather than just the answer requested. In responding to the previous question about problem number 4, the child might try to presuppose the difficulties of the requester and respond, "5/8; I converted to 8ths after solving the problem in 16ths." School-age children who provide specific information and process explanations are more likely to be high achievers (Peterson & Swing, 1985).

The "reasoning, judging, and predicting" function includes explaining a process ("When you get lost, you should find a police officer"), recognizing causal relationships ("The bridge fell because it was weak"), recognizing problems and solutions ("This box is too small; get another one"), drawing conclusions ("We couldn't finish the project because there wasn't enough glue"), and anticipating results ("If we pull this cord, the bell should ring"). In general, problem-solving tasks, such as designing or building an object, will elicit this function (Staab, 1983). Problem solving includes predicting, testing hypotheses, and drawing conclusions.

Finally, the "imagining and projecting" function includes projecting feeling onto others ("I think Carlos is afraid of the ghost") and imagining events in real life or fantasy ("I'm captain of the spaceship *Izits*. All aboard"). This function can be elicited by fantasy play (Staab, 1983).

Many activities can be projected into imaginings by asking children to imagine that they are some character in a story or what they would do in a particular situation. With older children, different situations can be role-played.

To be successful, children must be able to use all of these language functions with some facility. As noted, activities can be designed to aid this growth.

Talking With Children

Language input is important for later output, and adult interactions with children must facilitate language growth and learning. In a nonthreatening way, whenever possible, the speech-language pathologist should observe and comment on the use of language by teachers and parents. Teachers are often unaware of the effect their language has on the processing of children with language impairment. For example, teachers' oral directions may contain a large proportion of figurative expressions and indirect requests (Lazar et al., 1989).

Teachers' responsiveness to the initiations of children with delayed language is below an optimal level (Pecyna-Rhyner, Lehr, & Pudlas, 1990). In general, teachers respond infrequently and, often, in a manner that terminates the interaction. The teacher's frequent use of directives also may limit child-teacher interactions.

The speech-language pathologist can efficiently introduce teachers, aides, and parents to facilitative conversational techniques at in-service training sessions or parent meetings. She should help teachers, aides, and parents understand the importance of adult modeling and responding to communicative behaviors. She should attempt to decrease the directive style of some parents and teachers in favor of a more conversational approach.

The speech-language pathologist can provide teachers, aides, and parents with examples of good interactive styles. A handout, such as that in Table 11.10,

TABLE 11.10
Guide for parents' and teachers' interactive style

---

1. Talk about things in which the child is interested.

2. Follow the child's lead. Reply to the child's initiations and comments. Share his excitement.

3. Don't ask too many questions. If you must, use questions such as *how did/do...*, *why did/do...*, and *what happened...* that result in longer explanatory answers.

4. Encourage the child to ask questions. Respond openly and honestly. If you don't want to answer a question, say so and explain why. (*I don't think I want to answer that question; it's very personal.*)

5. Use a pleasant tone of voice. You need not be a comedian, but you can be light and humorous. Children love it when adults are a little silly.

6. Don't be judgmental or make fun of a child's language. If you are overly critical of the child's language or try to "shotgun" all errors, he will stop talking to you.

7. Allow enough time for the child to respond.

8. Treat the child with courtesy by not interrupting when he is talking.

9. Include the child in family and classroom discussions. Encourage participation and listen to his ideas.

10. Be accepting of the child and of the child's language. Hugs and acceptance can go a long way.

11. Provide opportunities for the child to use language and to have that language work for him to accomplish his goals.

---

is often helpful. She should stress the importance of different facilitator behaviors and the need to tailor techniques to the child's individual style and language level.

Whenever possible, she should review these techniques and use them in demonstration with the individual child. Teachers, aides, and parents then can attempt certain facilitative behaviors while the speech-language pathologist observes.

Peers as facilitators.   Classmates developing normally can serve well as models and can be taught strategies that promote interaction (Goldstein & Strain, 1988; Handekman, Harris, Kristoff, Fuentes, & Alessandri, 1991; Odom, Hoyson, Jamieson, & Strain, 1985). Sociodramatic or replica play can provide a basis for interaction for preschoolers. With school-age children, many alternative activities can foster interaction and carryover (Hazel, 1990).

Training young children with language impairment to play with toys has little effect on social interaction (Kohl, Beckman, & Swenson-Pierce, 1984). Targeting social skills, such as inviting others to play, is more effective (Kohler & Fowler, 1985).

Classmates developing normally can be taught to increase communication interaction using a few simple steps. Specific techniques for cuing and prompting can be taught but are relatively inffective and time-consuming to teach (Goldstein & Wickstrom, 1986). The fewer stratgies taught, the better (Goldstein & ferrell, 1987).

One effective method, presented in Table 11.11, is to teach interactive strategies rather than teaching techniques to the peer developing normally and then to prompt and reinforce these strategies (Goldstein & Strain, 1988). This approach can increase interactions and on-topic responses by children with language impairment (Goldstein & Ferrell, 1987; Goldstein & Wickstrom, 1986). Peer strategies reportedly continue when teacher prompts decline.

School-age peers can be encouraged to interact through cooperative learning, homework monitoring, and language contracts (Hazel, 1990). Cooperative learning fosters interdependence and individual acountability while encouraging face-to-face interactions and interpersonal skills (D. Johnson, R. Johnson, & Holubee, 1984). Students with different language abilities are paired for classroom language projects and rewarded for group achievement (Danserean, 1987).

Homework monitoring is another paired activity. A child who has the skills needed to accomplish the assignment helps a child with language impairment. The speech-language pathologist works with both to help them complete their homework, uses role play to teach the tutor and tutored roles to the tutoring peers, and critiques role-played interactions between the tutors. In addition, she monitors the peers when actual tutoring begins.

Finally, language contracts can be used to decrease inappropriate language behavior (Hazel, 1990). Both the child with language impairment and the classroom peers must be able to identify the behavior and understand the need to decrease its occurrence. The contract with the class defines the behavior and

TABLE 11.11
Training peers as facilitators in preschool classrooms

Step 1: Teach peer to interact.
　　Introduction
　　　　Explain purpose: To help friend "talk" better.
　　　　Model with another adult.
　　Direct instruction.
　　　　Children rehearse and adults critique.
　　　　　　Adults take role of child with disabilities.
　　　　Posters provide reminders.

Step 2: Prompt and reinforce use of strategies taught. Gradual change with less adult input and fewer peer facilitators and more children with disabilities.
　　Teacher prompts ("Remember to have your friend look at you first." "Remember to point.").
　　　　Adults should try not to interrupt too much—Inhibits children.
　　　　　　Whisper or point to posters.

Source: Adapted from Goldstein, H., & Strain, P. S. (1988). Peers as communication intervention agents: Some new strategies and research findings. *Topics in Language Disorders, 9*(1), 44–59.

specifies the cues to reduce the behavior and to elicit a more desirable behavior. It is helpful in eliciting peer cooperation that the class be solicited for suggestions for decreasing the behavior. The contract is reviewed periodically and peers reinforced for success.

INSTITUTING A CLASSROOM MODEL

The most difficult aspect of the classroom model is its initial institution. The transition from pull-out service to classroom-based service takes careful planning. Central to success is the resolution of the following issues:

Training of the speech-language pathologist

Training of other professionals

Establishment of a clear source of authority and responsibility for intervention

Administrative support in the form of adequate space, scheduled time slots, and financial commitment (L. Miller, 1989)

Identification criteria for students to receive services based not on standardized test scores, but on classroom language processing and use (L. Miller, 1989)

Responsibility for IEPs (L. Miller, 1989)

The task of changing an entire model of intervention seems overwhelming. It may take 3-5 years to implement fully a collaborative classroom intervention model. The process is one of evolution, not a solitary event (Ferguson, 1992b). It is essential, therefore, to begin slowly and to prepare parents and other professionals for the change.

The final model will vary with student needs and teacher/speech-language pathologist flexibility (Brandel, 1992). The teacher and the speech-language pathologist will need to consult for general language activities and for specific language support of individual children.

First, the individual speech-language pathologist must train herself. This training includes education in the use of a functional conversational approach and in the school curriculum (Montgomery, 1992b). This text provides one step in that education. Workshops, convention presentations, observation, and further professional reading are also essential. In addition, the speech-language pathologist should role-play the use of various techniques because they differ considerably from the more traditional behavioral patterns. The speech-language pathologist might begin by using core curricular materials in intervention (Moore-Brown, 1991).

Classroom teachers can help the speech-language pathologist become familiar with small and large group instruction. Possibly, the speech-language pathologist could spend an hour per week in some group activity within a classroom.

Several alternative models for collaboration are available (Russell & Kaderavek, 1993). Peer coaching and co-teaching seem especially promising. In peer coaching, the speech-language pathologist and the classroom teacher work as a team, coaching each other through observation and feedback, commenting on effective teaching strategies (Schmidt & Rodgers-Rhyme, 1988). In co-teaching, each professional focuses on his or her component of instruction on the basis of the curriculum goals of the class. The teacher and the speech-language pathologist jointly determine student needs, develop goals and objectives and activities to meet them, implement these plans, and evaluate progress (Holzhauser-Peters & Andrin-Husemann, 1990).

Second, the speech-language pathologist must train other people. The initial purpose of this training is to educate teachers and administrators about the need for classroom intervention. This is best accomplished with in-service training stressing (a) the importance of the environment for nonimpaired language learning, (b) questions of generalization, (c) the verbal nature of the classroom, (d) the practicality and efficiency of classroom intervention strategies, and (e) the need for and desirability of team approaches.

Administrators may be reluctant to change current one-on-one pull-out services. A more functional classroom model can be presented relative to inclusion, whole language, and efficacy (Moore-Brown, 1991). It is also important to remember that some children still will require pull-out services for special skills training. Collaborative teaching is better suited to training of general communication skills (Borsch & Oaks, 1992). Goals and objectives, probably modest at first, should be established prior to implementation (Dyer et al., 1991). At each step in implementation, administrators need to be kept informed of progress.

Once convinced of the need for such a model of intervention, the teachers can begin to learn specific intervention techniques. These techniques may be introduced in in-service training, with individual instruction to follow. Videotaped lessons including children with language impairment are excellent training vehicles to demonstrate the use of various techniques. Professionals conducting the training should be credible, knowledgeable, and practical. Appropriate materials and hands-on experience are essential to teacher training.

Third, clear lines of authority for language intervention must be established. It is vital to the success of this model that roles and responsibilities, as well as authority, be clearly established. This step requires administrative support and a definite statement of policy. New roles and responsibilities should be written into the curriculum, budget, and job descriptions.

Fourth, administrative support in the form of space, scheduled time, and necessary financial outlays must be established. It is too easy for administrators to declare a change in procedures without giving adequate support to ensure success.

The biggest single impediment to implementation is the lack of time (Montgomery, 1992a). The speech-language pathologist and the classroom teacher must allow time each week to discuss each child's success and to review targets and techniques. Unfortunately, administrators often are unwilling to grant time for these conferences. My experience is that these meetings often occur over lunch or during breaks in the schedule. Although this arrangement is less than optimum, it does allow these essential interactions to occur. A scheduled meeting time of at least a half hour per week is preferred.

Administrators also have difficulty seeing the need to lessen dependence on standardized measures of language. Language test scores offer a quantifiable measure of behavior that can be used for determinations of student needs and progress. Yet, similar measurement can be made against the curriculum and from conversational samples. The implementation of this step requires the joint educational effort of the speech-language pathologist and the classroom teacher.

Finally, IEPs will need to be written or modified to reflect the change in service delivery. Other members of the intervention team, including parents, will need to be educated on the rationale for such changes. Parents usually accept the classroom model when shown the increased service that their child will receive if the classroom teacher is also a language trainer. Many parents are also happy with the decreased amount of pull-out time.

The implementation phase should progress slowly and carefully because it is new to both the speech-language pathologist and the classroom teacher. At first, one child in one classroom can be targeted. This can gradually be expanded to include several children in this classroom or one child in each of several classrooms.

The selection of the first classroom is critical. The speech-language pathologist might begin with her best friend on the faculty, someone willing to learn, grow, and make mistakes (Moore-Brown, 1991). Teacher training should include speech-language pathologist critiques of teacher use of training techniques. A checklist can ensure objectivity. It might be best for teachers to begin by attempting to integrate a child's newly acquired skills into the daily routine, rather than trying to teach new language skills (Dyer et al., 1991).

The first class taught by the speech-language pathologist should, likewise, begin cautiously. One goal with one lesson is recommended (Ferguson, 1992a). Later, individual IEP goals can be introduced through focused lessons with the whole class.

Undoubtedly, there will be problems in initiating classroom intervention. The speech-language pathologist is advised to choose the initial child and classroom carefully to ensure some measure of success and to minimize friction with the classroom teacher. Once the speech-language pathologist and the teacher begin to experience success, other teachers will be more willing to adopt the model.

There will always be administrators, classroom teachers, and/or parents who refuse to accept or cooperate with the implementation of the classroom model. Rather than become discouraged, the speech-language pathologist should work with those individuals who accept the model and continue to try to educate those who do not. Usually, success with a few children is all that is needed to convince the foot-draggers. The key to success is "establishing a good rapport among the people involved" (Borsch & Oaks, 1992, p. 368).

CONCLUSION

Functional environmental approaches, as represented by the classroom model, are among the most progressive trends evidenced today (McCormick, 1986). In many school districts throughout Canada and the United States, this model is becoming a reality. Some districts are mandating the change from above, whereas others are experiencing a quiet revolution from below. No change as radical as this one can be accomplished without some difficulties.

The role of the speech-language pathologist is changing. In many cases, speech-language pathologists are being asked to implement intervention models for which they have minimal training. Although such requests are expected in a professional field that is changing and growing as rapidly as speech-language pathology, it does highlight the need for continuing professional education.

Still, the speech-language pathologist is the language expert responsible for identifying children with language impairments and for implementing intervention. In this new role of consultant, the speech-language pathologist enhances this intervention process through others.

12 Assessment of Children Who Are Presymbolic and Minimally Symbolic

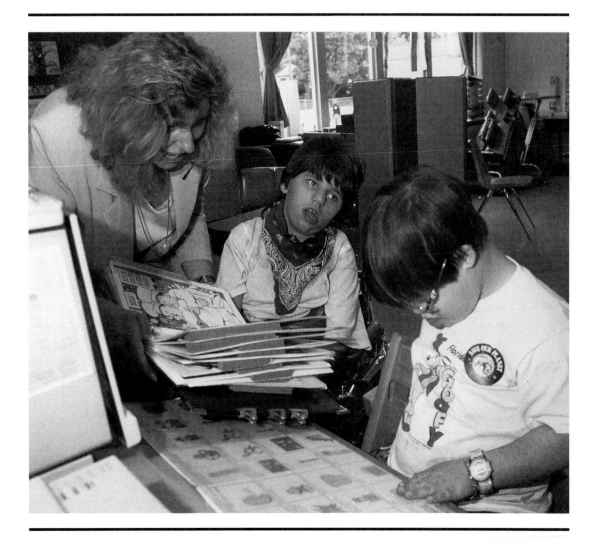

C hildren communicating at a level below 2 years of age have unique needs. The language and communication skills of these children may be extremely limited. Often, the goal of intervention is the *initiation* of effective communication. Such children may have rudimentary communication skills or use only single-symbol or short multisymbol communication. Because of their special circumstance and their increased need for functional intervention, these children represent a special case of intervention.

It is often difficult to decide when to intervene with very young children. One possibility might be to consider a child for communication and language assessment when he is one standard deviation or more below his age bracket on standardized tests and/or 6 months below chronological age in language production (Olswang & Bain, 1991). Children with syndromes or conditions that put them at risk for developing language impairments also should be assessed early and often to monitor communication and language development. Children with many types of language impairment, such as SLI and LLD, and those with behavioral disorders may exhibit early delay (Olswang & Bain, 1991; Theadore et al., 1990).

Early intervention is crucial for many reasons, including delay prevention, neural maturation, and socioemotional development (L. Baker & Cantwell, 1984; Beitchman, 1985; Prizant & Wetherby, 1988b; Sameroff & Chandler, 1975). Early intervention appears to be especially important for children with some underlying brain dysfunction, because it is widely held that the brain is more flexible in early childhood, and thus new neural pathways can be formed. Social factors are also important because communication problems can exacerbate social interactional problems that may exist between the child and the caregiver(s) (Garfin & Lord, 1986).

Children who are *presymbolic* do not use conventional signs, words, or pictures for communication. They may possess no recognizable communication system or may use gestures, such as pointing or touching or moving objects. Children who are *minimally symbolic* use some visual, verbal, or tactile symbols alone or in combination. These functioning levels may be the result of a disabling condition, such as mental retardation or deafness, a delay in the onset of language, or a language impairment. In this chapter, we address a number of issues relative to the assessment of children who are presymbolic and minimally symbolic.

Intervention with children who are presymbolic and minimally symbolic usually focuses on initial communication, presymbolic skills, lexical growth, and/or early symbol combination rules. At this level, it is especially important for training to incorporate functional procedures that will actively induce generalization (Spradlin & Siegel, 1982).

The needs of this population are discussed first. Next, a brief history of intervention with this population is explored to better understand current methodology. Finally, an integrated functional model is introduced, and assessment procedures for children who are presymbolic and minimally symbolic are discussed. In this section, we also briefly touch on issues relative to assessment for augmentative communication.

NEEDS OF CHILDREN WHO ARE PRESYMBOLIC AND MINIMALLY SYMBOLIC

Assessment and intervention should address the needs of children who are presymbolic or minimally symbolic while being cautiously mindful of presymbolic development provided by children developing normally. In this section, we explore both the needs of children with language impairment and the development of children developing normally.

Children Who Are Presymbolic Language Impaired

Children who are presymbolic and minimally symbolic are a very diverse group representing a variety of etiological and diagnostic labels. Their one common trait is the lack of or minimal ability to use symbols. An early difficulty with communication, such as lack of responsiveness, may result in a less than optimal language-learning environment. These children also may experience cognitive and/or sensory difficulties that impede the development of symbol-referent associations.

As with children developing normally, the interactional patterns of children with language impairment and their caregivers are important for the development of communication. Frequently, due to a lack of responding, the interactions of the children with their caregivers are less than optimal (Miranda & Donnellan, 1986; Rieke & Lewis, 1984). There may be a lack of appropriate verbal interactions. Caregivers may be directive, providing little opportunity for the children to engage in verbal or vocal give-and-take (Nakamura & Newhoff, 1982). Such directives typically elicit few verbal responses from the children (Prizant & Rentschler, 1983; Semmel, Peck, Haring, & Theimer, 1984).

It is important to note that the breakdown of communicative interaction is not the fault of any one communicative partner. Parents of such children usually respond to them in ways that are age appropriate but reflect the lack of responsiveness by the children. There may be a cycle in which caregivers gradually initiate and respond less as their children do.

For similar reasons, extended institutionalization also results in general deterioration of language abilities (Phillips & Balthazar, 1979; Shane, Lipshultz, & Shane, 1982). The most frequent verbal behaviors of institutional staff are directives. These behaviors result in the fewest client verbalizations. In turn, when clients do verbalize, they often are ignored by staff or receive nonverbal staff responses (Tizard, Cooperman, Joseph, & Tizard, 1972).

In the classroom, children with multiple disabilities have few opportunities to initiate communication (Guess & Siegel-Causey, 1985; Houghton, Bronicki, & Guess, 1987). Teachers are usually highly directive.

In home, institutional, or educational settings, there may be little motivation to develop more appropriate communication. Many daily activities are predictable routines. In addition, the caregivers may anticipate the children's needs. Thus, the children have little need to make requests, ask questions, or comment

(Calculator, 1988b). In this situation, the child may initiate very little communication or exhibit immature or idiosyncratic communication patterns. Idiosyncratic patterns are individualistic and do not generalize beyond such children and their immediate communication environment.

Children who are presymbolic and minimally symbolic with language impairment and residing in a nonresponsive communication environment or one that offers little opportunity to communicate are at risk for failure to develop useful presymbolic communication systems. Useful communication would, in turn, provide the motivation for learning symbols. This situation may be very different from the language-learning environment of children developing normally, which can serve as an intervention model.

Children Developing Normally

The cognitive and social knowledge of 12-month-old children developing normally is evident in the things they talk about and in their use of language. Cognitively, these children have been acquiring the ability to *represent* or re-present reality within their minds. These images stand for concepts, as linguistic symbols will do later.

Children spend the first year learning about the physical constancy and functions of objects and about object permanence, disappearance, and reappearance (Bloom & Lahey, 1978). More important, they learn means-ends or that an object or a person can be used to attain something else (Bates, Bretherton, Shore, & McNew, 1983). A gesture, vocalization, or verbalization can summon aid. Finally, children learn that certain sound sequences are paired consistently with certain entities to represent these entities. It is within the conversational context of children and caregivers that children acquire these words and their cognitive knowledge.

From birth, caregivers interpret children's nonvocal and vocal responses as meaningful. They treat children as conversational partners (Newson, 1979; Tronick, Als, & Adamson, 1979). Gradually, children learn patterns of conversational exchange (Kaye, 1979).

Throughout the first 2 years, children's behavior becomes more goal-oriented and more deliberate. At first, children's behavior is unintentional, although it may convey information about their condition or draw attention to them. By about 8 months, children's nonvocal behaviors have been conventionalized into a recognizable system of gestures (Bates et al., 1983).

With the use of gestures, children demonstrate a definite intention to communicate with their partners by considering these partners in their behavior. The child uses gestures to participate actively in reciprocal interactions, to repair communication breakdown, and to signal emotional states (Dunst & Lowe, 1986; Greenspan, 1988; Prizant & Wetherby, 1988a). First, children secure their partner's attention and then gesture and possibly vocalize (Scoville, 1983).

Gestures enable children to request, signal notice, ask questions, and offer objects. First words or symbols develop to fill these communicative functions (Bruner, 1978a; Bullowa, 1979).

By the time children developing normally use their first word, they have a well-established communication system. Intentionality merges with other developments in cognition and in social interactional abilities.

Children's first words are symbols for what they know (Palermo, 1982). Early meanings relate to objects, actions, locations, and descriptors. Usually, children talk about entities within their own world that they can manipulate and that are immediate. In other words, children *map* their cognitive knowledge onto language (K. Roberts & Horowitz, 1986).

Communication development is the result of interaction between the child, the caregiver(s), and the environment. This interaction becomes increasingly more effective as the child's behavior becomes more interpretable and the adult learns to respond better and to facilitate communication. Table 12.1 presents an overall developmental framework for early communication.

TOWARD A MODEL OF ASSESSMENT AND INTERVENTION

A model of assessment and intervention might reflect both the premises of this text and the history of assessment and intervention with the presymbolic and

TABLE 12.1
Possible presymbolic skills for assessment and training

Presymbolic Skills	Rational

Sensory skills: Any and all modalities
  Startle and notice
  Search for stimuli
  Localization to stimuli
  Following moving stimuli
	Locate and train use of various sensory modalities for communication input and output.

Motor imitation
  Gross motor imitation
  Fine motor including facial and vocal Imitation
  Imitation with objects
  Deferred imitation
	Learn Piagetian early cognitive skill. Later used as mode of training for other skills.
	Learn facial and vocal imitation to be used for speech.

Object permanence	Learn Piagetian cognitive skill
Turn taking with motor and vocal imitation	Gain early communication skill
Functional use of objects	Establish early meanings
Means-ends	Learn to control environment, communicate
Communicative gestures	
Receptive language and symbol recognition	Recognize symbol value

Sound imitation
  Vocal shaping
  Vocal sequencing
	Gain prerequisites to speech

Source: Compiled from Bricker & Bricker (1974); Hanna, Lippert, & Harris (1982); Horstmeier & MacDonald (1978b); Manolson (1985); Owens (1982c)

minimally symbolic population. To comprehend such a model fully, it is necessary to understand past and current models of assessment and intervention.

A Brief History of Therapy Models

Prior to the early 1960s, intervention efforts with children who are presymbolic and minimally symbolic stressed a language stimulation approach. Direct intervention services were very limited. The stimulation approach was followed in the late 1960s by a behavioral paradigm that was, in turn, replaced by a more cognitive and sociocommunicative design. Early behavioral approaches stressed speech as the means of production with little regard for presymbolic learning. The cognitive and sociocommunicative designs stressed selected presymbolic skills that were assumed necessary prerequisites for symbol use. Displeasure with the results of all of these methods led to a communication-first approach in which initial communication is established at some level and then altered toward a more symbolic communication system.

Although each approach has been able to demonstrate success with some children with language impairment, intervention with clients who are increasingly more severely involved has brought into question the efficacy of each approach. Even with these many approaches, children who are minimally symbolic "often fail to use language responses spontaneously in appropriate situations" (Wulz, Hall, & Klein, 1983, p. 2).

Currently, communication-training programs for children who are presymbolic and minimally symbolic reflect two general intervention strategies: presymbolic training and communication training. In the first, children are taught presymbolic skills prior to the introduction of symbolic communication (Bricker & Bricker, 1974; MacDonald et al., 1974). Presymbolic training usually includes cognitive, perceptual, social, and/or communicative targets identified as significant in the acquisition of symbol use by children developing normally. The presymbolic approach has been used most frequently and most successfully with young children who exhibit mild/moderate retardation.

Cognitive presymbolic training might include motor imitation, object permanence, symbolic play, and means-end. These skills represent important presymbolic cognitive abilities that the Swiss educator Jean Piaget and his followers recognized. It is reasoned that *object permanence,* or recognition that an object exists even when no longer visible, is a necessary step in the development of symbol use. First, the child learns to hold visual images in the mind, and then more abstract symbols. Unfortunately, the complex nature of the cognition-language relationship makes the value statements about such training tentative at best (Rice, 1983). The relationship of language and the specific cognitive areas mentioned is correlational, and skill attainment may be evidenced initially in either language or cognition (Kelly & Dale, 1989). Perceptual targets are usually awareness and recognition of sound and symbol production and symbol discrimination. Social and communicative targets could consist of nonvocal and vocal turn taking, eye contact, and gestures.

The specific behaviors selected for training vary in number, kind, and scope with the various commercially available training procedures (Horstmeier and MacDonald, 1978a; Manolson, 1985; McLean & Snyder-McLean, 1978; Owens, 1982c). This diversity reflects differing opinions on the relative worth of certain presymbolic behaviors. In general, a greater number of training targets reflects an attempt to include more presymbolic skills while also increasing the number of small or incremented training steps as an aid for children with more severe language impairment.

In recent years, a communication-first approach has evolved in which initial emphasis is on the establishment of a communication system that can be expanded later toward symbol use (Keogh & Reichle, 1985; Reichle, Piche-Cragoe, Sigafoos, & Doss, 1988; Sternberg, McNerney, & Pegnatore, 1985; Sternberg, Pegnatore, & Hill, 1983; Stillman & Battle, 1984; Stremel-Campbell, Johnson-Dorn, Guida, & Udell, 1984; D. Yoder, 1985). Proponents of this approach reason that communication training, especially with young children, should occur during the first 6 years of life, when the brain is experiencing its greatest physiological growth, rather than waiting until presymbolic skills have been learned (Wilbur, 1987).

The communication-first approach attempts to establish an early *signal* system, such as touch, to enhance the child's opportunities for interaction. One of the most promising methods of initiating this system is through *behavior chain interruption* strategies, in which a pleasurable activity, such as rocking or listening to music, is stopped and the child must signal to have it begin again (Goetz, Gee, & Sailor, 1985).

Proponents of the communication-first approach usually consider the presymbolic approach to be a *wait-until-the-client-is-ready* approach. The communication-first approach reflects (a) the frustration of many speech-language pathologists with the slow rate of client progress in acquiring presymbolic skills, (b) the realization that many clients communicate prior to acquiring language and prior to professional intervention, and (c) an acceptance that some clients may never communicate symbolically.

It is reasoned that insufficient data are available to exclude children from communication intervention while presymbolic training occurs. As noted, the relationship between cognition and language is correlational at best, not causal (Kelly & Dale, 1989).

Even though individuals who are presymbolic and have language impairment pass through the same Piagetian sensorimotor stages as do children developing normally, less congruence occurs within each stage (Kangas & Lloyd, 1988). Children with language impairment may exhibit behaviors from more than one stage. In addition, a disparity is found in some children with language impairment between sociocognitive level and language performance (Cardoso-Martins, Mervis, & Mervis, 1985; Cunningham, Glenn, Wilkinson, & Sloper, 1985; L. Smith & von Tetzchner, 1986; Thal & Bates, 1988). For example, late talkers begin combining gestures prior to combining words; children developing normally combine both at about the same time.

Piagetian measures must be applied cautiously because they rely heavily on experience that may be altered significantly for children with language impairment. The relationship of cognition to language must be questioned even more when applied to presymbolic adolescents and adults (Calculator, 1988a; Snyder-McLean, Etter-Schroeder, & Rogers, 1986). Speech-language pathologists must be cautious not to overextend normative data.

In recent years, there has been a recognition that fewer presymbolic behaviors than originally believed are necessary for symbol use and that some augmentative communication systems can be implemented successfully with little or no presymbolic training (Carr & Durand, 1985; Horner & Budd, 1985; Keogh & Reichle, 1985; Reichle & Yoder, 1985; Rice, 1983). **Augmentative communication** systems (e.g., signs, gestures, communication boards, computer-assisted devices) support, enhance, or augment the communication of children who do not speak (Beukelman, Yorkston, & Dowden, 1985). In general, speech-language pathologists use these systems with clients for whom the vocal-verbal mode of communication is dysfunctional, the symbol-referent relationship is difficult to establish, or the need to communicate is seemingly nonexistent.

The presymbolic skills and communication-first approaches are not mutually exclusive, and aspects of each may be incorporated into an integrated model. It is important to focus on the goal of symbol use to communicate. The purpose of this chapter is to bring the many intervention approaches together into a unified whole that reflects a functional approach based on the children's actual needs.

An Integrated Functional Model

Traditional speech-language clinical services rely primarily on isolated therapy within a segregated climate (Sternat, Nietupski, Messina, Lyon, & Brown, 1977). More appropriate than such "episodic intervention" for children who are presymbolic and minimally symbolic (L. Brown, Nietupski, & Hamre-Nietupski, 1976) is a 24-hour per day, sustained service delivery model (Falvey, Bishop, Grenot-Sheyer, & Coots, 1988; Graham, 1976; Halle, 1987; Kopchick & Lloyd, 1976). In the remainder of this chapter, assessment and intervention techniques that support this goal are described.

A functional model of intervention targets each child's present communication system and presymbolic and symbolic behaviors within many natural communication environments throughout the day. This approach also targets the communication behaviors of each child's primary caregivers who serve as natural interactional partners. The goal is to establish communicative environments that target the child's specific needs.

The speech-language pathologist's roles, as one of many communication partners, are to interact clinically with the child and to train other language facilitators within the classroom, unit, home, or community residence. Thus, the speech-language pathologist becomes both direct service provider and collaborator/consultant. As such, she designs the individual communication intervention plan with input from others, modifies that plan as necessary, provides in-service training for the professional and paraprofessional staff, trains each child-caregiver dyad, and maintains records.

The trainers or language facilitators are crucial to this integrated functional approach, and several commercially available language-training programs for children who are presymbolic and minimally symbolic use caregiver-trainers, such as parents (Horstmeier & MacDonald, 1978, 1978b; Manolson, 1985; Owens, 1982c). Child-caregiver conversational interactions are natural environments for language acquisition, and as many primary caregivers as possible should be enlisted as change agents.

As language facilitators, these caregivers are also clients of the speech-language pathologist, and their behavior should be monitored closely. Caregiver behaviors can be modified through training, modeling, role playing, and feedback (McNaughton & Light, 1989; Owens et al., 1987).

Training for the child who is presymbolic might use the dual approach mentioned previously, consisting of a primary thrust to establish an initial communication system and a secondary program of prerequisite skills training. Figure 12.1 is a diagram of this approach. An initial signal communication system is

FIGURE 12.1
Dual intervention approach with children who are presymbolic

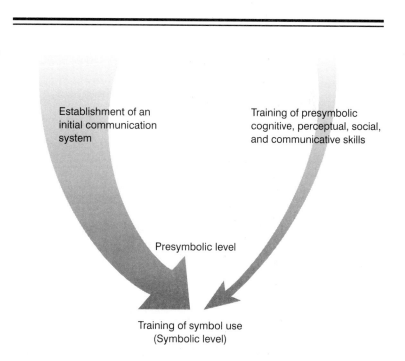

Establishment of an initial communication system

Training of presymbolic cognitive, perceptual, social, and communicative skills

Presymbolic level

Training of symbol use
(Symbolic level)

The primary presymbolic approach establishes an initial communication system, whereas the secondary approach teaches skills believed essential to symbol use. These two approaches join at the symbolic level in which the child is taught to use symbols within the context of the previously established communication system.

instituted and continually modified for each child, while training the prerequisite skills necessary for modification of that communication system to more conventional symbols, such as spoken words, signs, or pictured symbols, occurs. Social and cognitive skills are trained while the child's communication skills continue to improve, although not every child will progress to symbol use.

Content should reflect the child's environment and the entities the child knows and/or may desire. For example, presymbolic individuals learn symbols taught within the context of requests more rapidly than those taught as labels (Litt & Schreibman, 1982; Reichle, Rogers, & Barrett, 1984; Saunders & Sailor, 1979; Stafford, Sundberg, & Braam, 1978). The resultant communication becomes more purposeful and is reinforced by natural contingencies, rather than by learned reinforcers.

In summary, an integrated functional intervention approach offers instruction within natural conversational contexts in everyday activities, emphasizing introduction of a communication system and acquisition of presymbolic skills. Caregivers fulfill the role of language facilitators under the guidance of the speech-language pathologist. The vehicle for change is the child-caregiver interaction.

Evaluation: Getting the Whole Picture

The purpose of an evaluation is twofold: to identify and understand the nature of the problem, and to provide some preliminary guidance for intervention (Prizant & Wetherby, 1988b). The goal is to describe the child's present interactive system as thoroughly as possible.

The evaluation process is part science and part art. Although systematic procedures are used to gather data, it is the speech-language pathologist's creative or artistic skill that synthesizes this information into a useful whole and designs the appropriate intervention procedures. A variety of methods, including direct observation, caregiver interviews and questionnaires, observation including behavior scaling and rating, direct testing, and sampling, are used to attain an accurate description of each child's unique competencies within each communication context.

Communication intervention requires both training of the child and adaptation by the child's environment (Cirrin & Rowland, 1985; Donnellan, Mirenda, Mesaros, & Fassbender, 1984; Prizant & Wetherby, 1988a; Simeonsson, Olley, & Rosenthal, 1987; Vicker, 1985). If children change their behavior but environmental expectations do not change accordingly, then the children may have little or no opportunity to use these new behaviors. For example, if people in the environment do not expect a child to use a communication board, there will be little chance for the child's behavior to generalize. Therefore, the speech-language pathologist is interested in evaluating the child's abilities and needs and also the communication expectations and demands of the communication environment and the interaction of the child and the environment.

The Child's Abilities and Needs

The speech-language pathologist is interested primarily in the child's current communication system, including the mode of communication, and in the level of presymbolic and/or symbolic functioning. A holistic description of the child's communication abilities and needs requires a variety of data collection methods. Of interest are the manner and content of both social and nonsocial communication.

With children who are presymbolic and minimally symbolic, it is essential that a variety of collection methods be used to obtain an adequately diverse sample of each child's communication system. For example, observation may provide examples of the commenting or declaring intention but fail to elicit negative requests or protests (Coggins et al., 1987). In contrast, elicitation tasks may yield protesting but little commenting.

The child may have a rich and varied, albeit idiosyncratic, communication system. Several forms of presymbolic communication are listed in Table 12.2. Some forms may be situationally controlled. Only by using various methods to

TABLE 12.2
Examples of presymbolic communication

Generalized movements and changes in muscle tone
   Excitement in response to stimulation or in anticipation of an event
   Squirms and resists physical contact
   Changes in muscle tone in response to soothing touch or voice, in reaction to sudden
      stimuli, or in preparation to act

Vocalizations
   Calls to attract or direct another's attention
   Laughs or coos in response to pleasurable stimulation
   Cries in reaction to discomfort

Facial expressions
   Smiles in response to familiar person, object, or event
   Grimaces in reaction to unpleasant or unexpected sensation

Orientation
   Looks toward or points to person or object to seek or direct attention
   Looks away from person or object to indicate disinterest or refusal
   Looks toward suddenly appearing familiar or novel person, object, or event

Pause
   Ceases moving in anticipation of coming event
   Pauses to await service provider's instruction or to allow service provider to take turn

Touching, manipulating, or moving with another person
   Holds or grabs another for comfort
   Takes or directs another's hand to something
   Manipulates service provider into position to start an activity or interactive "game"
   Touches or pulls service provider to gain attention
   Pushes away or lets go to terminate an interaction
   Moves with or follows the movements of another person

TABLE 12.2, *continued*

Acting on objects and using objects to interact with others

  Reaches toward, leans toward, touches, gets, picks up, activates, drops, or pushes away
    object to indicate interest or disinterest

  Extends, touches, or places object to show to another or to request another's action

  Holds out hands to prepare to receive object

Assuming positions and going to places

  Holds up arms to be picked up, holds out hands to initiate "game," leans back on swing
    to be pushed

  Stands by sink to request drink, goes to cabinet to request material stored there

Conventional gestures

  Waves to greet

  Nods to indicate assent or refusal

Depictive actions

  Pantomimes throwing to indicate, "throw ball"

  Sniffs to indicate smelling flowers

  Makes sounds similar to those made by animals and objects to make reference to them

  Draws picture to describe or request activity

Withdrawal

  Pulls away or moves away to avoid interaction or activity

  Curls up, lies on floor to avoid interaction or activity

Aggressive and self-injurious behavior

  Hits, scratches, bites, or spits at service provider to protest action or in response to frus-
    tration

  Throws or destroys objects to protest action or in response to frustration

  Hits, bites, or otherwise harms self or threatens to harm self to protest action, in
    response to frustration, or in reaction to pain or discomfort

Source: From *Enhancing Nonsymbolic Communication Interactions Among Learners With Severe Disabilities* (p. 7) by E. Siegel-Causey and D. Guess. 1989. Baltimore, MD: Paul H. Brookes Publishing Co. Copyright 1989 by Paul H. Brookes Publishing Co. Reprinted by permission.

collect data from a number of sources can the speech-language pathologist hope to gain a complete description.

The child's presymbolic and/or symbolic functioning also should be fully described (Peck & Schuler, 1987). Table 12.3 presents presymbolic behaviors that a number of intervention specialists and programs consider important for assessment and training. Not all professionals agree on which presymbolic behaviors to target (J. Miller & Chapman, 1984). Each speech-language pathologist should add or delete presymbolic behaviors on the basis of the literature and her experience with the presymbolic population.

The assessment of presymbolic abilities is important even if children are possible candidates for augmentative communication systems. A number of tools offer effective guidelines for selecting the most appropriate augmentative system for a particular child on the basis of the child's abilities (Calculator, 1988c; Chapman & Miller, 1980; House & Rogerson, 1984; Musselwhite & St. Louis, 1982; Owens & House, 1984; Shane & Bashir, 1980).

TABLE 12.3
Possible presymbolic progressions for assessment

Means-end/tool use
- uses a tool that is contiguous with the goal as a means to obtain the goal (e.g., pulls string tied to object; pulls cloth under object)
- uses a tool that is noncontiguous with the goal as a means to obtain the goal (e.g., rakes in object with stick; moves chair in position and climbs on chair to obtain object on shelf)

Causality/communicative intent
- touches adult's hand or object to recreate spectacle
- uses gestural or vocal signal to regulate adult's behavior or to direct adult's attention
- discovers the source of an action (e.g., how to activate a mechanical toy; looks for the source of a thrown object)

Gestural/vocal imitation
- takes turns after adult imitates child's behavior or in familiar social routines
- imitates vocal or gestural behavior initiated by adult
- imitates a behavior at a much later time in the absence of the original model

Schemes for relating to objects/symbolic play
- explores the physical properties of objects
- uses recognitory gestures on realistic objects (e.g., combs own hair; brushes own teeth; eats from spoon)
- uses pretend schemes with miniature objects toward self (e.g., rolls toy car; drinks from doll's cup; pounds toy hammer)
- uses pretend schemes toward others (e.g., feeds doll with bottle; combs mother's hair)
- uses multiple pretend schemes in sequence (e.g., stirs pretend food in pan; pours food onto dish; and feeds doll)

Social relatedness/expression of emotion
- expresses emotions of joy, fear, and anger in appropriate situations or in response to adult's emotional expression
- responds differentially to strangers and caregivers
- uses gestural or vocal signals to establish closeness (e.g., pulls on adult's leg and reaches up to be picked up)
- knows how to get adult to react (e.g., to make adult laugh and make adult angry)
- expresses emotions of empathy, shame, guilt, affection, and defiance

Language comprehension
- uses nonlinguistic response strategies, including situational routines, contextual clues, intonation, gestures, and facial expression
- comprehends the meaning of single words (e.g., person names, object names, actions)
- comprehends multiword utterances based on semantic relations (e.g., action + object; agent + action; attribute + object)

Language production
- uses consistent preverbal forms tied to the context
- uses single word approximations or intoned jargon to encode dynamic, changing states, or objects that can be acted upon by the child
- uses multiword utterances to encode semantic relations (e.g., action + object; attribute + object)

Source: Prizant, B. M., & Wetherby, A. M. (1988a). Providing services to children with autism (ages 0 to 2 years) and their families. *Topics in Language Disorders, 9*(1), 1-23. Reprinted with permission.

Symbolic assessment should include more than a list of the symbols the child uses. The range of functions these symbols represents is important, regardless of the means or manner of communication. Various researchers suggest different combinations of illocutionary functions, such as requesting information or making comments (Page, 1982; Wexler, Blau, Dore, & Leslie, 1982); semantic functions, such as agent + action and negative + X (MacDonald, 1978a); or a combination of both (Owens, 1982b). Symbols are acquired initially to fulfill illocutionary functions already in children's repertoires. Children also treat symbols as representing various semantic functions that form building blocks for early multisymbol utterances. Table 12.4 presents some common semantic and illocutionary functions found in initial symbolic communication. Definitions are listed in Appendix L.

Questionnaire and interview.   The speech-language pathologist can ascertain initially the manner and content of the child's communication and some indication of functioning level by questionnaire and/or interview and by observation. Responses can enhance the validity of later testing. Of interest are the child's actual skills, rather than an age equivalency, which is of minimal value in making intervention decisions.

Questionnaires or scales often comprise a portion of published language intervention programs (Hanna, Lippert, & Harris, 1982; MacDonald, 1978b; Owens, 1982a) and can be modified to conform to the speech-language pathologist's model of initial language training. Table 12.5 presents questions of primary interest collected from a number of sources.

TABLE 12.4
Semantic and illocutionary functions of early symbolic communication

Semantic Functions	Illocutionary Functions
Nomination	Answer
This/that + Nomination	Question or requesting information
Location	Reply
X + Location	Elicitation
Negation	Continuant
Negation + X	Declaration
Modification (Types:	Practice or repeat
Attribution, possession, and recurrence)	Name or label
Modifier + X	Command, demand, request, protest
Notice	
Notice + X	
Action (signaled by agent, action, or object)	
Agent + action	
Action + object	

Source: Compiled from Dore (1975); MacDonald (1978a); Owens (1982c)

TABLE 12.5
Questionnaire or interview content for children who are presymbolic or minimally symbolic

How does the child communicate primarily?
    Does the child use vocalizations, gestures, postures, eye contact, or other means of communication?
    Who understands the child's communication efforts?
Does the child play alone or with others?
Does the child demonstrate any turn-taking behaviors?
Does the child enjoy making sounds? How often does the child make sounds?
Does the child ever initiate communication? How? In which situations?
Which situations seem to be high communication contexts?
Which caregivers seem to engage in the most interaction with the child?
Does the child
    Make wants known?
    Request help?
    Point to objects or actions, name, or both?
    Request information?
    Seek attention?
    Demonstrate emotion?
    Protest?

Source: Compiled from Calculator (1988a); MacDonald (1978b); Owens & Rogerson (1988)

Because children who are presymbolic or minimally symbolic can provide little information on questionnaires, caregivers are encouraged to participate in the intervention process. Questionnaire administration also provides an opportunity to acquaint caregivers with presymbolic skills that are of interest, though not readily obvious. The Oliver (MacDonald, 1978b), a caregiver inventory, actually instructs caregivers to engage in some test exercises with the child, thus providing valuable data for later testing.

Some scales attempt to establish a developmental age (Bzoch & League, 1971; Sacks & Young, 1982) by asking questions relative to skills acquired at various age levels. Generally, these tools do not weight scores in terms of the importance of these behaviors for later training. Thus, all behaviors appear equally important, which, of course, they are not. Nevertheless, such developmental scales can be helpful when normative age equivalencies are required.

For children using symbols, the speech-language pathologist will want to collect an initial lexicon. Caregivers can draw on their experience to provide a list of words or signs used. Checklists of possible symbols yield more responses from caregivers than do blank forms or even categorical inventories that give category names, such as nouns and personal names (Morrow, Mirenda, Beukelman, & Yorkston, 1993).

Observation.   Through structured observation, the speech-language pathologist attempts to describe the communicative environment of the child. Descriptive factors include the amount of time the child spends in certain environments, the frequency of communication in these environments, and the partners, activities, and objects present (Carlson, 1981). Both familiar routines and less structured contexts might be observed in order to note differing behaviors (Theadore et al., 1990).

One important aspect of evaluation is determining the communicative intention of the child's behaviors, whether appropriate, inappropriate, or anywhere in between. It is not the behavior itself, but its relationship to the context, that indicates communication. Unlike symbols, signals, such as gestures, almost always require the context for interpretation (Ogletree, 1993). Of interest is the range of intentions exhibited. Children with autism may have a very limited range of communicative functions (Wetherby & Prizant, 1989).

Communication behaviors are consistent, identifiable responses associated with environmental events or with the child's physical or emotional state. Children with sensory, mental, and/or physiological impairments often do not use clearly recognizable communication (G. Clark & Seifer, 1982; Odom, 1983). The child who turns away from another person or becomes self-abusive or increases self-stimulation when someone approaches is communicating a desire not to communicate. Some communication may be unrecognizable as such and may be misinterpreted (Houghton et al., 1987).

Communication behaviors may be message-specific, each communicating a single message, or may communicate a variety of messages (Iwata, Dorsey, Slifer, Bauman, & Richman, 1982; Schuler & Goetz, 1981). For example, loud vocalizations may signal attention getting or several functions, such as attention getting, desire for an object, and/or need for assistance. Communication also may be intentional or unintentional, depending on whether the listener is considered. The degree of intentionality and conventionality, as well as the sophistication of the signal itself, may vary with different functions and/or contexts.

Requesting is an important skill that enables children to regulate other people by asking for entities or for information. Along with other ways of regulating other people's behavior, such as protesting, requesting is relatively easy and develops early, even for children with autism (Wetherby, 1986). In contrast, referencing joint attending is more difficult and develops later (Cirrin & Rowland, 1985; Curcio, 1978; Greenwald & Leonard, 1979; Labato, Barrera, & Feldman, 1981; McLean & Snyder-McLean, 1987, 1988a, in press; Smith & von Tetzchner, 1986; Wetherby & Prutting, 1984; Wetherby, Yonclas, & Bryan, 1989).

A wide variety of methods is acceptable for requesting objects and actions—for example, gestures, vocalizations, and verbalizations. In general, the more specific the child's request, the more effective the child is in eliciting a response. In assessing the child who exhibits little or no requesting, the speech-language pathologist should ask the following questions (Olswang, Kriegsmann, & Mastergeorge, 1982):

How does the child code requests?

Does the child attempt to regulate the behavior of other people or appear to have the desire to do so?

Does the child's behavior indicate a recognition that other people can act as agents?

Are opportunities for requesting available?

How do caregivers encourage and respond to requests?

Requesting will be severely limited if the child sees no need to engage in the behavior or if there is little opportunity to do so.

The two aspects of the environment for the speech-language pathologist to monitor are the child's elicited and spontaneous requests, along with the activities in which they occur, and the caregiver antecedents used in eliciting requests. She can code children's requesting behaviors and caregiver's eliciting behaviors as in Table 12.6.

Intentional or social communication is persistent, typically addressed to and modified for the receiver, and awaits a response. Such communication may be signaled by establishing eye contact, awaiting a turn, responding, interrupting, moving to a conspicuous position or toward the receiver, and/or stopping when the goal is reached. Even self-injurious behavior may signal a message, such as a desire to escape or a feeling like "Leave me alone; I don't want to do this" (Carr, Newson, and Binkhoff, 1980).

TABLE 12.6
Observation of requesting behaviors

Child Request Behaviors

Types

    Spontaneous request—Child initiated, not preceded by verbal or nonverbal adult behavior.

    Elicited request—Child produces request following adult verbal or nonverbal elicitation.

Intention

    Request for objects/people—Names or points to object/person, directing listener to provide.

    Requests for action—Child directs listener to perform in a certain manner.

    Requests for information—Uses rising intonation or *wh-* word to direct listener to provide information.

Adult Elicitation Behaviors

    Direct model—Adult directs child to produce model provided ("Tell me, 'open door.'").

    Direct question—Adult asks question that elicits request ("What do you want?").

    Obstacle presentation—Adult gives command or direct verbal instruction, but some obstacle, such as a missing piece or broken object, is provided ("Get some candy" [jar sealed tightly]).

    General statement—Adult gives a verbal comment that refers in a general way to some object or activity that the child might want to request ("I have some funny books over here").

Source: Adapted from Olswang, L., Kriegsmann, E., & Mastergeorge, A. (1982). Facilitating functional requesting in pragmatically impaired children. *Language, Speech, and Hearing Services in Schools, 13,* 202–222.

In contrast, unintentional or nonsocial communication, such as speaking when no one is present, does not consider the receiver. Situational responses, such as an eye blink following a loud noise, also are considered unintentional communication unless the child interacts in some way with the receiver.

Behaviors may be classified along several continuums. One continuum might begin with nonintentional behavior—the type of behavior state communication, such as crying, seen in young infants—and progress through conventional communication (Dunst, Lowe, & Bartholomew, 1990). Another continuum might have gestural communication at one extreme and verbal at the other, noting stages of intentionality (Wetherby & Prizant, 1990). Gestural behavior may be dichotomized as contact/motoric and distal/signal (Atlas & Lapadis, 1988; Curcio, 1978; McLean & Snyder-McLean, 1987; McLean, Snyder-McLean, Brady, & Etter, 1991). These continuums are summarized in Table 12.7.

Finally, random or stereotypic behaviors, such as incessant rocking, that do not seem to be related to environmental events or to the child's state, appear to be noncommunicative (although this is not always the case). Some professionals contend that all behaviors have some functional message value (Schuler & Goetz, 1981; Watzlawick, Beavin, & Jackson, 1967).

In the past, intervention has begun with the elimination of inappropriate, unconventional, idiosyncratic, or aberrant behavior, ignoring the communication potential of these behaviors and their role in the limited communication repertoires of some children. These behaviors may be used by some children to communicate intent (Carr & Durand, 1985; Donnellan et al., 1984; Wetherby & Prutting, 1984). Through systematic observation, the speech-language pathologist can form initial tentative hypotheses regarding intentions. In turn, she can confirm these hypotheses by systematic and meticulous manipulation of antecedent and/or consequent events during testing.

The speech-language pathologist can record hypotheses regarding the child's intentions on a simple form similar to Figure 12.2 (Donnellan et al., 1984). Although designed for aberrant behavior, the form can be adapted and other child behaviors listed across the top. The communicative functions or intentions on the left are derived from a number of taxonomies of the intentions of children developing normally. Facilitator hypotheses of intent are marked in the space corresponding to the behavior and to the possible intention. In the examples shown, tantruming is believed to signal an intention to attract attention, and touching an object may signal a desire for some item.

For children using conventional symbols, the speech-language pathologist will want to observe turn taking, presupposition in the novelty of topics introduced by the child, and initiation and response. She will want to note perseverative behavior, echolalia, and reenactment (Dawson & Adams, 1984; Dawson & Galpert, 1986; Prizant & Rydell, 1984; Sigman & Ungerer, 1984; Wetherby & Prutting, 1984). In reenactment, the original event or part of it may be used to represent the event. Thus, the child might say, "Once upon a time," to mean, "I want you to read to me." This manner of representation is found in some children with autism.

TABLE 12.7
Stages in the development of intentionality

Stage	Behavior	Example
Perlocutionary (Nonpurposeful)		
Preintentional	Reflexive behavior that expresses the inner state (wet, tired) and serves as signal for adult who interprets it. Not directed at others; no anticipation of outcome.	Cry, posture change, coo, facial expression (smile, frown)
Unintentional-intentional	Behavior is intentional or goal-oriented (reaching for a mobile) but is not intended to be communicative. Again, serve as signals that adults interpret. Not directed at others; no anticipation of outcome.	Reach for object, look at or regard object, fuss
Illocutionary (Purposeful)		
Nonconventional	Nonconventional gestures, usually *physical contact, used with intent* of affecting adult. Demonstrates intention to communicate by eliciting behavior, checking adult attending, and anticipating outcomes. Persistence or frustration if goal unmet.	Tug, push away, pull (Proto-imperatives)
Conventional	Convention (standard) gestures and vocalization used with intention of affecting adult's behavior. Greater persistence.	Alternating gaze, hand object, point, wave, shake head, nod
Concrete	Limited use of iconic symbols *at some distance from the referent* to represent the environment. Range of intentions. May be accompanied by vocalization.	Point, reach, offer, request assistance, request information, sign
Symbolic/locutionary		
Abstract	Limited use of arbitrary symbols, used individually, to represent the environment. Some idiosyncratic symbols. Limited to the here and now. Still heavy reliance on gestures and vocalization.	Symbols
Formal	Rule-bound linear symbol combinations; referent need not be present. Language is primary means of communicating.	Combinations of symbols

Source: Adapted from Bates, Camaioni, & Volterra (1975); McLean & Snyder-McLean (1988b); Prizant (1984)

FUNCTIONS	AGGRESSION	BIZARRE VERBALIZATIONS	INAPP. ORAL / ANAL BEHAVIOR	PERSEVERATIVE RITUALS	SELF-INJURIOUS BEHAVIOR	SELF-STIMULATION BEHAVIOR	TANTRUM	FACIAL EXPRESSION	GAZE AVERSION	GAZING / STARING	GESTURING / POINTING	HUGGING / KISSING	MASTURBATION	OBJECT MANIPULATION	PROXIMITY POSITIONING	PUSHING / PULLING	REACHING / PULLING	RUNNING / GRABBING	TOUCHING	DELAYED ECHOLALIA	IMMEDIATE ECHOLALIA	LAUGHING / GIGGLING	SCREAMING / YELLING	SWEARING	VERBAL / PHYSICAL THREATS	WHINING / CRYING	COMPLEX SIGN / APPROX.	COMPLEX SPEECH / APPROX.	ONE WORD SIGN / APPROX.	ONE WORD SPEECH / APPROX.	PICTURE / WRITTEN WORD
I. Interactive																															
A. Requests for Attention							X																								
Social interaction																															
Play interactions																															
Affection																															
Permission to engage in an activity																															
Action by Receiver																															
Assistance																															
Information / classification																															
Objects																		X													
Food																															
B. Negations																															
Protest																															
Refusal																															
Cessation																															
C. Declarations / comments																															
About events / actions																															
About objects / persons																															
About errors / mistakes																															
Affirmation																															
Greeting																															
Humor																															
D. Declarations about feelings																															
Anticipation																															
Boredom																															
Confusion																															
Fear																															
Frustration																															
Hurt feelings																															
Pain																															
Pleasure																															
II. Non-interactive																															
A. Self-regulation																															
B. Rehearsal																															
C. Habitual																															
D. Relaxation/ Tension release																															

This form can be adapted to list the individual child's behaviors across the top. Hypotheses regarding the illocutionary functions of these behaviors can be recorded in the appropriate space.

FIGURE 12.2

Functions of children's behavior

Source: Donnellan, A., Mirenda, P., Mesaros, R., & Fassbender, L. (1984). Analyzing the communicative functions of aberrant behavior. *Journal of the Association for Persons with Severe Handicaps, 9,* 210–222. Reprinted with permission.

Direct testing. The purpose of direct testing is to determine the optimum input and output modes for communication, the desirability of an augmentative system of communication and the selection of type, and the presymbolic or symbolic functioning level of the child. This process is ongoing and may tax the creativity of even the best speech-language pathologist because of the difficulty in testing some children.

If the child already has some type of rudimentary communication system, the speech-language pathologist attempts to describe this system as accurately as possible. Initially, the speech-language pathologist is interested in input and output means. The three primary expressive and receptive modes of communication are manual/visual, vocal/verbal/auditory, and tactile. Manual/visual means include gestures, signs, body movement, and/or visual contact or pointing. Vocal/verbal/auditory means include intonation, speech sounds, phonetically consistent forms, and/or spoken words. Tactile means include touch, signing in the hand, and physical manipulation, such as moving a partner's hand to a desired object. A skillful communicator uses a combination of methods, depending on context. Some children with language impairment rely on one mode primarily or on different input and output modes. For example, a child may understand and comply with single words or short phrases received auditorily, but rely on a gestural form of expressive communication.

For children who are very low functioning presymbolic, the speech-language pathologist assesses each of the three means for consistent responding and for focused or directed behavior. The speech-language pathologist should assess also the oral mechanism for motor development and control (Morris, 1982; Morris & Klein, 1987; Sleight & Niman, 1984). Part of the evaluation may include a probe to determine the difficulty in establishing an initial communication system.

As mentioned earlier in this chapter, communication can be established by a behavior chain interruption method in which some pleasurable behavior, such as listening to music, is interrupted (Goetz et al., 1985). During the evaluation, the speech-language pathologist can attempt to determine activities pleasurable to the child that she can use in this training. These activities may include rocking, listening to music, eating or drinking, or playing with some toy. Physical rocking, in which the child is cradled, has been used very successfully to establish initial communication (Sternberg et al., 1983; Sternberg et al., 1985). Through this pleasurable activity, the child can build a consistent responding behavior to signal for the rocking to continue.

During testing, the speech-language pathologist can confirm hypotheses about illocutionary function formed during observation. The speech-language pathologist can manipulate events that precede and follow the behaviors in question and note the effect of these changes on the behavior's frequency and intensity. Changes in the behavior should indicate some relationship between the behavior and the environment. For example, if the speech-language pathologist suspects that rocking signals requesting of objects, she might give objects in the immediate context to the child when rocking occurs and observe the result.

Formal direct testing of age-related communication can be accomplished by using any number of infant communication or development measures (Bayley, 1969; Boyd, Stauber, & Bluma, 1977; Griffith & Sanford, 1975; Rogers, D'Eugenio,

Brown, Donovan, & Lynch, 1978; Song et al., 1980). Many items are not appropriate for older children and may have little application to their experiences. Such instruments also may be difficult to use with children with multiple disabilities. For example, the child with cerebral palsy may be unable to exhibit many of the motor behaviors listed. Necessary modifications in testing procedures may preclude the outright use of a test's age norms. At best, these instruments provide only a gross estimate of the child's overall communication abilities. Table 12.8 presents several assessment tools for children who are presymbolic and minimally symbolic.

TABLE 12.8
Assessment tools for children who are presymbolic and minimally symbolic

Interview and Observation

Bangs, T., and Dodson, S. (1979). *Birth to three developmental scales*. Allen, TX: DLM.	Through observation determine level of functioning in direction following, motor and verbal imitation, object and picture naming, and pointing.
Bzock, K., and League, R. (1978). *Receptive expressive emergent language test*. Austin, TX: Pro-Ed.	Norm referenced caregiver interview for 0-36 months. Receptive and expressive.
Coplan, J. (1987). *Early language milestone scale*. Tulsa, OK: Modern Education Corp.	Norm referenced screening scale for 0-36 months. Forty-two items take approximately 5 minutes to administer.
Hanna, R., Lippert, E., and Harris, A. (1982). *Developmental communication curriculum inventory*. San Antonio, TX: Psychological Corp.	Caregiver questionnaire *and direct assessment tool* for child. Assesses four levels: Prelinguistic, symbolic, symbolic relationships, and complex symbolic relationships.
Klein, M., and D. Briggs, M. H. (1987). *Observation of communicative interactions*. Los Angeles: California State University, Mother-infant Communication Project.	Scales the caregiver's response to the infant's communication cues in ten categories.
MacArthur communicative development inventory: Infants. San Diego: San Diego State University, Center for Research in Language.	Parental checklist format used to assess understanding, comprehension, production of words, and vocabulary.
MacDonald, J., and Gillette, Y. (1988). *Ecological communication system (ECO)*. San Antonio, TX: Psychological Corp.	Interactive scales focusing on social play, communication, language, and conversation of child and caregiver. Looks for balance in the interaction.
Owens, R. (1982a). *Caregiver interview and environmental observation*. San Antonio, TX: Psychological Corp.	Interview and observational tool used to establish approximate functioning level for further testing, manner and location of communication, and communication partners.
Owens, R. (1982c). *Diagnostic interactional survey*. San Antonio, TX: Psychological Corp.	Observational tool used to rate the quality of a ten-minute child-caregiver interaction.
Wetherby, A. and Prizant, B. (1991a). *Communication and symbolic behavior scales*. Chicago: Riverside.	Norm referenced scales for 9-24 months using caregiver questionnaire *and direct sampling* of verbal and nonverbal behaviors and observation of play.

Functional- or behavioral-level data from questionnaires, interviews, and observations provide initial data for evaluating actual presymbolic or symbolic skills through direct testing. Certain commercially available instruments assess varying numbers of presymbolic and symbolic behaviors (Hanna et al., 1982; Horstmeier & MacDonald, 1978b; MacDonald, 1978a; Owens, 1982b; Rescorla, 1989). Most of these tools were created by modifying developmental scales to reflect more accurately the population being tested and the skills specifically needed for symbolic communication. Because the speech-language pathologist is

Testing and Sampling

Connard, P. (1984). *Preverbal assessment intervention profile.* Austin, TX: Pro-Ed.	Designed for profoundly and multiply handicapped to assess early (stages I-III) Piagetian skills.
Dunst, C. (1980). *A clinical and educational manual for use with the Uzgiris and Hunt Scales of infant psychological development.* Austin, TX: Pro-Ed.	Procedural guidelines for determining overall sensorimotor development based on testing and observation.
Fewell, R. and Langley, M. (1984). *Developmental Activities Screening Inventory.* Austin, TX: Pro-Ed.	Direct testing of skills such as means-ends and causality for those functioning between 0-60 months. Adaptations for the visually impaired.
Horstmeier, D., and MacDonald, J. (1978b). *Environmental prelanguage battery.* San Antonio, TX: Psychological Corp.	Direct assessment tool used in a play format assisted by caregivers. Assesses attending, object permanence, functional use, imitation, receptive language, and one- and two-word imitation and production.
MacDonald, J. (1978a). *Environmental language inventory.* San Antonio, TX: Psychological Corp.	Direct assessment tool for early semantic categories in two-, three-, and four-word utterances in imitation, conversation, and play.
Olswang, L., Stoel-Gammon, C., Coggins, T., and Carpenter, R. (1987). *Assessing prelinguistic behaviors in developmentally young children.* Seattle, WA: University of Washington Press.	Scales cognitive antecedents to word meaning, play, intentions, language comprehension, and language production.
Owens, R. (1982b). *Developmental assessment tool.* San Antonio, TX: Psychological Corp.	Direct assessment tool used to determine level of functioning in attending, imitation, turn-taking, object permanence, means, gestures, receptive language, sound production, and semantic and illocutionary functions of early symbols.
Riley, A. (1984). *Evaluating acquired skills in communication.* Tucson, AZ: Communication Skill Builders.	Evaluates skills from 3 months to 8 years at prelinguistic, receptive/expressive I, and receptive/expressive II levels.
Rossetti, L. M. (1990). *Rosetti infant-toddler language scale.* East Moline, IL: LinguiSystems.	Criterion referenced scale for 0-36 months covering interaction and attachment, gestures, pragmatics, play, comprehension, and expression.
Stillman, R. (1978). *Callier-Azusa scale.* Dallas: University of Texas, Callier Center for Communication Disorders.	Direct assessment tool designed for children who are deaf-blind.

interested in not only the skill level of the child but also the ease of teaching presymbolic skills, a necessary portion of the assessment should include teaching.

The Ordinal Scales of Psychological Development (Uzgiris & Hunt, 1975), based on a Piagetian model of early cognitive development, and their adaptation by Dunst (1980) are stage-oriented assessment tools. Behaviors tested help to place the child in one of the sensorimotor stages of cognitive development. Other tests use age-based developmental indices. Most evaluative tools will need to be adapted for the child's specific limitations. Others, such as the Callier-Azusa Scale (Stillman, 1978), are designed for children with multiple disabilities. Because these tools are based on a hierarchical model of development, the results describe general cognitive functioning and suggest goals for further training. The speech-language pathologist can choose subtests most directly related to presymbolic development, such as those that relate to turn taking, gestures, means-ends, intentionality, and imitation (McLean & Snyder-McLean, 1988b).

No specific skills, such as the imitative behavior of clapping hands, will aid in the development of symbols. Hand clapping is one example of a larger behavioral class of imitation. The speech-language pathologist is more interested in the presence or absence of these general classes of behavior, and she probes overall conceptual development of these classes.

There is little guidance for selecting intervention activities on the basis of presymbolic performance. Figure 12.3 provides a decision matrix that might offer some aid (Crais & Roberts, 1991). It is a decision framework, not an absolute.

Assessments may tax the best creative methods. However, even stereotypic or perseverative behavior can be useful if the speech-language pathologist can elicit this behavior within a few seconds of her model. The speech-language pathologist who knows she can elicit this behavior is able to control the behavior for training purposes, such as modifying it.

She should encourage caregivers to attend the evaluation and to assist by providing suggestions and actual test items from the child's environment, such as toys or grooming items. The presence of both the caregiver and familiar objects enhances the validity of the testing procedure. Often, children who are presymbolic and minimally symbolic have very concrete meanings for symbols or demonstrate very ritualized behavior. A cup may not be *cup* for the child unless it is the one used every day. This information would be unavailable without the caregiver's presence, and the speech-language pathologist might assume that the child does not know the symbol *cup*.

Assessment for augmentative communication. There may be no single good assessment for augmentative communication use. Certain minimal presymbolic skills seem necessary, however, for use of some augmentative communication systems. The level of functioning necessary depends on the system selected. In short, the more symbolic the system, the higher cognitive skill involved. For example, some forms of gestural signaling may be accomplished at a relatively young developmental age when compared to speaking or signing.

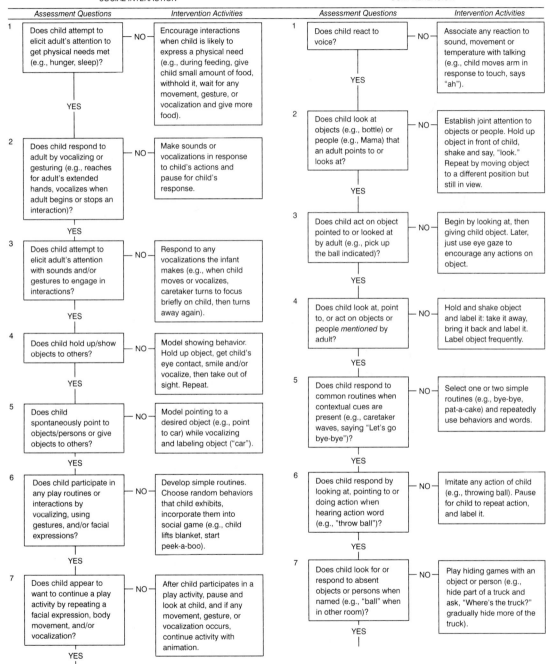

FIGURE 12.3
Decision making in training target selection

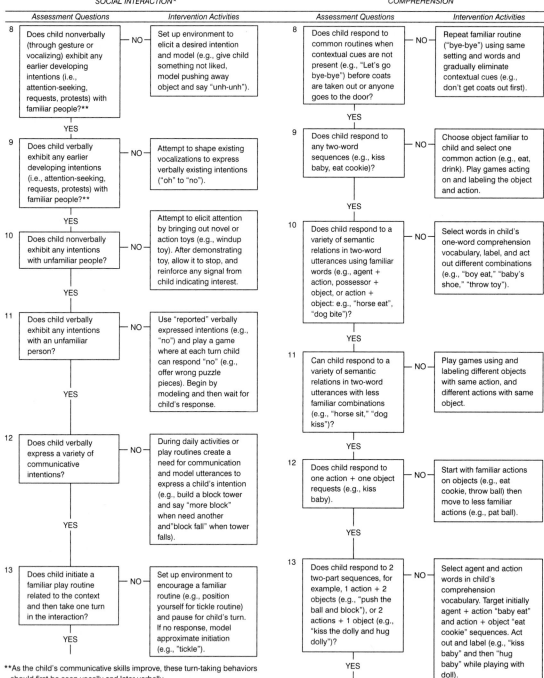

SOCIAL INTERACTION*

Assessment Questions	Intervention Activities
8 Does child nonverbally (through gesture or vocalizing) exhibit any earlier developing intentions (i.e., attention-seeking, requests, protests) with familiar people?** — NO →	Set up environment to elicit a desired intention and model (e.g., give child something not liked, model pushing away object and say "unh-unh").
YES ↓	
9 Does child verbally exhibit any earlier developing intentions (i.e., attention-seeking, requests, protests) with familiar people?** — NO →	Attempt to shape existing vocalizations to express verbally existing intentions ("oh" to "no").
YES ↓	
10 Does child nonverbally exhibit any intentions with unfamiliar people? — NO →	Attempt to elicit attention by bringing out novel or action toys (e.g., windup toy). After demonstrating toy, allow it to stop, and reinforce any signal from child indicating interest.
YES ↓	
11 Does child verbally exhibit any intentions with an unfamiliar person? — NO →	Use "reported" verbally expressed intentions (e.g., "no") and play a game where at each turn child can respond "no" (e.g., offer wrong puzzle pieces). Begin by modeling and then wait for child's response.
YES ↓	
12 Does child verbally express a variety of communicative intentions? — NO →	During daily activities or play routines create a need for communication and model utterances to express a child's intention (e.g., build a block tower and say "more block" when need another and "block fall" when tower falls).
YES ↓	
13 Does child initiate a familiar play routine related to the context and then take one turn in the interaction? — NO →	Set up environment to encourage a familiar routine (e.g., position yourself for tickle routine) and pause for child's turn. If no response, model approximate initiation (e.g., "tickle").
YES ↓	

**As the child's communicative skills improve, these turn-taking behaviors should first be seen vocally and later verbally.

COMPREHENSION

Assessment Questions	Intervention Activities
8 Does child respond to common routines when contextual cues are not present (e.g., "Let's go bye-bye") before coats are taken out or anyone goes to the door? — NO →	Repeat familiar routine ("bye-bye") using same setting and words and gradually eliminate contextual cues (e.g., don't get coats out first).
YES ↓	
9 Does child respond to any two-word sequences (e.g., kiss baby, eat cookie)? — NO →	Choose object familiar to child and select one common action (e.g., eat, drink). Play games acting on and labeling the object and action.
YES ↓	
10 Does child respond to a variety of semantic relations in two-word utterances using familiar words (e.g., agent + action, possessor + object, or action + object: e.g., "horse eat", "dog bite")? — NO →	Select words in child's one-word comprehension vocabulary, label, and act out different combinations (e.g., "boy eat," "baby's shoe," "throw toy").
YES ↓	
11 Can child respond to a variety of semantic relations in two-word utterances with less familiar combinations (e.g., "horse sit," "dog kiss")? — NO →	Play games using and labeling different objects with same action, and different actions with same object.
YES ↓	
12 Does child respond to one action + one object requests (e.g., kiss baby). — NO →	Start with familiar actions on objects (e.g., eat cookie, throw ball) then move to less familiar actions (e.g., pat ball).
YES ↓	
13 Does child respond to 2 two-part sequences, for example, 1 action + 2 objects (e.g., "push the ball and block"), or 2 actions + 1 object (e.g., "kiss the dolly and hug dolly")? — NO →	Select agent and action words in child's comprehension vocabulary. Target initially agent + action "baby eat" and action + object "eat cookie" sequences. Act out and label (e.g., "kiss baby" and then "hug baby" while playing with doll).
YES ↓	

FIGURE 12.3, *continued*

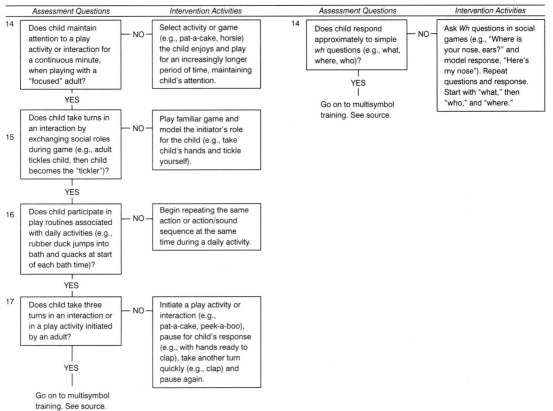

SOCIAL INTERACTION*

Assessment Questions	Intervention Activities
14 Does child maintain attention to a play activity or interaction for a continuous minute, when playing with a "focused" adult?	—NO— Select activity or game (e.g., pat-a-cake, horsie) the child enjoys and play for an increasingly longer period of time, maintaining child's attention.
YES	
15 Does child take turns in an interaction by exchanging social roles during game (e.g., adult tickles child, then child becomes the "tickler")?	—NO— Play familiar game and model the initiator's role for the child (e.g., take child's hands and tickle yourself).
YES	
16 Does child participate in play routines associated with daily activities (e.g., rubber duck jumps into bath and quacks at start of each bath time)?	—NO— Begin repeating the same action or action/sound sequence at the same time during a daily activity.
YES	
17 Does child take three turns in an interaction or in a play activity initiated by an adult?	—NO— Initiate a play activity or interaction (e.g., pat-a-cake, peek-a-boo), pause for child's response (e.g., with hands ready to clap), take another turn quickly (e.g., clap) and pause again.
YES	
Go on to multisymbol training. See source.	

COMPREHENSION

Assessment Questions	Intervention Activities
14 Does child respond approximately to simple *wh* questions (e.g., what, where, who)?	—NO— Ask *Wh* questions in social games (e.g., "Where is your nose, ears?" and model response, "Here's my nose"). Repeat questions and response. Start with "what," then "who," and "where."
YES	
Go on to multisymbol training. See source.	

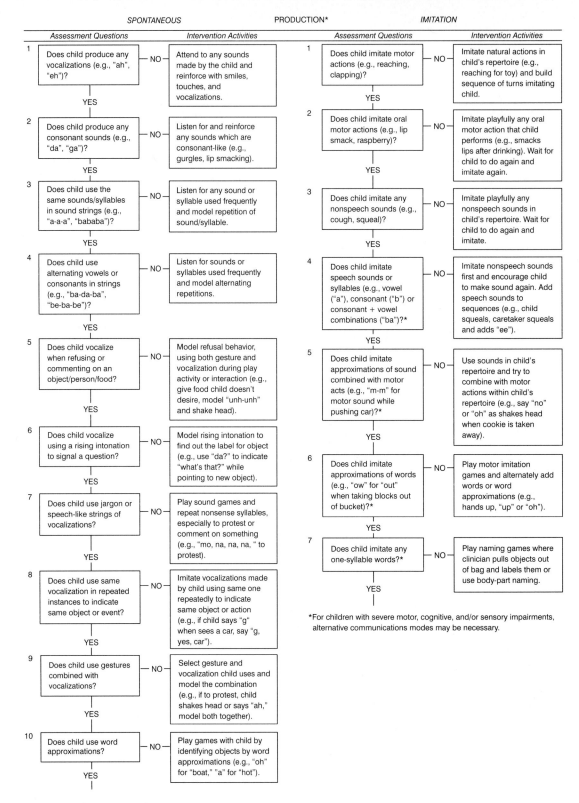

SPONTANEOUS   **PRODUCTION***   **IMITATION**

	Assessment Questions		Intervention Activities
1	Does child produce any vocalizations (e.g., "ah", "eh")?	NO	Attend to any sounds made by the child and reinforce with smiles, touches, and vocalizations.
	YES		
2	Does child produce any consonant sounds (e.g., "da", "ga")?	NO	Listen for and reinforce any sounds which are consonant-like (e.g., gurgles, lip smacking).
	YES		
3	Does child use the same sounds/syllables in sound strings (e.g., "a-a-a", "bababa")?	NO	Listen for any sound or syllable used frequently and model repetition of sound/syllable.
	YES		
4	Does child use alternating vowels or consonants in strings (e.g., "ba-da-ba", "be-ba-be")?	NO	Listen for sounds or syllables used frequently and model alternating repetitions.
	YES		
5	Does child vocalize when refusing or commenting on an object/person/food?	NO	Model refusal behavior, using both gesture and vocalization during play activity or interaction (e.g., give food child doesn't desire, model "unh-unh" and shake head).
	YES		
6	Does child vocalize using a rising intonation to signal a question?	NO	Model rising intonation to find out the label for object (e.g., use "da?" to indicate "what's that?" while pointing to new object).
	YES		
7	Does child use jargon or speech-like strings of vocalizations?	NO	Play sound games and repeat nonsense syllables, especially to protest or comment on something (e.g., "mo, na, na, na, " to protest).
	YES		
8	Does child use same vocalization in repeated instances to indicate same object or event?	NO	Imitate vocalizations made by child using same one repeatedly to indicate same object or action (e.g., if child says "g" when sees a car, say "g, yes, car").
	YES		
9	Does child use gestures combined with vocalizations?	NO	Select gesture and vocalization child uses and model the combination (e.g., if to protest, child shakes head or says "ah," model both together).
	YES		
10	Does child use word approximations?	NO	Play games with child by identifying objects by word approximations (e.g., "oh" for "boat," "a" for "hot").
	YES		

	Assessment Questions		Intervention Activities
1	Does child imitate motor actions (e.g., reaching, clapping)?	NO	Imitate natural actions in child's repertoire (e.g., reaching for toy) and build sequence of turns imitating child.
	YES		
2	Does child imitate oral motor actions (e.g., lip smack, raspberry)?	NO	Imitate playfully any oral motor action that child performs (e.g., smacks lips after drinking). Wait for child to do again and imitate again.
	YES		
3	Does child imitate any nonspeech sounds (e.g., cough, squeal)?	NO	Imitate playfully any nonspeech sounds in child's repertoire. Wait for child to do again and imitate.
	YES		
4	Does child imitate speech sounds or syllables (e.g., vowel ("a"), consonant ("b") or consonant + vowel combinations ("ba")?*	NO	Imitate nonspeech sounds first and encourage child to make sound again. Add speech sounds to sequences (e.g., child squeals, caretaker squeals and adds "ee").
	YES		
5	Does child imitate approximations of sound combined with motor acts (e.g., "m-m" for motor sound while pushing car)?*	NO	Use sounds in child's repertoire and try to combine with motor actions within child's repertoire (e.g., say "no" or "oh" as shakes head when cookie is taken away).
	YES		
6	Does child imitate approximations of words (e.g., "ow" for "out" when taking blocks out of bucket)?*	NO	Play motor imitation games and alternately add words or word approximations (e.g., hands up, "up" or "oh").
	YES		
7	Does child imitate any one-syllable words?*	NO	Play naming games where clinician pulls objects out of bag and labels them or use body-part naming.
	YES		

*For children with severe motor, cognitive, and/or sensory impairments, alternative communications modes may be necessary.

FIGURE 12.3, *continued*

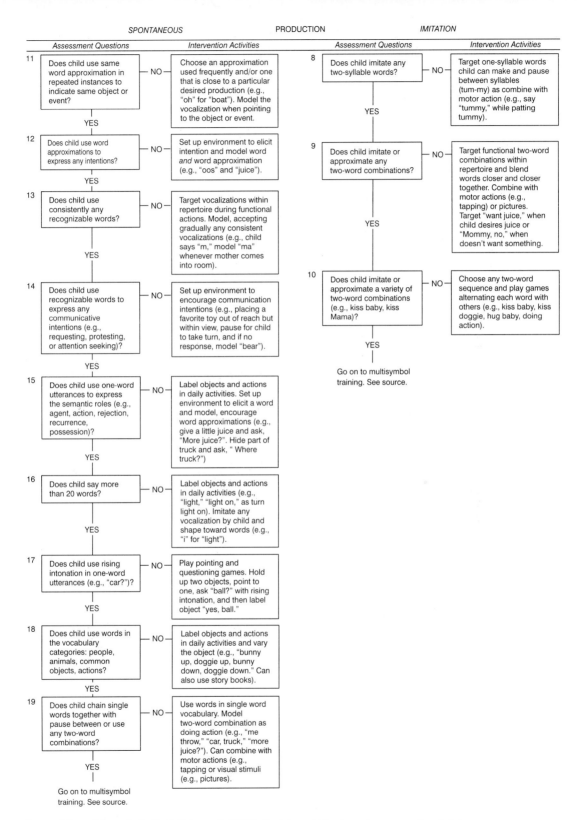

SPONTANEOUS   PRODUCTION   IMITATION

Assessment Questions	Intervention Activities

11 Does child use same word approximation in repeated instances to indicate same object or event? — NO → Choose an approximation used frequently and/or one that is close to a particular desired production (e.g., "oh" for "boat"). Model the vocalization when pointing to the object or event.

YES

12 Does child use word approximations to express any intentions? — NO → Set up environment to elicit intention and model word *and* word approximation (e.g., "oos" and "juice").

YES

13 Does child use consistently any recognizable words? — NO → Target vocalizations within repertoire during functional actions. Model, accepting gradually any consistent vocalizations (e.g., child says "m," model "ma" whenever mother comes into room).

YES

14 Does child use recognizable words to express any communicative intentions (e.g., requesting, protesting, or attention seeking)? — NO → Set up environment to encourage communication intentions (e.g., placing a favorite toy out of reach but within view, pause for child to take turn, and if no response, model "bear").

YES

15 Does child use one-word utterances to express the semantic roles (e.g., agent, action, rejection, recurrence, possession)? — NO → Label objects and actions in daily activities. Set up environment to elicit a word and model, encourage word approximations (e.g., give a little juice and ask, "More juice?". Hide part of truck and ask, " Where truck?")

YES

16 Does child say more than 20 words? — NO → Label objects and actions in daily activities (e.g., "light," "light on," as turn light on). Imitate any vocalization by child and shape toward words (e.g., "i" for "light").

YES

17 Does child use rising intonation in one-word utterances (e.g., "car?")? — NO → Play pointing and questioning games. Hold up two objects, point to one, ask "ball?" with rising intonation, and then label object "yes, ball."

YES

18 Does child use words in the vocabulary categories: people, animals, common objects, actions? — NO → Label objects and actions in daily activities and vary the object (e.g., "bunny up, doggie up, bunny down, doggie down." Can also use story books).

YES

19 Does child chain single words together with pause between or use any two-word combinations? — NO → Use words in single word vocabulary. Model two-word combination as doing action (e.g., "me throw," "car, truck," "more juice?"). Can combine with motor actions (e.g., tapping or visual stimuli (e.g., pictures).

YES

Go on to multisymbol training. See source.

Assessment Questions	Intervention Activities

8 Does child imitate any two-syllable words? — NO → Target one-syllable words child can make and pause between syllables (tum-my) as combine with motor action (e.g., say "tummy," while patting tummy).

YES

9 Does child imitate or approximate any two-word combinations? — NO → Target functional two-word combinations within repertoire and blend words closer and closer together. Combine with motor actions (e.g., tapping) or pictures. Target "want juice," when child desires juice or "Mommy, no," when doesn't want something.

YES

10 Does child imitate or approximate a variety of two-word combinations (e.g., kiss baby, kiss Mama)? — NO → Choose any two-word sequence and play games alternating each word with others (e.g., kiss baby, kiss doggie, hug baby, doing action).

YES

Go on to multisymbol training. See source.

Source: Adapted from Crais, E., & Roberts, J. (1991). Decision making in assessment and early intervention planning. *Language, Speech, and Hearing Services in Schools, 22,* 19-30. Printed with permission.

Cognitive abilities are especially important for the size and quality of the augmentative repertoire that the child will develop (Silverman, 1989). Cognitive functioning alone, however, does not predict success, especially with gestural communication (McLean et al., 1991). Although late Piagetian sensorimotor stages IV and early V are correlated with true symbol use, this correlation should not preclude augmentative instruction at a less than symbolic level that is useful to the child (Calculator, 1988c). Means-ends, pretend play, functional use of objects, and an awareness of symbols, such as a stop sign, seem important for symbol use (Mirenda & Schuler, 1988).

The speech-language pathologist frequently assesses social skills, such as turn taking, eye contact, joint attending, receptive language, and gesturing, when considering a child for an augmentative communication system. Many early non-symbolic forms of communication are listed in Table 12.2. Receptive language skills seem necessary for augmentative system generalization (Goosens, 1984; Hurlbut, Iwata, & Green, 1982).

The speech-language pathologist may classify gestures as coverbal for those that occur with verbalization, or paraverbal for those that occur without; contact or distal; signaling emotional state, attitude, or station; referential, referring to an object or event; or iconic, replicating some entity with hand shapes or movements (McLean et al., 1991; Yorkston & Dowden, 1984). Individuals with severe to profound mental retardation using only contact gestures demonstrate some early requesting and protesting intentions, while those using distal gestures demonstrate both these imperative-type intentions and early declarative intentions (McLean et al., 1991). As a group, those using only contact gestures also initiate communication less frequently and produce fewer wordlike vocalizations. If intentionality is not evident, then it might be best to begin training with very limited gestures, such as requesting or protesting (Prizant & Wetherby, 1985; Schuler & Prizant, 1987).

Assessments for augmentative communication should include a physical evaluation of manual dexterity, range and accuracy of movement, physical placement, oral-peripheral structure and functioning, and visual acuity. Observing hand movements in daily tasks may be more helpful than isolated movement tasks when evaluating manual dexterity. Various systems should be tried to determine those best suited to the child. It is not unusual to find children communicating via a number of augmentative modes simultaneously.

Although the decision process involved in selecting or designing an augmentative system for a child is a first step, the assessment does not need to be (Reichle & Karlan, 1985). A test-teach-test model, in which the child attempts to learn various systems while being assessed, seems promising (Reichle et al., 1988).

Sampling.   Most measures of presymbolic or minimally symbolic communication emphasize language form, rather than communication (Wetherby & Prizant, 1991b). Sampling is needed, therefore, as a supplement (Wetherby & Prizant, 1989). Structured situations may be used to elicit a variety of functions by enticing communication (Coggins et al., 1987; Prizant & Wetherby, 1988b; Wetherby

& Rodriguez, 1992). Table 12.9 presents some possible structured situations. It may be best to intersperse different functions to keep the child's interest and reduce potential perseveration.

At a symbolic level, whether verbal or through some augmentative means, the speech-language pathologist is interested in the number of symbols in the child's lexicon and in the variety of semantic and illocutionary functions the child

TABLE 12.9
Structured situations for eliciting communication

Declaring
Adult looks through some books with the child.
Adult gives the child four blocks to drop into a can. Immediately on completion, adult hands the child a small doll.
Adult rolls a ball to the child. After a few returns, adult substitutes a different toy and rolls it.
Adult takes item from box, such as a marker, and offers one to child. Adult replaces her marker after drawing and also places a strange object in the box, takes another marker, and hands the box to the child. A plastic spider has been used but might scare some children too much. A cotton ball could be placed in a food item.
Adult has a mechanical item move behind her but visible to the child. Adult operates switch unknown to child.

Greeting
On meeting child, adult awaits greeting. If not forthcoming after 5 seconds, adult greets the child.
Adult waves hello and good-bye to objects as they are removed from or replaced in containers. After doing this three or four times, the adult removes or replaces without doing it.

Protesting
Adult holds a disliked food item near the child or hands it to the child.
Adult places the child's hands in a cold, wet, or sticky substance, such as pudding, glue, or Jell-O.
Adult offers child a choice of two items, then hands the wrong one.

Requesting action
Adult initiates a pleasurable game or action, then stops and waits.
Adult blows up a balloon and slowly deflates it, then holds it to her mouth and waits or hands it to the child and waits.
Adult plays Give-Me-Five, in which child slaps adult's hands. When tables turn, adult waits.

Requesting assistance
Adult activates a wind-up toy, lets it run down, then hands it to the child.
Adult opens a jar of bubbles, blows some, then closes the jar tightly and gives it to the child.
While the child is watching, adult places a desired food item in a clear jar that the child cannot open, and then places the container in front of the child.

Requesting item
Adult eats a desired food item without offering any to the child.
Adult places two glasses on the table and declares thirst, pours juice for self, and then places pitcher out of child's reach.

Source: Adapted from McLean, Snyder-McLean, Brady, & Etter (1991); Wetherby, Cain, Yoncias, & Walker (1988); Wetherby & Prizant, 1990; Wetherby & Rodriguez (1992)

displays. The relative merits of sampling and more formalized testing are discussed in Chapter 4.

The speech-language pathologist collects a conversational sample and rates each utterance for the semantic and illocutionary functions found in early child language (MacDonald, 1978a; Owens, 1982b). Although such categories may be inappropriate for older children with retardation, they do suggest a standard set of functions with which to begin (Leonard, Steckol, & Panther, 1983). Normative distributions are not available for these functions, which are usually situationally related. Of greater interest is the range of functions the child uses.

The speech-language pathologist collects samples by observing everyday activities or routines with the child's primary caregivers, such as teachers, parents, and classroom aides. Children engaged in familiar, meaningful activities with age-appropriate materials are likely to interact more and to produce more language than do children in other situations.

Analysis can be accomplished at the utterance level. For children who speak, an *utterance* consists of one or more symbols separated from other symbols by a pause, a drop in the voice, or an inhalation. Children using augmentative communication may look at their partner or pause between utterances. Whatever the mode of transmission, the speech-language pathologist records and rates each utterance for both semantic and illocutionary function and for the number of symbols used. Appendix L provides definitions of the most common functions listed in Table 12.4. A form such as Figure 12.4 may be helpful for recording and analyzing the data. The speech-language pathologist records the number of symbols per utterance under the appropriate functions demonstrated by the utterance.

Repetitive utterances, such as "baby baby," may function as single-symbol utterances. If this is suspected, the speech-language pathologist should credit the child with only one symbol for that utterance. Likewise, certain combinations may function as single-symbol utterances. The child may repeatedly produce "dog here" yet not use either symbol independently or in combination with other symbols. If this is suspected, it can be confirmed by the caregivers or through observation, and the utterance rated accordingly.

The speech-language pathologist then uses the total number of symbols and the total number of utterances within each function from Figure 12.4 to compute the mean length of utterance (MLU) of each function. Of interest are the range of semantic and illocutionary functions and the length and means of communicating each (Caro & Snell, 1989; Owens, 1982a). She can use the results as follows to select training objectives (Owens, 1982d):

Teach relevant functions that do not occur.

Provide opportunities for low-frequency functions to occur.

Teach longer forms for functions with low MLUs.

Reduce or modify stereotypic, perseverative, or echolalic utterances that seem nonfunctional.

FIGURE 12.4

Utterances	SEMANTIC FUNCTIONS											ILLOCUTIONARY FUNCTIONS								FORM				TYPE		
	Nom.	L.	Neg	P.	Att.	R.	Not.	O.	Act.	Ag+	+Ob	A.	Q.	R.	D.	P.	N.	S.	O.	Ges.	Sig.	Voc.	Ver.	Init.	Resp
1. BALL	1																1			1			1	1	
2. (WANT) BALL									2		2							2		1			1	2	
3. (THROW) BALL									2		2							2		1			1	2	2
4. THROW ME		2							2									2			2		2	2	
5. WANT THAT?	2												2							2			2	2	2
6. NO THAT			2															2		2			2	2	
7. MORE THROW						2												2					2	2	
8. BALL?	1												1										2	2	
9. THROW BALL ME		3							3		3							3		3			3	3	
44.																									
45.																									
46.																									
47.																									
48.																									
50.																									
OVERALL TOTAL (Words)	4	5	2	0	0	2	0	0	9	0	7	0	3	0	0	0	1	13	0	9	2	0	16	13	4
TOTAL NO. OF UTT.	3	2	1	0	0	1	0	0	4	0	3	0	2	0	0	0	1	6	0	6	1	0	9	7	2
MLU by functions (Divide total words by total utterances)	1.3	2.5	2	0	0	2	0	0	2.3	0	2.3	0	1.5	0	0	0	1	2.2	0	1.5	2	0	1.8	1.9	2

Nom. = Nomination
L. = Location
Neg. = Negation
P. = Possession
Att. = Attribution

R. = Recurrence
Not. = Notice
O. = Other
Act. = Action
Ag+ = Agent + Action

+Ob = Action + Object
A. = Answer
Q. = Question
R. = Reply
D. = Declaration

P. = Practice
N. = Name
S. = Suggestion, Command, Demand, Request
O. = Other

Ges. = Gesture
Sig. = Sign
Voc. = Vocalization
Ver. = Verbalization
Init. = Initiate

Resp. = Respond

In the first utterance, the child pointed at the object and said one symbol ("Ball") clearly a semantic *Nominative* and an illocutionary *Name*. Utterances 4 ("Throw me"), 6 ("No that") and 7 ("More throw") are two-symbol examples of the semantic rules *X + Locative*, *Negative + X* and *Recurrent + X*, respectively. At the two-symbol level, these semantic functions are expanded by adding another symbol. This format applies to the first seven semantic functions. In contrast, utterance 3 ("Throw ball") is an example of a different type. The *Agent, Action*, and *Object* categories are expanded by combining categories. Thus, utterance 3 is an example of a two-symbol *Action* and a two-symbol *Object*. Utterance 2 is similar. Utterance 9 represents a combination of *X + Locative* and *Action + Object*. Utterance 9 represents a combination of *X + Locative* and *Action + Object*, a three-category combination scored under each appropriate category. In all utterances gestures support the communication but language is the primary form of communication. Gestured portions of an utterance are in parentheses. If more than one form is used, the verbal symbol is underlined.

FIGURE 12.4

Functional analysis of a language sample of a child who is minimally symbolic

Source: Adapted from Owens, R. (1978). *Speech acts in the early language of non-delayed and retarded children: A taxonomy and distributional study.* Unpublished doctoral dissertation, Ohio State University, Columbus.

Such detailed collection and analysis procedures are very time-consuming, but they are necessary for children who are presymbolic and early symbolic and who may exhibit a low incidence of communicative behavior and use inappropriate and unconventional signal systems.

The speech-language pathologist may collect semantic functions within a structured format by using conversational and/or imitative cues to elicit function-specific two-, three-, and four-word utterances (MacDonald, 1978a). Although less naturalistic than sampling, these techniques can elicit a broader range of functions than may be possible within interactional samples. She then can compare these data with the spontaneous sample.

The Communication Environment

The speech-language pathologist is interested in more than just the functioning level of the child. Given the effect of context—both linguistic and nonlinguistic—on communication, the speech-language pathologist must evaluate also the communication potential of the child's natural environment (Caro & Snell, 1989). Again, she gathers initial information through interviews with caregivers and by observation. Of interest are the situations, activities, and locations that are high-communication contexts and the child's communication behavior in each. The speech-language pathologist is interested also in identifying caregivers who evoke the most communication from the child and in describing their behaviors, especially the communication demands they place on the child (Mahoney & Weller, 1980). The ideal environment is one that nourishes development and enhances generalization (Haring, Roger, Lee, Breen, & Gaylord-Ross, 1986). The child should have ample opportunities to express himself and to make choices (Falvey, McLean, & Rosenberg, 1988).

The speech-language pathologist may wish to conduct a four-step survey of the child's communication needs and uses (L. Brown et al., 1979; D. Yoder, 1985). First, she describes the functionally most relevant and least restrictive communication environments, at present and in the foreseeable future. These might include the classroom or the home. Second, she divides these environments into subenvironments by the most relevant and functional activities in each, such as snacktime or bathing. Third, she determines the skills needed to participate in each activity. Fourth, the speech-language pathologist describes how each activity and/or environment may be adapted to allow or enhance the child's participation. This process provides the data needed to design intervention programs to teach interactional skills and environmental adaptation.

The Interaction of Child and Environment

Although the child and the environment are important in themselves, the data gathered from each are most meaningful when we consider how each affects the other. Communication is an interaction between the child and the caregivers, and learning can be measured only by the effect the child's newly acquired behaviors have on the environment of which these caregivers are a part. For maximum generalization, the child's caregivers must become language facilitators. "If one member of a [caregiver-child] dyad undergoes developmental change, the other is also likely to do so" (Bronfenbrenner, 1979, p. 65).

In determining the language facilitator potential of each caregiver, the speech-language pathologist first must determine the quality of the interaction between the child and the caregiver. The speech-language pathologist then can, when appropriate, suggest modifications in the caregiver's behavior that may, in turn, change the child's communicative behavior. For example, the caregiver who demonstrates a relatively directive style, such as anticipating the child's needs or talking incessantly, might be instructed to wait for the child's request for assistance and to pause for verbal and nonverbal turns by the child.

Several observational tools are available, including the Observation of Communication Interactions (OCI) Scale (Klein & Briggs, 1987), the Parent-Infant Interaction Scale (G. Clark & Seifer, 1982), and the Diagnostic Interactional Survey (DIS) (Owens, 1982c). If the child is presymbolic, the speech-language pathologist is interested in the manner in which partners perceive the child's behavior (Ogletree, 1993). For children using symbols, the speech-language pathologist would want to note caregiver responsiveness and consistency and the adjustments caregivers make for the child's developmental level and emotional state (Greenspan, 1988; Ogletree, 1993; Tiegerman & Siperstein, 1984). The appropriateness of caregiver verbal models is also important.

Qualitative judgments of child-caregiver interaction might be based on the presence or absence of certain behaviors by both individuals. Behaviors to observe include the caregivers' uses of natural reinforcement, physical proximity, imitation of the child's behaviors, expansion, reply/extension, and content appropriate to the child's experience and functioning level. The child might be rated for attending to the interaction, referencing or signaling notice, physical proximity, and vocal/verbal responding. The presence of these 10 characteristics has been associated with subjective judgments of quality interaction (Russo & Owens, 1982). Although useful, such prepackaged scales might overlook information valuable for any specific child-caregiver dyad. A more descriptive scale that delineates child strategies for engagement, termination, and re-engagement and the primary modes of signaling might be more useful (Wilcox & Campbell, 1983).

In general, children who are presymbolic engage in a greater frequency and higher level of communication when they initiate interactions. The child's level of responding in both adult-initiated and child-initiated interactions might be described, noting vocalizations, limb movements, and facial and body postures (J. Norris & Hoffman, 1990a).

Another rating system, ECOmaps, evaluates social play, turn taking, nonverbal communication, language, and conversation within the interaction by using a 1-9 scale (MacDonald & Carroll, 1992a; MacDonald & Gillette, 1982). These areas are evaluated in three contexts: play with objects, play with people alone, and spontaneous interactions during caregiving. In addition, the speech-language pathologist engages the child in interaction and notes differences between this interaction and that with the caregiver. The scales rate actual behavior or an approximate percentage of the time that each interactant engages in the specific behaviors listed. Results allow for an estimate of communication match for that behavior; severe inequities signal a potential mismatch. If the caregiver is rated 9 on "initiates contact" and the child receives only 1, the inequity in this area requires intervention. A progressive match in which the caregiver is monitoring the child's performance and modeling slightly above that level is more desirable. The Teaching Strategies ECOmap rates the caregiver's use of events and strategies the child needs to communicate at a higher level. Finally, the Problems ECOmap identifies specific potential interactional problems.

CONCLUSION

Prior to initiating therapy and throughout the intervention process, the speech-language pathologist must conduct a thorough evaluation of the child's communication system and environment. A variety of data collection procedures is needed to attain an adequate description. Of interest is the child's present communication system and potential for modification and the child's presymbolic or early symbolic level of functioning. The speech-language pathologist will want to identify the communication characteristics of the child's environment and of the child-caregiver interaction and to describe the communication behaviors of all primary caregivers. She would continue to monitor these variables throughout intervention to ensure the child's performance at the optimum communication level.

The goal of a truly functional communication training program necessitates a thorough understanding of the dynamics of the child-caregiver interaction. From initial contact with the child, it is critical that the speech-language pathologist consider the contextual variables that affect communication and that are, in turn, affected by it.

13 Intervention with Children Who Are Presymbolic and Minimally Symbolic

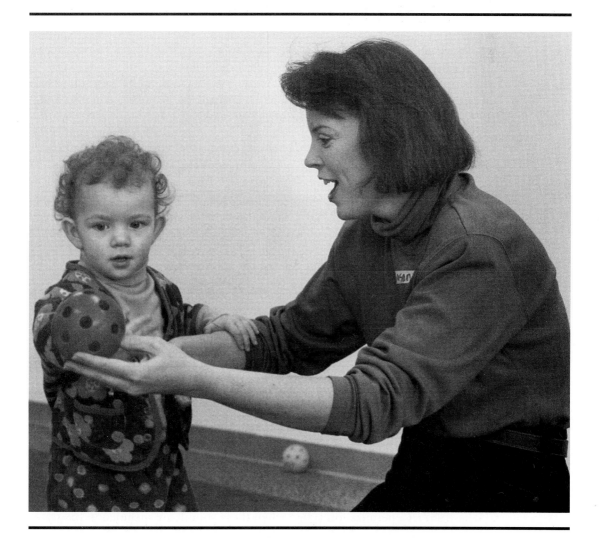

I ntervention with children who are presymbolic and minimally symbolic can follow many of the principles emphasized throughout this book by being naturalistic, functional, and developmentally appropriate. The child's intervention plan should be based on and should address the needs of all three major areas assessed—child-related variables, environmental variables, and interactional variables—within an overall integrated functional approach. In this section we discuss strategies and techniques applicable to each area.

AN INTEGRATED FUNCTIONAL INTERVENTION MODEL

As noted, "lack of generalization of newly acquired responses from instructional contexts to spontaneous use in actual settings has been another shortcoming of operant instruction" (P. Hunt & Goetz, 1988, p. 59). Progress will be minimal unless the family, classroom, and everyday contexts are of primary concern and central to intervention (Caro & Snell, 1989; Dunst et al., 1990; Guess, Keogh, & Sailor, 1978; Harris, 1975).

It is essential that caregivers be involved in the training. "The child affects and is affected by the entire family system" (Bristol, 1985, p. 49). Therefore, the speech-language pathologist must work at the level of the dyad, rather than the individual child. Communication is a cooperative venture. A child cannot be taught to communicate by him- or herself.

Ideally, the speech-language pathologist sees the child daily for individual or group therapy within a classroom or unit setting with the caregiver. If this arrangement is not possible, the caregiver should attend at least once a week. When this attendance is not possible, the speech-language pathologist can inform the caregiver about the training through detailed reports and instructions, and she can train the caregiver periodically in evening group sessions.

The speech-language pathologist can observe the teachers and aides in the natural classroom environment and make suggestions for improving the quality of the child-caregiver interaction. With instructional staff, training can occur at in-service sessions or in direct instruction following the brief observation and data review sessions in the classroom environment. Each caregiver should maintain a record of all formal training for review, along with the speech-language pathologist's records, when making decisions about the intervention plan. Staff also should participate in assessments and in setting intervention goals (McNaughton & Light, 1989).

All language facilitators should be trained to recognize the communication intentions of the child's behaviors, to implement the training program, and to assess the functionality and practicality of intervention methods, materials, and adaptations (Falvey, McLean, & Rosenberg, 1988). Strategies for facilitating communication should be stressed.

As noted previously, natural settings contain naturally arising stimuli, such as materials, partners, and physical surroundings, that influence communication (Halle, 1987). Generalization is best when these stimuli are included in the training. The poor generalization skills of children with autism—a result of stimulus overselectivity, prompt dependence, and perseverance of routines—suggests that training in the actual use environment is essential (Donnellan & Mirenda, 1983; Koegel, Rincover, & Egel, 1982; Mirenda & Schuler, 1988; Nietupski, Hamre-Nietupski, Clancy, & Veerhusen, 1986).

Similarly, natural environments usually contain sequences of behavior, rather than isolated instances. Skill training can be clustered so that the consequence of one behavior is the cue for the next (Guess & Helmstetter, 1986). In this way, training is more like everyday events and less repetitive and more varied.

The speech-language pathologist may use contrived instructional settings effectively, especially if there is concurrent instruction in the natural environment (Glennen & Calculator, 1985; Nietupski et al., 1986). For best generalization, the simulated environment should be varied to reflect the natural environment, and instruction in the simulated and natural environments should occur as close as possible in time (Nietupski et al., 1986).

Consistent routines and expected daily schedules within the natural environment enhance communication by providing redundancy that cues interactions (vanDijk, 1985). Behaviors associated with each activity become signals for that activity and natural environmental cues for communication (Snell & Zirpoli, 1987).

Training may focus on either expanding the breadth of communication behaviors, such as increasing the number of illocutionary functions or the number of means of expressing current functions, or increasing developmental complexity, such as moving from nonintentional to intentional communication or from presymbolic to symbolic. Idiosyncratic means of communication can be replaced gradually by more conventional means (Carr & Durand, 1985; Donnellan et al., 1984; Schuler & Prizant, 1987; M. Smith, 1985).

As noted elsewhere in this chapter, this environment must be an interactive one, involving encouraging turn taking, recognizing and responding to the child's communication, and creating opportunities for the child to communicate (Cirrin & Rowland, 1985; Vicker, 1985). For many children who are presymbolic, the need to communicate has been eliminated (MacDonald, 1985). Children need to have choices that influence their environment in order to increase their communication skills and independence (Glennen & Calculator, 1985; Guess, Benson, & Siegel-Causey, 1985; Klein et al., 1981; Shevin & Klein, 1984).

Activities within each child's various interactional environments form the bases for communication and training. Communication and language training occur at natural junctures within these ongoing activities (Rowland & Schweigert, 1989a, 1989b). Three intervention techniques are beneficial: incidental teaching, stimulation, and formal training (Owens, 1982d).

Incidental Teaching

Incidental teaching is a strategy that arises naturally within the child's and caregiver's daily activities or in unstructured situations. In this child-directed strategy, the child controls the focus of the interaction by signaling interest. While enhancing these naturally occurring communication interactions, the caregiver trains or strengthens presymbolic or early symbolic behaviors. In other words, the behavior is trained within the child's daily activities in which it would naturally appear. For example, the child learning about object permanence could encounter natural teaching situations while bathing with nonfloating soap or while searching for misplaced toys. *Incidental teaching is not formal training disguised as fun.* Hidden training, such as preschool action songs, may be just as irrelevant to the context and to the child as formal training, although action songs in another context can aid in valuable concept development.

The caregiver's tasks are to be aware of the learning potential within each situation and to structure events to enhance learning. Caregiver input to the child should match or lead slightly the complexity of the child's language (Owens, 1982d; Prizant & Schuler, 1987). In unstructured activities, such as free play, the child's expressed interest is the key. Caregivers can learn to follow the child's lead and to incorporate training into these interests. Table 13.1 presents examples of incidental teaching.

A number of studies have reported success, albeit limited, in the use of incidental techniques. For example, institutionalized adolescents increased their verbal initiations for food at meals following a delaying procedure in which the trainer awaited client signals (Halle et al., 1979). In addition, teacher use of the procedures spread to other settings. Similar results have been reported with the use of sign (Oliver & Halle, 1982). Adolescents with autism have been taught object labels within a lunch preparation activity in a kitchen area (McGee et al., 1983).

Ongoing activities and routines serve as the context for training. As an active participant, the child affects real outcomes directly related to the content of communication. Behavior directly related to outcomes is easier to learn than behavior taught through drills (Hunt & Goetz, 1988; Koegel & Williams, 1980; Litt & Schreibman, 1982; Saunders & Sailor, 1979; Stafford et al., 1978).

TABLE 13.1
Examples of incidental teaching

Type of Training	Example
Establishing eye contact	During feeding, the child looks at the facilitator in order to receive a spoonful of food.
Object permanence	While bathing, the facilitator "loses" nonfloating soap in the bath water and states, "Oh, I lost the soap; can you find it?"
Imitation with objects	During daily living skills training, the child imitates the facilitator's use of a comb.
Requesting gesture	At snacktime, the child requests a special snack from those on the table.
Symbol recognition	The child picks out clothes named during dressing.

Unfortunately, this incidental aspect of training is most difficult for caregivers to comprehend. Although it is relatively easy to train caregivers to engage in formal training with children, and it is relatively easy for these caregivers to adapt the training to other environments, it is not as easy for them to adapt the training to less structured, informal, everyday activities unless directly taught these behaviors (Alpert & Rogers-Warren, 1984; Salzberg & Villani, 1983).

The speech-language pathologist can assist caregivers in using incidental techniques by following these suggestions:

1. Keep the training procedures simple.
2. Role-play potential situations with the caregiver.
3. Target a few frequently occurring everyday situations, rather than try to cover every possible situation.
4. Do not require record keeping of incidental teaching.
5. Demonstrate in the actual environment or within real situations.

Caregivers are overwhelmed easily by the plethora of training advice to be used in numerous different potential teaching situations.

After a review of incidental teaching research, Warren and Kaiser (1986b) concluded, "Incidental teaching (a) teaches target skills effectively in the natural environment; (b) typically results in generalization of those skills across settings, time, and persons; and (c) results in gains in the formal and functional aspects of language" (p. 296). Incidental teaching is useful for generalization and for relevancy of training. Without such techniques, the 24-hour-a-day approach is impossible.

Incidental teaching is "ecologically sound." It is more likely than other methods to meet the needs of the family or classroom because it incorporates their daily routines where skills are taught and used.

Many caregivers express reservations about their ability to implement formal training and to make the assumed time commitment. Thus, incidental teaching is a practical response to the need for more child instruction and more useful child-caregiver interaction.

Warren and Kaiser (1986b) further concluded, "Because research with mentally retarded children is limited . . . the extent to which incidental teaching can remediate serious communication deficits . . . is less clear" (p. 296). This concern is addressed by using the two additional teaching strategies of stimulation and formal training in conjunction with incidental teaching.

Stimulation

Stimulation, the way caregivers interact with the child, should be just slightly more complex than the child's functioning to serve as a model. The child will learn best, according to the minimal discrepancy principle, when the model is far enough above her or his competency level to maintain interest but not so far as to frustrate (J. Hunt, 1961). Our best guide is the communication behavior of mothers of nonimpaired infants.

These mothers treat their children as conversational partners who exhibit meaningful communication. After addressing their children, these mothers usually wait for a response and treat any following behavior as meaningful. The mothers use a variety of techniques, such as exaggerated movements, to gain and maintain their children's interest.

Caregivers must expect and be alert for the child's communication and must structure situations to encourage it. Once communication occurs, caregivers provide appropriate models and feedback and allow the child to make choices that can affect change (Owens, 1982d; Page, 1982; Tapajna & Finn-Scardine, 1981). Even peers developing normally can serve as excellent language stimulation models (D. Cole, Vandercook, & Rynders, 1987). Table 13.2 presents some suggested stimulation techniques.

Because research has not identified which behaviors are the most effective, caregivers should use as many as are practical. It is best for caregivers to change their own behavior slowly, possibly incorporating one or two techniques and waiting until these feel comfortable before using more. It will not be necessary to use all of the stimulation techniques with every child. Small changes in the current method of interacting, such as increasing the number of verbalizations addressed to the child, may have dramatic effects (Owens et al., 1987). Augmentative sym-

TABLE 13.2
Suggested stimulation techniques for children who are presymbolic and minimally symbolic

Presymbolic Children
  Speak in short sentences of three to five words containing one or two syllables each.
  Speak about entities in the immediate context.
  Speak slowly with pauses and emphasize content words.
  Use self-talk and parallel talk to describe your own and the child's actions, respectively.
  Gesture or use simple signs when it may aid comprehension.
  Allow time for the child to respond even though she or he may not.
  Establish a communication position vis-à-vis the child's face that is comfortable for the
      child and that demonstrates a genuine interest in the child's communication efforts.
  Maintain the child's attention by varying the intensity and pitch of your verbalizations.

Minimally Symbolic Children
In addition to the techniques above:
  Attend to all symbolic initiations.
  Gently correct with feedback.
  Expand the child's communication into a more mature form.
  Reply to the child's communication with a relevant and appropriate comment.
  Do not ask too many adultlike questions. They are difficult to process.

Source: Adapted from Owens, R. (1982d). From the *Program for the Acquisition of Language with the Severely Impaired (PALS),* Copyright © 1982 by The Psychological Corporation. Reproduced by permission. All rights reserved.

bols, such as signs, can be learned singly, possibly in a "signs of the week" program (Spragle & Micucci, 1990).

Formal Training

Formal training, a third strategy, occurs a few brief times daily. The speech-language pathologist monitors this training closely for content, procedures, and the child's progress. She analyzes each skill to be taught for antecedent and consequent events and constructs a hierarchy that includes the steps needed for successful completion. With children who are presymbolic, especially those above preschool age, it is essential that training hierarchies consist of small increments of change. This necessitates a task analysis approach that reflects the child's individual style and sequence of learning, the individual cues necessary, reinforcers, success criteria, and content.

Generalization will be affected by the content selected and by the manner and sequence of formal training. Content or training items and the location of training should come from the child's natural environment. It does little good to train requesting of cookies if the child is unable to have refined sugar or, on a larger scale, to train requesting if the child has little opportunity to use this behavior. The speech-language pathologist must analyze the child's communication environment to determine whether there are natural opportunities for the behavior to occur.

The reinforcement should reflect the child's environment in order to aid generalization. Parents should be trained to respond as naturally as possible. Conversational replies may be best. Consequences, such as "Good talking," occur infrequently in the child's daily interactions and provide little conversational input beyond their reinforcing quality. Conversational responding, such as "Um-hm, that is a horsie, big horsie," is more appropriate and aids generalization to conversation because of its inherent conversational nature.

Child development studies have demonstrated the reinforcing power and teaching potential of *expansion, extension,* and *imitation,* discussed in Chapter 9. *Expansion* is a more adult model of the child's utterance that maintains the child's word order. If the child says, "That bes horsie," the facilitator might respond by expanding to "Um-hm, that is a horsie." In contrast, an *extension* is a reply to the content or topic of the child's utterance. In the previous example, the facilitator might extend to, "Um-hm, Uncle Ed has a horse." Finally, *imitation* is a whole or partial repetition of the child's utterance. In response to, "That bes horsie," the facilitator might repeat, "That bes horsie," or simply say, "Horsie." All three provide feedback on acceptability of the child's utterance within a conversational context. Similar responses can be used with the child's presymbolic behaviors, such as imitating a child's action or expanding it into a more complex action.

CHILD TRAINING

As in assessment, training should focus on both the child's communication system and presymbolic or early symbolic skills. The communication system is expanded and moved ever closer to symbolic communication while the child is learning presymbolic cognitive, social, and communicative skills.

Establishing and Expanding the Communication System

Many older training programs began with the punishment of self-injurious and self-stimulatory behaviors. Facilitators should be careful to note the signal value to the child of these excess behaviors before beginning intervention. In addition to possibly using self-injurious and self-stimulatory behavior in initial communication, the speech-language pathologist can rely on additional techniques, such as behavior chain interruption.

Self-Injurious and Self-Stimulatory Behaviors

Self-injurious, tantruming, and aggressive behavior may signal either frustration and a desire to escape or a call for attention (Carr & Durand, 1985). Although excess behavior cannot be allowed to continue to the child's detriment, punishment should be paired with reinforcement of less destructive, more socially acceptable communication behaviors. To the degree that such behavior signals escape, attention getting, or demand, the frequency should decrease with the learning of more socially acceptable methods of signaling this information (Carr, 1979; Carr & Durand, 1985; Carr & Lovaas, 1982; Donnellan et al., 1984; Durand, 1982; Durand & Kishi, 1986; Horner & Budd, 1983, 1985; L. Meyer & Evans, 1986; Reichle, 1990; Robinson & Owens, in press).

Self-stimulatory behaviors can be treated differently and used as reinforcers for behaviors that are less likely to occur. The child is allowed to engage in self-stimulatory behavior when the speech-language pathologist elicits a social or communication behavior. This training is an application of the *Premack Principle,* which states that a behavior that is highly likely to occur acts as a reinforcer for one less likely to occur.

The child's limited repertoire of behaviors may be expanded through gradual modification or the introduction of more appropriate alternative behaviors to signal intentions. The speech-language pathologist must decide whether to maintain the child's present method of signaling intentions, modify it, or train new signals. In general, such signals may be maintained if they are not part of a perseverative pattern, if their intention is easily discernible, and if they do not call undue attention to the child (Reichle et al., 1988). It is important that the signal be clearly differentiated from others and socially appropriate (Theadore et al., 1990).The speech-language pathologist must find ways to prompt or cue the acceptable communicative behavior prior to the inception of excess behavior in order to decrease and control the excess behavior. It must be stressed that not all excess behavior is socially motivated and, therefore, amenable to reduction with the introduction of functional communication.

Behavior Chain Interruption

Interruption strategies have been used effectively with individuals with severe mental retardation and multiple disabilities (Romer & Schoenberg, 1991). Establishment of a communication system might begin with behavior chain interruption strategies, such as the *resonance training* mentioned in Chapter 12. In resonance training, the facilitator cradles the child and rocks slowly while speaking about the action. This training should not be attempted without consultation with the physical therapist to ensure that handling and positioning are optimal. A large mirror in front of the pair provides feedback on the child's reaction.

Initially, the facilitator is interested primarily in child responses that signal the child's realization that someone has intruded on his space. The child may try to help the facilitator rock by pushing in the direction of the rocking. Although such behavior signals compliance and acceptance, this movement should not serve as a signal when the rocking stops, because it is part of the movement itself (L. Sternberg, 1984). The pushing is, however, an indication that the child is motivated to signal, and the facilitator physically prompts a signal, such as touching her foot or tapping the floor. The prompted signal is followed by continuation of the rocking and the facilitator's talking about the activity. The prompt is faded gradually.

After several sessions in which the child has signaled for the activity to continue, the facilitator changes the criterion and will not begin rocking initially until the child signals. The facilitator and the child assume the rocking posture but do nothing until the child signals. At first, this signal probably will need to be prompted. More important than the signal is the lesson that through communication the child can affect the environment. Development of other related behaviors may occur. For example, the child may produce repetitive actions with objects. The child also should begin to indicate recognition of the facilitator and familiar objects.

As the facilitator moves from a cradling position to a side-by-side or facing one, she is in a better position later to attempt such training as physical imitation, an important presymbolic skill. This phase of training is called *coactive movement*. With fewer and fewer prompts, the child learns to follow an increasingly diverse set of facilitator behaviors, beginning with rocking.

The facilitator can attempt similar behavior chain interruption training with any behavior pleasurable to the child, such as listening to music. The behavior is interrupted and a signal prompted for it to resume (Goetz et al., 1985; P. Hunt, Goetz, Alwell, & Sailor, 1986). Once the signal is used consistently, training moves to initiation. Interruption strategies can be used within a number of pleasurable routines and expanded to include passively blocking a child from the next action, delaying presentation of an item needed for task completion, placing needed items out of reach, and removing needed items (P. Hunt & Goetz, 1988).

Close physical proximity, touching, and a gentle, pleasant manner and voice may help establish an initial communication system. If the child does not respond well to touching or to close proximity, initial assessment and training may have to focus on toleration and desensitization, which usually are accomplished by pairing touching with a pleasurable or reinforcing stimulus.

The child may respond with any of the means already mentioned. With one child, a primitive communication system using eye contact with a spoon to signal "Feed me" was established in a few hours. In another case, a primitive signal system within resonance training was established in only 45 seconds.

The speech-language pathologist can expand the communication system to include environmental *tangible symbols* (Rowland & Schweigert, 1989a), signals, and gestures, such as having the child reach for, touch, or look at common objects prior to beginning everyday activities in which they will be used. For example, she might require the child to look at or touch a toothbrush before brushing. The toothbrush becomes a tangible symbol for brushing and later can signal that activity. Initially, to avoid confusion, the toothbrush used to signal may be the one actually used for brushing, but later brushes should be separate to preserve the signal quality of the nonused one. The object becomes a sign for the event.

Anticipation shelves may be used in which each daily activity is represented by related objects arranged sequentially in boxes on a shelf (L. Sternberg, 1984). At the beginning of each activity, the child removes the sign from its box. After the activity is completed, the child places the tangible symbol into a "done" box. Gradually, the tangible symbol and the event become associated. At the next level of training, the child uses the tangible symbol to initiate the event. Even at the tangible symbol level, success requires at least sensorimotor stage III functioning by the child (L. Sternberg, 1984). The child is using a primitive augmentative communication system.

The speech-language pathologist must be careful at this point in training to ensure that the child engages in communication interaction using the tangible symbols, not just in associational tasks. The objects should be used also to request, protest, and signal notice (Rowland & Schweigert, 1989b).

Presymbolic Training

Obviously, not every behavior of the child developing normally is an appropriate training target. Nor should the speech-language pathologist assume that infant development scales identify the skills that children with language impairment need. These scales often include a variety of activities, many unrelated to symbol use. The speech-language pathologist should select presymbolic targets judiciously, choosing those that affect communication and symbol use. A long list of prerequisites actually may prevent children who are presymbolic from learning to communicate (Wulz et al., 1983).

Although some children who are presymbolic may attain initial language skills when trained first on prerequisite cognitive behaviors, such as means-ends and object permanence, rather than on language alone (Kahn, 1982), the precise presymbolic skills to teach have not been identified. Therefore, each speech-language pathologist must consider "which developmental behaviors and what sequences of mastery" (Switzy, Rotatori, Miller, & Freagon, 1979, p. 169) by determining her own theoretical position.

The speech-language pathologist can determine presymbolic targets by beginning with skills important for the language development of children developing normally, such as means-ends, turn taking, and gestures, and modifying these targets on the basis of some training rationale (Table 13.3) (McLean & Sny-

TABLE 13.3
Determining presymbolic training targets

Presymbolic Cognitive and Social Skills	+	Client Communication Needs	=	Training Targets
Object permanence		Semantic knowledge of objects		Functional use of objects. Appearance, disappearance, and reappearance of objects.
Means-ends		Semantic knowledge of objects		Repeat action with pleasurable outcome. Object manipulation. Indirect means, such as pulling string or winding toy. Tool use.
Gestures		Influence others		Generic (basic, constant) behaviors used to signal. Hierarchy from contact to distal signals. Range of signals.
Turn taking		Interact with others		Joint action routines—Ritualized pattern with a specific theme, following a logical sequence in which each participant plays a specific role, with specific response expectations essential to successful completion

Source: Adapted from McLean, J., & Snyder-McLean, L. (1988b, September). *Assessment and treatment of communicative competencies among clients with severe/profound developmental disabilities.* Workshop presented by Craig Developmental Disabilities Service Office and State University of New York, Genesseo.

der-McLean, 1988b). Each possible presymbolic target should be evaluated on the basis of how it will facilitate the development of symbol use for a specific child.

A general hierarchy of presymbolic skill training was presented in Chapter 12. Even within presymbolic training, such communication skills as turn taking and gestures are targeted. Several commercially available programs also provide extensive information (Bricker & Bricker, 1974; Hanna et al., 1982; Horstmeier & MacDonald, 1978b; Manolson, 1985; Owens, 1982d). Although programs differ on particulars, it generally is accepted that the child should be functioning at Piagetian sensorimotor stage late IV or early V when symbols are introduced (Calculator, 1988c; Owens & Rogerson, 1988).

All training is considered in relation to the three strategies of incidental teaching, stimulation, and formal training. The speech-language pathologist and the other language trainers must keep accurate records of the child's performance and continually adjust the training to meet the child's changing abilities and needs.

Training procedures and sequences mentioned are equally applicable, whether the child's ultimate form of communication is speech, an augmentative system, or a combination. Recognition and receptive training with augmentative systems can begin at a relatively low level of presymbolic functioning. Presymbolic training is not ignored, however, because augmentative symbol systems require a level of cognitive functioning at least as high as that for verbal symbols.

Symbolic Training

Symbolic training is superimposed on a gestural, gestural-vocal, or augmentative base trained previously. At the symbolic level, the dual nature of training in communication and prerequisite skills becomes one as the child's communication system becomes more symbolic in nature.

Symbols should be taught for referents that are established clearly in the client's meaning system. Attempts to teach referential concepts and symbols simultaneously may confuse the child (Romski & Sevcik, 1989). He may associate the symbol with the teaching context, rather than with the referent.

It is important that symbolic training remain functional and fulfill a broad range of communication intentions, whether the means of transmission is verbal or augmentative. All too often, training deteriorates to the child's responding to such cues as, "What's this?" in the hope that the response will be used spontaneously on some future occasion.

Initially, each lexical item should correspond to a specific pragmatic function. General symbols, such as *want, more,* and *no,* might be used. Specific symbols, such as *juice* or *hot,* also may be trained, but they, too, should be function-specific. Children who are minimally symbolic have difficulty generalizing the use of a symbol across several illocutionary functions (Calculator & Delaney, 1986; LaMarre & Holland, 1985).

Careful selection of individual symbols requires a study of the child's environment that is sensitive to the child's needs. Whether the child is using an augmentative or a verbal communication mode, the speech-language pathologist should select vocabulary that is "individualized, functional, and dynamic" (Yorkston, Honsinger, Dowden, & Marriner, 1989, p. 102). Vocabulary should enhance the child's functioning in multiple environments frequently throughout the day, be age appropriate, and be valued by both the child and the caregivers (L. Brown et al., 1988). Vocabulary is dynamic and should be updated continually as the child and the child's environment, knowledge, and needs change (Beukelman, McGinnis, & Morrow, 1991). The lexicon should be "open-ended," capable of modification (Blau, 1983; Carlson, 1981).

Standardized vocabulary lists do not provide a sufficiently thorough lexicon for the individual child. Such lists, if adopted, are inefficient because they contain many words that are rarely used (Holland, 1975; Karlan & Lloyd, 1983; Lahey & Bloom, 1977; Yorkston, Smith, & Beukelman, 1990).

Even lists of the most frequently used words of peers who are nondisabled may be of little value in vocabulary selection because they include such words as *to, a, it, am,* and *and* (Beukelman, Jones, & Rowan, 1989) that are abstract and difficult to teach, especially at the single-symbol level of communication. Lexicons based on frequency of occurrence by the individual child within different natural communication contexts may yield a short but highly useful list of symbols.

The child should be involved in vocabulary selection to the best of his abilities. The speech-language pathologist can observe daily activities and "script" them for possible vocabulary needed (Carlson, 1981). Caregivers, too, can suggest vocabulary. The speech-language pathologist should be careful to select symbols that reflect the child's needs. If symbols chosen relate only to basic needs, however, the system's use will be very restricted (Morrow et al., 1993). Table 13.4 is a list of the words most commonly selected by caregivers.

Too often, training concentrates on limited use of nouns, ignoring the rich presymbolic functional communication of children developing normally. It is assumed by trainers that nouns are easier to learn and more functional than other types of words (Beukelman et al., 1991). Social-regulative terms, such as *please, thank you, excuse me, I'm sorry, I'm finished, be quiet, stop, help, more, good, yes, no, I want, hello,* and *good-bye,* also can be learned easily and can increase normalization of communication (Adamson, Romski, Deffenbach, & Sevcik, 1992; Buzolich, King, & Baroody, 1991). Symbols such as *please, thank you,* and *toilet* may reflect caregiver desires, however, and have little relevance for the child. Symbols learned but not used by the child are of little value; thus, the need for such words must be established first.

The speech-language pathologist can use a combination of the gestural intentions already present and verbal and nonverbal cues to vary the child's behavior. For example, symbols are first trained in imitation to cues, such as, "Say ___ " ("Sign ___," "Point to ___," etc.), when the child demonstrates an interest in or desire for an entity. This verbal cue is accompanied by a nod that signals the child to respond. The trainer also may prompt by beginning the response for the child.

Verbal imitative cues should be minimized and decreased as soon as possible to decrease possible dependence. This reduction is especially true for children with autism who may develop echolalia. Child-initiated communication may not occur unless it is planned.

The verbal cue "Say" ("Sign," "Point to") can be faded gradually and the response shifted to the visual nodding cue. The child now will respond with the name after the trainer names the object and nods. Gradually, the verbal model is faded. Because the child will name in response to a nod, he can be cued in other ways to get a range of illocutionary and semantic functions. It is possible to train a variety of functions for each symbol, thus increasing the child's repertoire.

Words, signs, and visual symbols are learned faster for requesting than for labeling (J. Goodman & Remington, 1993). General symbols for *want* or *more* have broad application and will occur frequently, thus enhancing generalization to the transfer environment (Reichle, 1990; Stremel-Campbell et al., 1984). More explicit symbols, such as "hamburger," place less burden for interpretation on the listener but have narrower application than do vaguer general symbols. General symbols can be paired with object and event names to form longer utterances, such as "Want juice" or "More book."

TABLE 13.4
Most common caregiver selected words for training

afraid	close	goodbye	library	popcorn	take
alone	coat	grandfather	lie (down)	potatoes	talk
alphabet	coke	grandma	little	pretty	teacher
am	cold	grandmother	living room	pull	telephone
apple	comb	grandpa	love	purple	thank you
applesauce	come	grapes	mad	push	thirsty
are	computer	green	magazine	puzzle	tired
arm	cookie	grits	make	radio	toast
bad	crazy	ham	McDonald's	read	toilet
ball	cry	hamburger	meat	record player	toothbrush
banana	dad	hand	medicine	red	toothpaste
bathroom	dance	happy	milk	restaurant	towel
bedroom	dining room	has	mom	ride	truck
behind	dirty	hat	mouth	roast beef	t-shirt
beside	doctor	head	need	root beer	turn
between	down	hear	no	run	tv
bicycle	draw	hello	nose	sad	ugly
big	drink	help	numbers	school	under
black	ears	home	oatmeal	see	underwear
blanket	eat	hospital	on	shirt	up
blocks	eggs	hot	open	shoes	upset
blue	elbow	hotdog	orange	shorts	walk
boat	empty	how	outside	sick	want
book	eyes	hungry	over	sing	was
break	fall	hurry	pancakes	sit	water
broken	fat	hurt	pants	sleep	were
brown	feel	I	paper	smell	wet
bus	fight	ice cream	park	soap	what
buy	fish	in	pear	socks	when
cake	fix	is	peas	soft drink	where
candy	foot	jeans	pencil	soup	who
car	french fries	juice	pie	spaghetti	why
carrots	funny	kiss	pizza	stand	work
carry	game	kitchen	plane	stomach	write
cereal	give	knee	play	stop	yellow
chest	gloves	know	playground	store	yes
chicken	go	laugh	please	supermarket	yuck
church	good	leg	poor	sweater	zoo

Source: Morrow, D. R., Mirenda, P., Beukelman, D. R., & Yorkston, K. M. (1993). Vocabulary selection for augmentative communication systems: A comparison of three techniques. *American Journal of Speech-Language Pathology, 2*(2), 19-30. Printed with permission.

Initially, the speech-language pathologist should require both gestures and verbalizations of the child because there is often a lack of correspondence between the two with young learners (Baer, Williams, Osnes, & Stokes, 1984; Guevremont, Osnes, & Stokes, 1986a, 1986b). Unless the child chains the verbal and nonverbal behaviors, correspondence between the two may not occur. Through training that uses two items, one desirable and one not, the child can learn to make specific requests for the desirable one (Piche-Cragoe, Reichle, & Sigafoos, 1986).

The trainer modifies intonation and gestures that accompany a single symbol to model a variety of functions. For example, "cup" said while pushing it away might indicate a semantic function of negation and an illocutionary function of protest or command. Such a behavior might be termed a *negative command* or *protest*. The trainer might cue questioning by saying, "Guess what's behind my back," and prompting questions. Responses such as *Doggie?* or *Drink?* would fulfill a *nominative question* function.

Speech-language pathologists should target also a variety of semantic functions. Routinely they train agent and object symbols while giving less attention to other categories, such as action (K. Chapman & Terrell, 1988). Initially, children use action-related symbols called *protoverbs*. These verblike symbols, which accompany specific actions the children perform, include *up, down, no, on-here, inside, there, get-down, bye-bye, night-night,* and *out* (Barrett, 1983; Benedict, 1979; E. Clark, 1979). Gradually, each symbol acquires broader meaning and becomes decontextualized.

Multisymbol combinations should be trained gradually. It is vital that the child not be introduced to too many new training targets simultaneously. Lexical items should be learned prior to being taught in symbol combinations (Mineo & Goldstein, 1990). At this point, receptive comprehension and expressive production seem to be mutually beneficial, and it might be best that the child has many exposures to the semantic pattern targeted, such as agent + action, prior to requiring comprehension or production (Goldstein, 1985; Smeets & Striefel, 1976).

A matrix training format, illustrated in Figure 10.4, may be useful for presentation (H. Goldstein, 1983, 1985; H. Goldstein, Angelo, & Mousetis, 1987). Children are able to generalize to combinations of symbols not explicitly taught.

Modified Milieu Approach

Within the classroom, a modified version of the milieu or mand-model approach described in Chapter 8 can be used with children who are presymbolic to teach them requesting and commenting or declaring (Warren, Yoder, Gazdag, Kim, & Jones, 1993). The techniques generalize across different materials, settings, teachers, and interactive styles.

Requesting and commenting have been targeted because these are the earliest developing intentions and the most frequent illocutionary functions in the presymbolic period (Bates, O'Connell, & Shore, 1987; Wetherby, Cain, Yonclas, & Walker, 1988). In addition, these are the building blocks for later symbolic communication (Bruner, Roy, & Ratner, 1980; Snow, 1989).

As the severity of a child's language impairment increases, there are fewer and fewer opportunities for prelinguistic communication and thus fewer opportunities to teach (Brooks-Gunn & Lewis, 1984; P. Yoder, 1987; P. Yoder & Feagans, 1988). The milieu approach uses naturally occurring situations and prompts child responses to those situations.

The environment is arranged so that the child can select a toy for play. The adult follows the child's lead with the toy and initiates familiar turn-taking games. Within this activity, the trainer uses the techniques described in Table 13.5.

Classroom modeling alone may be a superior strategy to modeling in individual pull-out sessions for early symbolic training (Wilcox et al., 1991). In classrooms are more opportunities for activities and more conversational partners, and the routine lends itself to more scriptlike scaffolding of communication.

Augmentative Communication

The use of augmentative systems can improve speech intelligibility, increase communication initiations, and improve overall communication skills (Calculator & D'Altilio-Luchko, 1983; Glennen & Calculator, 1985; Hurlbut et al., 1982; Kouri, 1989; Kraat, 1985; Pecyna, 1984, 1988; Reichle & Karlan, 1985; Romski, Sevcik, & Joyner, 1984; Romski, White, Millen, & Rumbaugh, 1984). Although data are difficult to obtain, it is estimated that as high as 25% of those with severe and profound mental retardation use sign to communicate (Bryen, Goldman, & Quinlisk-Gill, 1988). Others may use communication boards or electronic augmentative systems.

Augmentative communication systems can be divided into two categories: unaided and aided. *Unaided systems* consist of sign systems, such as American Sign Language or Signed English, and gesture systems, such as American Indian Signs. *Aided systems* use some piece of equipment to assist communication. These usually are classified as non-electronic and electronic. Non-electronic devices include several types of communication boards as diverse as wallet foldouts, wheelchair-mounted trays, and Plexiglas windows containing pictures or symbols. Textured shapes, such as from corrugated cardboard, sponge, sandpaper, rubber stair treads, plastic mesh, quilt with stitching, fur, carpet, and towel, have been used effectively with children with severe/profound mental retardation and multiple disabilities (Murray-Branch, Udavari-Solner, & Bailey, 1991). Electronic devices are as diverse as simple lights above selected symbols and computer-assisted systems with simultaneous voice and audio output. Even a portable transistor radio can be modified to produce an oscillating tone as an attention-getting device (T. King, 1991).

One method of augmentative communication—facilitated communication—should be mentioned here, although it will not be discussed in detail. *Facilitated communication* is a spelling method of communication developed primarily for children with severe cerebral palsy and adapted for children with autism (Crossley & McDonald, 1980). It aids the child in overcoming neuromotor difficulties that inhibit speech and, some believe, may be at the heart of autism (Crossley, 1988).

TABLE 13.5
Techniques in a modified milieu approach

Requesting

Prompt-Free Approach: Hold up a highly desirable item, obtain eye contact, and wait, gazing at the child with raised eyebrows and quizzical look.

If child produces request correctly, respond to illocutionary function of the utterance with a comment, possibly a semantically related two-word utterance, and give the item to the child.

If no response or incorrect response, provide assistance to complete.

If no eye contact previously, say, "Look at me." Recue.

If no response or incorrect response, provide a verbal/sign/graphic (picture on communication board) model.

If no response again, provide physical assistance to sign or point.

Prompted Approach: Either stop activity and ask, "What do you want? or hold item needed to resume an activity and ask, "Do you want this?"
Wait.

If child produces request correctly, respond to illocutionary function of the utterance with a comment, possibly a semantically related two-word utterance, and obtain the item for the child.

If no response, incorrect response, or incomplete response, provide assistance to complete.

If no eye contact previously, say, "Look at me." Recue.

If no response or incorrect response, provide a verbal/sign/graphic model and a physical pointing model toward the object.

If no response again, provide physical assistance to sign, point to symbol, or point to the object.

If incomplete response, say "What?"

Commenting

Frequently model commenting. Focus on what the child is attending to (joint attending) and verbalize ("Wow" or "Good" or "Yuck"). Cue child to imitate with, "Say ___," or, "You say it."

If child imitates, respond conversationally.

Fade model as spontaneous use increases.

Physically back away and attend elsewhere as novel items are introduced. Respond to child's vocalizations as if they attract your attention.

Labeling

Establish joint attending with the child and verbalize the name of the item of focus.

If child imitates label, respond to the illocutionary function of the utterance and expand into semantically related two-word utterance.

If label incorrect, give corrective feedback ("No, that's a horse"). Cue the child to imitate.

Respond to spontaneous utterances by expanding or extending the utterance.

Source: Adapted from Kozleski (1991); Warren, Yoder, Gazdag, Kim, & Jones (1993); Wilcox, Kouri, & Caswell (1991)

The child is taught to type with minimal physical support from a facilitator, first hand-over-hand or hand-at-wrist, progressing through touch to independent functioning (Biklen, Morton, Gold, Berrigan, & Swaminathan, 1992). Ideally, the facilitator does not guide the child to the target letters, but rather supports the child's hand and pulls the child's hand back after each letter is touched. Support is faded as soon as the child begins to use the aid successfully. Training begins with structured practice, such as object names, question-answer, crossword puzzles, and matching games, and progresses to conversation.

Although many claims of success have been made (Biklen, 1990, 1992a, 1992b; Biklen & Schubert, 1991; Crossley, 1988), detractors are quick to note the lack of stringent research criteria (Calculator, 1992a, 1992b). Most children using facilitated communication had acquired literary skills first but had no way of demonstrating them (Crossley & Remington-Gurney, 1992). In this way, these children are very different from the children who are presymbolic and minimally symbolic discussed in this chapter. Facilitated communication "is not by itself the answer to severe communication problems" (Crossley & Remington-Gurney, 1992, p. 42), but unfortunately, its reported success has led to unrealistic expectations for some presymbolic clients.

The ease in learning augmentative communication systems depends on the child's overall developmental and communication level, the system chosen, and the training method (Mirenda & Locke, 1989; Mizuko, 1987; Pecyna, 1984). Although the exact level of development necessary for a truly functional communication system is unknown, this factor should not be ignored even for low-level gestural systems.

Symbol transparency or "guessability" is one consideration in system selection and training. In general, the more a representation or symbol resembles the real object, the more transparent it is (C. Clark, 1981; Ecklund & Reichle, 1987; Hurlbut et al., 1982; Mirenda & Locke, 1989; Mizuko, 1987; Sevcik & Romski, 1986; Vanderheiden & Lloyd, 1986). Thus, pictures or manual signs that resemble their referents are more transparent and easier to learn. Figure 13.1 presents the order of graphic augmentative systems by transparency.

Readers should note the seemingly illogical location of miniature objects in this figure. Children who are presymbolic may not see miniatures as representing real objects (Vanderheiden & Lloyd, 1986). It is also important to remember that whereas whole systems may be more or less transparent, individual signs or symbols vary greatly (Bloomberg, Karlan, & Lloyd, 1990). In addition, it should be noted that judgments of transparency by children developing normally and by adults do not necessarily reflect the perceptions of children who are presymbolic and have language impairment (Bloomberg et al., 1990; Dunham, 1989). Young children especially do not make the same types of associations as adults (Bruno & Goehl, 1991). For example, an adult might associate *candle* with light, but a child might associate it with Christmas. Nor does the level of transparency correlate with the task of learning to use a symbol system or with specific skills needed for learning such as visual perception (Sevcik, Romski, & Wilkinson, 1991).

Other determiners of the ease of manual sign learning are symmetry, inclusion of a portion of the body, and concreteness. In general, signs are easier to

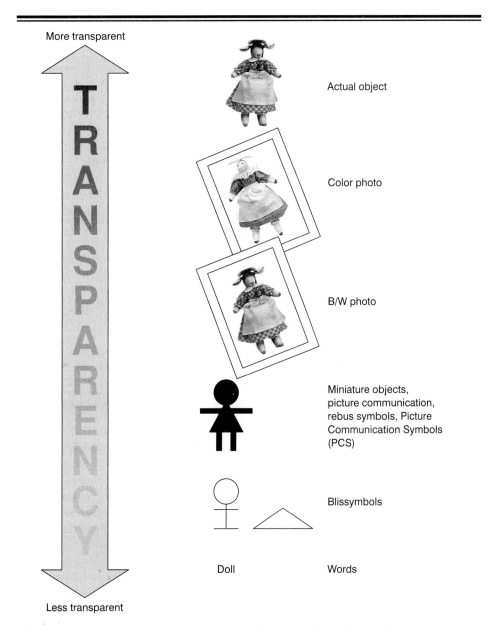

More transparent

T
R
A
N
S
P
A
R
E
N
C
Y

Actual object

Color photo

B/W photo

Miniature objects, picture communication, rebus symbols, Picture Communication Symbols (PCS)

Blissymbols

Doll

Words

Less transparent

More transparent or more guessable visual systems are easier to learn than are less transparent ones.

FIGURE 13.1
Transparency of graphic augmentative communication systems
Source: Bloomberg, Karlan, & Lloyd (1990); Burroughs, Albritton, Eaton, & Montague (1990); Mirenda & Locke (1989)

learn if both hands move symmetrically and the body is touched in some way, and if the signs are concrete rather than abstract (Kohl, 1981). Even though bilateral arm movements develop earlier than unilateral, they still may be very difficult for someone with motoric involvement (Keogh & Sugden, 1985). For children with mental retardation, the easiest signs to imitate are also the easiest to learn to produce, although there seems to be no effect on receptive language (Kiernan, 1984).

Intervention.   Often, the concept that symbols have a function is the most difficult aspect of training for children who are presymbolic (Romski, Sevcik, & Pate, 1988). The cognitive-linguistic relationship is not clearly understood for children with severe/profound mental retardation (Reichle & Karlan, 1985). Initial contact between the symbol and the client might be by chance. Children with severe/profound mental retardation and sensory impairments can be taught to relate textured shapes with their referents in this manner (Murray-Branch et al., 1991). When the child accidentally touches the shape, he is given the referent. Gradually, the child makes the association, and his behavior becomes more purposeful. The size of the shape is reduced as the child becomes better able to discriminate. Next, requesting is trained by using a physical prompting technique.

Children must learn that they can affect change through symbol use. The speech-language pathologist can encourage the child to select a representation or symbol of a desired item to gain some control of his world. Initially, the child selects the one representation or symbol presented. Foils, such as an uninteresting item or a blank picture, then are introduced. Two-item choices are trained next. The facilitator might use a modified vending machine device using light, sound, and symbol cues to train children to choose from among several desired items (Romski et al., 1988). In similar fashion, a child might use eye contact with a television or stereo to signal a request for TV or music, respectively.

Once communication is established with other people, the maintenance of that interaction can be attributed to the reciprocity inherent in communication (Kohler & Fowler, 1985). In other words, the reciprocal nature of communication is reinforcing for both partners.

Children with more severe or multiple disabilities may have difficulty moving from gestural communication to abstract symbols. These children have difficulty with the one-to-one relational concept of symbol-to-referent. This learning is made more difficult by the simultaneous shift from context-bound gestural systems to more context-free symbols.

For children using aided systems, the transition to symbols might begin with the easier task of match-to-sample (Saunders & Spradlin, 1989). In match-to-sample, the child picks from an available group of objects, pictures, or symbols the one that matches the "sample" held by the trainer. Two discrimination tasks are involved in matching: first, discriminating the choice from the others available in the group; second, matching the sample and the choice, a successive task and the more difficult of the two (Carter & Eckerman, 1975). Obviously, matching an object, such as a ball, to another sample object would be easier than matching a picture or symbol to an object. Before moving to this more symbolic task, the speech-language pathologist should ensure that the child can match both objects to objects and pictures or symbols to their like members.

Mentioned previously, tangible symbols, or representations in the form of objects or pictures with a clear perceptual relationship to the referent, can form a link between gestural and symbolic systems of communication. Actual objects or identifiable packaging might be used. Between the actual object and the color photo levels of transparency on Figure 13.1, the following three levels of representation might exist (Rowland & Schweigert, 1989a):

1. Associated objects, such as a shoelace to represent a shoe
2. Shared feature objects, such as a cookie refrigerator magnet to represent a real cookie
3. Artificial associations in which an object appears on the communication board and also is attached to the referent, such as a wooden apple on the cafeteria door to represent meals

A *cue-pause-point* method (McMorrow, Fox, Faw, & Bittle, 1987) has been effective in teaching responsive use of signs (Fox, Kyle, Faw, & Bittle, 1988). In this method, the child is taught a signed answer and then must await the appropriate question. Pauses are used at critical points to encourage responding. Table 13.6. presents the training steps in sequence. As the prompts are removed systematically, the signs are maintained and generalized to novel questions.

To forestall the child's learning of responsive communication behaviors only, the speech-language pathologist can train requesting, mentioned previously, and commenting. Commenting allows the user to convey an attitude or opinion and includes expressions such as *wow, yuck, fun, I don't like this,* and *great.* These can be learned first through modeling, then by direct cuing ("You could say ___"), and finally by indirect cuing ("What would you say?") (Buzolich et al.,

TABLE 13.6
Cue-pause-point method for teaching responsive use of signs

Step I:	Ask a question, such as, "What's that?" "Where's ___?" or, "What do we eat with?" Present signed answer. Pause prompt: Hold finger up to prevent signing until cued again.
Step II:	Ask a question, such as, "Where's ___?" or, "What do we eat with?" Point prompt: Point to object that answers question.
Step III:	If incorrect response to Step II, train object or item name by sign imitation.
Step IV:	If correct in Step II, cover the object and repeat Step II.

Provide feedback at each step.

Source: Adapted from Foxx, Kyle, Faw, & Bittle (1988); McMorrow, Fox, Faw, & Bittle (1987)

1991). Finally, eye contact, a nod, and/or an expectant delay can be used as mentioned previously.

Generalization.   As with other aspects of communication training, there is often a lack of generalization of augmentative system use. This problem may result from (a) facilitator-centered or -controlled training, (b) unintelligibility of the child's system as used, (c) the precedence within training of the system over the communication process, (d) nonuse of natural settings, and (e) nonusers' lack of response in the natural environment (Calculator, 1988b). One survey of children with severe/profound mental retardation who were learning signing found that augmentative training (a) frequently ignored receptive comprehension, (b) was taught primarily through imitation while rarely encouraging spontaneous use, (c) was rarely taught in meaningful situations outside the therapy setting, and (d) often chose vocabulary that was irrelevant to ongoing activities and interests of the child (Bryen et al., 1988). The result was that on average after 3 years of training, the children had only four signs they produced spontaneously. In general, children with severe/profound mental retardation and multiple disabilities learn augmentative communication very slowly and exhibit poor generalization skills (Siegel-Causey, Ernst, & Guess, 1987).

Intervention should focus on encouraging flexible use of various modes of communication (Downing & Siegel-Causey, 1988). Instead, as in verbal symbolic training, the means of transmission and/or the code often is taught separately from the communication function of the symbols. The goal of training becomes learning the system, rather than optimizing communication. This inflexibility is obvious when a child who is nonspeaking is required to rely on an augmentative response, such as signing "no" when a head shake would suffice.

Targets should be functional, such as requesting aid or objects from other people, rejecting or protesting, and commenting (L. Brown et al., 1984; Calculator & Jorgensen, 1991; Reichle, 1990; Reichle et al., 1984). Thus, the child learns to control acquisition and refusal of specific entities within the environment. In general, requesting is easier to train than are the other functions (Reichle et al., 1988). The child might touch desired items to signal a request (Klein et al., 1981). Both preferred and nonpreferred items should be offered so that the child must make an active choice. Otherwise, the signal becomes a general request, rather than a discriminating one (Reichle, 1990). Once a choice is made, the facilitator can probe the child's choice by offering two items: the requested one and another. The speech-language pathologist can expand requesting behaviors with the use of a generalized request signal, such as *want* or *more*. She can place the printed symbol for *want* or *more* before the child as he reaches for desired items. The child touches the signal in the process of reaching for the item.

The child might signal protest or rejection by pushing away unwanted objects (Stremel-Campbell et al., 1984). An instructional prompt to touch a rejection or protest signal can be delivered prior to offering items that are predictably refused (Reichle, 1990). The child might be taught also to use a general rejection signal (*no*) in different situations (Keogh & Reichle, 1985). The comment function can be taught by using object names or labels (Koegh & Reichle, 1985). Initially, commenting serves a notice function that directs the attention of others and may be signaled by a generalized "look" or "notice me" signal. For ease of learning, separate lexical items should be used for different functions.

Vocabulary size can be increased by the flexible use of multimodality responding, including gestures, nods, signs, pictures, and vocal-verbal behaviors (Mirenda & Schuler, 1988; Morrow et al., 1993). If the child can shake his head "no," there is no reason at the onset of augmentative system use for him to be forced to use a symbol or sign to replace it. Children developing normally use many modes of communicating.

Multimodality communication may be more difficult for some children because of the different memory tasks involved (Iacono, Mirenda, & Beukelman, 1993). Pictures and visual symbols require recognitory memory; signs and speech require recall memory (Bristow & Fristoe, 1984; Kiernan, 1983).

Symbols used for many illocutionary functions can give the child a very flexible system (Owens, 1982d). Children developing normally use a small core vocabulary in just such a way. The 25 most frequently used words of preschoolers make up 45.1% of what they say (Beukelman et al., 1989). Too often, augmentative communication users exhibit a limited range of illocutionary functions (Light, 1988).

Training should stress both receptive comprehension and expressive production. Learning symbol use in one mode, such as production, does not ensure transfer to another, such as comprehension. In general, expressive learning of signs is best for symbols previously known receptively in speech (Clarke, 1987; Light, Remington, Clarke, & Watson, 1989). The reverse is not true (Remington & Clarke, 1983). Children tend to overselect the visual model in expressive training and to ignore the verbal name for the symbol they are being taught to express. This problem can be overcome by training receptive use first or by using differential sign training in which the cue alternates between a verbal-visual cue and a verbal-only one (Remington & Clarke, 1993a, 1993b).

Because generalization from simulated environments to the transfer or natural environment is difficult for many presymbolic clients, augmentative communication systems should be trained within a wide variety of functional activities as these naturally occur in the transfer environment (Calculator, 1985, 1988b; Calculator & Jorgensen, 1991; Falvey, 1986; Falvey, Bishop et al., 1988; Guess & Helmstetter, 1986; Kangas & Lloyd, 1988; Light, Collier, & Parnes, 1985; Orelove & Sobsey, 1987, Siegel-Causey & Downing, 1987). When trained within everyday activities, communication becomes relevant to the child's world (Nietupski, Scheutz, & Ockwood, 1980). Generalization is especially difficult for children with severe/profound mental retardation (Snell & Browder, 1986). Unfortunately, training, even with augmentative systems, too often consists of unnatural, out-of-context, mass-trial formats (Helmstetter & Guess, 1987).

The spontaneous use of augmentative systems can be a problem for both the user and the communication partner or nonuser. Compared with speakers, augmentative users have fewer conversational partners and engage in shorter exchanges (Kraat, 1985). Caregivers may know few signs and use them only infrequently outside training (Bryen et al., 1988; Bryen & McGinley, 1991). If the child only uses the system with the speech-language pathologist, then she becomes a discriminative stimulus for system use (Stremel-Campbell & Campbell, 1985).

Although augmentative systems can improve the quality of the communication, at present most users still have considerable delay as they produce their responses. Production time can be decreased for aided systems by the placement of items on a communication board, by the vocabulary selected, by careful analysis of the child-device interface, and by multimodality responding.

For more advanced children, especially those with motoric difficulties, who are able to type their messages, communication can be painfully slow. Studies of speed increase have focused on lessening the necessary keystrokes in any given message (Higginbothom, 1992). Computer-generated prediction systems that attempt to complete a child's electronically generated message on the basis of the most frequent words used have been effective in enhancing augmentative system use and in shortening transmission time (Newell et al., 1992). Other methods of decreasing the time include abbreviated or encoded strategies, such as prestored prefixes and suffixes and lexicons (Creech, 1989; Goodenough-Trepagnier, & Prather, 1981; Goodenough-Trepagnier, Tarry, & Prather, 1982; Schwejda, 1986; Swiffin, Arnott, Pickering, & Newell, 1987; Vanderheiden & Kelso, 1987; Woltosz, 1988).

In general, the nonuser partner assumes a disproportionate responsibility for the conversation (Buzolich & Wiemann, 1988; Farrier, Yorkston, Marriner, & Beukelman, 1985). Nonuser behavior often is based on nonuser assumptions of user competence. Although the system output seems to affect such assumptions very little, the length of the user messages is significant in judgments of competence (Hoag & Bedrosian, 1992). With little expectation that the user will participate, nonusers may talk around the user, fall into a yes-no probing strategy, answer their own questions or comment before the user can answer, use less mature language, and anticipate a response and preempt (Calculator & Dollaghan, 1982; Goosens & Kraat, 1985; Shane et al., 1982). These modifications cause the user to lose control of the conversation. In turn, the child may underfunction or behave as if he is much more limited.

This underfunctioning is reported frequently for augmentative communication users (Calculator, 1985; Houghton et al., 1987). It is the result of insufficient motivation to communicate, which may be caused by a lack of opportunity or reason to communicate or by a lack of responsiveness by nonusers. The child adopts a pattern of passivity and learned helplessness (Basil, 1992; Kraat, 1985; Light, 1988; D. Yoder, 1984).

Nonuser partners can change their behavior, but doing so requires that the speech-language pathologist instruct them in the use of the augmentative system too (Calculator & D'Altilio-Luchko, 1983). Instruction is especially important if the expectations and demands of the environment are dissimilar from those used in teaching the user. The speech-language pathologist can teach even peers who are preschool nonusers to become good partners and to initiate, turn take, and respond (Goldstein & Ferrell, 1987). She also can effectively and efficiently train and integrate caregivers into the training process through a combination of in-service and direct training and by including them in the assessment and goal-setting process (McNaughton & Light, 1989).

After only a few short sessions in which caregivers are taught via demonstrations and role playing to facilitate communication, they are able to decrease their control of communication effectively, to initiate less, to respond more, to use more open-ended questions, and to wait for the child to initiate or respond (Basil, 1992; Light, Dattilo, English, Gutierrez, & Hartz, 1992). More importantly, these changes can generalize to everyday interactions, especially with follow-up by the speech-language pathologist.

The speech-language pathologist should encourage use of the child's augmentative communication system whenever possible throughout the day by using incidental and stimulation techniques. She reinforces both the child and the caregivers for augmentative system usage. In general, the more the child and the caregivers use the system, the more it will generalize. The key to successful learning and use is a system that is easy to use, an ability by the child to be understood, and a motivation to imitate and use the system in response to natural cues in everyday contexts (Halle, 1987; McGregor, Young, Gerak, Thomas, & Vogelsberg, 1992; Rotholz, Berkowitz, & Burberry, 1989).

COMMUNICATION ENVIRONMENT MANIPULATION

The speech-language pathologist can modify the child's communication environment in several ways to enhance communication and training. The environment can scaffold both natural and contrived opportunities for learning. After a thorough analysis of the communication demands placed on the child, she identifies high and low communication contexts by location, activities, and communication partners.

High communication contexts are encouraged and increased. Modifications would change the interactional quality between the child and the environment. For example, the child's daily routine might be changed to provide more opportunities to interact with a certain classroom aide with whom the child vocalizes frequently. These high-communication contexts often offer ideal opportunities for incidental teaching. For example, the aide mentioned might be trained to elicit a variety of vocalizations from the child within their daily routine. Because the child is communicating at a high level, presumably because the context is reinforcing, the speech-language pathologist can change the manner of that communication and modify the context to enhance communication training while leaving the interaction intact.

The facilitator modifies or eliminates low communication contexts. For example, the child's communication behavior may elicit no response from the school bus aide. The facilitator might instruct this person in a few simple methods of conversational responding to increase the communication learning potential of this situation. If the child spends long periods each day in solitary play, these times might be eliminated or changed to parallel group play.

INTERACTIONAL CHANGES

As noted in the previous section, caregivers can become effective agents of change for presymbolic and minimally symbolic individuals if trained and monitored appropriately (Baker, 1976; Heifetz, 1980; Owens et al., 1987; Salzberg & Villani, 1983). Caregivers will need guidance to help them redefine their perceptions of their child's abilities (Sameroff & Feise, 1990). This change of attitude may require helping caregivers reassess communication breakdowns and identify subtle ways in which their child may be communicating. Caregivers should be encouraged to alter nonfacilitative strategies. Initial caregiver training might begin with the following three principles (MacDonald, 1985):

1. Everyone engages in some form of communication.
2. Every communication occurrence has the potential for reciprocity.
3. Expectation of one partner affects motivation of the other to initiate communication.

Children's language development is greatly influenced by the interactive style of adults in the child's environment. Children learn to the extent to which they communicate in contexts that support these endeavors and are reciprocal and balanced (MacDonald & Carroll, 1992b).

Possible targets for caregiver interactional training might include learning to abandon her or his own agenda and to follow the child's lead, to establish joint attention and action, to give the child the freedom to make meaningful choices, to balance turn taking with no one partner dominating, to be less directive, to respond in a semantically and pragmatically contingent manner, and to use a variety of illocutionary functions and a child lexicon (Dobe, 1989; Holton, 1987; MacDonald, 1989; MacDonald & Carroll, 1992b; Manolson, 1985; Theadore et al., 1990; J. Young, 1988). Essentially, the adult is learning to fine-tune her or his communication for the abilities of the child. Possible changes in caregiver behaviors are listed in Table 13.7.

Even minimum instruction in training techniques is beneficial and enables some caregivers to adopt suitable teaching strategies spontaneously (Cheseldine & McConkey, 1979). Feedback from the speech-language pathologist regarding the application of newly acquired teaching skills, however, is the critical element (Polk, Schilmoeller, Emboy, Holman, & Baer, 1976; Salzberg & Villani, 1983). Caregivers cannot be expected to function in a vacuum with little input from the speech-language pathologist.

The speech-language pathologist can train caregivers to perform formal training, elicit trained responses, and provide appropriate language input for the

TABLE 13.7
Possible changes in caregiver behavior as a result of training

Balancing conversational partnership with child
  Physically prompt child to take a turn.
  Wait expectantly.
  Allow enough time for child's turn.
  Follow the child's lead.
  Respond in meaningful ways to keep the conversation going.
Matching the child's linguistic abilities
  Respond to movements and sounds with similar ones.
  Expand one-word utterances to two words or short phrases.
  Add something to the child's turn that is slightly more mature.
  Act like the child in interactions.
Responding contingently
  Respond to even the slightest behaviors.
  Pay attention to appropriate behavior while ignoring immature or disruptive behavior.
  Respond immediately to imitated behaviors.
  Be fun to be with; be a reinforcer.
Being nondirective
  Limit questions and directives to authentic ones.
  Wait and expect.
  Match child's language and cognitive level.
  Engage child in conversations of more than one turn.
  Follow child's lead but expect that he will follow yours on occasion.
Becoming emotionally attached
  Balance your turns for length.
  Match the child's interest and communication.
  Respond sensitively.
  Share the lead, be nondirective.
  Enjoy your time together.
  Reduce stress by focusing on play, not achievement.
  Avoid negative judgments.
  Concentrate on keeping the interaction going, rather than on correcting the child.

Source: Adapted from MacDonald, J., & Carroll, J. (1992b). A social partnership model for assessing early communication development: An interaction model for preconversational children. *Language, Speech, and Hearing Services in Schools, 23,* 113–124.

child. Training caregivers to provide structured formal training has been very successful (MacDonald et al., 1974; Salzberg & Villani, 1983).

The caregiver can elicit trained responses within the home or classroom through environmental manipulation (McNaughton & Light, 1989; Wulz et al., 1983). After the child is taught to respond to *need to communicate* situations, the caregiver restructures needs-meeting situations within daily routines so that the child's needs are not anticipated but are dependent on the communication behavior. The behavior becomes situationally dependent and makes sense in context, rather than dependent on a verbal prompt from the facilitator (Halle, 1987).

Child-caregiver interactions may be restructured formally to encourage and require communication (Horstmeier & MacDonald, 1978a). The caregivers can structure elicitation situations, such as turn-taking games, choice-making, enticement with desirable items, and assistance requesting (McNaughton & Light, 1989). Once a skill is learned, the child is required to use that skill to attain desired entities or privileges for which it was not formerly required. Previously accepted behaviors are no longer sufficient.

Children may omit the initial step of obtaining their partner's attention when necessary prior to communicating. A two-step procedure of attention getting and message transmission is difficult to teach (Sobsey & Reichle, 1986). Children assume that other people will always attend when they communicate if this is the training situation. It may be difficult for the child to discriminate between situations that require attention getting and those that do not.

A strategy of *waiting*, or time delay, has been used effectively to enhance spontaneous use of trained communication behaviors (Charhop, Schreibman, & Thebodeau, 1985; Gobbi, Cipani, Hudson, & Lapenta-Neudeck, 1986). This procedure is most effective when the child desires some item or has to communicate to complete a task. The presence of a language trainer also may act as a nonlinguistic cue to stimulate production (Carr & Kologinsky, 1983).

Interactive routines in which the child has some expectation from past events offer an opportunity to create a need to communicate (McLean et al., 1991). The facilitator can wait as the child anticipates and hopefully signals.

Other effective strategies for child initiation are *introduction of novel elements*, *oversight*, and *sabotage* (McLean & Snyder-McLean, 1988b). Novel items usually spark a notice of referential response. Oversight is simply forgetting to complete some task or to add a crucial step, such as intentionally leaving the peanut butter out of a peanut butter sandwich. Finally, sabotage is the introduction of challenging actions or events that prevent some activity, such as tying shoes together prior to giving them to the child to put on. The goal is for the child to request assistance.

Finally, the stimulation behaviors discussed previously can be a helpful guide for caregiver interactional behaviors. The following are additional conversational suggestions (MacDonald & Gillette, 1986):

Structure the activity for give-and-take.

Follow the child's lead.

Imitate the child.

WAIT for the child to take a turn.

SIGNAL the child to take a turn.

Chain responses by using turnabouts, in which a turn includes both a response to the child's turn, as well as a cue for the child to take another turn.

Summary

Communication training should be ongoing for children who are presymbolic and minimally symbolic. Caregivers should administer training under the speech-language pathologist's direction and guidance. Throughout the day within each child's natural communication environment, caregivers use the three intervention techniques of incidental teaching, stimulation, and formal training. An effective program must target the child's behaviors, environmental factors, and the child-caregiver interaction.

CONCLUSION

Children who are presymbolic and minimally symbolic have special needs that often relate to the very purposes for communication. If these children are going to communicate more effectively, there must be a reason for doing so. In addition, the environment must provide models and respond to the child appropriately. Initial communication training cannot be an isolated affair; by its nature, communication is central to all human interactions. Communication will not generalize to the everyday use environment unless that environment becomes a facilitative one for such behavior. Only an integrated, functional intervention that targets both the child and the environment can hope to change effectively the child's current behavior.

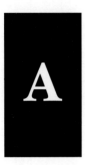

Language Test Content

TABLE A.1
Language test content

Category	Feature	ACLC	Bankson	Berko	CELI	ITPA	Miller-Yoder	NSST	OLSIDI	OLSIST	PLST	SICD	TACL	TSA	TSA-Screening	Assign. Struc. Stage	DSS	DST	LSAT
Nouns	Possessives			×	×	×	×	×									×	×	×
	Plural (reg.)	×	×	×	×	×	×	×	×			×	×			×	×	×	×
	Plural (irreg.)	×		×	×	×	×					×					×	×	×
	Derivational Suffix			×	×	×						×	×	×		×			
Verbs	Present	×	×		×	×	×	×			×	×	×				×	×	×
	Present Participle	×	×	×								×	×			×	×	×	×
	Present Progressive	×	×	×	×	×	×	×	×			×	×			×	×	×	×
	Past (reg.)		×	×	×	×	×		×	×	×	×	×			×	×	×	×
	Past (irreg.)		×	×	×	×			×	×		×	×			×	×	×	×
	Future		×		×	×	×	×		×		×	×	×		×	×	×	×
	Present Perfect		×		×		×					×	×			×	×	×	×
	Past Perfect				×											×	×	×	×
	Past Progressive								×	×						×	×	×	×
	Present Perfect Prog.				×									×		×	×		
	Passive								×	×	×	×	×	×		×	×		
	Modals				×				×	×			×	×		×	×	×	×
	Copula				×				×	×	×	×	×	×		×	×	×	×
	Auxiliary Verbs				×			×	×	×	×	×	×			×	×	×	×
	Third Per. Sing. (reg.)		×		×	×	×		×	×		×	×			×	×	×	×
	Third Per. Sing. (irreg.)		×		×				×	×									
	Infinitives/Gerunds				×				×	×			×				×		×
Pronouns	Subject Pronouns	×			×	×		×	×	×	×	×	×			×	×	×	×
	Object Pronouns	×			×		×	×		×	×	×	×			×	×	×	
	Possessive: Nom./Deter.	×			×	×		×	×	×	×	×	×			×	×	×	×
	Indefinite Pronouns				×												×		
	Reflexive Pronouns				×	×	×	×	×			×	×			*	×		
Adjectival	Adjectives	×	×	×	×	×	×					×	×			×	×	×	×
	Demonstratives				×			×				×				×	×	×	×
	Articles				×				×	×			×	×		×	×	×	×
	Comparatives		×	×	×	×						×	×						
	Superlatives		×	×	×							×	×						
Adverbs	Adverbs				×							×	×					×	×
Prepositions	Prepositions	×	×		×	×	×	×	×	×		×				×		×	×
Clausal	Wh-Questions						×	×		×	×		×				×	×	×
	Yes/No Questions				×			×	×	×		×	×	×		×	×	×	×
	Embedding				×				×	×		×	×	×		*	×		×
	Coordinated/Conjunction				×				×	×		×		×		*	×	×	×
	Negatives		×		×		×	×	×	×		×	×	×		×	×	×	×
	"Do" Insertions				×				×	×						×	×	×	×
Other	Response to Commands		×								×	×							
	Quantity		×								×	×	×					×	
	Body Parts		×									×							
	Common Nouns	×	×		×	×		×				×	×					×	×
	Color		×		×		×				×	×	×						
	Categorization		×																
	Miscellaneous		×	×							×					*			×

*Miller's Complex Sentence Development rating format.

Source: Language Test Content: A Comparative Study by R. Owens, M. Haney, V. Giesow, L. Dooley, and R. Kelly, 1983. *Language, Speech, and Hearing Services in Schools, 14,* 7–21. Reprinted with permission.

A-2

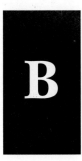

B

Phonological Development

TABLE B.1
Phonological development

Phonological Aspect	Age in months						
	24	36	48	60	72	84	96
Word shapes Consonant clusters (CC)	CV, VC, CVC	CV, VC, CVC, CC__ __CC	CV, VC, CVC, CC__, __CC, CC__CC	CV, VC, CVC, CC__, __CC, CC__CC	CV, VC, CVC, CC__, __CC, CC__CC	CV, VC, CVC, CC__, __CC, CC__CC	CV, VC, CVC, CC__, __CC, CC__CC
Number of syllables	2-syllable	2-syllable	3-syllable	3+ syllable	3+ syllable	3+ syllable	3+ syllable
Speech sounds Vowels	one each - high, low, front, back	i,ε,ʌ,ə,u,o, ɔ,ɑ,ɑɪ,ɑʊ,ɪ	i,ɪ,eɪ,ε,æ ʌ,ə,u,U,oU,o, ɔ,ɑ,ɑɪ,ɑʊ,ɪ	i,ɪ,eɪ,ε,æ ʌ,ə,u,U,oU,o, ɔ,ɑ,ɑɪ,ɑʊ,ɔɪ	All (including 3 & ɚ)	All	All
Consonants							
Nasals	/m,n/(I,F)	/m,n/(I,F)	/m,n/(I,F)	/m,n/(I,F)	/m,n/(I,F)	/m,n/(I,F),/ŋ/(F)	/m,n/(I,F),/ŋ/(F')
Glides	/w,j/	/w,j/	/w,j/	/w,j/	/w,j/	/w,j/	/w,j/
Stops	/b,t,d,g/(I), /p,k/(I,F)	/t,d/(I), /p,b,k,g/(I,F)	/t,d/(I), /p,b,k,g/(I,F)	/t,d/(I), /p,b,k,g/(I,F)	/p,b,t,d,k,g/(I,F)	/p,b,t,d,k,g/(I,F)	/p,b,t,d,k,g/(I,F)
Fricatives	/f,s/(I,F)	/f,s/(I,F),/h/(I)	/f,s,z,ʃ/(I,F), /h/(I)	/f,v,s,z,ʃ/(I,F), /h/(I)	/f,v,s,z,ʃ,ʒ,ð/ (I,F),/h/(I)	/f,v,s,z,ʃ,ʒ,ð/ (I,F),/h/(I)	/f,v,s,z,ʃ,ʒ,θ,ð/ (I,F),/h/(I)
Affricatives			/dʒ/(I,F)	/tʃ,dʒ/(I,F)	/tʃ,dʒ/(I,F)	/tʃ,dʒ/(I,F)	/tʃ,dʒ/(I,F)
Liquides				/r/(I,F),/l/(I)	/r/(I,F),/l/(I)	/r/(I,F),/l/(I)	/r,l/(I,F)

Source: Shriberg, L. D. (1993). Four new speech and prosody–voice measures for genetics research and other studies of developmental phonological disorders. *Journal of Speech and Hearing Research, 36,* 105–140.

C

Considerations for Children with LEP and Different Dialects

Most regional and ethnic dialects differ only slightly from the standard or are used by a limited number of individuals. Three ethnic dialects, however, represent rather large segments of the U.S. population and have some very important differences with Standard American English. These dialects are Black English, Hispanic or Latino English, and Asian English. Black English is used primarily by working–class African Americans in the urban northern United States and rural African Americans in the South. Not every African American uses Black English, and not everyone who uses it is African American.

Hispanic or Latino English and Asian English are probably misnomers. Hispanic English, as used here, is a composite of the English used by many speakers who are bilingual and learned English as a second language. Individual variations represent the age of learning and level of mastery, the Spanish dialect used, socioeconomic status, and where the person lives in the United States. Asian English is also a composite, but of bilingual speakers of Asian who learned English as a second language. As such, Asian English probably does not exist except to simplify our discussion. Asians speak many languages, and each has a different effect on the learning of English. In addition to the original language learned, other individual differences may reflect the same factors as those of Hispanic English. Each dialect is discussed in some detail. Where possible, information has been reduced to tables to aid presentation. Each dialect is compared with Standard American English, an idealized norm uninfluenced by the dialectal differences each person possesses.

Black English

Black English reflects the complex racial and economic history of the United States and the migration of African Americans from the rural South to the urban North after World War II. Regional differences exist to some degree. The major variations between Standard American English and Black English in phonology, syntax, and morphology are presented in Tables C.1 and C.2.

Hispanic English

Speakers who are bilingual may move back and forth between both languages in a process called *code switching*. The amount of code switching depends on the speaker's mastery of the two languages and on the audience being addressed. Of course, a great deal of code switching makes the speaker's English incomprehensible to the listener who is monolingual American English.

Most characteristics of Hispanic English reflect interference points, or points where the two languages differ, thus making learning somewhat more difficult. For example, the speaker of Hispanic English may continue to use the Spanish possessive form in which the owner is preceded by the entity owned, as in "the dress of Mary." The major variations between Standard American English and Hispanic English in phonology, syntax, and morphology are presented in Tables C.3 and C.4.

Asian English

Chinese culture and language have for centuries influenced all other Asian cultures and languages. Other cultures, such as that of the Indian subcontinents, have influenced nearby Asian neighbors. Colonial occupation, especially by the French in Indochina, also has influenced the culture and language of the affected region.

The most widely used languages—Chinese, Filipino, Japanese, Khmer, Korean, Laotian, and Vietnamese—represent only a portion of the languages of the area. Each language contains many dialects and has distinct linguistic features. It is therefore impossible to speak of an Asian English dialect. Instead, I shall attempt to describe the major overall differences between Asian English and Standard American English. These major differences in phonology, syntax, and morphology are listed in Tables C.5 and C.6.

TABLE C.1
Phonemic contrasts between Black English and Standard American English

SAE Phonemes	Position in Word		
	Initial	**Medial**	**Final**[*]
/p/		Unaspirated /p/	Unaspirated /p/
/n/			Reliance on preceding nasalized vowel
/w/	Omitted in specific words (*I 'as, too!*)		
/b/		Unreleased /b/	Unreleased /b/
/g/		Unreleased /g/	Unreleased /g/
/k/		Unaspirated /k/	Unaspirated /k/
/d/	Omitted in specific words (*I 'on't know*)	Unreleased /d/	Unreleased /d/
/ŋ/		/n/	/n/
/t/		Unaspirated /t/	Unaspirated /t/
/l/		Omitted before labial consonants (help-hep)	"uh" following a vowel (*Bill-Biuh*)
/r/		Omitted or /ə/	Omitted or prolonged vowel or glide
/θ/	Unaspirated /t/ or /f/	Unaspirated /t/ or /f/ between vowels	Unaspirated /t/ or /f/ (*bath-baf*)
/v/	Sometimes /b/	/b/ before /m/ and /n/	Sometimes /b/
/ð/	/d/	/d/ or /v/ between vowels	/d/, /v/, /f/
/z/		Omitted or replaced by /d/ before nasal sound (*wasn't-wud'n*)	

Blends
/str/ becomes /skr/
/ʃr/ becomes /str/
/θr/ becomes /θ/
/pr/ becomes /p/
/br/ becomes /b/
/kr/ becomes /k/
/gr/ becomes /g/

Final Consonant Clusters (second consonant omitted when these clusters occur at the end of a word)

/sk/	/nd/	/sp/
/ft/	/ld/	/dʒ d/
/st/	/sd/	/nt/

[*] Note weakening of final consonants.

Source: Data drawn from Fasold & Wolfram (1970); Labov (1972); F. Weiner & Lewnau (1979); R. Williams & Wolfram (1977)

TABLE C.2
Grammatical contrasts between Black English and Standard American English

Black English Grammatical Structure	SAE Grammatical Structure
Possessive -'s	
Nonobligatory where word position expresses possession.	Oblicatory regardless of position.
Get *mother* coat.	Get mother*'s* coat.
It be mother's.	It's mother*'s*.
Plural -s	
Nonobligatory with numerical quantifier.	Obligatory regardless of numerical quantifier.
He got ten *dollar*.	He has ten dollars.
Look at the cats.	Look at the cats.
Regular past -ed	
Nonobligatory; reduced as consonant cluster.	Obligatory.
Yesterday, I *walk* to school.	Yesterday, I walk*ed* to school.
Irregular past	
Case by case, some verbs inflected, others not.	All irregular verbs inflected.
I *see* him last week.	I *saw* him last week.
Regular present tense third person singular -s	
Nonobligatory.	Obligatory.
She *eat* too much.	She eat*s* too much.
Irregular present tense third person singular -s	
Nonobligatory.	Obligatory.
He *do* my job.	He *does* my job.
Indefinite *an*	
Use of indefinite *a*.	Use of *an* before nouns beginning with a vowel.
He ride in *a* airplane.	He rode in *an* airplane.
Pronouns	
Pronominal apposition: pronoun immediately follows noun.	Pronoun used elsewhere in sentence or in other sentence; not in apposition.
Momma *she* mad. She . . .	Momma is mad. *She* . . .
Future tense	
More frequent use of *be going to* (gonna).	More frequent use of *will*.
I *be going to* dance tonight.	I *will* dance tonight.

I *gonna* dance tonight.	I *am going to* dance tonight.
Omit *will* preceding *be*.	Obligatory use of *will*.
I *be* home later.	I *will* (I'll) *be* home later.
Negation	
Triple negative.	Absence of triple negative.
Nobody don't never like me.	*No* one ever likes me.
Use of *ain't*.	*Ain't* is unacceptable form.
I *ain't* going.	I'*m not* going.
Modals	
Double modals for such forms as might, *could*, and *should*.	Single modal use.
I *might could* go.	I *might be able to* go.
Questions	
Same form for direct and indirect.	Different forms for direct and indirect.
What *it is*?	What *is it*?
Do you know what *it is*?	Do you know what *it is*?
Relative pronouns	
Nonobligatory in most cases.	Nonobligatory with *that* only.
He the one stole it.	He's the one *who* stole it.
It the one you like.	It's the one (that) you like.
Conditional *if*	
Use of *do* for conditional *if*.	Use of *if*.
I ask *did* she go.	I asked *if* she went.
Perfect construction	
Been used for action in the distant past.	*Been* not used.
He *been* gone.	He left a long time ago.
Copula	
Nonobligatory when contractible.	Obligatory in contractible and uncontractible forms.
He sick.	He's sick.
Habitual or general state	
Marked with uninflected *be*.	Nonuse of *be*; verb inflected.
She *be* workin'.	She's *working* now.

Source: Data drawn from Baratz (1969); Fasold & Wolfram (1970); R. Williams & Wolfram (1977)

TABLE C.3
Phonemic contrasts between Hispanic English and Standard American English

	Position in Word		
SAE Phonemes	**Initial**	**Medial**	**Final[*]**
/p/	Unaspirated /p/		Omitted or weakened
/m/			Omitted
/w/	/hu/		Omitted
/b/			Omitted, distorted, or /p/
/g/			Omitted, distorted, or /k/
/k/	Unaspirated or /g/		Omitted, distorted, or /g/
/f/			Omitted
/d/		Dentalized	Omitted, distorted, or /t/
/ŋ/	/n/	/d/	/n/ (*sing-sin*)
/j/	/dʒ/		
/t/			Omitted
/ʃ/	/tʃ/	/s/, /tʃ/	/tʃ/ (*wish-which*)
/tʃ/	/ʃ/ (*chair-share*)	/ʃ/	/ʃ/ (*watch-wash*)
/r/	Distorted	Distorted	Distorted
/dʒ/	/d/	/j/	/ʃ/
/θ/	/t/, /s/ (*thin-tin, sin*)	Omitted	/ʃ/, /t/, /s/
/v/	/b/ (*vat-bat*)	/b/	Distorted
/z/	/s/ (*zip-sip*)	/s/ (*razor-racer*)	/s/
/ð/	/d/ (*then-den*)	/d/, /θ/, /v/ (*lather-ladder*)	/d/

Blends
/skw/ becomes /eskw/[*]
/sl/ becomes /esl/[*]
/st/ becomes /est/[*]

Vowels
/I/ becomes /i/ (*bit-beet*)

[*] Separates cluster into two syllables.

Source: Data drawn from J. Sawyer (1973); F. Weiner & Lewnau (1979); F. Williams, Cairns, & Cairns (1971)

TABLE C.4
Grammatical contrasts between Hispanic English and Standard American English

Hispanic English Grammatical Structure	SAE Grammatical Structure
Possessive -'s	
Use postnoun modifier.	Postnoun modifer used only rarely.
This is the homework *of my brother*.	This is my brother*'s* homework.
Article used with body parts.	Possessive pronoun used with body parts.
I cut *the* finger.	I cut *my* finger.
Plural -s	
Nonobligatory.	Obligatory, excluding exceptions.
The *girl* are playing.	The *girls* are playing.
The *sheep* are playing.	The *sheep* are playing.
Regular past -ed	
Nonobligatory, especially when understood.	Obligatory.
I *talk* to her yesterday.	I *talked* to her yesterday.
Regular third person singular present tense -s	
Nonobligatory.	Obligatory.
She *eat* too much.	She *eats* too much.
Articles	
Often omitted.	Usually obligatory.
I am going to store.	I am going to *the* store.
I am going to school.	I am going to school.
Subject pronouns	
Omitted when subject has been identified in the previous sentence.	Obligatory.
Father is happy. Bought a new car.	Father is happy. *He* bought a new car.
Future tense	
Use *go + to*.	Use *be + going to*.
I *go to* dance.	I *am going to* the dance.
Negation	
Use *no* before the verb.	Use *not* (preceded by auxiliary verb where appropriate).
She *no* eat candy.	She does *not* eat candy.
Question	
Intonation: no noun-verb inversion.	Noun-verb inversion usually.
Maria is going?	*Is Maria* going?
Copula	
Occasional use of *have*.	Use of *be*.
I *have* ten years.	I *am* ten years old.
Negative imperatives	
No used for *don't*.	*Don't* used.
No throw stones.	*Don't* throw stones.
Do insertion	
Nonobligatory in questions.	Obligatory when no auxiliary verb.
You like ice cream?	*Do* you like ice cream?
Comparatives	
More frequent use of longer form (more).	More frequent use of shorter -er.
He is *more* tall.	He is tall*er*.

Source: Data drawn from Davis (1972); O. Taylor (1986)

TABLE C.5
Phonemic contrasts between Asian English and Standard American English

SAE Phonemes	Position in Word		
	Initial	**Medial**	**Final**
/p/	/b/[****]	/b/[****]	Omission
/s/	Distortion[*]	Distortion[*]	Omission
/z/	/s/[**]	/s/[**]	Omission
/t/	Distortion[*]	Distortion[*]	Omission
/tʃ/	/ʃ/[****]	/ʃ/[****]	Omission
/ʃ/	/s/[**]	/s/[**]	Omission
/r/, /l/	Confusion[***]	Confusion[***]	Omission
/θ/	/s/	/s/	Omission
/dʒ/	/d/ or /z/[****]	/d/ or /z/[****]	Omission
/v/	/f/[***]	/f/[***]	Omission
	/w/[**]	/w/[**]	Omission
/ð/	/z/[*]	/z/[*]	Omission
	/d/[****]	/d/[****]	Omission

Blends
Addition of /ə/ between consonants[***]
Omission of final consonant clusters[****]

Vowels
Shortening or lengthening of vowels (seat-sit, it-eat[*])
Difficulty with /I/, /ɔ/, and /æ/, and substitution of /e/ for /æ/[**]
Difficulty with /I/, /æ/, /ɔ/, and /ə/[****]

[*] Mandarin dialect of Chinese only
[**] Cantonese dialect of Chinese only
[***] Mandarin, Cantonese, and Japanese
[****] Vietnamese only

Source: Adapted from Cheng, L. (1987). Cross–cultural and linguistic considerations in working with Asian populations. *Asha, 29*(6), 33–39.

TABLE C.6
Grammatical contrasts between Asian English and Standard American English

Asian English Grammatical Structure	SAE Grammatical Structure
Plural -*s*	
Not used with numerical adjective: *three cat*	Used regardless of numerical adjective: *three cats*
Used with irregular plural: *the sheeps*	Not used with irregular plural: *the sheep*
Auxiliaries *to be* **and** *to do*	
Omission: *I going home. She not want eat.*	Obligatory and inflected in the present progressive
Uninflected: *I is going. She do not want eat.*	form: *I am going home. She does not want to eat.*
Verb have	
Omission.	Obligatory and inflected: *You have been here. He has*
You been here.	*one.*
Uninflected.	
He have one.	
Past tense -*ed*	
Omission: *He talk yesterday.*	Obligatory, nonovergeneralization, and single-
Overgeneralization: *I eated yesterday.*	marking: *He talked yesterday. I ate yesterday. She*
Double-marking: *She didn't ate.*	*didn't eat.*
Interrogative	
Nonreversal: *You're late?*	Reversal and obligatory auxiliary: *Are you late? Do*
Omitted auxiliary: *You like ice cream?*	*you like ice cream?*
Perfect marker	
Omission: *I have write letter.*	Obligatory: *I have written a letter.*
Verb-noun agreement	
Nonagreement: *He go to school. You goes to school.*	Agreement: *He goes to school. You go to school.*
Article	
Omission: *Please give gift.*	Obligatory with certain nouns: Please give the gift.
Overgeneralization: *She go the school.*	She went to school.
Preposition	
Misuse: *I am in home.*	Obligatory specific use: *I am at home. He goes by bus.*
Omission: *He go bus.*	
Pronoun	
Subjective/objective confusion: *Him go quickly.*	Subjective/objective distinction: *He gave it to her.*
Possessive confusion: *It him book.*	Possessive distinction: *It's his book.*
Demonstrative	
Confusion: *I like those horse.*	Singular/plural distinction: *I like that horse.*
Conjunction	
Omission: *You I go together.*	Obligatory use between last two items in a series: *You*
Negation	*and I are going together. Mary, John, and Carol went.*
Double-marking: *I didn't see nobody.*	Single obligatory marking: *I didn't see anybody. He*
Simplified form: *He no come.*	*didn't come.*
Word order	
Adjective following noun	Most noun modifiers precede noun: *new clothes.*
(Vietnamese): *clothes new.*	
Possessive following noun	Possessive precedes noun: *her dress.*
(Vietnamese): *dress her.*	
Omission of object with transitive verb: *I want.*	Use of direct object with most transitive verbs: *I*
	want it.

Source: Adapted from Cheng, L. (1987). Cross–cultural and linguistic considerations in working with Asian populations. *Asha, 29*(6), 33–39.

D

Language Tests for Children with LEP and Different Dialects

TABLE D.1
Screening and diagnostic instruments

Name	Description	Cost	Publisher
All India Institute of Medical Sciences: Aphasias Diagnostic Test Battery, Aphasia Screening Test Battery, Test of Auditory Comprehension of Language, Test of Articulation *Subhash Bhatnagar*	Batteries developed to identify and diagnose speech and language impairments in the Hindi population.	Nominal cost for duplication	Subhash Bhatnagar Department of Speech Pathology and Audiology Marquette University Milwaukee, WI 53233 (414) 224-7349
Assessment of Phonological Processes—Spanish *Barbara Hodson*	An instrument to identify broad error patterns in unintelligible utterances while de-emphasizing dialectal differences or normal developmental variations.	Manual and forms $50.00 Objects for Spanish version $31.95	Los Amigos Research Associates 7035 Galewood San Diego, CA 92120 (619) 286-3162 Imaginart 307 Arizona St. Bisbee, AZ 85603 (800) 828-1376 Fax: (800) 432-5134

Name	Description	Cost	Publisher
Bilingual Aphasia Test *Michel Paradis*	A measure for evaluating residual abilities in each of an aphasic patient's languages. The test has been translated into 40 different languages and 60 language pairs.	Text $45.00 Single-language test $34.00 Adapted test (language-specific) $17.50	L. Erlbaum Associates, Inc. 365 Broadway Hillsdale, NJ 07642 (201) 666-4110
Bilingual Health and Developmental History Questionnaire *Christina Gomez-Valdez*	An interviewing questionnaire for use with parents who are Spanish-speaking. Used to obtain information about their child's developmental milestones. Questions are listed in both English and Spanish.	Instruction booklet and 30 copies of questionnaire $16.50	Los Amigos Research Associates 7035 Galewood San Diego, CA 92120-1908 (619) 286-3162
Bilingual Home Inventory	A bilingual instrument to use when interviewing parents of handicapped children and youth to determine appropriate educational objectives for students' homes and communities. Available in English/Spanish, English/Portuguese, and/ English/Philipino.	$9.00	Dr. Herbert Grossman, Director Bilingual/Multicultural Special Education Programs Division of Special Education and Rehabilitation Services San Jose State University San Jose, CA 95192 (408) 277-9160
Bilingual Language Proficiency Questionnaire *Larry J. Mattes* *George Santiago*	A parent interview questionnaire used to obtain information about development and functional use of a variety of speech and language skills among bilingual Spanish-English children. Items are listed in both English and Spanish.	Instruction booklet and 30 record forms $16.50	Los Amigos Research Associates 7035 Galewood San Diego, CA 92120-1908 (619) 286-3162
Bilingual Syntax Measure I and II (BSM I + BSM II) (Medida de Sintaxis Bilingual) *Marina K. Burt* *Heidi C. Dulog*	A normed measure of syntactic mastery in both English and Spanish for children 1st–2nd grade (BSM I) and 3rd–12th grade (BSM II). Uses cartoon-type pictures and questions to elicit language samples.	Complete BSM I + BSM II $565.00 BSM I $282.50 BSM II $282.50	The Psychological Corp. 555 Academic Court San Antonio, TX 78203-2498 (800) 228-0752

Boehm Test of Basic Concepts-Revised *Ann E. Boehm*	A test designed to measure children's understanding of basic concepts. Available in Spanish.	Examination Kit $68.50	The Psychological Corp. 555 Academic Court San Antonio, TX 78203-2498 (800) 228-0752
Brigance Diagnostic Assessment of Basic Skills, Portugese Edition	A bilingual Portuguese adaptation of the Brigance Test.	$40.00	Dr. Herbert Grossman, Director Bilingual/Multicultural Special Education Programs Division of Special Education and Rehabilitation Services San Jose State University San Jose, CA 95192 (408) 277-9160
Cartoon Conversation Scales	A measure designed to assess intellectual development in any language without bias. Designed to test for gifted or special education placement.	Complete $79.00	CTB/McGraw-Hill Del Monte Research Park Monterey, CA 93940 (800) 538-9547 (408) 649-8400
Chinese Oral Proficiency Test	Chinese-English exam for testing oral comprehension and word associations in children grades K–6.	Test Packet and 30 Answer Sheets $2.95	The National Hispanic University 255 East 14th Street Oakland, CA 94606 (415) 451-0511
EICIRCO Assessment Series	An assessment instrument that tests comprehension of simple mathematical concepts and basic linguistic structures in Spanish and English. An additional language screen for facility in Spanish is also available. Test was developed for Spanish-speaking children from Mexican-American, Puerto Rican, and Cuban backgrounds.	Test Booklets (30) $428.85 Language Check $10.00	CTB/McGraw-Hill Del Monte Research Park Monterey, CA 93940 (800) 538-9547 (408) 649-8400
Comprehensive Identification Process (CIP)—Spanish Edition *R. Reid Zehrbach*	Designed to identify children (2½–5½ years) who may be eligible for special preschool programming.	Screening Kit $145.00 Components also available separately.	Scholastic Testing Service, Inc., Dept. E. 480 Meyer Road Bensenville, IL 60106 (708) 766-7150
Compton Phonological Assessment of Foreign Accent *Arthur J. Compton*	A step approach for analyzing the speech of non-native English speakers. Analysis is derived from a sampling of speech sounds	Complete Set $45.00 Additional Response Booklets (25) $16.00	Carousel House 212 Arguello Blvd. San Francisco, CA 94118 (800) LANGUAGE (415) 921-0629

Name	Description	Cost	Publisher
Compton Phonological Assessment of Foreign Accent (continued)	on single words, phrases, sentences, oral reading and conversation.		
Compton Speech and Language Screening Evaluation: Spanish Adaptation *Arthur J. Compton* *Marlaine Kline*	Screen provides an estimate of speech and language development in young Spanish-speaking children (3–6 years). Assesses comprehension and production.	Complete Set $50.00 Additional Response Forms (25) $10.00	Carousel House 212 Arguello Blvd. San Francisco, CA 94118 (800) LANGUAGE (415) 921-0629
Developmental Assessment of Spanish Grammar (DASG) *Allen S. Toronto*	A language analysis procedure for Spanish-speaking children adapted from the Developmental Sentence Scoring (DSS) procedure.	N/A	The procedure is detailed in a journal article: Toronto, A. S. (1976). Developmental assessment of Spanish grammar. Journal of Speech and Hearing Disorders, 41(2), 150–171.
Dos Amigos Verbal Language Scale *Donald Critchlow*	Norm referenced assessment of cognitive levels of language functioning in both English and Spanish among individual students between the ages of 5 and 13 years.	Complete Set $25.00	Academic Therapy Publications 20 Commercial Blvd. Novato, CA 94949-6191 (415) 883-3314 (800) 422-7249
Examen de Afasia Multilingue (MAE-S) *G. J. Ray* *A. L. Benton*	Seven subtests evaluate the severity of Aphasia in Spanish-speaking individuals.	Complete Kit $168.00	The Psychological Corp 555 Academic Court San Antonio, TX 78204-2498 (800) 228-0752
Examines Para Diagnosticar Impedimentos de Afasia *Joseph S. Keenan* *Esther G. Brassell*	An adaptation of the Aphasia Language Performance Scale (ALPS) used to assess 9 areas of language functioning in individuals grade 7 through adult who are Spanish-speaking. Performance is evaluated and reported in terms of language competency, not normative values.	$38.00	Pinnacle Press P. O. Box 210663 Nashville, TN 37221-0663 (615) 646-8483
Expressive One-Word Picture Vocabulary Test—Revised (EOWPVT-R), Spanish *Morrison F. Gardner*	This companion to the Receptive One-Word establishes the quality and quantity of a child's vocabulary and the fluency in English of a bilingual child. For Spanish-speaking children 2 to 12 years. Translation.	Complete (EOW-PVT-R) $75.00	Academic Therapy Publications 20 Commercial Blvd. Novato, CA 94949-6191 (415) 883-3314 (800) 422-7249

Expressive One-Word Picture Vocabulary Test Upper Extension (EOW-PVT-UE), Spanish	Normed measure of ability to name pictures similar to the EOWPVT-R. For Spanish-speaking children ages 12 to 16 years. Translation.	Complete (EOWPVT-UE) $65.00	Academic Therapy Publications 20 Commercial Blvd. Novato, CA 94949-6191 (415) 883-3314 (800) 422-7249
Goodenough-Harris Drawing Test *Florence L. Goodenough* *Dale B. Harris*	A nonverbal tool for assessing cognitive ability in children (3–15 years). Can be used with non-English speaking children and can be administered individually or in groups.	Complete Kit $78.50	The Psychological Corp. 555 Academic Court San Antonio, TX 78204-2498 (800) 228-0752
Human Figures Drawing Test (HFDT) *Eloy Gonzales*	A measure of nonverbal conceptual ability of children (5–10 years). Can be used when assessing non-English speakers. Cognitive maturity is evaluated by analyzing drawings of human figures.	Complete Kit $39.00	Pro-Ed 8700 Shoal Creek Blvd. Austin, TX 78757-6897 (512) 451-3246 Fax: (512) 451-8542
Language Assessment Scales	Test for determining oral language ability in English and Spanish. Available at three levels—PreLAS (preschoolers), LASI (K–5), and LAS II (grades 6–12).	Complete Kit $69.00	CTB/McGraw-Hill Del Monte Research Park Monterey, CA 93940 (800) 538-9547 (408) 649-8400
Language Proficiency Test *Joan E. Garard* *Gloria Weinstock*	Measure assesses wide range of English language abilities for adolescents to adults. Specifically designed for students using ESL. Optional translation for Spanish, German, French, Tagalog, and Japanese.	Complete Kit $45.00	Academic Therapy Publications 20 Commercial Blvd. Novato, CA 94949-6191 (415) 883-3314 (800) 422-7249
Leiter International Performance Scale (LIPS)	Widely used noncultural, nonverbal test of intelligence. Follows match-to-sample format.	Complete Kit $610.00	Slosson Educational Publication Inc. P. O. Box 280 East Aurora, NY 14052 (800) 828-4800 Fax: (716) 655-3840
Lindamood Auditory Conceptualization Test—Spanish *Charles H. Lindamood* *Patricia C. Lindamood*	Criterion-referenced test of auditory perception and conceptualization of speech sounds. Spanish version of examiner's cue sheet is available.	Complete Program $81.00	Riverside Publishers 8420 Bryn Mawr Ave. Chicago, IL 60631 (800) 767-8378

Name	Description	Cost	Publisher
Look Listen and Tell, a Language Screening Instrument for Indian Children	Instrument was developed for use as a language screening device for Native American children (3–7 years). Designed to be used by child-care workers with no formal training in speech-language pathology.	$3.00	Southwest Communication Resources, Inc. P. O. Box 788 Bernalillo, NM 87004 (505) 867-3396
Medida Espanola de Articulacion (Spanish Articulation Measure) *Marilyn Aldrich-Mason* *Blanche Figueroa-Smith* *Mary Martinez-Hinshaw*	Tool to assess early acquisition of phonemes in Spanish.	Consult publisher for current price.	San Ysidro School District 4350 Otay Mesa Road San Ysidro, CA 92073 (619) 428-4476
Multicultural Vocabulary Test *Gerald Trudeau*	Test of expressive vocabulary in English and Spanish which uses body parts as stimulus items. For children aged 3 to 12 years.	$35.00	Los Amigos Research Associates 7035 Galewood San Diego, CA 92120 (619) 286-3162
PAL Oral Language Dominance Measure *Rosa Apodaca*	Test uses picture responses to determine oral language proficiency in English and/or Spanish.	$9.00	El Paso Public Schools P. O. Box 2100 El Paso, TX 79998 (915) 779-4056
Parent as a Teacher Inventory (PAAT)—Spanish Edition *Robert D. Strom*	Instrument used with parents of children age 3–9 years to obtain information on the parent-child interactive system.	Set $45.50	Scholastic Testing Service, Inc., Dept. E 480 Meyer Road Bensenville, IL 60106 (708) 766-7150
Peabody Picture Vocabulary Test (Spanish Version)	A test of receptive vocabulary development in Spanish. A translation.	Complete Kit $74.95	American Guidance Service P.O. Box 99 Circle Pines, MN 55014-1796 (800) 328-2560
Preschool Language Assessment Instrument (PLAI): The Language of Learning in Practice—Spanish Language Edition. *Marian Blank* *Susan Rose* *Laura Berlin*	Test assesses the ability of 3–6 year olds to name, imitate, sequence, match, define, predict, remember information, problem solve, and describe. Information obtained provides insight into how children handle language demands.	Complete Kit $66.00	The Psychological Corp. 555 Academic Court San Antonio, TX 78204-2498 (800) 228-0752

Preschool Language Scale (PLS-3), Spanish *Irie Lee Zimmerman* *Violette G. Steiner* *Roberta Evatt Pond*	Diagnostic measure of receptive and expressive language, with items measuring grammar, vocabulary, memory, attention span and temporal/special relations. Record forms are available in English or Spanish (Mexican-American).	Complete PLS Starter Kit Examiner's manual $12.50 12 forms $22.00 May be used with pictures available in English version.	The Psychological Corp. 555 Academic Court San Antonio, TX 78204-2498 (800) 228-0752
Proficiency in Oral English Communication: An accent assessment battery, revised edition.	Series of comprehensive subtests for articulation, information, auditory discrimination, pragmatics, and language. Use with adolescents or adults.	Complete POEC Kit $79.95	LDS and Associates 11142 Wickford Dr. Santa Anna, CA 92705 (714) 838-6002 Fax: (714) 573-0314
Prueba De Lectura y Lenguaje Escrito (PLLE) *Donald D. Hammill* *Stephen C. Larsen* *J. Lee Weiderholt* *Joanne Fountain-Shambers*	A test of reading and writing in Spanish.	$62.00	Pro-Ed 8700 Shoal Creek Blvd. Austin, TX 78757-6897 (512) 451-3246 Fax: (512) 451-8542
Prueba Del Desarrollo Inical Del Lenguaje (PDIL) *Wayne P. Hresko* *D. Kim Reid* *Donald D. Hammill*	A test of spoken language in Spanish.	$49.00	Pro-Ed 8700 Shoal Creek Blvd. Austin, TX 78757-6897 (512) 451-3246 Fax: (512) 451-8542
Pruebas de Expresion Oral y Percepcion de le Lengua Espanola (PEOPLE) *Sharon Mares*	A bilingual assessment tool intended to be administered by bilingual speech-language pathologists to children of Mexican descent (6 and 10 years).	$5.00	Los Angeles County Office of Education Kit Carson School, Resource Room, Rm. 2 3530 W. 147th Street Hawthorne, CA 90250 (213) 676-0121 (213) 676-0122
Receptive One-Word Picture Vocabulary (ROWPVT) *Morrison F. Gardner*	This companion to the EOWPV assesses the ability of children (2–12 years) to match an object of concept with its name for determining receptive vocabulary skills. Spanish translation.	Complete Test Kit $65.00	Academic Therapy Publications 20 Commercial Blvd. Novato, CA 94949-6191 (415) 883-3314 (800) 422-7249

Name	Description	Cost	Publisher
Receptive One-Word Picture Vocabulary Test Upper Extension (ROW-PVT-UE) Spanish	Normed measure for ages 12 to 16 that assesses ability to match a picture with its name. Spanish translation.	Complete ROW-PVT-UE $65.00	Academic Therapy Publications 20 Commercial Blvd. Novato, CA 94949-6191 (415) 883-3314 (800) 422-7249
Screening Kit of Language Development (SKOLD) *Lynn S. Bliss* *Doris V. Allen*	Normed measure of preschool language development, including separate norms for speakers of Black English.	Complete SKOLD-$55.00	Slosson Educational Publications, Inc. P. O. Box 280 East Aurora, NY 14052 (800) 828-4800 Fax: (716) 655-3840
Spanish Articulation Measures *Larry J. Mattes*	A criterion-referenced test which includes spontaneous and elicited tasks to assess production of speech sounds and use of phonological processes. For school-aged Spanish-speaking children.	Complete Kit $39.00	The Speech Bin, Inc. 1965 Twenty-fifth Ave. Vero Beach, FL 32960 (800) 4-SPEECH FAX: (407) 770-0006
Spanish Expressive Vocabulary Test *Leticia Valdivia* *Trish Lopez* *Donald R. Omark*	Normed measure that uses pictures to elicit vocabulary from children who are Spanish-speaking or bilingual, grades K–6. Mexican-American norms may be inappropriate for other Spanish-speaking children.	$40.00	Los Amigos Research Associates 7035 Galewood San Diego, CA 92120-1908 (619) 286-3162
Spanish Language Assessment Procedures: A Communication Skills Inventory (Revised and Expanded) (SLAP) *Larry J. Mattes*	Normed measure for children 5 to 8 years to assess both structural and functional aspects of Spanish communication, including articulation, vocabulary, sentence structure, and verbal reasoning.	Complete Kit $65.00	Los Amigos Research Associates 7035 Galewood San Diego, CA 92120-1908 (619) 286-3162
Spanish Language Synthetic Sentence Identification (SSI-S) Developed and recorded by: *Jerger*	Ten sets of synthetic sentences in Spanish, with accompanying instructional and response cards. Scoring forms provided are in English. Available with both contra- and ipsilateral competing messages.	Reel to Reel or Cassette Tapes $42.00	Auditec of St. Louis 330 Selma Avenue St. Louis, MO 63119 (314) 962-5890

Spanish Oral Language Screening Instrument	A screening instrument in Spanish-English for determining language skills in Spanish-speaking children, grades K–6.	$2.95	The National Hispanic University 255 East 14th Street Oakland, CA 94606 (415) 451-0511
Spanish Test for Assessing Morphological Production (STAMP) *T. M. Nugent* *K. G. Shipley* *D. O. Provencio*	Normed measure for children 5 to 8 years to assess production of Spanish morphemics through sentence completion.	Complete Kit $56.00	Academic Communication Associates Dept. 84-F 4149 Avenida de la Plata P. O. Box 586249 Oceanside, CA 92058-6249
Spotting Language Problems: Pragmatic Criteria for Language Screening *Jack S. Damico* *John W. Oller*	A language screening instrument which uses a pragmatic approach. For English speaking, bilingual and/or limited English proficient children. In-service training suggestions for teachers are also provided.	$30.00	Los Amigos Research Associates 7035 Galewood San Diego, CA 92120-1908 (619) 286-3162
SRT and Discrimination Lists—French Recorded by: *Auditec*	Tapes of a list of words for speech reception threshold testing and for speech discrimination testing in French.	Reel to Reel $38.00 Cassette $32.00	Auditec of St. Louis 330 Selma Avenue St. Louis, MO 63119 (314) 962-5890
SRT and Discrimination Lists—Spanish Recorded by: *Auditec* SRT words developed by: *Pasco*	Tapes of lists of words in Spanish for speech reception threshold and speech discrimination testing. One recording contains two forms of 36 trisyllable words for SRT, and four lists of bisyllable words for speech discrimination. Also included are two lists of monosyllables.	SRT & Discrimination (Reel to Reel) $38.00 Monosyllables (Reel to Reel) $34.00 SRT & Discrimination (Cassette) $32.00 Monosyllables (Cassette) $24.50	Auditec of St. Louis 330 Selma Avenue St. Louis, MO 63119 (314) 962-5890
Structure Photographic Expressive Language Test-II, preschool *Ellen O'Hara Werner* *Janet Dawson Krescheck.*	Test of expressive language for standard English or Black English, or Spanish speakers. Versions for preschoolers or elementary age children.	Both Tests $46.00 Preschool Only $37.00	Janelle Publications P. O. Box 12 Sandwich, IL 60548 (312) 552-7771
System of Multicultural Pluralistic Assessment (SOMPA) *Jane R. Mercer* *June F. Lewis*	A system for assessing cognitive and sensorimotor abilities and adaptive behavior of children (5–11 years).	Complete SOMPA Kit (includes ABIC) $99.00 Components also available separately.	The Psychological Corporation P. O. Box 9954 San Antonio, TX 78204-2498 (800) 228-0752

Name	Description	Cost	Publisher
System of Multicultural Pluralistic Assessment (SOMPA) (continued)	Components include a parent interview in English or Spanish, student assessment materials, and the Adaptive Behavior Inventory for Children (ABIC). Normative data are provided for Black, Hispanic and White Children.		
Test for Auditory Comprehension of Language: English and Spanish Forms (Revised) *Elizabeth Carrow*	Norm referenced test designed for use with children 3.0 to 6.11 measures receptive language problems in English or Spanish. Spanish translation.	Complete TACL-R $144.00	Riverside Publishers 8420 Bryn Mawr Ave. Chicago, IL 60631 (800) 767-8378
Test of Nonverbal Intelligence: A Language Free Measure of Cognitive Ability, second edition. *Linda Brown* *Rita J. Sherbenou* *Susan K. Johnson*	Norm-reference test designed for use with individuals 5.0 to 85.11 to measure intelligence, aptitude, and reasoning without the use of reading, writing, or speaking.	Complete TNI-2 $129.00	Pro-Ed 8700 Shoal Creek Blvd. Austin, TX 78757-6897 (512) 451-3246 Fax: (512) 451-8542
Texas-Acevedo Screening of Speech and Language *Mary Ann Acevedo*	An English-Spanish articulation and language screening test for English- or Spanish-speaking children (3 to 6 years).	Free–furnished only to Head Start programs, preschools or others who provide screening services at no cost to clients	Vision, Hearing and Speech Services Bureau of Bureau of Maternal and Child Health Texas Department of Health 1100 West 49th Street Austin, TX 78756 (512) 458-7111
Woodcock Language Proficiency Battery (Spanish Form) *Richard W. Woodcock*	Battery measures three components of language proficiency: oral, reading, and written language.	$159.00	Riverside Publishers 8420 Bryn Mawr Ave. Chicago, IL 60631 (800) 767-8378
Woodcock-Munoz language Survey (Spanish Form)	Measure of cognitive-academic language proficiency (CALP) in four areas of vocabulary, verbal analysis, letter-word identification, and diction. Comes with IBM or Apple	Complete Kit $129.00	Riverside Publishers 8420 Bryn Mawr Ave. Chicago, IL 60631 (800) 767-8378

Zuni Articulation Test	Adapted Zuni alphabet book for use as a stimulus book for articulation testing. Picture and word stimuli for sounds in initial and medial positions are provided. Several pictures are presented for each sound.	Contact the School District for current information on training and availability of the test.	Zuni Public School District Speech and Language Therapy Program P. O. Drawer A Zuni, NM 87327
Zuni Language Screening Instrument	Measure designed to quickly evaluate language proficiency in the Zuni language for children in grades kindergarten through 12. Both receptive and expressive language are measured, and a language sample can be obtained. Instructions and age-appropriate language samples have been taped in Zuni.	Contact the School District for current information on training and availability of the test.	Zuni Public School District Speech and Language Therapy Program P. O. Drawer A Zuni, NM 87327

Source: Deal, V., & Rodriguez, V. (1987). *Resource guide to multicultural tests and materials in communicative disorders.* Rockville, MD: American Speech–Language–Hearing Association. Revised and expanded by R. Owens (1994).

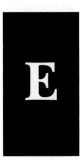

E

Form for Reporting the Language Skills of Children with LEP and Different Dialects

TABLE E.1
Reporting language skills of children with LEP and different dialects

ASSESSMENT INSTRUMENT FOR MULTICULTURAL CLIENTS

CLIENT'S NAME: _____ AGE: _____

SEX: _____ SCHOOL GRADE: _____

1. Evaluator of L1* _____ Date _____
   (name of SLS or Interpreter)***

If Interpreter, check whether:
Family Member _____ Other _____

2. Evaluator of L2** _____ Date _____
   (name of SLS)

3. Evaluator of Dialect _____ Date _____
   (name of SLS)

Nonnative English Speaker

1. Spanish-influenced English _____
2. Asian-influenced English _____
3. Other _____

Nonstandard English Speaker

4. African-influenced English _____
5. Appalachian-influenced English _____
6. Other _____

UTILIZATION OF THE ASSESSMENT INSTRUMENT

1. The following assessment instrument can be used to evaluate the communicative proficiency of both LEP as well as nonstandard speakers of English. In particular, this model allows for the determination and recording of a client's (a) linguistic deficiencies vs. differences, (b) appropriate vs. inappropriate use of language, and (c) the quantity of nonnative or nonstandard English utterances.

2. At a minimum, obtain at least two relatively short language samples; if possible, obtain three samples in different situations.

3. Play back the language samples as frequently as is necessary in order to obtain the relevant information concerning the student's communication skills. As you do so, listen intently for each facet of the assessment instrument.

* L1 = Native Language
** L2 = Acquired Language/English
*** SLS = Speech-Language Specialist

4. If necessary or desired, you may use a standard test, particularly an articulation test of your choice, to supplement the information obtained through the language samples.

AURAL/ORAL COMMUNICATIVE ASSESSMENTS

Check if Accomplished

_____ 1. Pragmatic Language Samples: Obtain samples of language usage in at least two different situations and, if possible, with two different testers in each of the situations. Note and discuss the following:

_____   A. Clinic: intelligibility of the sample..............page 4a
         and the quantity of dialect/language
         differences..page 4b

_____   B. Other: compare to clinic sample

_____ 2. Evaluate client's use of segmentals. By subjective or objective testing, note and discuss the phonological and morphosyntactic utterances you observe that are inappropriate for the language/dialect being assessed. See morphosyntactic summary ....page 6

_____ 3. Evaluate client's use of suprasegmentals and body language ....page 4c

_____ 4. Evaluate client's voice and fluency patterns ....page 4d

_____ 5. Evaluate client's auditory acuity and comprehension...page 5e

_____ 6. Use of Language in the Classroom (if appropriate). Ascertain from teacher: ....page 7

         (1) intelligibility of the speaker;

         (2) amount of dialect/language differences used by child;

         (3) his/her knowledge and use of standard language rules in the classroom;

         (4) the child's auditory comprehension in L1 and L2

A-28

SUMMARY OF RESULTS

Circle the Appropriate Number

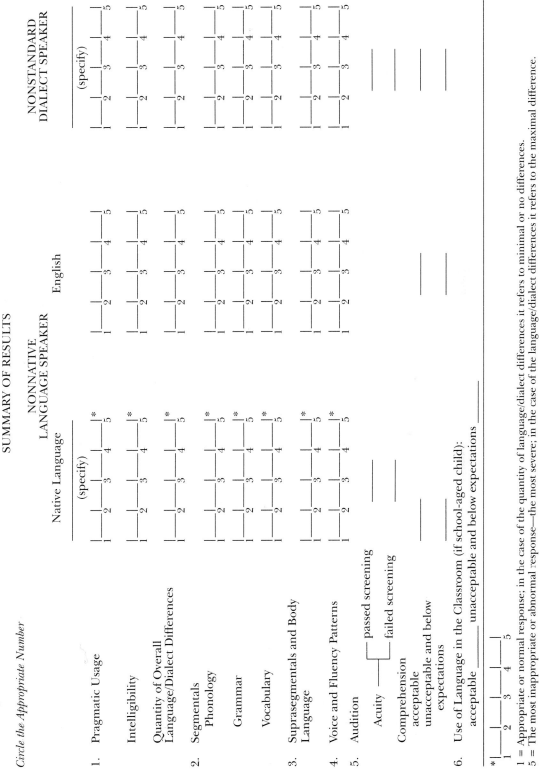

	NONNATIVE LANGUAGE SPEAKER		NONSTANDARD DIALECT SPEAKER
	Native Language (specify) ___	English	(specify) ___
1. Pragmatic Usage	1 2 3 4 5*	1 2 3 4 5	1 2 3 4 5
Intelligibility	1 2 3 4 5*	1 2 3 4 5	1 2 3 4 5
Quantity of Overall Language/Dialect Differences	1 2 3 4 5*	1 2 3 4 5	1 2 3 4 5
2. Segmentals Phonology	1 2 3 4 5*	1 2 3 4 5	1 2 3 4 5
Grammar	1 2 3 4 5*	1 2 3 4 5	1 2 3 4 5
Vocabulary	1 2 3 4 5*	1 2 3 4 5	1 2 3 4 5
3. Suprasegmentals and Body Language	1 2 3 4 5*	1 2 3 4 5	1 2 3 4 5
4. Voice and Fluency Patterns	1 2 3 4 5*	1 2 3 4 5	1 2 3 4 5

5. Audition

Acuity ⎯⎯ passed screening ___
        failed screening ___

Comprehension
acceptable ___
unacceptable and below expectations ___

6. Use of Language in the Classroom (if school-aged child):
acceptable ___ unacceptable and below expectations ___

*| 1 — 2 — 3 — 4 — 5 |

1 = Appropriate or normal response; in the case of the quantity of language/dialect differences it refers to minimal or no differences.
5 = The most inappropriate or abnormal response—the most severe; in the case of the language/dialect differences it refers to the maximal difference.

A-29

FOR THE SPEECH-LANGUAGE SPECIALIST

Native Language (L1), Acquired English (L2), Nonstandard Dialect (D)

(a) INTELLIGIBILITY

L1   L2   D

____ ____ ____
____ ____ ____
____ ____ ____
____ ____ ____
____ ____ ____

1. Standard pronunciation, with no trace of "different" accent or dialect.
2. No conspicuous mispronunciations but would not be taken for a native speaker because of some subtle prosodic differences.
3. Marked accent and occasional mispronunciations which do not interfere with understanding.
4. Accent or prosody not appropriate to dialect/language being assessed and leading to occasional misunderstanding.
5. Frequent gross errors and a very heavy accent making understanding difficult.

(b) AMOUNT OF DIALECT/LANGUAGE DIFFERENCES NOTED WHEN SPEAKER IS USING "STANDARD" ENGLISH. Estimate the amount of dialect/language differences on the following scales (minimum or none to maximum) (Circle the appropriate number.)

|—|—|—|—|—|
1 2 3 4 5
Phonology

|—|—|—|—|—|
1 2 3 4 5
Grammar

|—|—|—|—|—|
1 2 3 4 5
Vocabulary

|—|—|—|—|—|
1 2 3 4 5
Prosody

|—|—|—|—|—|
1 2 3 4 5
Body Lang.

|—|—|—|—|—|
1 2 3 4 5
Over-all

(c) SUPRASEGMENTALS OR PROSODY

L1   L2   D

____ ____ ____
____ ____ ____
____ ____ ____
____ ____ ____
____ ____ ____
____ ____ ____
____ ____ ____

1. Appropriate
2. Stress pattern is unusual*
3. Intonation pattern is unusual
4. Inflection pattern is unusual
5. Loudness pattern is unusual
6. Pitch pattern is unusual
7. Other _____

BODY LANGUAGE

L1   L2   D

____ ____ ____
____ ____ ____
____ ____ ____
____ ____ ____
____ ____ ____
____ ____ ____

1. Appropriate
2. Eye contact pattern is unusual
3. Eye movement pattern is unusual
4. A body movement pattern is unusual
5. Spacial relationship is unusual
6. Other _____

(d) VOICE PATTERNS

L1   L2   D

____ ____ ____
____ ____ ____
____ ____ ____
____ ____ ____
____ ____ ____
____ ____ ____

1. Appropriate
2. Harshness seems to be abnormal*
3. Breathiness seems to be abnormal
4. Loudness seems to be abnormal
5. Pitch seems to be abnormal
6. Other _____

FLUENCY PATTERNS

L1   L2   D

____ ____ ____
____ ____ ____
____ ____ ____
____ ____ ____
____ ____ ____

1. Appropriate
2. Speech very slow and uneven
3. Speech more hesitant and jerky than a native speaker of the same age.
4. Abnormal number of repetitions, prolongations, or stoppages in speech pattern.
5. Other _____

*Whenever the terms *unusual* or *abnormal* are noted, discuss in detail the reasons for the notations. These terms suggest that the utterance is inappropriate for the language/dialect being assessed.

(e) AUDITORY ACUITY: passed screening _____ failed screening _____

(f) AUDITORY COMPREHENSION

L1   L2   D

_____ _____ _____ 1. Understands everything in both formal and colloquial speech expected of a native speaker of the same age.

_____ _____ _____ 2. Understands everything in conversation except for colloquial speech.

_____ _____ _____ 3. Understands somewhat simplified speech directed to him, with some repetition and rephrasing.

_____ _____ _____ 4. Understands only slow, very simple speech on concrete topics; requires considerably more repetition and rephrasing than would be expected of a native speaker of the same age.

_____ _____ _____ 5. Understands too little for the simplest type of conversations.

MORPHOSYNTACTIC ANALYSIS (from language sample)

Note the client's nonnative (acquired English) or nonstandard grammatical patterns; also rate the client on the accompanying grammar scale.

1. Morphologic Problems

L1   L2   D

_____ _____ _____ a. noun forms

_____ _____ _____ b. adjective

_____ _____ _____ c. verb forms

_____ _____ _____ d. adverb

2. Syntactic Problems

L1   L2   D

_____ _____ _____ a. word order

_____ _____ _____ b. questions

_____ _____ _____ c. negation

_____ _____ _____ d. prepositions

_____ _____ _____ e. pronouns

_____ _____ _____ f. subject-verb

_____ _____ _____ g. present for future

3. Grammar Scale:

L1   L2   D

_____ _____ _____ 1. Normal standard English grammar.

_____ _____ _____ 2. Few errors, with no patterns of failure, but still lacking full control over grammar that is expected of that age.

_____ _____ _____ 3. Occasional errors showing imperfect control of some grammatical patterns but no weakness that causes misunderstanding.

_____ _____ _____ 4. Frequent errors showing lack of control of some major patterns and causing more misunderstanding than would be expected for a native speaker of that age level.

_____ _____ _____ 5. Grammar almost entirely inaccurate except in common phrases.

FOR THE CLASSROOM TEACHER

Please Check and Discuss Any Information of Relevance

Child's Name _____ Age _____ Sex _____

Address _____

Grade Level _____

School _____

Address _____

CHILD IS:

Nonnative English Speaker
1. Spanish-influenced English _____
2. Asian-influenced English _____
3. Other _____

Nonstandard English Speaker
4. African-influenced English _____
5. Appalachian-influenced English _____
6. Other _____

Discuss:

Intelligibility (Understandability) of the Child

Amount of Dialect/Language Differences Used by Child in the Classroom

Estimate the amount of dialect/language differences (from minimal or none to maximum on following scales

1—2—3—4—5	1—2—3—4—5	1—2—3—4—5	1—2—3—4—5	1—2—3—4—5	1—2—3—4—5
Phonology or Articulation Usage	Grammar	Vocabulary	Prosody or Speech Rhythm	Body Lang. or use of Body when Talking	Over-all

USE OF LANGUAGE IN THE CLASSROOM

1. Appropriate
2. Opening or closing a conversation is unusual.
3. Turn-taking during conversations is unusual.
4. Interruptions are unusual.
5. Silence as a communicative device is unusual.
6. Laughter as a communicative device is unusual.
7. Appropriate types of conversation are unusual.
8. Humor and when to use it is unusual.
9. Nonverbal behavior that accompanies conversation is unusual.
10. Logical ordering of events during discourse is unusual.
11. Other: _____

AUDITORY COMPREHENSION IN THE CLASSROOM

1. Understands everything in both formal and colloquial speech expected of a native speaker of the same age.
2. Understands everything in conversation except for colloquial speech.
3. Understands somewhat simplified speech directed to him, with some repetition and rephrasing.
4. Understands only slow, very simple speech on concrete topics; requires considerably more repetition and rephrasing than would be expected of a native speaker of the same age.
5. Understands too little for the simplest type of conversations.

Source: Adler, S. (1991). Assessment of language proficiency in limited English proficient speakers: Implications for the speech-language pathologist. *Language, Speech, and Hearing Services in Schools, 22,* 12–18. Reprinted with permission.

A-32

F

Language Analysis Methods

ASSIGNING STRUCTURAL STAGE/COMPLEX SENTENCE DEVELOPMENT

In Assigning Structural Stage, Miller (J. Miller, 1981) proposes a three-tiered analysis that includes MLU, percentage correct of Brown's 14 morphemes, and sentence analysis. These three measures enable the speech-language pathologist to determine the stage of development and to describe the forms used. Although less precise than Developmental Sentence Scoring (DSS), Assigning Structural Stage is more descriptive and prescriptive in nature. After determining the child's stage of language development, the speech-language pathologist can target linguistic forms in the next stage (Prutting, 1979).

Analysis begins by collecting a language sample. The speech-language pathologist collects 50–100 utterances or 15 minutes of conversation, whichever is larger, from the child for analysis. Unlike DSS, these utterances do not have to be sentences. First, she calculates MLU to determine the stage of development and the approximate language age of the child. MLU calculation is discussed in Chapter 6.

After she has determined MLU, the speech-language pathologist decides on the analysis method to follow. She may choose Assigning Structural Stage and/or Complex Sentence Development. If the MLU of the child is below 3.0, the speech-language pathologist uses only Assigning Structural Stage. If the child's MLU is above 4.5, she uses only Complex Sentence Development. For MLUs of 3.0 to 4.5, she uses both procedures.

In Assigning Structural Stage, the speech-language pathologist calculates the percentage correct for Brown's 14 morphemes. A minimum number of occurrences or possibilities of occurrence are needed before the speech-language pathologist can decide on consistency or inconsistency of use or nonuse. The child should attempt a morpheme at least four times before a percentage correct figure is calculated.

The percentage correct value is determined by dividing the number of correct appearances by the total number of obligatory contexts. After calculating the percentage correct, the speech-language pathologist again can attempt to describe the child's stage of language development.

Next, she analyzes each utterance within four possible categories of noun phrase, verb phrase, and negative and interrogative development. Utterances are divided into noun and verb phrases where applicable, and each phrase is assigned to the stage of development that best describes its structures. Negative or interrogative utterances are further assigned to stages representing their level of development.

The speech-language pathologist should be familiar with the information Miller (J. Miller, 1981) presents for each stage of development. Some of this information is presented in Table 6.16, although Miller presents a great deal more. The analysis process is demonstrated here by using some of the information in Table 6.16. Consider the child's utterance, "Want a big doggie." The noun phrase "a big doggie" has been expanded by the addition of an article and an adjective to the noun. This noun phrase occurs in the object position of the sentence. Expansion of the noun phrase only in the object position is an example of stage II (see intrasentence column of Table 1.16). Therefore, this sentence represents noun phrase development characteristic of stage II. The verb phrase is unelaborated, and no subject is present. This represents stage I development. No analysis is required for negative or interrogative forms.

Complex Sentence Development is used similarly, but different samples and categories are used for analysis. Analysis is based on a 15-minute sample of the child's communication, rather than on 50 utterances. For children with MLUs between 3.0 and 4.5, these samples can overlap. Five aspects of complex sentences are noted: percentage of both conjoined and embedded sentences within the sample, type of embedding, conjoining, conjunctions, and the number of different conjunctions. At each stage, development is described by the forms exhibited by 50-90% and by greater than 90% of the children.

Limited data from Complex Sentence Development are incorporated into Table 6.16. By post-stage V, 90% of children should be using *and* within a 15-minute sample. To complete a full analysis, the speech-language pathologist should consult Complex Sentence Development (J. Miller, 1981).

Each sentence is analyzed by using Assigning Structural Stage or Complex Sentence Development or both, and the data are summarized. Most likely, the child will exhibit language forms in each stage of development. Now, the speech-language pathologist must use her skill.

Even mature language users occasionally use language forms that are characteristic of less mature learning. Adults use many one-word utterances everyday. These forms are not the most characteristic forms, however, and the speech-language pathologist must gather a summary of overall language form to determine most accurately the user's abilities. It is the same with the child with language impairment. The speech-language pathologist determines those behaviors that are most characteristic of the child. These might be behaviors at a particular stage that the child uses most frequently or behaviors that represent the highest attainment level. The speech-language pathologist must make this determination.

All data from the two analysis methods—Assigning Structural Stage and Complex Sentence Development—are combined to place the child's language form within a stage or stages of development and to describe the child's language form. The child functioning well below age expectancy may need intervention.

DEVELOPMENTAL SENTENCE SCORING

Developmental Sentence Scoring, the process discussed in *Developmental Sentence Analysis* (L. Lee, 1974), is one of the most widely used and popular methods for assessing children's syntactic and morphologic development. Even so, DSS requires considerable study by the speech-language pathologist to score language samples correctly. Although the instructions are explicit and straightforward, they require a thorough understanding of English syntax and morphology. Because the scale does not evaluate many aspects of children's language, it should be only one aspect of an evaluation battery.

In the following section I discuss the primary aspects of DSS and its most common problems. This survey cannot take the place of a thorough reading of DSS procedures and actual practice with the instrument.

To rate a sample of child language, the speech-language pathologist collects 50 different consecutive *sentences*. No speaker uses full sentences all the time. Therefore, utterances that do not qualify as sentences simply are omitted, and the remainder collected until 50 consecutive sentences are amassed. DSS analysis should not be undertaken if less than 50% of the child's utterances are sentences.

Because the sample should include 50 different consecutive sentences, repeated sentences are discarded unless some change occurs. Run-on sentences of several independent clauses joined by conjunctions are segmented so that no more than two independent clauses are joined. For example, the following run-on should be divided as noted:

> [We went to the zoo, and I saw monkeys,] [and we had a picnic, and I ate a hot dog,] [and I fed pigeons, and we came home on the bus .]

The *and* at the beginning of each sentence ("*and* we had. . ., *and* I fed. . .") would not be scored. A sentence may have more than one *and* if the word does not link clauses, but rather is used for compound subjects, verbs, or objects, for example:

> Tom, Mary, *and* John were throwing *and* kicking beach balls *and* soccer balls.

Sentences that begin with a conjunction, such as "Because I falled down," are included in the sample, but the conjunction itself should not be scored because it does not link clauses.

Each sentence is rated on the basis of eight grammatical categories and assigned a score of 1–8 points in the applicable categories. The categories and point values are given in Table F.1. Each structure demonstrated in the sentence is scored each time it occurs. For example, sentence 1 in Table F.2, "I don't know what I like," contains the word *I* twice. Therefore, the word receives a score of 1 twice under personal pronouns, in addition to other points.

TABLE F.1
Developmental sentence scoring categories and point values

Score	Indefinite Pronouns or Noun Modifiers	Personal Pronouns	Main Verbs	Secondary Verbs
1	it, this, that	1st and 2nd person: I, me, my, mine, you, your(s)	A. Uninflected verb: I *see* you. b. copula, is or 's: *It's* red. C. is + verb + ing: He *is coming*.	
2		3rd person: he, him, his, she, her, hers	A. -s and -ed: *plays, played* B. irregular past: *ate, saw* C. Copula: *am, are, was, were* D. Auxiliary *am, are, was, were*	Five early-developing infinitives: I wan*na* see (want *to see*) I'm gon*na* see (going *to see*) I got*ta* see (got *to see*) Lem*me* [to] see (let me [*to*] *see*) Let's [to] play (let [us *to*] *play*)
3	A. no, some, more, all, lot(s), one(s), two (etc.), other(s), another B. something, somebody, someone	A. Plurals: we, us, our(s), they, them, their B. these, those		Non-complementing infinitives: I stopped *to play*. I'm afraid *to look*. It's hard *to do that*.
4	nothing, nobody, none, no one		A. can, will, may + verb: *may go* B. Obligatory do + verb: *don't go* C. emphatic do + verb: I *do see*.	Participle, present or past: I see a boy *running* I found the toy *broken*.

Score	Negatives	Conjunctions	Interrogative Reversals	Wh Questions
1	it, this, that + copula or auxiliary is, 's, + not: It's *not* mine. This is *not* a dog. That *is not* moving.		Reversal of copula: *Isn't it* red? *Were they* there?	
2				A. who, what, what + noun: *Who* am I? *What is* he eating? *What book* are you reading? B. where, how many, how much, what . . . do. what . . . for *Where* did it go? *How much* do you want? *What* is he *doing*? What is a hammer *for*?
3		and		
4	can't, don't		Reversal of auxiliary be: *Is he* coming? *Isn't he* coming? *Was he* going? *Wasn't he* going?	

Sentences that would be acceptable mature forms are given an additional point called a *sentence point*. The sentence point should only be awarded when the sentence is syntactically and semantically correct by mature standards. The following would not receive a sentence point:

Carol and me went to the store.

Nobody didn't go.

I got six pencils in my desk.

TABLE F.1, *continued*

Score	Indefinite Pronouns or Noun Modifiers	Personal Pronouns	Main Verbs	Secondary Verbs
5		Reflexives: myself, yourself, himself, herself, itself, themselves		A. Early infinitival complements with differing subjects in kernels: I want you *to come*. Let him [*to*] *see*. B. Later infinitival complements: I had *to go*. I told him *to go*. I tried *to go*. He ought *to go*. C. Obligatory deletions: Make it [*to*] *go*. I'd better [*to*] *go*. D. Infinitive with wh-word: I know what *to get*. I know how *to do* it.
6		A. Wh-pronouns: who, which, whose, whom, what, that, how many, how much I know *who* came. That's *what* I said. B. Wh-word + infinitive: I know *what* to do. I know *who(m)* to take	A. could, would, should, might + verb: *might come, could be* B. Obligatory does, did + verb C. Emphatic does, did + verb	

In Table F.2, sentence 2, "What do you like?" receives a score of 4; it does not receive a sentence point because it is not an acceptable mature sentence. Sentence 3, "I don't know," does receive the sentence point.

Attempt markers and incomplete markers may be awarded for structures. An *attempt marker*—a line or hyphen in place of a score—is awarded when a structure is attempted but incorrect. Naturally, as in sentence 4, "He bes happy," the sentence cannot receive a sentence point. Surface structures that are conversationally appropriate but incomplete receive the incomplete marker *inc* in place of a score. If the structure is conversationally acceptable, it receives a sentence

Score	Negatives	Conjunctions	Interrogative Reversals	Wh Questions
5	isn't, won't	A. but B. so, and so, so that C. or, if		when, how, how + adjective *When* shall I come? *How* do you do it? *How big* is it?
6		because	A. Obligatory do, does, did: *Do they* run? *Does it* bite? *Didn't it* hurt? B. Reversal of modal: *Can you* play? *Won't it* hurt? *Shall I* sit down? C. Tag question: It's fun, *isn't it?* It isn't fun, *is it?*	

point. For example, in the following exchange, the child's response would receive an incomplete for the main verb.

SP–LANG PATH: Who let the guinea pig out?
CHILD: I didn't. [I didn't (let him out).]

Attempt and incomplete markers are difficult to use and confusing for those not familiar with DSS. They do not affect the score and are meant to aid the speech-language pathologist in deciding where to begin intervention. This decision can be made on the basis of other data and these markers omitted.

The point value of each sentence is totaled and added to the value for every other sentence. This overall total is divided by the number of sentences (usually

TABLE F.1, *continued*

Score	Indefinite Pronouns or Noun Modifiers	Personal Pronouns	Main Verbs	Secondary Verbs
7	A. any, anything, anybody, anyone B. every, everything, everybody, everyone C. both, few, many, each, several, most, least, much, next, first, last, second (etc.)	(his) own, one, oneself, whichever, whoever, whatever Take *whatever* you like.	A. Passive with *get*, any tense Passive with *be*, any tense B. must, shall + verb: *must come* C. have + verb + en: *I've eaten* D. have got: I*'ve got* it.	Passive infinitival complement: With *get*: I have *to get dressed.* I don't want to *get hurt.* With *be*: I want *to be pulled.* It's going *to be locked.*
8			A. have been + verb + ing had been + verb + ing B. modal + have + verb + en: *may have eaten* C. modal + be + verb + ing: *could be playing* D. Other auxiliary combinations: *should have been sleeping*	Gerund: *Swinging* is fun. I like *fishing.* He started *laughing.*

50) to yield a score. The speech-language pathologist must remember that this value is a DSS score, not an MLU. The two values are very different.

She then applies the DSS score to a table of ages and scores to compare the child's performance with that of other children at that age. Figure F.1 shows the average scores (50th percentile) for each age and the scores for the 10th, 25th, 75th, and 90th percentiles. For example, an average score for a 4-year-old would be approximately 7.3. Only the highest 10% of 4-year-olds would receive a score of 9.0 (90th percentile).

Score	Negatives	Conjunctions	Interrogative Reversals	Wh Questions
7	All other negatives: A. Uncontracted negatives: I can *not* go. He has *not* gone. B. Pronoun-auxiliary or pronoun-copula contraction: I'm *not* coming. He's *not* here. C. Auxiliary-negative or copula-negative contraction: He *wasn't* going. He *hasn't* been seen. It *couldn't* be mine. They *aren't* big.			why, what if, how come, how about + gerund *Why* are you crying? *What if* I won't do it? *How come* he is crying? *How about* coming with me?
8		A. where, when, how, while, whether (or not), till, until, unless, since, before, after, for, as, as + adjective + as, as if, like, that, than: I know *where* you are. Don't come *till* I call. B. Obligatory deletions: I run faster *than* you [run]. I'm *as big as* a man [is big]. It looks *like* a dog [looks]. C. Elliptical deletions (score 0): That's *why* [I took it]. I know *how*. [*I can do it*]. D. *Wh-words* + infinitive: I know how to do it.	A. Reversal of auxiliary have: *Has he seen you?* B. Reversal with two or three auxiliaries: *Has he been eating? Couldn't he have waited? Could he have been crying? Wouldn't he have been going?*	whose, which, which + noun *Whose* cat is that? *Which book* do you want?

Source: Lee, L. (1974). *Developmental sentence analysis* (pp. 134–135). Evanston, IL: Northwestern University Press. Copyright © 1974 by Northwestern University. Reprinted with permission.

TABLE F.2
Language sample analysis using developmental sentence scoring

Developmental sentence scoring form

Name:
D.O.B.:
D.O.K.:
C.A.:
Score

	Indefinite Pronouns	Personal Pronouns	Main Verbs	Secondary Verbs	Negatives	Conjunctions	Interrogative Reversals	Wh Questions	Sentence Point	Total
I don't know what I like		1,1,6	4,1		4				1	18
What you like?		1	1					2		4
I don't know		1	4		4				1	10
He bes happy		2	inc							2

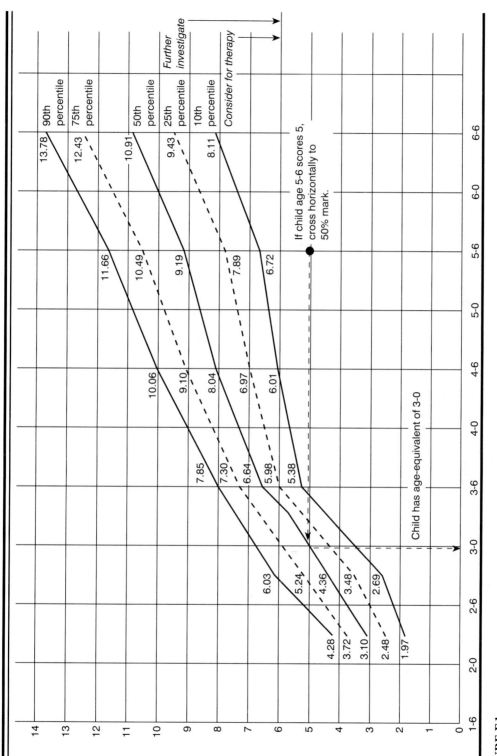

FIGURE F.1

DSS expected scores and ages

Source: Lee, L. (1974). *Developmental sentence analysis.* Evanston, IL: Northwestern University Press. Reprinted with permission.

A-43

According to the instructions, children whose scores place them below the 10th percentile should be considered for therapy. Therefore, a 4-year-old who scores below 4.7 should be considered for therapy.

An age equivalent for the child placing below the 10th percentile can be determined by noting the point at which the horizontal line for the child's score crosses the diagonal 50th-percentile line. At this age, the child's score is an average score. For example, the child aged 5 1/2 who receives an average score of 5.0 points is well below the 10th percentile for that age and needs intervention. The age equivalent would be found by following the 5.0 line to the left until it intersects the diagonal 50th-percentile line. This occurs at an age of 3 years. Thus, the child's age equivalent is approximately 3 years.

Age equivalence, if needed, can be found in the same way for children, such as those with mental retardation, who may exceed the age norm ceiling of 6 1/2 years. Obviously, the percentile values are not relevant.

Language delay in years can be determined by subtracting the age equivalent from the child's chronological age. In the previous example, the child's language delay is approximately 2 1/2 years. Although this value means little for the direction of therapy, it does provide a score for those people, such as administrators, who demand such data, and it can be used as an index of change over time. The same precautions for such statistics given in Chapter 3 apply.

The most common problems encountered with DSS are associated with determination of grammatical units and with scoring (Lively, 1984). These problems are discussed briefly in the following section. Readers can refer to Lively (1984) and Hughes, Fey, and Long (1992) for a more thorough discussion.

Scoring adverbs as indefinite pronouns/noun modifiers.   Words such as *first, last,* and *everywhere* that tell the manner or place of an action are adverbs ("Let's do this *first*") and should not be scored as indefinite pronoun/noun modifiers. In contrast, other words, especially numbers, should be scored when they do function as indefinite pronoun/noun modifiers, as in the following:

Can I have *one*?

I have *two* dolls.

No one don't like me.

Personal pronoun/*wh-* conjunction/*wh-* question confusion.   *Wh-* words may be used as personal pronouns (score 6) or as conjunctions (score 8). The distinction can be clarified by remembering that a complete clause will follow the conjunction.

I want the one *that* talks.	(Pronoun, because "talks" is not a complete clause.)
He told us *that* we could shovel his driveway.	(Conjunction, because "we could shovel his driveway" is a complete clause.)
I know *what* you want.	(Pronoun, because "you want" is not a complete clause.)
What do you want?	(Wh-question)

Main verbs. All uninflected or unmarked verbs receive a score of 1. Regular and irregular inflected verbs receive some other score.

I *like* ice cream.	(Uninflected = 1)
She *likes* ice cream.	(Inflected = 2)
She *ate* ice cream.	(Inflected = 2)

Incorrect attempts, such as using *got* for *have*, receive an attempt score. The verb *do* as a main verb receives a 1 or 2. As an auxiliary, it receives a 4 if uninflected and a 6 if inflected. The modal auxiliary verbs *can, will,* and *may* are scored in the same manner.

Do it for me.	(Uninflected main verb = 1)
I *did* my homework.	(Inflected main verb = 2)
I *do* like ice cream.	(Uninflected auxiliary = 4)
I *did* like ice cream.	(Inflected auxiliary = 6)
He *does* like ice cream.	(Inflected auxiliary = 6)
I *can* swim.	(Uninflected modal = 4)
I *could* swim.	(Inflected modal = 6)

In contrast, the modal auxiliaries *must* and *shall* are always scored as 7. The perfect tense forms of *have + verb (en)* also receive a 7. All sentences with two or more auxiliaries, as in "He could have gone," receive an 8.

Passive sentences present a special case, and speech-language pathologists should refer to L. Lee (1974).

Compound sentences can be very difficult, especially if material is omitted. With compound verbs, each is scored. If the auxiliary is omitted, both verbs still should receive the full score.

I *was singing* and *dancing*.	(The second "was" is omitted and understood, so each verb receives a score of 2.)

If, on the other hand, the main verb is omitted, only the complete form is scored and the other abbreviated or elliptical form receives an incomplete score.

I *did* complete my lesson, but Carol *didn't*.	(The second "did" receives an incomplete score, whereas the first received a 6.)

Secondary verbs. The chief error in this category is in identifying the infinitive. Often the signal word *to* is omitted. If the child uses *gonna, wanna, gotta, lemme,* or *let's,* the infinitive is scored as 2. Other infinitives receive a 5 if the subject of the infinitive is different from the subject of the main verb.

I wanna go.	(Score as 2.)
I want to go.	(Score as 2.)

I want her to go.	(Different subjects = 5)
Make the car (to) go.	(The subject is understood to be "you" and car is "to go," so score the infinitive as 5.)

The form *be* + *verb(en)* in the present tense is scored as copula plus adjective unless the agentive prepositional is explicit. In the past form *was/were* + *verb(en)*, it is scored as passive as long as it makes sense when the agentive phrase is added.

The door is broken.	(Score as 1)
The glass is broken by the cat.	(Score as 7)
The glass was broken (by the cat).	(Score as 7)
The girl was lost.	(Score as 2)

Negatives.   The only negative to receive a score of 1 is the *this/that/it* + *is/'s not* form. All other forms of this combination receive a higher score. Any other subject or auxiliary verb receives a score of 7.

It is not yours.	("It is not" = 1)
It's not yours.	("It's not" = 1)
It isn't yours.	("It isn't" = 5)
You *can't* do it.	("Can't" = 7)

Conjunctions.   Score the conjunction *then* as 3 for *and then* even though the *and* is omitted, as long as two independent clauses are joined.

Interrogative reversals.   Speech-language pathologists often overlook interrogative reversals when scoring *wh-* questions. Tag questions, except those ending in *huh, okay, eh,* and the like, receive a score of 6.

Sentence point.   If the child *has been interrupted* in mid-sentence but has produced the subject and the predicate of the sentence and this stem is grammatically acceptable, the partial sentence should be scored and given a sentence point.

Obviously, Developmental Sentence Scoring is a very complex analysis system, not to be attempted without a thorough knowledge of both English syntax and DSS procedures. Unfortunately, the child's score offers little direction for intervention, although Lee suggests appropriate places at which to begin intervention based primarily on the percentage of correct production. The hierarchy presented in Table F.1 offers only limited guidance and omits many important structures. This type of problem seems inherent in any analysis system that reduces complex behavior to point values.

Modification for Children with LEP and Different Dialects

The nature of the DSS makes it an inappropriate tool to use for assessing the language abilities of children with LEP and different dialects. Some advances have been made in this area. Black English Sentence Scoring (BESS) is a promising attempt to maintain the DSS format while measuring Black English usage. The scoring criteria, a sample scoring, and means and standard deviations are listed in Tables F.3, F.4, and F.5 respectively.

Summary

DSS is a good quantitative measure, although no data are available on the relationship of DSS scores to the type and extent of a child's language impairment (Hughes et al., 1992). Even when matched with peers on the basis of MLU, chil-

TABLE F.3
Black English sentence scoring categories and point values

	Indefinite Pronouns or Noun Modifiers	**Personal Pronouns**	**Main Verbs**	**Secondary Verbs**
1	– these/this: *these* many.	– mine's/my, you/your: That *you* book? – y'all (plural *you*) – me/I (in compound subj.): Me and my brother went in it.	– Ø copula *is, am, are*: That boy my friend. Or hypercorrect: I'm is six. – Ø aux *be* + Ving: The girl singin'. – locational *go* or existential *it's*: Here *go* some lights. *It's* two dimes stuck on the table. – *got* as uninflected *have*: You gotta take it home.	
2		– he, she (in apposition): My brother, *he* bigger than you. – they/he: They my uncle. – he, he's/his: He's name is Terry. – she, she's/her	– third person singular and regular past tense markers deleted. – have/has: It have money on it. – Regularization of -s and -ed: Trudy and my sister hides. (hypercorrect) – Aux was/were: We *was gon'* rob some money. – Irreg. past tense–Uninflected: He *find* the money; Past form as participle: We *have went*: Participle as past form: He *done* it first.	– I'm, I'mon, I'ma pronunciation of I'm gonna + V: I'm play. I'ma be tired. – *go* pronunciation of gonna: His nose go bleed. – fixin' to (used like gonna): I'm fixin' to take him to jail.

	Negatives	Conjunctions	Interrogative Reversal	Wh- Questions
1	– it, this, that + Ø copula/aux + not/ain't: That *not* mine. It *ain't* on?		– rising intonation with deleted or unreversed copula: You my friend? Where the gas at? What this is? – is/are: Derrick, is you?	
2				– who, what, what + noun (with deleted aux or copula) – where, how many, how much, what . . . do, what . . . for (with deleted aux or copula): Where the man? – Wh- Qs formed without interrogative reversal: What that is?

dren with language impairments tend to have more difficulty with the main verb and pronoun categories and may have difficulty with secondary verbs, negatives, and conjunctions (J. Johnston & Kamhi, 1984; Liles & Watt, 1984; Leonard, 1972). DSS has shown great resiliency and has been modified for speakers of Black English, expanded to 6- to 10-year-olds, and converted to a computerized version (Hughes, Low, Fey, & Alsop, 1990; Long & Fey, 1991; N. Nelson & Hyter, 1990; Stephens, Dallman, & Montgomery, 1988).

Language Assessment, Remediation, and Screening Procedure (LARSP)

The Language Assessment, Remediation, and Screening Procedure (LARSP) (Crystal et al., 1976) is used more widely in England, Canada, and Australia than in the United States. More psycholinguistic in nature than the other methods

	Indefinite Pronouns or Noun Modifiers	Personal Pronouns	Main Verbs	Secondary Verbs
3	– *no* (when 2nd or 3rd neg. marker): He don't like me *no* more.	– we, they (in apposition): The boys, *they* got in trouble. – they/their: *They* name is Tanya and Bryan. – them/they or their: I know what *them* is. One of 'em name is Caesar. – them/those: *them* kids.		
4	– nothing, nobody, none, no one (when 2nd or 3rd neg. marker): Ain't nobody got none.		– Ø modal *will* or *'ll*: I be five when my birthday come. – don't + verb (3rd pers. sing.): My mama, she don't like it. – *do* uninflected: *Do* he still have it? (Score inc. in My sister *do*.) – Ø *do* in Qs: You still have it? – ain't (as copula or aux): Ain't no dirt in it. Nobody ain't got no more. – can't, don't, won't as preposed neg. aux.: Can't nobody do it. – could/can: He could climb that tree.	– Participate with deleted -en: She has a state name Tennessee. (phonological cluster reduction rule) – I found the toy broke. (morphological difference)

included in this appendix, LARSP analyzes language on the basis of phrase and sentence structure and on the number of elements found in the child's utterances. These values relate to seven stages of language development, mostly in the preschool years.

The speech-language pathologist collects 30 minutes of the child's speech from two different 15-minute activities. In the first, the child plays with a familiar adult; in the second, the child and the adult participate in a dialogue.

All utterances are included in the analysis, describing what the child can or cannot do. Therefore, all utterances are transcribed with intonations and pauses

	Negatives	Conjunctions	Interrogative Reversals	Wh- Questions
3		– and plus – Ø and (when into-nation makes sen-tence combination clear): He pointed his finger at him, (with rising intona-tion) he pointed his finger at him (with falling intonation).		
4	– don't (with 3rd pers. sing. as 2nd or 3rd neg. mark-er): He *don't* want none. No, nobody *don't* live with me. – can't, don't (as pre-posed aux): Can't nobody make me. – Ø copula/aux + not + V: My mama *not* gonna pick me up today. He *not* a baby. – ain't (as negative copula or aux. *be*): He *ain't* my friend.		– Ø auxiliary be: My voice gonna come out of here? You gonna tell my mama? – was/were: Was you throwin' rocks?	

indicated. Important nonlinguistic information is included to aid analysis. The speech-language pathologist uses the following markers when transcribing:

( )	Parentheses, placed around unintelligible speech, may be left blank, may signal the possible number of syllables, or may guess at the unintelligible por-tion by placing words within.
?	A question mark is placed before any word for which the transcriptional accuracy is in doubt. This occurs when two listeners disagree.
*	Asterisks are placed around speakers' words that overlap.

Indefinite Pronouns or Noun Modifiers	Personal Pronouns	Main Verbs	Secondary Verbs
5	– personal datives me, him, her: I'm gonna buy *me* some candy. He make *him* a lot of 'em. – reflexives: hisself, theirselves, themself, theyselves.		– Deleted *to* in infinitival complements: My grandma tell me stay away from him. I like go shopping. My mommy used do it.
6	– what (in apposition): My voice gonna come out of here *what* I said on that book? – what/that or who: He's the one *what* I told you about. – Deleted relative pronoun: I saw a little girl was on the street.	– did + nt + verb (when 2nd or 3rd neg. marker: Nobody didn't do it. – could, would, should + nt + verb (preposed neg. aux): Couldn't nobody do it. – Ø contracted could or would (phonol. deletions): You('d) burn your head off. – might/will: Who might be the baby?	

(())	Double parentheses are placed around interjections or repairs that do not disturb the flow of communication.

Analysis is accomplished on a worksheet and transferred to the Profile Chart shown in Table F.6. First, synchronic analysis is accomplished in Sections A, B, and C. In-depth analysis is accomplished by using the developmental stage portion of the chart. The authors recommend that the total analysis be completed by using eight separate scans of the transcript.

	Negatives	Conjunctions	Interrogative Reversal	Wh- Questions
5	– won't (as preposed aux): *Won't* nobody help him.	– for/so: The dog make too much noise for they won't catch many fish. – conditional *and*: You do that *and* I'm gonna smack you. – *if* with phrase deletions: He lookin' if he see the money. – aux. inversion in indirect Qs (instead of *if*): She ask me do he want some more.		– when, how (with deleted aux, copula or do): How you do this?
6		– or either, or neither (as disjunctives): He will go *or either* he will stay. He told her that he wouldn't be bad *or neither* get in trouble. – preposed why phrase (with because): Why he's in here, cause baby scared the dog.	– Ø do: You know that one with the tractor? Where you work? You got blue eyes? – do (with 3rd pers. sing.) Do he still have it? – Ø or unreversed modal: Now, what else I be doin? Why you can't talk on that? – Tag question with ain't: It gonna be fun, ain't it?	

In Scan I, the speech-language pathologist removes for later analysis all utterances that cannot be analyzed. These are of two types: unanalyzed and problematic. Unanalyzed utterances may be wholly unintelligible, may consist of symbolic noise, such as truck or airplane sounds, or may be *deviant* sentences. Deviant sentences are utterances that are structurally inadmissible in adult grammar and are not part of the expected grammatical development of children developing normally. Problematic utterances include incomplete sentences that do not represent expected grammatical development, and ambiguous sentences that may be interpreted in two different ways on the basis of the communication situation. The number of utterances within each category is tallied and placed in

Indefinite Pronouns or Noun Modifiers	Personal Pronouns	Main Verbs	Secondary Verbs
7 – many a: *Many* a people likes to give him a nickel		– passive verb + en with *getting* (aux. deleted): Leroy *getting* dressed. – passive verb ± be ± en: One is name Brick. They named Chief and JoJo. – done + verb + en (completive aspect): I *done tried*. – ± (neg.) aux. + supposed: He don't supposed to do it. What toy you supposed to play with? – ± have ± verb ± en: We seen him already. He have made him mad.	– Passive with phonological deletions: I'm be dressed up real cute. I'ma be tired. She gonna be surprise, ain't she? I want it cut on.
8		– invariant *be*: My daddy know I skip school 'cause I be home with him. He be mad when somebody leave him home. – double modals: We might could come. – other expanded aux. forms: He be done jumped out the tub. He been going. (*have* has undergone phonological deletion) You shouldn't did that. – remote past aspect: She been whuptin' the baby. I been wanted this.	– gerund with *go to*, *got to*, *start to*: When I cry, she goes to whipping me. He started to crying. He got to thinking.

	Negatives	Conjunctions	Interrogative Reversal	Wh- Questions
7	– ain't (for have + not) ± uninflected V: I *ain't* taste any. – ain't (for did + not) ± uninflected V: Yesterday, he *ain't* go to school. I ain't found Marge in the school. – couldn't, wouldn't, shouldn't (as preposed aux) – wasn't/weren't: The brakes wasn't workin' right. – weren't/wasn't: There weren't no money. – uncontracted, uninflected neg. aux.: Lester *do not* like it.			– why, what if, how come (with deleted or unreversed aux. copula or do, or with got): Why she turn that way? Hey, why you got a dress on mama?
8		– less'n (for unless) – to/till: I didn't get to sleep *to* I had to come in the morning. – ± as + adjective + as: He sock Leroy in the arm hard as he could.	– deleted have: He seen it? How you been? What you been doing? – have with 3rd pers. sing.: Have he seen you?	– whose, which, which + noun (with deleted aux. copula or do) – who/whose: Who this bed? Who baby is that?

Source: From *Black English Sentence Scoring: Development and Use as a Tool for Nonbiased Assessment* by N. W. Nelson and Y. D. Hyter. 1990. Unpublished manuscript. Western Michigan University, Kalamazoo. Copyright 1990 by N. W. Nelson. Reprinted by permission.

TABLE F.4
Language sample analysis using Black English sentence scoring

Name   Eric
Age   4:0
Date   May 31, 1993   DSS   3.73   BESS   6.55

	Indef. Pron.	Pers. Pron.	Prim. Verb	Sec. Verb	Neg.	Conj.	Inter. Rev.	WH Ques.	Sent. Point	Total
1. That the food that grandma ate.	1	6	1 / -, 2						1[c] / 0	11[b] / 9[a]
2. I goin' to nursery school.		1	1 / -						1 / 0	3 / 1
3. I putting my sister on a motorcycle.	.	1, 1	1 / -						1 / 0	4 / 2
4. I listening.		1	1 / -						1 / 0	3 / 1
5. I watched him yesterday.		1, 2	2						1	6
6. I like these.		1, 3	1						1	6
7. I push all these buttons, ok?	3	1, 3	4 / -						1 / 0	12 / 7
8. They try catch me.		3, 1	2 / -	5 / -					1 / 0	12 / 4
9. I had a spoon.		1	2						1	4
10. Who this on the phone?	1		1 / -				1 / -	2. / -	1 / 0	6 / 1
11. Where the gun?			1 / -				1 / -	2 / -	1 / 0	5 / 0

Total DSS for this partial sample:
    41 divided by 11 = 3.73
Total BESS for this partial sample:
    72 divided by 11 = 6.55

[a] Sentence total for DSS.
[b] Sentence total for BESS.
[c] Point earned for BESS but not DSS. (Numbers above DSS attempt markers (—) represent credit awarded for BESS but not DSS.)

Source: Nelson, N. W., & Hyter, Y. D. (1990). *Black English sentence scoring and use as a tool for nonbiased assessment.* Unpublished manuscript, Western Michigan University, Kalamazoo. Reprinted by permission.

A-55

TABLE F.5
Means and standard deviations for DSS and BESS

Age Range	N	Mean DSS	SD	Mean Bess	SD
3:0–3:6	8	5.63	0.91	7.44	1.15
3:6–4:0	8	5.73	1.04	7.71	0.98
4:0–4:6	8	7.47	1.58	9.33	1.26
4:6–5:0	8	7.51	1.68	8.85	1.48
5:0–5:6	8	8.86	1.93	10.79	1.92
5:6–6:0	8	8.31	2.04	10.02	2.16
6:0–6:6	8	9.12	2.43	11.08	1.61
6:6–7:0	8	9.47	1.72	11.17	2.17

Source: Nelson, N. W., & Hyter, Y. D. (1990). *Black English sentence scoring and use as a tool for nonbiased assessment.* Unpublished manuscript, Western Michigan University, Kalamazoo. Reprinted by permission.

Section A of the Profile Chart. With these utterances identified, the subsequent scans are less problematic.

Scan 2, recorded in Sections B and C, establishes the proportion of spontaneous to responsive utterances and analyzes the type of each. The type of response depends on the type of stimulus sentence. LARSP distinguishes between question stimuli and others.

Normal responses may be classified as *elliptical major sentences,* in which shared information is omitted; *full major sentences;* or *minor sentences* consisting of single word answers, such as *yes/no.* In addition, elliptical sentences are rated by the number of elements included in each. Abnormal responses may demonstrate either structural deviance, in which a mismatch occurs between the expected structural pattern of the response and the one produced, or *zero response,* in which a response is expected but not received. Other responses are classified as *repetitions* of the other speaker or *problems.* The problems category is an *other* category for those utterances that do not fit anywhere else. The number of each type of response is recorded in Section B in the type of response column and in the stimulus row.

Spontaneous utterances are divided into *novel* sentences and *full self-repetitions.* The number of utterances within each category is recorded in the appropriate space on the Profile Chart.

Scan 3 is for sentence connectivity. Each type is tabulated and counted. The four types include *intonation,* in which emphasis or stress indicates old or contrasting information; *vocabulary replacement,* in which another word other than a pronoun replaces the old information; *common sense semantic connection,* in which sequencing provides connectivity; and *grammatical links,* such as adverbs, cross-referenced articles and pronouns, and ellipses.

Scans 4–7 are more grammatical in nature and include coordination and subordination, clause structure, phrase structure, and word structure, respectively. Scans 5, 6, and 7 provide the most information on structure. Information regarding the number of each type of structure is recorded under the most appropriate

TABLE F.6
LARSP profile chart

| Name | | Age | | Sample date | | Type | |

A Unanalyzed / Problematic

A	**Unanalyzed**			**Problematic**		
	1 Unintelligible	2 Symbolic Noise	3 Deviant	1 Incomplete	2 Ambiguous	3 Stereotypes

B Responses

					Normal Response					Abnormal		
					Major							
				Elliptical								
Stimulus Type	Totals	Repetitions	1	2	3+	Reduced	Full	Minor	Structural	θ	Problems
☐ Questions											
☐ Others											

C Spontaneous

D Reactions

		General	Structural	θ	Other	Problems

Stage I (0:9–1:6)

Minor	Responses		Vocatives		Other		Problems	
Major	*Comm.*	*Quest.*	*Statement*					
	"V"	"Q"	"V"	"N"	Other		Problems	

Stage II (1:6–2:0)

Conn.		Clause				Phrase		Word
	VX	QX	SV	AX	DN	VV	-ing
			SO	VO	Adj N	V part	pl
			SC	VC	NN	Int X	
			Neg X	Other	PrN	Other	-ed

Stage III (2:0–2:6)

	X + S:NP	X + V:VP	X + C:NP	X + O:NP	X + A:AP		
	VXY	QXY	SVC	VCA	D Adj N	Cop	-en
			SVO	VOA	Adj Adj N		3s
	let XY	VS(X)	SVA	VO$_d$O$_i$	Pr DN	Aux$_O^M$	
	do XY		Neg XY	Other	Pron$_O^P$	Other	gen

Stage IV (2:6–3:0)

	XY + S:NP	XY + V:VP	XY+C:NP	XY+O:NP	XY+A:AP		n't
	+ S	QVS	SVOA	AAXY	NP Pr NP	Neg V	cop
		QXY+	SVCA	Other	Pr D Adj N	Neg X	aux
	VXY+	VS(X+)	SVO$_d$O$_i$		cX	2 Aux	
		tag	SVOC		XcX	Other	

Stage V (3:0–3:6)

and	Coord.	Coord.	Coord.	1	1+	Postmod. clause	1	1+	-est
c	Other	Other	Subord. A	1	1+				-er
s			S	C	O				
Other			Comparative			Postmod. phrase	1+		-ly

Stage VI (3:6–4:6)

	(+)				(–)				
NP	VP	Clause	Conn.	Clause		NP		VP		Word
					Element				N V
Initiator	Complex	Passive	*and*	Ø	D	Pr	Pron^P	Aux^M Aux^O Cop	*irreg*
Coord.		Complement	c	⇆	DØ	PrØ			
		how	s	Concord	D⇆	Pr⇆	Ø	Ø	*reg*
		what							
Other								Ambiguous	

Stage VII (4:6 +)

Discourse		*Syntactic Comprehension*	
A Connectivity	*it*		
Comment Clause	*there*	*Style*	
Emphatic Order	Other		
Total No. Sentences		Mean No. Sentences Per Turn	Mean Sentence Length

Source: Crystal, D., Fletcher, P., & Garman, M. (1976, revised 1981). *The grammatical analysis of language disability.* New York: Elsevier. Reprinted with permission. Revised 1981.

stage next to the structures listed. Clausal and phrasal structure coding is listed in Table F.7. The stages represent seven theoretical levels of development of syntax and should not be confused with Brown's stages of development. Approximate ages for each stage are given in Table F.8. Crystal et al. (1976) provide descriptions and examples of each stage.

Morphological markers, or *word-structure patterns,* also are recorded on the right–hand side of the Profile Chart. These are not related to any specific stage. The coding for these markers is given in Table F.9.

Scan 8 involves only the utterances that are problems because of structural abnormalities. These may provide a key to disordered language.

Finally, three additional items of information are computed: the total number of sentences, the mean number of sentences per turn, and the mean sentence length in words. The total number of sentences includes all utterances, even repetitions, except for unanalyzed and problem utterances. The mean number of utterances per turn is found by combining the totals in Sections B and C and dividing this amount by the total of the conversational partner's stimulus types, found in Section B.

Conclusion

Although somewhat more specific than Assigning Structural Stage/Complex Sentence Development (J. Miller, 1981), LARSP is more theoretical and based on

TABLE F.7
LARSP clausal and phrasal structure coding

V	Verb
Q	Question word (*What, where*)
N	Noun
X	All elements that may co-occur with another element
S	Subject
C/O	Complement/object
A	Adverb (Usually location)
Neg	Negative word (*No, not*)
D	Demonstrative (Including possessive pronouns)
Adj	Adjective
Pr	Preposition
Part	Particle (*Out* as in *Come out*)
Y	Used with X to indicate any **two** elements of clause structure
NP	Noun phrase
VP	Verb phrase
Cop	Copula
Aux	Auxiliary verb (Not just *be*)
Pron	Pronoun
O_d	Direct object
O_i	Indirect object
Z	Use with X and Y to indicate any **three** elements of clause structure
c	Coordinating conjunction
s	Subordinating conjunction

TABLE F.8
LARSP stages and approximate ages

Stage I	9 mos.—1 yr. 6 mos.
Stage II	1 yr. 6 mos.—2 yrs.
Stage III	2 yrs.—2 yrs. 6 mos.
Stage IV	2 yrs. 6 mos.—3 yrs.
Stage V	3 yrs.—3 yrs. 6 mos.
Stage VI	3 yrs. 6 mos.—4 yrs. 6 mos.
Stage VII	4 yrs. 6 mos.—9 yrs.

older, more psycholinguistic models of language development. Although LARSP avoids the pitfalls of phrase structure-based grammars, it still adheres to the notion of elements added one at a time. It might be best to ignore the stage information but incorporate a portion of the analysis methodology, especially the phrasal and sentential structures. Responsive versus spontaneous data and the mean number of sentences per turn are also valuable.

Crystal et al. (1976) provide some interpretation of the results with regard to specific language impairments. Sketchy intervention programs are suggested for the patterns exhibited in the samples.

Systematic Analysis of Language Transcripts (SALT)

Systematic Analysis of Language Transcripts (SALT) (J. Miller & Chapman, 1985) is one of the most promising computer analysis methods available. Based on Assigning Structural Stage/Complex Sentence Development (J. Miller, 1981), SALT is designed for use with the IBM PC, the Apple II series, and Macintosh computers. Within limits, SALT analyzes morphemic, syntactic, and semantic aspects of a language sample.

The transcript is typed in standard English orthography. Time is critical for calculation of duration and pause times and must be noted. Each feature to be analyzed is signaled with a different marker. Therefore, it takes approximately 7 minutes for even the skilled user to enter each minute of conversation into the transcription format.

TABLE F.9
LARSP word–structure pattern codes

-ing	Present progressive *-ing*
pl	Plural *-s* marker
-ed	Past tense *-ed*
-en	Past participle *-en*
3s	Third person singular *-s*
gen	Possessive *-s*
n't	Contracted negative (is*n't*)
'cop	Contracted form of the copula (She*'s* happy)
'aux	Contracted form of the auxiliary *be* (He*'s* eating)
-est	Superlative *-est*
-er	Comparative *-er*
-ly	Adverbial suffix *-ly*

The speech-language pathologist can accomplish several types of analyses by using SALT. These types include utterance type; turn overlap and distribution; pause duration and number; utterances per minute and words per utterance; frequency of verbal and nonverbal data of interest, such as past tense; utterance length; type-token ratio; MLU; Brown's stages of development; expected age range of development; word and category lists; and other user-designated analysis.

Conclusion

SALT is a very promising and versatile analysis method that is easy for the speech-language pathologist to use after she becomes familiar with entering the transcript into the computer. As with other computer analysis methods, however, it is not the great panacea. At present, most results are a calculation of those features signaled by the speech-language pathologist when she enters the data. Thus, special care is required to ensure that features are signaled accurately.

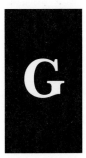

G

Selected English Morphological Prefixes and Suffixes

TABLE G.1
Prefixes and suffixes

Derivational		Inflectional
Prefixes	**Suffixes**	
a- (in, on, into, in a manner)	-able (ability, tendency, likelihood)	-ed (past)
bi- (twice, two)	-al (pertaining to, like, action, process)	-ing (at present)
de- (negative, descent, reversal)	-ance (action, state)	-s (plural)
ex- (out of, from, thoroughly)	-ation (denoting action in a noun)	-s (third person marker)
inter- (reciprocal between, together)	-en (used to form verbs from adjectives)	-'s (possession
mis- (ill, negative, wrong)	-ence (action, state)	
out- (extra, beyond, not)	-er (used as an agentive ending)	
over- (over)	-est (superlative)	
post- (behind, after)	-ful (full, tending)	
pre- (to, before)	-ible (ability, tendency, likelihood)	
pro- (in favor of)	-ish (belonging to)	
re- (again, backward motion)	-ism (doctrine, state, practice)	
semi- (half)	-ist (one who does something)	
super- (superior)	-ity (used for abstract nouns)	
trans- (across, beyond)	-ive (tendency or connection)	
tri- (three)	-ize (action, policy)	
un- (not, reversal)	-less (without)	
under- (under)	-ly (used to form adverbs)	
	-ment (action, product, means, state)	
	-ness (quality, state)	
	-or (used as an agentive ending)	
	-ous (full of, having, like)	
	-y (inclined to)	

H

Indirect Elicitation Techniques

There is an infinite variety of indirect elicitation techniques, although we tend to rely on two old favorites:

Tell me what you see.

Tell me in a whole sentence.

Here are a few conversational techniques that came to mind one day. The list is not exhaustive, merely illustrative.

Technique	Target	Example	
The emperor's new clothes	Negative statements	CLINICIAN:	Oh, Shirley, what beautiful yellow boots!
		CHILD:	I'm not wearing boots!
Pass it on	Requests for information	CLINICIAN:	John, do you know where Linda's project is?
		CHILD:	No.
		CLINICIAN:	Oh, see if she does?
		CHILD:	Linda, where's your project?
Violating routines ("Silly rabbit")	Imperatives, directives	CLINICIAN:	Here's your sandwich.
		CHILD:	Nothing in it.
		CLINICIAN:	Oh, you must like different sandwiches than I do. What do you want?
		CHILD:	Peanut butter.
		CLINICIAN:	How do I do it? (there's your opener)

Nonblabbermouth	Requests for information	CLINICIAN:	(Place interesting object in front of child) "Boy, is this neat."
		CHILD:	What is it?
		CLINICIAN:	A flibbideejibbit. (Now STOP. Don't give any-more info.)
		CHILD:	What's it do?
What I have	Request for action	CLINICIAN:	Oh, I can't wait to show you what I have in this bag. It's really neat. (Wait child out)
Guess what I did	Request for information, Past tense verbs	CLINICIAN:	Guess what I did yesterday in the park.
		CHILD:	Jogged? Picked flowers? Had a picnic?
Mumble	Contingent query	At height of an interesting story or punchline of a joke, clinician should mumble so that child does not receive message. If need-ed, increase pressure by asking questions on what was just said.	
Ask someone else	Request for infor-mation	CLINICIAN:	What do you need?
		CHILD:	Sugar.
		CLINICIAN:	I don't know where it is. Why don't you ask Sally where the sugar is.
Rule giving	Requests for objects	CLINICIAN:	I have the athletic equipment for recess. If you need some, just ask me.
		CHILD:	I want jump rope.
Request for assistance	Initiating conversation	CLINICIAN:	John, can you ask Keith to help me?
Modeling with meaningful intent	I want ___	CLINICIAN:	We have lots of colored paper for our project. Now let's see who needs some. I want a green one. (Take one and wait)
		CHILD:	I want blue.
"Screw up" #1	Locatives, Prepositions	CLINICIAN:	Can you help me dress this doll? (Place shoe on doll's head) How's that?
		CHILD:	No. The shoe goes *on* the doll's foot.
		CLINICIAN:	But now the foot's all gone.
		CHILD:	No. It's *in* the shoe.
"Screw up" #2	Negative statements	CLINICIAN:	Here's your snack. (Give child a pencil)
		CHILD:	That's not a snack.
Requests for topic	Statements	CLINICIAN:	Now let's talk about your birthday party. (Not shared information)
Expansion of child utterance into desired form	Infinitives	CHILD:	I want paste crayon.
		CLINICIAN:	You want crayon to *sing with*?
		CHILD:	No, to color.
		CLINICIAN:	What?
		CHILD:	I want crayon to color.

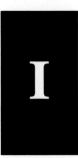

Intervention Activities and Language Targets

Targets

Activities	Nouns	Plurals	Verb tensing	Adjectives/descriptive words	Adverbs	Pronouns	Articles and/or demonstratives	Prepositions/spatial terms	Requests for objects	Requests for assistance	Requests for information	Negatives	Interrogatives	Following directions	Giving directions	Sequencing	Turn taking	Topic introduction and maintenance	Categorization	Register	Presupposition	Conversational repair	Variety of pragmatic features	Auditory processing and memory	Word association	Vocabulary
Barrier tasks	X		X	X				X						X	X	X					X			X		
Body tracing			X	X			X	X		X				X	X	X										X
Colorforms			X	X			X												X							
*Cooking	X	X	X	X				X	X	X	X		X	X	X											X
Describing pictures that others cannot see	X	X		X			X				X										X					
Dolls, clothing, and furniture	X	X		X				X												X						X
Dressing	X	X				X			X																	
Dress-up			X	X		X	X	X												X		X	X			
Explaining "how-to"	X	X	X	X	X		X	X				X		X	X	X		X			X					
Farm or zoo play	X	X		X								X						X	X		X					
Guiding others through an activity								X				X		X	X	X		X			X					
Treasure Hunt–"You're getting warmer. . ."														X	X						X					
Interviewing				X				X			X		X				X	X		X		X				
"I see something that's. . ."									X	X	X	X	X				X									
Jeopardy									X	X	X	X	X				X									
Kitchen play			X	X					X	X																
*Making things	X		X	X	X	X	X	X	X	X	X	X	X	X	X	X	X	X					X			X
Map following					X	X		X		X	X	X		X	X	X										X
Mime				X	X	X								X							X					
My "ME" book				X	X									X	X	X		X							X	
Music and action songs				X										X	X	X		X								

FIGURE I.1
Activities and targets

*See third page of table

A-66

Activity	1	2	3	4	5	6	7	8	9	10	11	12	13	14	15	16	17	18	19	20	21
Nature or science activity			X					X	X	X		X	X	X	X	X		X					X	X
Obstacle course		X	X				X		X			X	X	X	X								
Planning an activity		X	X	X	X	X	X										X			X				X
Planting seeds		X	X				X					X	X											X
Playhouse		X			X	X	X										X			X		
Playing teacher									X			X			X			X	X	X	X	
Pretend shopping	X	X						X	X	X	X			X	X	X				X			X
Puppet show												X				X			X		
Putting objects in order		X			X										X				X		
"Safety Town" (Safety curriculum for preschool and kindergarten)			X	X		X		X	X			X	X					X			X		X
Simon says											X	X	X							X	
Simulated restaurant						X		X		X				X		X	X	X		X			X
Sorting clothing	X	X				X				X				X							
Story-telling (true or make-believe)		X			X	X						X		X			X		X		
Telephone play				X	X		X	X	X			X	X	X	X	X	X	X			
TV commercials		X											X	X	X	X	X				
"Twenty questions" variations		X				X	X	X													
Washing dishes	X	X	X			X	X		X	X											
"What am I?"		X	X	X	X	X		X	X	X			X			X					
"What did you do when. . .?"		X		X	X	X	X		X		X			X			X				

* Possible cooking activities:
1. Cookies, cupcakes, muffins
2. Cornbread and butter
3. Edible honeybees—Mix 1/2 cup peanut butter, 1 T. plus 1/3 cup honey, 2 T. sesame seeds, and 2 T. toasted wheat germ. Roll into balls. Make stripes on the bee by dipping a toothpick in cocoa powder and pressing into ball. Use slivered almonds for wings.
4. English muffin pizzas
5. Fruit salad—Use a few vegetables just to confuse the issue and to elicit some language.
6. Ice cream sundaes
7. Instant pudding
8. Milkshakes—Lots of variations here, such as vanilla, chocolate, and banana (use real ones in the blender).
9. Peanut butter and jelly sandwiches.
10. Peanut butter balls—Mix 1/2 cup honey, 1/2 cup peanut butter, 1 cup dry milk, and 1 cup oatmeal. Roll into balls. Refrigerate.
11. Peanut butter "face" sandwiches—Make faces on the bread with a peanut butter base using raisins (eyes), peanut (nose), chocolate chips (mouth), and carrot slivers or coconut (hair).
12. Picnic lunch
13. Popcorn and popcorn balls

** Things to make:
1. Cereal box instrument—Use a strong cereal box with a circular hole cut in the face similar to the hole in a guitar. Stretch various size rubber bands around the box and tack them into wooden blocks that act as bridges.
2. Costumes from grocery bags—Cut eye holes or a hole for face. Cut arm holes if desired. Decorate bag. Slip over child.
3. Cowgirl and cowboy outfits from grocery bags—Bags can easily be cut to resemble vests and yokes. Be sure to fringe them. Add a bandanna and you have the outfit.
4. Decorate a shoebox "room" with scraps of wallpaper.
5. Food sculptures—Use shredded coconut or lettuce, raisins, peanuts, M & Ms, hot cinnamon candies, cheese strips, fruit halves, celery and carrot sticks, olives, marshmallows, gum drops, and toothpicks.
6. Holiday cards
7. Kites
8. Paper bag puppets
9. Paper butterflies
10. Paper flowers
11. Playdough—Mix 2 cups flour, 1 cup water, 1 T. salad oil, 1 cup salt, and food coloring.
12. Potato and sponge prints
13. Sachets—Cloves and crumbled bay leaves and cinnamon sticks in square of cloth. Pull ends of cloth together and tie with a ribbon.
14. Snowmen and snowwomen—Use styrofoam balls, pipecleaners, cloves, and toothpicks.
15. Stained glass windows—Cut out a cardboard mold. Tape aluminum foil over one side of the cut-out sections. Place this side down. Fill the holes with Elmer's glue. Swirl in food coloring. Allow to dry thoroughly. Peel foil. Hang in sunny window.

Note: A variety of language features can be elicited within these activities by using the indirect elicitation techniques in Appendix H and the nonlinguistic strategies in Chapter 9.

J

Analyzing Classroom Communication Breakdown

The following questions can serve as a guideline to the teacher in determining where students are failing in formal communicative interactions in the classroom. Several different interactions should be analyzed to get an overall perspective of the child's linguistic abilities, cognitive status, and communicative competence.

Language

Phonologic System

Has the child acquired the rules that govern the sounds of the language being used? (e.g., Does Jim make different articulation errors each time he speaks?)

How successful is the child in understanding spoken utterances? (e.g., Does Mary know that *cat* and *rat* are two different words?)

How successful is the child in producing spoken utterances? (e.g., To what degree is the child unintelligible?)

Semantic System

Is the child familiar with the vocabulary being used by the teacher? Has she or he heard these words before in similar situations? In different situations? (e.g., Does Joan know this is an angle without someone pointing to it?)

Do the vocabulary items have meaning for the child? Do the words have meaning only in specific contexts, or does the child understand the words in all contexts? (e.g., Does Keesha know what an angle is?)

Does the child have word-finding difficulties for familiar vocabulary items? For new words? (e.g., Are there hesitations or word substitutions when Jackie speaks?)

Syntactic System

Has the child acquired the rules that govern word order and other aspects of grammar? (e.g., Does Rang understand subject-verb agreement?)

Is the child familiar with the grammatical form being used by the teacher? Has she or he heard this form in similar situations? In different situations? (e.g., Does Diego know who is doing the hitting in the sentence "Mary was hit by Tom"?)

Is the grammatical form that is being used meaningful to the child? Does the child understand the relationships that exist among the lexical items in the utterance? (e.g., Does Maria know why the sentence "The desk stepped on my toes" is anomalous?)

Does the child have access to the grammatical form needed to express his response? (e.g., How adequately does Tommy express himself on a topic of his interest?)

Pragmatics—Functional Use or Intent?

Does the child know the rules for communicative intent that govern social interaction at home? At school? (e.g., Who talks when and under what conditions?)

Does the child know the rules for politeness?

Does the child know when to make eye contact?

Does the child know how close it is permissible to stand when talking with another person?

Does the child know when to raise his hand for recognition?

Does the child know that it is helpful to the learning process to request clarification of new information?

Does the child know how to interpret both direct and indirect requests?

Thinking

Information Processing

Is the child's attention span long enough to attend to a stimulus utterance or event? (e.g., Does Juwan watch the teacher when she holds up a pencil?)

Does the child attend to so many environmental stimuli that she or he is unable to focus on a single one? (e.g., Is Junko constantly turning to look when noises or movements occur?)

Is the child's sensory input reduced or distorted?

What is the length of the child's short-term memory? Is it long enough for the child to hold the utterance to decode it? (e.g., Can Mai–Ling remember a list of things to buy at the play store?)

Does the child spontaneously rehearse or use mnemonic devices to aid short-term memory? If the child does not rehearse spontaneously, can she or he be taught to use such strategies?

Does the child have a backlog of experiences against which to judge new information? (e.g., "Kay, have you ever been to a farm to see a cow?")

Is the child's long-term memory functionally accessible? (e.g., "Do you remember your phone number, Tim?")

Does the child form associations between new and previously stored information? Is the new information integrated with the old? (e.g., "What does this new ball look like? Isn't it just like the one we saw at the soccer game?)

Is retrieval from long-term memory impaired?

Does the child spontaneously evaluate the quality of the information received and the response being formulated?

Conceptual information

Has the child had enough previous experience to interpret conceptual notions correctly? (e.g., Has the child had experience with blocks of different shapes before being asked to classify them?)

If not, has the previous experience been deficient in the quantity of experiences or in the appropriateness or variety of concept instances?

Does the child have difficulty expressing the conceptual relationships required by the situation? (e.g., Has the child been given the language to use to talk about squares and rectangles?)

Integration and Association of Information

Is the child able to integrate new information into old, previously stored information?

Is the child able to make use of integrated or associated information provided by the teacher? (e.g., Can the child use analogies provided by the teacher?)

Is the child able to formulate a response that demonstrates that integration of information has taken place?

The consequence of going through an analysis of this sort is having the information needed to modify classroom interactions to make them better situations for learning. Modifications might be in teacher language, topics or content, and the context of the interaction. The assessment by the teacher can be developed into an ongoing activity that provides continuing feedback on the success of interactions as learning situations. For children with language disorders, such interactive assessment in the classroom setting provides the opportunity for linguistic experience appropriate to the level of functioning and in an amount that is not possible under traditional models of intervention.

Source: Vetter, D. (1982). Language Disorders and Schooling. *Topics in Language Disorders*, 2(4), 13-19. Reprinted with permission of Aspen Publishers, Inc., © 1982.

K

Use of Children's Literature in Preschool Classrooms

Book	Language use
Aardema, *Oh, Kojo! How Could You!*	Predicting, cause and effect, multicultural
Ahlberg, *Jolly Postman*	Predicting
Ahlberg, *Each Peach Pear Plum*	Rhyming, predicting, visual discrimination
Allard, *Miss Nelson Has a Field Day**	Predicting, cause and effect, emotions
Allard, *Miss Nelson Is Missing**	Predicting, cause and effect, reasoning
Allard, *Miss Nelson Is Back**	Predicting, cause and effect
Avery, *Everybody Has Feelings (Todos tenemos sentimientos)*	Emotions, multicultural
Barrett, *Cloudy With a Chance of Meatballs*	Metaphors, if/then conditional sentences, "s" words, humor
Baylor, *Everybody Needs a Rock*	Sequencing, pragmatic conversational skills, complex and compound sentences, pronouns, comparative and superlative
Brown, *Goodnight Moon*	Predicting, noun-verb agreement, plurals, multicultural
Byars, *Go and Hush the Baby*	Predicting
Carle, *The Very Hungry Caterpillar**	Sequencing, auditory memory
Carle, *Very Busy Spider**	Predicting
Cauley, *Goldilocks and The Three Bears*	Predicting
Cauley, *Jack and The Beanstalk*	Predicting
Charlip, *Fortunately*	Predicting, emotions, past tense

DePaola, *Pancakes for Breakfast**	Predicting, storytelling, sequencing, "-ing" verbs
DePaola, *Charlie Needs a Cloak*	Sequencing, vocabulary (words defined at end), past tense
Ga'g, *Millions of Cats*	Predicting
Galdone, *Henny Penny*	Predicting
Ginsburg, *Good Morning, Chick*	Past tense, chanting, demonstratives (*this, that*)
Hudson, *Jamal's Busy Day*	Importance of school, multicultural
Hutchins, *Don't Forget the Bacon*	Auditory memory, word play
Hutchins, *Goodnight Owl*	Predicting, chanting, regular past tense
Hutchins, *The Doorbell Rang**	Predicting, conversational skills, simple practical math
Hutchins, *The Surprise Party*	Predicting, auditory memory
Joslin/Sendak, *What Do You Say Dear*	Predicting
Kraus, *Leo the Late Bloomer*	Predicting, emotions
Lewin, *Jafta's Mother*	Emotions, multicultural, "s" words, noun-verb agreement
Martin, *Polar Bear, Polar Bear, What Do You Hear?*	Sequencing, "-ing" verbs, categorization, "p" & "b" sounds
McCauley, *Why the Chicken Crossed the Road*	Problem solving, inference, cause and effect, idioms and metaphors, temporal markers
Morninghouse, *Nightfeathers*	Poetry, multicultural
Munsch, *The Paper Bag Princes*	Predictable patterning, inference, logical sequencing, life skills, "th" words, final consonant blends
Numeroff, *If You Give a Mouse a Cookie*	Sequencing, auditory and visual memory, cause and effect, temporal markers, idioms
Numeroff, *If You Give a Moose a Muffin*	Sequencing, auditory and visual memory, cause and effect, temporal markers, idioms
Neitzel, *The Jacket I Wear in the Snow*	Sequencing, chanting, auditory memory
Peek, *Mary Wore Her Red Dress*	Predicting, color words, modifiers, "l" in initial and final positions, chanting, visual detail, sequencing
Piper, *Little Engine That Could*	Predicting
Sendak, *Chicken Soup with Rice*	Predicting, months, chanting
Shaw, *It Looked Like Spilt Milk*	Predicting, chanting
Sheer, *Rain Makes Applesauce*	Predicting
Vagin & Asch, *Here Comes the Cat!**	Predicting, chanting
Viorst, *Alexander and the Terrible, Horrible, No Good, Very Bad Day**	Categorization, inference, feelings, modifiers, functional vocabulary
Williams, *The Little Old Lady Who Was Not Afraid of Anything**	Predicting, chanting
Wood, *The Napping House**	"-ing" verbs, adjectives, synonyms, cause and effect
Zolotow, *Do You Know What I'll Do?*	Predicting
Zolotow, *Some Things Go Together*	Predicting, word associations, categorization
Zolotow, *Someday*	Predicting, future tense, initial "s" words

*Appropriate for Narrative enactment (Culatta, Horn, Theadore, & Sutherland, 1993)

Note: Special thanks to Montgomery (1992a) for giving me several entries.

L

Definitions of Illocutionary and Semantic Functions

Functions	Examples
Semantic	

Nomination — naming a person or object using a single- or multiword name or a demonstrative-plus as a name

Doggie, Choo-choo
This horsie

Location — marking spatial relationships. Utterances may contain single location words or two-word utterances containing an agent, action, or object plus a location word. The function can be demonstrated in response to *where* questions.

PARTNER: Where's Doggie?
CHILD:　　Chair.

Ball table, Doggie chair, Throw me, Throw here (X + locative)

Negation — marking of nonexistence, rejection, and denial using single negative words or a negative followed by another word (negative + X).

Nonexistence generally develops first and marks the absence of a once-present object.

All gone (count as a single word), Away, No milk (child drank it), All gone car (the ride is over), No

Rejection marks an attempt to prevent or to stop an event.

PARTNER: Time for bed.
CHILD:　　No (or No bed)
　　　　　　Stop it, No milk (pushes glass away)

Denial marks rejection of a proposition.

PARTNER: See the bear?
CHILD:　　No bear.

Functions	Examples
Modification	

Modification

Possession — appreciating that an object belongs to or is frequently associated with someone. Single-word utterances signal the owner's name. In two-word utterances, stress is usually on the initial word, the possessor.

Mine, My dollie, Johnnie bike (modifier + head)
Dollie (child clutches doll)

Attribution — using descriptors for properties not inherently part of the object.

Yukky, Big doggie, Little baby (modifier + head)

Recurrence — understanding that an object can reappear or an event can be reenacted.

More, More milk, 'Nuther cookie (modifier + head)

Notice — signaling that an object has appeared, an event has happened, or an attempt to gain attention.

Hi Mommy, Bye-bye, Look Jim

Action — marking an activity

Action — single-action words

Jump, Eat

Agent + Action — two-word signal that an animate initiated an activity.

Mommy throw, Doggie eat, Baby sleep

Action + Object—two-word signal that an animate or inanimate object was the recipient of action

Eat cookie, Throw ball

Illocutionary

Answer — child responds to questions. The questioner's behaviors are a cue for the child's response; the response probably would not be produced without this cue. The child's responses are cognitively related to the question, although they may be incorrect.

PARTNER (*holding doll*): What's this?
CHILD: Baby

PARTNER: Is this a mirror?
CHILD: No

Question — child asks for information or verification by addressing the other person verbally. The child's behavior is a stimulus or cue and indicates that he expects an answer. The child can ask himself questions when engaged in egocentric play.

CHILD: (*picks up toy telephone*): Phone?

CHILD: What this?

Reply — child makes meaningful response to the content of the other speaker's previous utterance, a verbal cue external to the child. The child may continue to build on the content and ignore the form of the utterance, such as responding to a word or thought in a question without answering the question. In many cases, the child will build on the content *and* respond with an appropriate form. This category does not include mere repetition.

PARTNER: Johnny, bring me the scissors. (command)
CHILD: No.
PARTNER: May I have the keys? (request)
CHILD: In a minute.
PARTNER: This is a cute dog. (declaration)
CHILD: My doggie.

Elicitation — child self-repeats in response to a request for repetition or clarification or in response to "Say *x*."

Continuant — child signals that he is listening and wants to continue the interchange or that he missed what was said.

Declaration — child makes a statement that is situationally related and for communication but is not in response to another speaker. The utterance is more like a commentary. Cues are internal or situational but not verbal. This category also includes situationally related phonemic exclamations.

CHILD: Kitty go. (declaration)
PARTNER: What?
CHILD: Kitty go.
PARTNER: Mary, say "ball."
CHILD: Ball. Uh-huh, Okay. I see, yes. What? Huh?

CHILD   (*playing game with mother and glances out*): It raining out.
CHILD   (*playing with car*): Car go up.
PARTNER: This is a cute doggie.
CHILD: My doggie. (reply) He lives in a house. (declaration)
PARTNER: This is a cute doggie.
CHILD: My doggie. (reply) I have kitty, too. (declaration)

Practice — repeats or imitates in whole or part what he or another person says with no change in intonation that would indicate a change of intent. In addition, internal replay without added new information is considered *practice*. This category also includes counting, singing, babbling, or rhyming behaviors in which the child seems to be experimenting or rehearsing.

Perseverative responses, even if the other person interjects an utterance between them, are considered *practice* as long as they do not mark discrete events or objects.

PARTNER: Ball.
CHILD: Ball.
PARTNER: See the red ball.
CHILD: Red ball.
PARTNER: See the red ball.
CHILD: See ball. (practice) Ball, ball, ball. (practice)

Name — child labels an object or event that is present, but the label is not in response to a question. This verbal behavior usually is accomplished by pointing or nodding.

CHILD   (*picks up ball*): Ball.
CHILD   (*points to ball*): That ball.

Suggestion, Command, Demand, Request — The primary function of the child's utterance is to influence another person's behavior by getting that person to do something or to give the child permission. The form may be imperative, declarative, or interrogative.

CHILD: Gimmie cookie.
CHILD: Stop that.
CHILD: Mommy.
CHILD: Throw ball. (*parent throws*)
          Throw ball. (*parent throws*) Throw ball.

Source: Adapted from Owens (1982)

Glossary

Assimilation. Phonological process in which a child changes one syllable to make it more like another, as in *doddie* (/dɔdi/) for *doggie*.

Augmentative communication. Communication other than verbal that may complement or supplement verbal means.

Construct validity. Accuracy with which or extent to which a measure describes or measures some trait or construct.

Content generalization. Carryover of the learned entity to untrained content.

Content validity. Faithfulness with which a sample or measure represents some attribute or behavior.

Context generalization. Carryover of the learned entity to novel situations.

Contingency. Relatedness of an utterance to the previous utterance. Contingency may relate to meaning (semantic contingency) and/or intention or purpose (pragmatic contingency) of the previous utterance.

Contingent query. Request for clarification.

Contrast training. Training method that teaches a child to discriminate between structures and situations that obligate use of the feature being trained and those features that do not.

Copula. Verb *to be,* used as a main verb.

Criterion validity. Effectiveness or accuracy with which a measure predicts success.

Deixis. Process of using the speaker's perspective as a reference.

Discriminative stimulus (S^D). A stimulus in the presence of which the trainee will be reinforced for a correct response. For example, in the presence of the phone ringing, one is reinforced for answering it by the party on the other end.

Ellipsis. Omission of known or shared information in subsequent utterances in which it would be redundant.

Generalization. Carryover of learning to untrained content and/or novel situations; an interaction of the learner, the learned content, and the context or environment.

Illocutionary function. Intention(s) of a speaker.

Incidental teaching. Training within everyday activities and contexts with everyday partners as teachers.

Internal consistency. Degree of relationship among items and the overall test.

Linguistic context. Verbal features of the context that precede, accompany, and follow a verbalization.

Minimal pairs. Two words that differ by only one phoneme that signals a difference of meaning.

Minimally symbolic. Highest level of functioning is the use of symbols singularly or in limited combinations.

Modal. Auxiliary or helping verb that expresses mood or a feeling toward the main verb. Examples: *may, might, must, will, should, could, would.*

Nonlinguistic context. Features of the context, other than linguistic ones, that precede, accompany, and follow a verbalization. The nonlinguistic context of an utterance or verbalization is what is happening in the environment at the time of the verbalization.

Presupposition. The speaker's assumption about the knowledge level of the listener or what the listener knows and needs to know.

Presymbolic. Prior to the use of symbols in the form of words, signs, pictures, and the like.

Reduplication. A phonological process in which a child changes one syllable in a two-syllable word to repeat another syllable, as in *mama* or *wawa* (water).

Referential communication. Speaker selects and verbally identifies attributes of an entity, thereby enabling the listener to identify the entity accurately.

Reliability. Repeatability of a measure, based on the accuracy or precision with which a sample, at one time, represents performance based on either a different but similar sample or the same sample at a different time.

Representativeness. Degree to which a sample reflects the general feature being measured.

Script. Basic sequential notion of familiar events.

Semantic function. Meaning(s) of a speaker.

Standard error of measure (SEm). The statistical error inherent in a score, representing the range that a score may indicate.

Story grammar. Organizational pattern of narratives.

Strategy-based intervention. Training that teaches the child information processing and problem-solving strategies.

Systems model. Intervention that targets the child's interactive systems or contexts.

Transparency. "Guessability" of an augmentative symbol.

T-units (minimal terminal units). A main clause plus any attached or embedded subordinate clause or nonclausal structure.

Turnabout. Contingent utterance that acknowledges the partner's previous utterance and cues the partner for the next response.

Validity. Effectiveness of a test in representing, describing, or predicting an attribute. A test's ability to assess what it purports to measure.

References

Abbeduto, L., Davies, B., Solesby, S., & Furman, L. (1991). Identifying the referents of spoken messages: Use of context and clarification requests by children with and without mental retardation. *American Journal on Mental Retardation, 95,* 551-562.

Abbeduto, L., Furman, L., & Davies, B. (1989). Relation between the receptive language and mental age of persons with mental retardation. *American Journal on Mental Retardation, 93,* 535-545.

Abkarian, G., Jones, A., & West, G. (1992). Young children's idiom comprehension: Trying to get the picture. *Journal of Speech and Hearing Research, 35,* 580-587.

Abramson, L. Y., Garber, J., & Seligman, M. E. P. (1980). Learned helplessness in humans: An attributional analysis. In J. Garber & M. E. P. Seligman (Eds.), *Human helplessness: Theory and applications.* New York: Academic Press.

Acevedo, M. A. (1986). Assessment instruments for minorities. In F. H. Bess, B. S. Clark, & H. R. Mitchell (Eds.), *Concerns for minority groups in communication disorders* (pp. 46-51). Rockville, MD: American Speech-Language-Hearing Association.

Ackerman, P., Dykman, R., & Gardner, M. (1990). Counting rate, naming rate, phonological sensitivity, and memory span: Major factors in dyslexia. *Journal of Learning Disabilities, 23,* 325-327.

Adams, M. (1990). *Beginning to read: Thinking and learning about print.* Cambridge: MIT Press.

Adamson, L. B., Romski, M. A., Deffenbach, K., & Sevcik, R. A. (1992). Symbol vocabulary and the focus of conversations: Augmenting language development for youth with mental retardation. *Journal of Speech and Hearing Research, 35,* 1333-1343.

Ad Hoc Committee on Service Delivery in the Schools, ASHA. (1993). Definitions of communication disorders and variations. *Asha, 35*(3)(Suppl. 10), 40-41.

Adler, S. (1973). Social class bases of language: A reexamination of socioeconomic, sociopsychological, and sociolinguistic factors. *Asha, 15*(1), 3-9.

Adler, S. (1988). A new job description and a new task for the public school clinician: Relating effectively to the nonstandard dialect speaker. *Language, Speech, and Hearing Services in Schools, 19,* 28–33.

Adler, S. (1990). Multicultural clients: Implications for the speech-language pathologist. *Language, Speech, and Hearing Services in Schools, 21,* 135-139.

Adler, S. (1991). Assessment of language proficiency in limited English proficient speakers: Implications for the speech-language specialist. *Language, Speech, and Hearing Services in Schools, 22,* 12-18.

Adler, S., & Birdsong, S. (1983). Reliability and validity of standardized testing tools used with poor children. *Topics in Language Disorders, 3*(3), 76-88.

Alamanza, H. P., & Mosley, W. J. (1980). Curriculum adaptations and modifications for culturally diverse handicapped children. *Exceptional Children, 48,* 808-814.

Albertini, J. (1980). The acquisition of five grammatical morphemes: Deviance or delay? *Proceedings from the Wisconsin Symposium on Research in Child Language Disorders, 1,* 94-111.

Allen, R. E., & Oliver, J. M. (1982). The effects of child maltreatment on language development. *Child Abuse and Neglect, 6,* 299-305.

Allen, R. E., & Wasserman, G. A. (1985). Origins of language delay in abused children. *Child Abuse and Neglect, 9,* 333-338.

Alley, G., & Deshler, D. (1979). *Teaching the learning disabled adolescent: Strategies and methods.* Denver: Love Publishing.

Alley, G. R., Deshler, D. D., & Warner, M. M. (1979). Identification of learning disabled adolescents. *Learning Disability Quarterly, 2,* 76–83.

Allington, R. L. (1983). The reading instruction provided readers of differing ability. *Elementary School Journal, 83,* 255-265.

Alpert, C., & Rogers–Warren, A. (1984). *Mothers as incidental language trainers of their language–disordered children.* Unpublished manuscript, University of Kansas, Lawrence.

Altwerger, B., Edelsky, C., & Flores, B. M. (1987). Whole language: What's new? *The Reading Teacher, 41,* 144-154.

Alvermann, D. (1983). Reading achievement and linguistic stages: A comparison of disabled readers and Chomsky's 6- to 10-year-olds. *Journal of Research Developments in Education, 16,* 26-31.

Ambert, A., & Dew, N. (1982). *Special education for exceptional bilingual students: A handbook for educators.* Dallas: Evaluation, Dissemination, and Assessment Center.

American Psychiatric Association (APA). (1987). *Diagnostic and statistical manual of mental disorders* (3rd ed. rev.). Washington, DC: Author.

American Speech-Language-Hearing Association. (1983). Position of the American Speech-Language-Hearing Association on social defects. *Asha, 25*(9), 23-25.

Ames, L. (1966). Children's stories. *Genetic Psychological Monographs, 73,* 307–311.

Anderson, G., & Nelson, N. (1988). Integrating language intervention and education in an alternate adolescent language classroom. *Seminars in Speech and Language, 9,* 341–353.

Anderson, N. B. (1991). Understanding cultural diversity. *American Journal of Speech-Language Pathology, 1*(3), 9-10.

Anderson, N. B. (1992). Understanding cultural diversity. *American Journal of Speech-Language Pathology, 1*(2), 11-12.

Anderson, R. C., & Davison, A. (1988). Conceptual and empirical bases of readability formulas. In G. Green & A. Davison (Eds.), *Linguistic complexity and text comprehension* (pp. 23-54). Hillsdale, NJ: Lawrence Erlbaum.

Anderson, R. C., Hiebert, E., Scott, J. A., & Wilkenson, I. A. (1985). *Becoming a nation of readers.* Washington, DC: National Institute of Education.

Andrews, J., Andrews, M., & Shearer, W. (1989). Parents' attitudes toward involvement in speech–language services. *Language, Speech, and Hearing Services in Schools, 20,* 391–399.

Andrews, N., & Fey, M. (1986). Analysis of the speech of phonologically impaired children in two sampling conditions. *Journal of Speech, Language, and Hearing Services in Schools, 17,* 187-198.

Anselmi, D., Tomasello, M., & Acunzo, M. (1986). Young children's responses to neutral and specific contingent queries. *Journal of Child Language, 13,* 135–144.

Applebee, A. N. (1978). *The child's concept of story.* Chicago: University of Chicago Press.

Aram, D. M. (1988). Language sequelae of unilateral brain lesions in children. In F. Plumb (Ed.), *Language, communication, and the brain* (pp. 171-197). New York: Raven.

Aram, D. M. (1991). Comments on specific language impairment as a clinical category. *Language, Speech, and Hearing Services in Schools, 22,* 84-87.

Aram, D. M., & Ekelman, B. L. (1987). Unilateral brain lesions in children: Performance on the Revised Token Test. *Brain and Language, 32,* 137-158.

Aram, D. M., & Ekelman, B. L. (1988). Scholastic aptitude and achievement among children with unilateral brain lesions. *Neuropsychologia, 26,* 903-916.

Aram, D. M., Ekelman, B. L., & Nation, J. E. (1984). Preschoolers with language disorders: 10 years later. *Journal of Speech and Hearing Research, 27,* 232-244.

Aram, D. M., Ekelman, B. L., & Whitaker, H. A. (1986). Spoken syntax in children with acquired unilateral hemispheric lesions. *Brain and Language, 27,* 75-100.

Aram, D. M., Ekelman, B. L., & Whitaker, H. A. (1987). Lexical retrieval in left and right brain lesioned children. *Brain and Language, 31,* 61-87.

Aram, D. M., Morris, R., & Hall, N. (1993). Clinical and research congruence in identifying children with specific language impairment. *Journal of Speech and Hearing Research, 36,* 580–591.

Aram, D. M., & Nation, J. E. (1975). Patterns of language behavior in children with developmental language disorders. *Journal of Speech and Hearing Research, 18,* 229-241.

Aram, D. M., & Nation, J. E. (1980). Preschool language disorders and subsequent language and academic difficulties. *Journal of Communication Disorders, 38,* 159-170.

Argyle, M., & Cook, M. (1976). *Gaze and mutual gaze.* Cambridge, MA: Harvard University Press.

Armbuster, B. B., Anderson, T. H., & Ostertag, J. (1987). Does text structure/summarization instruction facilitate learning from expository text? *Reading Research Quarterly, 22,* 331-346.

Armstrong, S. L., Gleitman, L., & Gleitman, H. (1983). What some concepts might not be. *Cognition, 13,* 263-308.

Arwood, E. (1983). *Pragmatism: Theory and application.* Rockville, MD: Aspen.

ASHA Position Paper. (1985, June). Clinical management of communicatively handicapped minority language populations. *Asha, 27*(6), 29–32.

Astington, J. W., & Olson, D. R. (1987, April). *Literacy and schooling: Learning to talk about thought.* Paper presented at the Annual Meeting of the American Educational Research Association, Washington, DC.

Atkins, C., & Cartwright, L. (1982). An investigation of the effectiveness of three elicitation procedures on Head Start children. *Language, Speech, and Hearing Services in Schools, 13,* 33–36.

Atkinson, R. H., & Longman, D. G. (1985). Sniglets: Give a twist to teenage and adult vocabulary instruction. *Journal of Reading, 29,* 103-105.

Atlas, J. A., & Lapadis, L. B. (1988). Symbolization levels in communicative behaviors of children showing pervasive developmental disorders. *Journal of Communication Disorders, 21,* 75-84.

Audet, L. R., & Hummel, L. J. (1990). A framework for assessment and treatment of language-learning disabled children with psychiatric disorders. *Topics in Language Disorders, 10*(4), 57-74.

Auer, J. C. (1984). *Bilingual conversation.* Amsterdam: John Benjamins.

Augustinos, M. (1987). Developmental effects of child abuse: Recent findings. *Child Abuse and Neglect, 11,* 15-27.

Baer, R., Williams, J., Osnes, P., & Stokes, T. (1984). Delayed reinforcement as an indiscriminable contingency in verbal/nonverbal correspondence training. *Journal of Applied Behavior Analysis, 17,* 29–44.

Baggett, P. (1979). Structurally equivalent stories in movies and text and the effect of medium on recall. *Journal of Verbal Learning and Verbal Behavior, 18,* 333-356.

Bailet, L. L. (1990). Spelling rule usage among students with learning disabilities and normally achieving students. *Journal of Learning Disabilities, 18,* 162-165.

Bain, B., Olswang, L., & Johnson, G. (1992). Language sampling for repeated measures with language-impaired preschoolers: Comparison of two procedures. *Topics in Language Disorders, 12*(2), 13-27.

Baker, B. (1976). Parent involvement in programming for the developmentally disabled child. In L. Lloyd (Ed.), *Communication assessment and intervention* (pp. 691–733). Baltimore: University Park Press.

Baker, B., Murphy, D., Heifitz, L., & Brightman, A. (1975). *Parents as teachers: Follow–up after 18 months.* Cambridge, MA: Behavioral Education Projects.

Baker, J. G., Ceci, S. J., & Hermann, D. (1987). Semantic structure and processing: Implications for the learning disabled child. In H. L. Swanson (Ed.), *Memory and learning disability: Advances in learning and behavioral disabilities.* Greenwich, CT: JAI.

Baker, L. (1982). An evaluation of the role of metacognitive deficits in learning disabilities. *Topics in Learning and Learning Disabilities, 2*(1), 27-35.

Baker, L., & Brown, A. L. (1984). Metacognitive skills and reading. In P. D. Pearson, M. Kamil, R. Barr, & P. Mosenthal (Eds.), *Handbook of reading research* (pp. 353–394). New York: Longman.

Baker, L., & Cantwell, D. (1984). Primary prevention of the psychiatric consequences of childhood communication disorders. *Journal of Preventative Psychiatry, 2*(1), 75–97.

Balota, D. A., & Duchek, J. (1989). Age-related differences in lexical access, spreading activation, and simple pronunciation. *Psychology and Aging, 3*, 84-93.

Baltaxe, C. A. (1977). Pragmatic deficits in the language of autistic adolescents. *Journal of Pediatric Psychology, 2*, 176-180.

Baltaxe, C. A., & Simmons, J. Q. (1983). Communication deficits in the adolescent and adult autistic. *Seminars in Speech and Language, 4*, 27-42.

Banch, J. (1989). Parent involvement: Phone home. *Principal, 68*(4), 48.

Bangs, T., & Dodson, S. (1979). Birth to Three Developmental Scales. Allen, TX: DLM.

Bankson, N. (1977). Bankson Language Screening Test. Baltimore: University Park Press.

Barbero, G. (1982). Failure-to-thrive. In M. H. Klaus, T. Leger, & M. A. Trause (Eds.), *Maternal attachment and mothering disorders: Pediatric round table: 1* (pp. 3-6). Skillman, NJ: Johnson & Johnson Baby Products.

Barnes, S., Gutfreund, M., Satterly, D., & Wells, G. (1983). Characteristics of adult speech which predict children's language development. *Journal of Child Development, 10*, 65–84.

Barrett, M. D. (1983a). The course of early lexical development: A review and an interpretation. *Early Child Development and Care, 11*, 19-32.

Barrett, M. D. (1983b). The early acquisition and development of the meanings of action–related words. In T. Seiler & W. Wannenmacher (Eds.), *Concept develop-*

ment and development of word meaning (pp. 191–209). New York: Springer Verlag.

Bartlett, E. (1976). Sizing things up: The acquisition of the meaning of dimensional adjectives. *Journal of Child Language, 3*, 205-219.

Bartolucci, G., Pierce, S., Streiner, D., & Eppel, P. T. (1976). Phonological investigation of verbal autistic and mentally retarded subjects. *Journal of Autism and Childhood Schizophrenia, 6*, 303-316.

Bashaw, W. L., & Anderson, H. E. (1968). Developmental study of the meaning of adverbial modifiers. *Journal of Educational Psychology, 58*, 111–118.

Bashir, A. (1987, June). *Language and curriculum.* Paper presented at the Language Learning Disabilities Institute, Emerson College, Boston.

Bashir, A. S. (1989). Language intervention and the curriculum. *Seminars in Speech and Language, 10*(3), 181-191.

Basil, C. (1992). Social interaction and learned helplessness in severely disabled children. *Augmentative and Alternative Communication, 8*, 188-199.

Bass, P. M. (1988, November). *Attention deficit disorder/Management in preschool, adolescent, and adult populations.* Paper presented at the Annual Conference of the American Speech-Language-Hearing Association, Boston.

Bates, E. (1976a). *Language and context: The acquisition of pragmatics.* New York: Academic Press.

Bates, E. (1976b). Pragmatics and sociolinguistics in child language. In D. Morehead & A. Morehead (Eds.), *Normal and deficient child language* (pp. 411–463). Baltimore: University Park Press.

Bates, E. (1979). *The emergence of symbols.* New York: Academic Press.

Bates, E., Bretherton, I., Shore, C., & McNew, S. (1983). Names, gestures, and objects: The role of context in the emergence of symbols. In K. Nelson (Ed.), *Children's language* (Vol. 4, pp. 59–123). Hillsdale, NJ: Lawrence Erlbaum.

Bates, E., Bretherton, I., & Snyder, L. (1988). *From first words to grammar: Individual differences and dissociable mechanisms.* New York: Cambridge University Press.

Bates, E., Camaioni, L., & Volterra, V. (1975). The acquisition of performatives prior to speech. *Merrill-Palmer Quarterly, 21*(3), 205–226.

Bates, E., & MacWhinney, B. (1982). Functionalist approaches to grammar. In E. Wanner & L. Gleitman (Eds.), *Language acquisition: The state of the art* (pp. 173–218). New York: Cambridge University Press.

Bates, E., O'Connell, B., & Shore, C. (1987). Language and communication in infancy. In J. Osofsky (Ed.), *Handbook of infant development* (pp. 149-203). New York: John Wiley.

Bates, E., Thal, D. J., Whitesell, K., Fenson, L., & Oakes, L. (1989). Integrating language and gesture in infancy. *Developmental Psychology, 25,* 1004-1019.

Bateson, M. (1975). Mother–infant exchanges: The epigenesis of conversational interaction. *Annals of the New York Academy of Sciences, 263,* 101–113.

Battles, D. (1990, March). *Black dialects.* Paper presented at the Spring Workshop of the Genesee Valley Speech–Language–Hearing Association, Rochester, NY.

Bauer, N. M., & Sapona, R. H. (1988). Facilitating communication as a basis for intervention for students with severe behavior disorders. *Journal of the Council for Children with Behavior Disorders, 13,* 280-287.

Baumann, J. F. (1983). Children's ability to comprehend main ideas in content textbooks. *Reading World, 22,* 322-331.

Baumann, J. F. (1984). The effectiveness of a direct instruction paradigm for teaching main idea comprehension. *Reading Research Quarterly, 20,* 93-115.

Baumann, J. F., & Stevenson, J. A. (1986). Teaching students to comprehend anaphoric relationships. In J. W. Irwin (Ed.), *Understanding and teaching cohesion comprehension* (pp. 95-124). Newark, DE: International Reading Association.

Bayley, N. (1969). The Bayley Scales of Infant Development. San Antonio: Psychological Corp.

Beastrom, S., & Rice, M. (1986, November). *Comprehension and production of the articles "a" and "the."* Paper presented at the Convention of the American Speech-Language-Hearing Association, Detroit.

Beck, I. L., McKeown, M. G., & Omanson, R. C. (1987). The effects and uses of diverse vocabulary instructional techniques. In M. G. McKeown & M. E. Curtis (Eds.), *The nature of vocabulary acquisition* (pp. 147–164). Hillsdale, NJ: Lawrence Erlbaum.

Beckwith, L., Cohen, S., Kopp, C., Parmelee, A., & Marcy, T. (1976). Caregiver–infant interaction and early cognitive development in preterm infants. *Child Development, 47,* 579–587.

Bedrosian, J. L. (1979, May). *Communicative performance of mentally retarded adults: A topic analysis.* Paper presented at the convention of the American Association on Mental Deficiency, Miami Beach, FL.

Bedrosian, J. L. (1982). *A sociolinguistic approach to communication skills: Assessment and treatment methodology for mentally retarded adults.* Unpublished doctoral dissertation, University of Wisconsin.

Bedrosian, J. L. (1985). An approach to developing conversational competence. In D. N. Ripich & F. M. Spinelli (Eds.), *School discourse problems* (pp. 231-255). San Diego: College–Hill.

Bedrosian, J. L. (1988). Adults who are mildly to moderately mentally retarded: Communicative performance, assessment, and intervention. In S. Calculator & J. Bedrosian (Eds.), *Communication assessment and intervention for adults with mental retardation* (pp. 265–307). San Diego: College–Hill.

Bedrosian, J. L. (1993). Making minds meet: Assessment of conversational topic in adults with mild to moderate mental retardation. *Topics in Language Disorders, 13*(3), 36-46.

Bedrosian, J. L., & Prutting, C. (1978). Communicative performance of mentally retarded adults in four conversational settings. *Journal of Speech and Hearing Research, 21,* 79-95.

Bedrosian, J. L., & Willis, T. (1987). Effects of treatment on the topic performance of a school–age child. *Language, Speech, and Hearing Services in Schools, 18,* 158–167.

Beeghly, M., Jernberg, E., & Burrows, E. (1989). *Validity of the Early Language Inventory (ELI) for use with 25–month-olds.* Paper presented at the Biennial Meeting of the Society for Research in Child Development.

Beilin, H. (1975). *Studies in the cognitive basis of language development.* New York: Academic Press.

Beitchman, J. H. (1985). Speech and language impairment and psychiatric risk: Toward a model of neurodevelopmental immaturity. *Psychiatric Clinics of North America, 8,* 721–735.

Bellugi, U., & Brown, R. (1964). The acquisition of language. *Monographs for the Society for Research in Child Development, 29*(No. 92).

Belmont, J. (1967). Long-term memory in mental retardation. In N. Ellis (Ed.), *International review of research in mental retardation* (Vol. 1, pp. 219–256). New York: Academic Press.

Bender, N., & Carlson, J. (1982). Prosocial behavior and perspective taking of mentally retarded and nonretarded children. *American Journal of Mental Deficiency, 86,* 361-366.

Benedict, H. (1979). Early lexical development: Comprehension and production. *Journal of Child Language, 6,* 183–200.

Benton, A. L. (1973). The measurement of aphasic disorders. In A. C. Velasquez (Ed.), *Aspectos patalogicos del lengage.* Lima, Peru: Centro Neuropsicologico.

Ben-Yishay, Y. (1985). *Rehabilitation of cognitive and perceptual deficits in persons with chronic brain damage: A comparative study.* Annual progress report. New York: New York University, Medical and Research Training Center for Head Trauma and Stroke.

Berger, J., & Cunningham, C. (1983). The development of early vocal behaviors and interactions in Down's syndrome and non-handicapped infant-mother pairs. *Developmental Psychology, 19,* 322-331.

Bernstein, D. (1986). The development of humor: Implications for assessment and intervention. *Topics in Language Disorders, 1*(4), 47-58.

Bernstein, D. (1989). Assessing children with limited English proficiency: Current prospectives. *Topics in Language Disorders, 9*(3), 15–20.

Bernstein, D., & Tiegerman, E. (1993). *Language and communication disorders in children.* New York: Merrill/Macmillan.

Bernstein, M. (1984). Non-linguistic responses to verbal instructions. *Journal of Child Language, 11,* 293-311.

Berry, J. W. (1980). Acculturation as varieties of adaptation. In A. M. Padilla (Ed.), *Acculturation: Theoretical models and some new findings* (pp. 9-26). Boulder, CO: Westview.

Berry, M. F., & Talbott, R. (1977). *Berry–Talbott developmental guide to the comprehension of grammar.* Rockford, IL: M. F. Berry.

Berthoff, A. E. (1981). *The making of meaning.* Upper Montclair, NJ: Boynton/Cook.

Beukelman, D. R., Jones, R., & Rowan, M. (1989). Frequency of word usage by non-disabled peers in integrated preschool programs. *Augmentative and Alternative Communication, 5,* 243-248.

Beukelman, D. R., McGinnis, J., & Morrow, D. (1991). Vocabulary selection in augmentative and alternative communication. *Augmentative and Alternative Communication, 7,* 171-185.

Beukelman, D. R., Yorkston, K., & Dowden, P. (1985). *Communication augmentation: A casebook of clinical management.* San Diego: College–Hill.

Biber, D. (1986). Spoken and written textual dimensions in English: Resolving the contradictory findings. *Language, 62,* 384–414.

Biklen, D. (1990). Communication unbound: Autism and praxis. *Harvard Educational Review, 60,* 291-314.

Biklen, D. (1992a). Facilitated communication: Biklen responds. *American Journal of Speech-Language Pathology, 1*(2), 21-22.

Biklen, D. (1992b). Typing to talk: Facilitated communication. *American Journal of Speech-Language Pathology, 1*(2), 15-17.

Biklen, D., Morton, M. W., Gold, D., Berrigan, C., & Swaminathan, S. (1992). Facilitated communication: Implications for individuals with autism. *Topics in Language Disorders, 12*(4), 1-28.

Biklen, D., & Schubert, A. (1991). New words: The communication of students with autism. *Remedial and Special Education, 12*(6), 46-57.

Bilovsky, D., & Share, J. (1975). The ITPA and Down's syndrome: An exploratory study. *American Journal of Mental Deficiency, 70,* 78-82.

Bilsky, L., Walker, N., & Sakales, S. (1983). Comprehension and recall of sentences by mentally retarded and nonretarded individuals. *American Journal of Mental Deficiency, 87,* 558-565.

Bishop, D. V. M. (1979). Comprehension in developmental language disorders. *Developmental Medicine and Child Neurology, 21,* 225-238.

Bishop, D. V. M. (1982). Comprehension of spoken, written, and signed sentences in childhood language disorders. *Journal of Child Psychology and Psychiatry, 23,* 1-20.

Bishop, D. V. M. (1985). Automated LARSP [Computer program]. Manchester, England: University of Manchester.

Bishop, D. V. M., & Adams, C. (1992). Comprehension problems in children with specific language impairments: Literal and inferential meaning. *Journal of Speech and Hearing Research, 35,* 119-129.

Bishop, D. V. M., & Edmundson, A. (1987). Language-impaired four year olds: Distinguishing transient from persistent impairment. *Journal of Speech and Hearing Disorders, 52,* 156-173.

Bittle, R. (1975). Improving parent-teacher communication through recorded telephone messages. *Journal of Educational Resources, 69*(3), 87-95.

Bjork, R. A., & Bjork, E. L. (1992). A new theory of disuse and an old theory of stimulus fluctuation. In A. F. Healy, S. M. Kosslyn, & R. M. Shiffrin (Eds.), *From learning processes to cognitive processes: Essays in honor of William K. Estes* (Vol. 2, pp. 35-67). Hillsdale, NJ: Lawrence Erlbaum.

Bjorkland, D., Ornstein, P., & Haig, J. (1975, April). *Development of organizational patterns in free recall: The effects of training in categorization.* Paper presented at the Biennial Meeting of the Society for Research in Child Development, Denver.

Blache, S., & Parsons, C. (1980). A linguistic approach to distinctive feature training. *Language, Speech, and Hearing Services in Schools, 4,* 203–207.

Blache, S., Parsons, C., & Humphreys, J. (1981). A minimal word–pair model for teaching the linguistic significance of distinctive feature properties. *Journal of Speech and Hearing Disorders, 46,* 291–295.

Blachman, B. (1984). Relationship of rapid naming ability and language analysis skills in kindergarten and first grade reading achievement. *Reading Research Quarterly, 13,* 223-253.

Black, J. B. (1985). An exposition on understanding expository text. In B. K. Britton & J. B. Black (Eds.), *Understanding expository text* (pp. 249–267). Hillsdale, NJ: Lawrence Erlbaum.

Blager, F. M., & Martin, H. P. (1976). Speech and language of abused children. In H. P. Martin (Ed.), *The abused child: A multidisciplinary approach to developmental issues and treatment* (pp. 83-92), Cambridge, MA: Ballinger.

Blake, I. (1984). *Language development in working–class black children: An examination of form, content, and use.* Unpublished doctoral dissertation, Columbia University, New York.

Blalock, J. (1981). Persistent problems and concerns of young adults with learning disabilities. In W. Cruickshank & A. Silvers (Eds.), *Bridges to tomorrow: The best of ACDL* (Vol. 1, pp. 35–56). Syracuse, NY: Syracuse University.

Blank, M., & Marquis, A. (1987). *Directing discourse: 80 situations for teaching meaningful conversations to children.* Tucson, AZ: Communication Skill Builders.

Blank, M., Rose, S., & Berlin, L. (1978). *The language of learning: The preschool years.* New York: Grune & Stratton.

Blau, A. (1983). Vocabulary selection in augmentative communication: Where do we begin? In H. Winitz (Ed.), *Treating language disorders: For clinicians by clinicians.* Baltimore: University Park Press.

Blau, A., Lahey, M., & Oleksiuk–Velez, A. (1984). Planning goals for intervention: Language testing or language sampling? *Exceptional Children, 51,* 78–79.

Blaxley, L., Clinker, M., & Warr–Leeper, G. (1983). Two language screening tests compared with Developmental Sentence Scoring. *Language, Speech, and Hearing Services in Schools, 14,* 38–46.

Bleile, K. M., & Wallach, H. (1992). A sociolinguistic investigation of the speech of African American preschoolers. *American Journal of Speech-Language Pathology, 1*(2), 54-62.

Bliss, L. S. (1987). "I can't talk anymore: My mouth doesn't want to." The developmental and clinical applications of modal auxiliaries. *Language, Speech, and Hearing Services in Schools, 18,* 72–79.

Bliss, L. S. (1989). Selected syntactic usage by language-impaired children. *Journal of Communication Disorders, 22,* 277-289.

Bliss, L. S. (1992). A comparison of tactful messages by children with and without language impairments. *Language, Speech, and Hearing Services in Schools, 23,* 343-347.

Bloom, L., & Lahey, M. (1978). *Language development and language disorders.* New York: John Wiley.

Bloom, L., Lahey, M., Hood, L., Lifter, K., & Fiess, K. (1980). Complex sentences: Acquisition of syntactic connectives and the semantic relations they encode. *Journal of Child Language, 7,* 235–261.

Bloom, L., Rocissano, L., & Hood, L. (1976). Adult–child discourse: Developmental interaction between information processing and linguistic knowledge. *Cognitive Psychology, 8,* 521–522.

Bloomberg, K., Karlan, G., & Lloyd, L. (1990). The comparative translucency of initial lexical items represented in five graphic symbol systems and sets. *Journal of Speech and Hearing Research, 33,* 717-725.

Bloome, D. (1985). Reading as a social process. *Language Arts, 62*(2), 134-142.

Bloome, D., Harris, O. L., & Ludlum, D. E. (1991). Reading and writing as sociocultural activities: Politics and pedagogy in the classroom. *Topics in Language Disorders, 11*(3), 14-27.

Boatner, M. T., Gates, J. E., & Makkai, A. (1975). *A dictionary of American idioms* (rev. ed.). Woodbury, NJ: Barron's.

Borgh, K., & Dickson, W. P. (1986, April). *The effects on children's writing of adding speech synthesis to a word processor.* Paper presented at the Annual Meeting of the American Educational Research Association, San Francisco.

Borkowski, J., & Cavanaugh, J. (1979). Maintenance and generalization of skills and strategies by the retarded. In N. Ellis (Ed.), *Handbook of mental deficiency: Psychological theory and research* (2nd ed., pp. 569–617). Hillsdale, NJ: Lawrence Erlbaum.

Borsch, J. C., & Oaks, R. (1992). Effective collaboration at Central Elementary School. *Language, Speech, and Hearing Services in Schools, 23,* 367-368.

Bower, G. H., Black, J. B., & Turner, T. J. (1979). Scripts in memory for text. *Cognitive Psychology, 11,* 177-220.

Bowers, P. G., Steffy, R. A., & Swanson, L. B. (1986). Naming speed, memory, and visual processing in reading disability. *Canadian Journal of Behavioral Science, 18,* 209-223.

Bowers, P. G., & Swanson, L. B. (1991). Naming speed deficits in reading disability: Multiple measures of a singular process. *Journal of Experimental Child Psychology, 51,* 195-219.

Bowman, S. (1984). A review of referential communication skills. *Australian Journal of Human Communication Disorders, 12,* 93–112.

Boyce, N., & Larson, V. L. (1983). *Adolescents' communication: Development and disorders.* Eau Claire, WI: Thinking Publications.

Boyd, R., Stauber, K., & Bluma, S. (1977). *The portage parent program: Instructor's manual.* Portage, WI: Cooperation Educational Service Agency 12.

Bracken, B. (1988). Rate and sequence of positive and negative poles in basic concept acquisition. *Language, Speech, and Hearing Services in Schools, 19,* 410–417.

Bradbury, B., & Lunzer, E. (1972). The learning of grammatical inflections in normal and subnormal children. *Journal of child psychology and psychiatry, 13,* 239-248.

Bradley, R., & Caldwell, B. (1976). The relation of infants' home environments to mental test performance at 54 months: A follow-up study. *Child Development, 47,* 1172–1174.

Bradley, L., & Bryant, P. (1985). *Rhyme and reason in reading and spelling.* Ann Arbor: University of Michigan Press.

Brandel, D. (1992). Collaboration: Full steam ahead with no prior experience! *Language, Speech, and Hearing Services in Schools, 23,* 369-370.

Bray, C., & Wiig, E. (1987). Let's Talk Inventory for Children. San Antonio: Psychological Corp.

Bray, N. (1979). Strategy production in the retarded. In N. Ellis (Ed.), *Handbook of mental deficiency: Psychological theory and research* (2nd ed., pp. 699–726). Hillsdale, NJ: Lawrence Erlbaum.

Bretherton, I., & Bates, E. (1984). The development of representation from 10 to 28 months: Differential stability of language and symbolic play. In R. N. Emde & R. H. Harmon (Eds.), *Continuities and discontinuities in development* (pp. 229–262). New York: Plenum.

Bretherton, I., & Beeghly, M. (1982). Talking about internal states: The acquisition of a theory of mind. *Developmental Psychology, 18*, 906-921.

Bricker, D. D. (1986). *Early education of at-risk and handicapped infants, toddlers, and preschool children.* Glenview, IL: Scott, Foresman.

Bricker, W., & Bricker, D. (1974). An early language training strategy. In R. L. Schiefelbusch & L. L. Lloyd (Eds.), *Language perspectives: Acquisition, retardation, and intervention* (pp. 431–468). Baltimore: University Park Press.

Bricker, W., Heal, L., Bricker, D. D., Hayes, W., & Larsen, L. (1969). Discrimination learning and learning set with institutionalized retarded children. *American Journal of Mental Deficiency, 74*, 242-248.

Bridge, C. A., Belmore, S. M., Moskow, S. P., Cohen, S. S., & Matthews, P. D. (1984). Topicalization and memory for main ideas in prose. *Journal of Reading Behavior, 16*(1), 61-80.

Bridge, C. A., Tierney, R., & Cera, M. (1977, December). *Inferential operations of children involved in discourse processing.* Paper presented to the National Reading Conference, New Orleans.

Bridges, A. (1980). SVO comprehension strategies revisited: The evidence of individual patterns of response. *Journal of Child Language, 7*, 89-104.

Briggs, C. (1984). Learning how to ask: Native meta communicative competence and the incompetence of field workers. *Language in Society, 13*, 1–28.

Brinton, B., & Fujiki, M. (1982). A comparison of request–response sequences in the discourse of normal and language–disordered children. *Journal of Speech and Hearing Disorders, 47*, 57–62.

Brinton, B., & Fujiki, M. (1989). *Conversational management with language-impaired children: Pragmatic assessment and intervention.* Rockville, MD: Aspen.

Brinton, B., & Fujiki, M. (1992). Setting the context for conversational language sampling. *Best Practices in School Speech Language Pathology, 2*, 9-19.

Brinton, B., Fujiki, M., & Sonnenberg, E. (1988). Responses to requests for clarification by linguistically normal and language–impaired children in conversation. *Journal of Speech and Hearing Disorders, 53*, 383–391.

Brinton, B., Fujiki, M., Winkler, E., & Loeb, D. (1986). Responses to requests for clarification in linguistically normal and language-impaired children. *Journal of Speech and Hearing Disorders, 51*, 370-378.

Bristol, M. (1985). Designing programs for young developmentally disabled children: A family systems approach to autism. *Remedial and Special Education, 6*(4), 46–53.

Bristol, M. (1988). Impact of autistic children on families. In B. Prizant & B. Schaechter (Eds.), *Autism: The emotional and social dimensions.* Boston: The Exceptional Parent.

Bristow, D., & Fristoe, M. (1984). Learning of Blissymbolics and manual signs. *Journal of Speech and Hearing Disorders, 49*, 145-151.

Britton, B., & Black, J. (Eds.). (1985). *Understanding expository text.* Hillsdale, NJ: Lawrence Erlbaum.

Broen, P. A., & Westman, M. J. (1990). Project parent: A preschool speech program implemented through parents. *Journal of Speech and Hearing Disorders, 55*, 495-502.

Bromley, K. D. (1984). Teaching idioms. *The Reading Teacher, 38*, 272-276.

Bronfenbrenner, V. (1979). *The ecology of human development.* Cambridge, MA: Harvard University Press.

Brooks-Gunn, J., & Lewis, M. (1984). Material responsivity in interactions with handicapped infants. *Child Development, 55*, 782-793.

Brophy, J. E. (1983). Research on the self–fulfilling prophecy and teacher expectations. *Journal of Educational Psychology, 75*, 631–661.

Brotherton, P. (1979). Speaking and not speaking: Processes for translating ideas into speech. In A. Siegman & S. Feldstein (Eds.), *Of speech and time.* Hillsdale, NJ: Lawrence Erlbaum.

Brown, A. L. (1974). The role of strategic memory in retardate memory. In N. R. Ellis (Ed.), *International review of research in mental retardation* (Vol. 7, pp. 55-111). New York: Academic Press.

Brown, A. L. (1978). Knowing when, where, and how to remember: A problem of metacognition. In R. Glaser (Ed.), *Advances in instructional psychology* (Vol. 1). Hillsdale, NJ: Lawrence Erlbaum.

Brown, A. L. (1980). Metacognitive development and reading. In R. J. Spiro, B. C. Bruce, & W. F. Brewer (Eds.), *Theoretical issues in reading comprehension.* Hillsdale, NJ: Lawrence Erlbaum.

Brown, A. L. (1982). Learning to learn how to read. In J. Langer & T. Smith–Burke (Eds.), *Reader meets author, bridging the gap: A psycholinguistic and social linguistic perspective* (pp. 26–54). Newark, DE: International Reading Association.

Brown, A. L., & Campione, J. C. (1984). Three faces of transfer: Implications for early competence, individual differences, and instruction. In M. Lamb, A. Brown, & B. Rogoff (Eds.), *Advances in developmental psychology* (Vol. 3, pp. 143-192). Hillsdale, NJ: Lawrence Erlbaum.

Brown, A. L., Campione, J. C., & Day, J. D. (1981). Learning to learn: On training students to learn from texts. *Educational Research, 10*, 14-21.

Brown, A. L., & Day, J. D. (1983). Macrorules for summarizing texts: The development of expertise. *Journal of Verbal Learning and Verbal Behavior, 22*, 1-14.

Brown, A. L., & Palincsar, A. S. (1982). Inducing strategic learning from texts by means of informed, self-control training. *Topics in Learning and Learning Disabilities, 2*, 1-17.

Brown, A. L., & Smiley, S. S. (1977). Rating the importance of structural units of prose passage: A problem of metacognitive development. *Child Development, 48*, 1-8.

Brown, G., Anderson, A., Shillcock, R., & Yule, G. (1984). *Talking talk: Strategies for production and assessment.* Cambridge, UK: Cambridge University Press.

Brown, J. (1989). The truth about scores children achieve on tests. *Language, Speech, and Hearing Services in Schools, 20*, 366–371.

Brown, L., Branston, M., Hamre–Nietupski, S., Pumpian, I., Certo, N., & Gruenewald, L. (1979). A strategy for developing chronological age appropriate and functional curricular content for severely handicapped adolescents and young adults. *Journal of Special Education, 13*, 81–90.

Brown, L., Nietupski, J., & Hamre–Nietupski, S. (1976). Criterion of ultimate functioning. In M. Thomas (Ed.), *Hey, don't forget about me! Education's investment in the severely, profoundly and multiply handicapped* (pp. 16–35). Reston, VA: Division of Mental Retardation, Council for Exceptional Children.

Brown, L., Shiraga, B., Rogan, P., York, J., Zanella Albright, K., McCarthy, E., Loomis, R., & Van–Deventer, P. (1988). The "why" question in instruction programs for people who are severely intellectually disabled. In S. Calculator & J. Bedrosian (Eds.), *Communication assessment and intervention for adults with mental retardation* (pp. 139–153). San Diego: College–Hill.

Brown, L., Sweet, M., Shiraga, B., York, J., Zanella, K., & Rogan, P. (1984). *Educational programs for students with severe handicaps* (Vol. 14). Madison, WI: Madison Metropolitan School District.

Brown, R. (1973). *A first language: The early stages.* Cambridge, MA: Harvard University Press.

Browne, K., & Sagi, S. (1988). Mother-infant interaction and attachment in physically abusing families. *Journal of Reproductive and Infant Psychology, 6*, 163-182.

Bruner, J. (1975). The ontogenesis of speech acts. *Journal of Child Language, 2*, 1–20.

Bruner, J. (1978a). *Acquiring the uses of language.* Paper presented as Berlyne Memorial Lecture, University of Toronto.

Bruner, J. (1978b). On prelinguistic prerequisites of speech. In R. N. Campbell & P. T. Smith (Eds.), *Recent advances in the psychology of language* (pp. 199–214). New York: Plenum.

Bruner, J., Roy, C., & Ratner, N. (1980). The beginnings of request. In K. E. Nelson (Ed.), *Children's language* (Vol. 3, pp. 91-138). New York: Garner.

Bruno, J., & Goehl, H. (1991). Comparison of picture and word association performance in adults and preliterate children. *Augmentative and Alternative Communication, 7*, 70-79.

Bryan, J. H. (1981). Social behaviors of learning disabled children. In J. Gottlieb & S. Strichart (Eds.), *Developmental theory and research in learning disabilities.* Baltimore: University Park Press.

Bryan, T., Donahue, M., & Pearl, R. (1981). Learning disabled children's peer interaction during a small group problem–solving task. *Learning Disability Quarterly, 4*, 13–22.

Bryan, T., Donahue, M., Pearl, R., & Herzog, A. (1981). *Mother–learning disabled child conversational interactions during a problem–solving task.* Chicago: Chicago Institute for the Study of Learning Disabilities.

Bryen, D., Goldman, A., & Quinlisk-Gill, S. (1988). Sign language with students with severe/profound mental retardation: How effective is it? *Education and Training in Mental Retardation, 23*, 129-137.

Bryen, D., & Joyce, D. (1985). Language intervention with the severely handicapped: A decade of research. *Journal of Special Education, 19*, 7–39.

Bryen, D., & McGinley, V. (1991). Sign language input to community residents with mental retardation. *Education and Training in Mental Retardation, 26*, 207-214.

Bryson, C. (1970). Systematic identification of perceptual disabilities in autistic children. *Perceptual and Motor Skills, 31*, 239-246.

Buium, N., Rynders, J., & Turnure, J. (1974). Early maternal linguistic environment of normal and non-normal language-learning children. *American Journal of Mental Deficiency, 79*, 52-58.

Bullowa, M. (1979). Introduction; Prelinguistic communication: A field for scientific research. In M. Bullowa (Ed.), *Before speech* (pp. 1–62). New York: Cambridge University Press.

Bunce, B. (1989). Using a barrier game format to improve children's referential communication skills. *Journal of Speech and Hearing Disorders, 54*, 33–43.

Bunce, B., Ruder, K., & Ruder, C. (1985). Using the miniature linguistic system in teaching syntax: Two case studies. *Journal of Speech and Hearing Disorders, 50*, 247–253.

Burke, A. E., Crenshaw, D. A., Green, J., Schlosser, M. A., & Strocchia-Rivera, L. (1989). Influence of verbal ability on the expression of aggression in physically abused children. *Journal of the American Academy of Child and Adolescent Psychiatry, 28,* 215-218.

Burr, D., & Rohr, A. (1978). Patterns of psycholinguistic development in the severely mentally retarded: A hypothesis. *Social Biology, 25,* 15-22.

Burroughs, J., Albritton, E., Eaton, B., & Montagne, J. (1990). A comparative study of language delayed preschool children's ability to recall symbols from two symbol systems. *Augmentative and Alternative Communication, 6,* 202-206.

Butkowsky, I. S., & Willows, D. M. (1980). Cognitive-motivational characteristics of children varying in reading ability: Evidence for learned helplessness in poor readers. *Journal of Educational Psychology, 72,* 408-422.

Butler, K. (1986). *Language disorders in children.* Austin, TX: Pro-Ed.

Butler, K. (1993, November). *Toward a model of dynamic assessment: Application to speech.* Paper presented at the Annual Convention of the American Speech-Language-Hearing Association, Anaheim, CA.

Butler-Hinz, S., Caplan, D., & Waters, G. (1990). Characteristics of syntactic comprehension deficits following closed head injury versus left cerebrovascular accident. *Journal of Speech and Hearing Research, 33,* 269-280.

Butterfield, E., Wambold, C., & Belmont, J. (1973). On the theory and practice of improving short-term memory. *American Journal of Mental Deficiency, 77,* 654-669.

Buttrill, J., Niizawa, J., Biemer, C., Takahashi, C., & Hearn, S. (1989). Serving the language learning disabled adolescent: A strategies–based model. *Language, Speech, and Hearing Services in Schools, 20,* 185–204.

Buzock, K., & League, R. (1978). Receptive Expressive Emergent Language Test. Austin, TX: Pro–Ed.

Buzolich, M., King, J., & Baroody, S. (1991). Acquisition of the commenting function among system users. *Augmentative and Alternative Communication, 7,* 88-99.

Buzolich, M., & Wiemann, J. (1988). Turn–taking in atypical conversations: The case of the speaker–augmented communicator dyad. *Journal of Speech and Hearing Research, 31,* 3–18.

Bybee, J., & Slobin, D. (1982). Rules and schemas in the development of the English past tense. *Language, 58,* 265-289.

Bzoch, K., & League, R. (1971). *Assessing language skills in infancy.* Baltimore: University Park Press.

Calculator, S. (1985). Describing and treating discourse problems in mentally retarded children: The myth of mental retardese. In D. Ripich & F. Spinelli (Eds.), *School discourse problems* (pp. 125–147). San Diego: College–Hill.

Calculator, S. N. (1988a). Exploring the language of adults with mental retardation. In S. Calculator & J. Bedrosian (Eds.), *Communication assessment and intervention for adults with mental retardation* (pp. 95–106). San Diego: College–Hill.

Calculator, S. N. (1988b). Promoting the acquisition and generalization of conversational skills by individuals with severe disabilities. *Augmentative and Alternative Communication, 4,* 94–103.

Calculator, S. N. (1988c). Teaching functional communication skills to adults with mental retardation. In S. Calculator & J. Bedrosian (Eds.), *Communication assessment and intervention for adults with mental retardation* (pp. 309-338). San Diego: College-Hill.

Calculator, S. N. (1992a). Facilitated communication: Calculator responds. *American Journal of Speech-Language Pathology, 1*(2), 23-24.

Calculator, S. N. (1992b). Perhaps the emperor has clothes after all: A response to Biklen. *American Journal of Speech-Language Pathology, 1*(2), 18-20.

Calculator, S. N., & D'Altilio–Luchko, C. (1983). Evaluating the effectiveness of a communication board training program. *Journal of Speech and Hearing Disorders, 48,* 185–192.

Calculator, S. N., & Delaney, D. (1986). Comparison of nonspeaking and speaking mentally retarded adults' clarification strategies. *Journal of Speech and Hearing Research, 51,* 252–259.

Calculator, S. N., & Dollaghan, C. (1982). The use of communication boards in a residential setting: An evaluation. *Journal of Speech and Hearing Disorders, 47,* 281-287.

Calculator, S. N., & Jorgensen, C. M. (1991). Integrating AAC instruction into regular education settings: Expounding on best practices. *Augmentative and Alternative Communication, 7,* 204-214.

Calfee, R., & Calfee, K. (1981). *Interactive reading assessment systems.* Unpublished manuscript, Stanford University. (Available from authors)

Calvert, M. B., & Murray, S. L. (1985). Environmental Communication Profile: An assessment procedure. In C. S. Simon (Ed.), *Communication skills and classroom success: Assessment of language-learning disabled students* (pp. 135-165). Austin, TX: Pro-Ed.

Camarata, S. M., Hughes, C., & Ruhl, K. (1988). Mild/moderate behaviorally disordered students: A population at risk for language disorders. *Language, Speech, and Hearing Services in Schools, 19,* 191–200.

Camarata, S. M., & Nelson, K. E. (in press). Treatment efficiency as a function of target selection in the remediation of child language disorders. *Clinical Linguistics and Phonetics.*

Camarata, S. M., Nelson, K. E., Welsh, J., Butkowski, L., Harmer, M., & Camarata, M. (1991, October). The effects of treatment procedures on normal language acquisition [abstract]. *Asha,* p. 152.

Cambourne, B. (1988). *The whole story: Natural learning and the acquisition of literacy in the classroom.* New York: Scholastic.

Cambourne, B., & Turbill, J. (1987). *Coping with chaos.* Portsmouth, NH: Heinemann.

Campbell, B., & Grieve, R. (1978). Social and attentional aspects of echolalia in highly echolalic mentally retarded persons. *American Journal of Mental Deficiency, 82,* 414-416.

Campbell, L. R. (1993). Maintaining the integrity of home linguistic varieties: Black English vernacular. *American Journal of Speech-Language Pathology, 2*(1), 11-12.

Campbell, S. B. (1985). Hyperactivity in preschoolers: Correlates and prognostic implications *Clinical Psychology Review, 5,* 405-428.

Campbell, T., & Shriberg, L. (1982). Associations among pragmatic functions, linguistic stress, and natural phonetic processes in speech-delayed children. *Journal of Speech and Hearing Disorders, 25,* 547-553.

Campbell, T. F., & Dollaghan, C. A. (1990). Expressive language recovery in severely brain-injured children and adolescents. *Journal of Speech and Hearing Disorders, 55,* 567-581.

Campbell, T. F., & Dollaghan, C. A. (1992). A method for obtaining listener judgments of spontaneously produced language: Social validation through direct magnitude estimation. *Topics in Language Disorders, 12,*(2), 42-55.

Cantwell, D. P., Baker, L., & Rutter, M. (1978). A comparative study of infantile autism and specific developmental receptive language disorder, IV: Analysis of syntax and language function. *Journal of Child Psychology and Psychiatry, 19,* 351-363.

Capelli, C. A., Nakagawa, N., & Madden, C. M. (1990). How children understand sarcasm: The role of context and intonation. *Child Development, 61,* 1824–1841.

Caramazza, A., Grober, E., Garvey, C., & Yates, J. (1977). Comprehension of anaphoric pronouns. *Journal of Verbal Learning and Verbal Behavior, 16,* 601–609.

Cardoso–Martins, C., Mervis, C., & Mervis, C. (1985). Early vocabulary acquisition by children with Down's syndrome. *American Journal of Mental Deficiency, 90,* 255–265.

Carey, S. (1978). The child as word learner. In M. Halle, J. Bresnan, & G. Miller (Eds.), *Language theory and psychological reality* (pp. 264–293). Cambridge: MIT Press.

Carey, S., & Bartlett, E. (1978). Acquiring a single new word. *Papers and Reports on Child Language Development, 15,* 17-29.

Carlisle, J. F. (1987). The use of morphological knowledge in spelling derived forms by learning disabled and normal students. *Annals of Dyslexia, 37,* 90-108.

Carlisle, J. F. (1988). Knowledge of derivational morphology and spelling ability in fourth, sixth, and eighth graders. *Applied Psycholinguistics, 9,* 247-266.

Carlson, F. (1981). A format for selecting vocabulary for the nonspeaking child. *Language, Speech, and Hearing Services in Schools, 12,* 140-145.

Carlson, V., Cicchetti, D., Barnett, D., & Braunwald, K. B. (1989). The development of disorganized/disoriented attachment in maltreated infants. *Developmental Psychology, 25,* 525-531.

Carni, E., & French, L. (1984). The acquisition of before and after reconsidered: What develops. *Journal of Experimental Child Psychology, 37,* 394-403.

Caro, P., & Snell, M. (1989). Characteristics of teaching communication to people with moderate and severe disabilities. *Education and Training in Mental Retardation, 29,* 63-77.

Carpenter, A., & Strong, J. (1988). Pragmatic development in normal children: Assessment of a testing protocol. *National Student Speech–Language–Hearing Association Journal, 12,* 40–49.

Carpenter, R., Mastergeorge, A., & Coggins, T. (1983). The acquisition of communicative intentions in infants eight to fifteen months of age. *Language and Speech, 26,* 101-116.

Carr, E. (1979). Teaching autistic children to use sign language: Some research issues. *Journal of Autism and Developmental Disorders, 9,* 345–359.

Carr, E., & Durand, V. (1985). Reducing behavior problems through functional communication training. *Journal of Applied Behavior Analysis, 18,* 111–126.

Carr, E., & Kologinsky, E. (1983). Acquisition of sign language by autistic children, II: Spontaneity and generalization. *Journal of Applied Behavior Analysis, 16,* 297–314.

Carr, E., & Lovaas, O. (1982). Contingent electric shock as a treatment for severe behavior problems. In S. Axelrod & J. Apsche (Eds.), *The effects of punishment on human behavior* (pp. 221–246). New York: Academic Press.

Carr, E., Newson, C., & Binkhoff, J. (1980). Escape as a factor in the aggressive behavior of two retarded children. *Journal of Applied Behavior Analysis, 13,* 101–117.

Carr, E., Schreibman, L., & Lovaas, O. (1975). Control of echolalic speech in psychotic children. *Journal of Abnormal Child Psychology, 3,* 331-351.

Carrow, E. (1973). Test for Auditory Comprehension of Language. Austin, TX: Urban Research Group.

Carrow, E. (1974). Carrow Elicited Language Inventory. Austin, TX: Learning Concepts.

Carrow–Woolfolk, E. (1985). Test of Auditory Comprehension of Language, Revised Edition. Allen, TX: DLM Teaching Resources.

Carson, J. (1987). *Tell me about your picture: Art activities to help children communicate.* Englewood Cliffs, NJ: Prentice–Hall.

Carter, D., & Eckerman, E. (1975). Symbolic matching by pigeons: Rate of learning complex discriminations predicted from simple discriminations. *Science, 187,* 662-664.

Casby, M. (1992). An intervention approach for naming problems in children. *American Journal of Speech-Language Pathology, 1*(3), 35-42.

Case, R. (1978). Intellectual development from birth to adulthood: A neo-Piagetian interpretation. In R. Siegler (Ed.), *Children's thinking: What develops?* (pp. 37–72). Hillsdale, NJ: Lawrence Erlbaum.

Catts, H. W. (1986). Speech production/phonological deficits in reading-disordered children. *Journal of Learning Disabilities, 19,* 504-508.

Catts, H. W. (1991). Facilitating phonological awareness: Role of speech-language pathologists. *Language, Speech, and Hearing Services in Schools, 22,* 196-203.

Catts, H. W., & Kamhi, A. G. (1986). The linguistic basis of reading disorders: Implications for the speech-language pathologist. *Language, Speech, and Hearing Services in Schools, 17,* 329-341.

Catts, H. W., & Kamhi, A. G. (1987). Intervention for reading disabilities. *Journal of Childhood Communication Disorders, 2*(1), 67–80.

Cazden, C. (1972). *Child language and education.* New York: Holt, Rinehart & Winston.

Ceci, S. (1983) Automatic and purposive semantic processing characteristics of normal and language/learning-disabled children. *Developmental Psychology, 19,* 427-439.

Chafe, W. (1970). *Meaning and the structure of language.* Chicago: University of Chicago Press.

Chai, D. T. (1967). *Communication of pronominal referents in ambiguous English sentences for children and adults* (Report No. 13). Ann Arbor: University of Michigan.

Chall, J. S., & Jacobs, V. A. (1984). Writing and reading in the elementary grades: Developmental trends among low SES children. In J. M. Jensen (Ed.), *Composing and comprehending* (pp. 93–104). Urbana, IL: Clearinghouse on Reading and Communication Skills.

Chall, J. S., Jacobs, V. A., & Baldwin, L. E. (1990). *The reading crisis: Why poor children fall behind.* Cambridge, MA: Harvard University Press.

Chamberlain, P., & Medinos–Landurand, P. (1991). Practical considerations for the assessment of LEP students with special needs. In E. V. Hamayan & J.

S. Damico (Eds.), *Limiting bias in the assessment of bilingual students* (pp. 112-156). Austin, TX: Pro-Ed.

Chaney, C. (1990). Evaluating the whole language approach to language arts: The pros and cons. *Language, Speech, and Hearing Services in Schools, 21,* 244-249.

Channell, R., & Ford, C. (1991). Four grammatical completion measures of language ability. *Language, Speech, and Hearing Services in Schools, 22,* 211-218.

Channell, R., & Peek, M. (1989). Four measures of vocabulary ability compared in older preschool children. *Language, Speech, and Hearing Services in Schools, 20,* 407–417.

Chapman, K., & Terrell, B. (1988). "Verb–alizing": Facilitating action word usage in young language–impaired children. *Topics in Language Disorders, 8*(2), 1–13.

Chapman, L. J. (1981, May). *The comprehension of anaphora.* Paper presented at the meeting of the International Reading Association, New Orleans.

Chapman, L. J. (1983). *Reading development and cohesion.* London: Heinemann.

Chapman, R. L. (1987). *A new dictionary of American slang.* New York: Harper & Row.

Chapman, R. S. (1981). Exploring children's communicative intents. In J. Miller (Ed.), *Assessing language production in children* (pp. 22–25). Baltimore: University Park Press.

Chapman, R. S., Kay-Raining Bird, E., & Schwartz, S. E. (1990). Fast mapping of words in event contexts by children with Down syndrome. *Journal of Speech and Hearing Disorders, 55,* 761-770.

Chapman, R. S., & Miller, J. (1980). Analyzing language and communication in the child. In R. Schiefelbusch (Ed.), *Nonspeech language and communication: Assessment and intervention* (pp. 159–195). Baltimore: University Park Press.

Chapman, R. S., Miller, J., MacKenzie, H., & Bedrosian, J. (1981, August). *Development of discourse skills in the second year of life.* Paper presented at the Second International Congress for the Study of Child Language, Vancouver.

Chapman, R. S., Schwartz, S. E., & Kay-Raining Bird, E. (1988, November). *Predicting comprehension of children with Down syndrome.* Paper presented at the Annual Convention of the American Speech-Language-Hearing Association, Boston.

Chappell, G. (1980). Oral language performance of upper elementary school students obtained via story reformulation. *Language, Speech, and Hearing Services in Schools, 11,* 236–250.

Charhop, M., Schreibman, L., & Thebodeau, M. (1985). Increasing spontaneous verbal responding in autistic children using time delay. *Journal of Applied Behavior Analysis, 18,* 155–166.

Charlop, M. (1986). Setting effects on the occurrence of autistic children's immediate echolalia. *Journal of Autism and Development Disorders, 16,* 473-483.

Cheng, L. (1987). Cross–cultural and linguistic considerations in working with Asian populations. *Asha, 29*(6), 33–38.

Cheseldine, S., & McConkey, R. (1979). Parental speech to young Down's syndrome children: An intervention study. *American Journal of Mental Deficiency, 83,* 612-620.

Chi, M., & Ceci, S. (1987). Content knowledge in memory development. *Advances in Child Development and Behavior, 20,* 91-143.

Christie, D., & Schumacher, G. (1975). Developmental trends in the abstraction and recall of relevant vs. irrelevant thematic information from connected verbal material. *Child Development, 46,* 598–602.

Cicchetti, D. (1987). Developmental psychopathology in infancy: Illustration from the study of maltreated youngsters. *Journal of Consulting and Clinical Psychology, 55,* 837-845.

Cicchetti, D., & Lynch, M. (1993). Toward an ecological/transactional model of community violence and child maltreatment: Consequences for children's development. *Psychiatry, 56.*

Cimorell, J. (1983). *Language facilitation, a complete cognitive therapy program.* Baltimore: University Park Press.

Cirrin, F. M. (1983). Lexical access in children and adults. *Developmental Psychology, 19,* 452-460.

Cirrin, F. M., & Rowland, C. M. (1985). Communicative assessment of nonverbal youths with severe/profound mental retardation. *Mental Retardation, 23,* 52-62.

Clahsen, H. (1989). The grammatical characterization of developmental aphasia. *Linguistics, 27,* 897-920.

Clancy, P. M. (1980). Referential choice in English and Japanese narrative discourse. In W. Chafe (Ed.), *The pear stories: Cognitive, cultural, and linguistic aspects of narrative production* (pp. 127-199). Norwood, NJ: Ablex.

Clancy, P. M., Jacobsen, T., & Silva, M. (1976). The acquisition of conjunction: A cross–linguistic study. *Papers and Reports in Child Language Development, 13,* 71–80.

Clark, C. H. (1981). Learning words using traditional orthography and the symbols of Rebus, Bliss, and Carrier. *Journal of Speech and Hearing Disorders, 46,* 191–196.

Clark, C. H. (1986). Instructional strategies to promote comprehension of normal and noncohesive tests. In J. W. Irwin (Ed.), *Understanding and teaching cohesion comprehension.* Newark, DE: International Reading Association.

Clark, E. V. (1973). Non–linguistic strategies and the acquisition of word meanings. *Cognition, 2,* 161–182.

Clark, E. V. (1978). Strategies for communicating. *Child Development, 49,* 953-959.

Clark, E. V. (1979). Building a vocabulary: Words for objects, actions, and relations. In P. Fletcher & M. Garman (Eds.), *Language acquisition* (pp. 149–160). New York: Cambridge University Press.

Clark, E. V. (1980). Here's the top: Nonlinguistic strategies in the acquisition of orientation terms. *Child Development, 51,* 329-338.

Clark, E. V., & Andersen, E. (1979). Spontaneous repairs: Awareness in the process of acquiring language. *Papers and Reports on Child Language Development, 16,* 1–12.

Clark, G., & Seifer, R. (1982). Facilitating mother–infant communication: A treatment model for high risk and developmentally delayed infants. *Infant Mental Health Journal, 4*(2), 67–81.

Clark, H. (1983). Making sense of nonce sense. In G. Flores d'Arcais & R. Jarvella (Eds.), *The process of language understanding* (pp. 297–332). New York: John Wiley.

Clark, H., & Clark, E. (1977). *Psychology and language: An introduction to psycholinguistics.* Orlando, FL: Harcourt Brace Jovanovich.

Clark, J. O. (1990). *Harrup's dictionary of English idioms.* London: Harrup.

Clarke, S. (1987). *An evaluation of the relationship between receptive speech and manual sign language with mentally handicapped children.* Unpublished doctoral dissertation, University of Southampton, UK.

Cochran, P. S., & Bull, G. L. (1991). Integrating word processing into language instruction. *Topics in Language Disorders, 11*(2), 31–49.

Cochrane, R. (1983). Language and the atmosphere of delight. In H. Winitz (Ed.), *Treating language disorders: For clinicians by clinicians* (pp. 143–162). Baltimore: University Park Press.

Coelho, C. A., Liles, B. Z., & Duffy, R. J. (1991). *Conversational patterns of aphasic, closed head injured, and normal speakers.* Paper presented at the 21st Annual Clinical Aphasiology Conference, Destin, FL.

Coggins, T. (1991). Bringing context back into assessment. *Topics in Language Disorders, 11*(4), 43-54.

Coggins, T., & Olswang, L. B. (1987). The pragmatics of generalization. *Seminars in Speech and Language, 8,* 283–302.

Coggins, T., Olswang, L., & Guthrie, J. (1987). Assessing communicative intents in young children: Low structured observation or elicitation tasks? *Journal of Speech and Hearing Disorders, 52,* 44-49.

Cohen, S. (1991). Adapting educational programs for students with head injuries. *Journal of Head Trauma Rehabilitation, 6,* 56-64.

Cole, D., Vandercook, T., & Rynders, J. (1987). Dyadic interactions between children with and without mental retardation: Effect of age discrepancy. *American Journal of Mental Deficiency, 92,* 194–202.

Cole, K. N., & Dale, P. (1986). Direct language instruction and interactive language instruction with language-delayed preschool children: A comparison study. *Journal of Speech and Hearing Research, 29,* 206-217.

Cole, K. N., Dale, P., & Mills, P. (1990). Defining language delay in young children by cognitive referencing: Are we saying more than we know? *Applied Psycholinguistics, 11,* 291-302.

Cole, K. N., Mills, P., & Dale, P. (1989). Examination of test–retest and split–half reliability for measures derived from language samples of young handicapped children. *Language, Speech, and Hearing Services in Schools, 20,* 259–268.

Cole, M., & Cole, J. (1981). *Effective intervention with the language impaired child.* Rockville, MD: Aspen.

Cole, P. (1982). *Language disorders in preschool children.* Englewood Cliffs, NJ: Prentice-Hall.

Cole, P., Harbert, W., Herman, G., & Sridhar, S. (1980). The acquisition of subjecthood. *Language, 56,* 719–743.

Coleman, M., & Gillberg, C. (1985). *The biology of the autistic syndrome.* New York: Praeger.

Coleman, R., & Rainwater, L. (1978). *Social standing in America.* New York: Basic Books.

Coley, J., & Gelman, S. (1989). The effect of object orientation and object type on children's interpretation of the word "big". *Child Development, 60,* 372-380.

Collins, A., Brown, J. S., & Larkin, K. M. (1980). Inference in text understanding. In R. J. Spiro, B. C. Bruce, & W. F. Brewer (Eds.), *Theoretical issues in reading comprehension* (pp. 385–407). Hillsdale, NJ: Lawrence Erlbaum.

Collins, W. (1983). Social antecedents, cognitive processing, and comprehension of social portrayals on television. In E. Higgins, D. Ruble, & W. Hartup (Eds.), *Social cognition and social development* (pp. 110–133). New York: Cambridge University Press.

Collins, W., Wellman, H., Keniston, A., & Westby, S. (1978). Age–related aspects of comprehension and inference from a television dramatic narrative. *Child Development, 49,* 389–399.

Condus, M. M., Marshall, K. L., & Miller, S. R. (1986). Effects of reference keyword mnemonic strategy on vocabulary acquisition and maintenance of learning-disabled children. *Journal of Learning Disabilities, 19,* 609–613.

Confal, K. L. (1993). Collaborative consultation for speech-language pathologists. *Topics in Language Disorders, 14*(1), 1–14.

Conklin, N. F., & Lourie, M. A. (1983). *A host of tongues: Language communities in the United States.* New York: Free Press.

Connard, P. (1984). Preverbal Assessment Intervention Profile. Austin, TX: Pro–Ed.

Connell, P. J. (1982). On training language rules. *Language, Speech, and Hearing Services in Schools, 13,* 231–240.

Connell, P. J. (1986a). Acquisition of semantic role by language-disordered children: Differences between production and comprehension. *Journal of Speech and Hearing Research, 29,* 366-374.

Connell, P. J. (1986b). Teaching subjecthood to language-disordered children. *Journal of Speech and Hearing Research, 29,* 481-493.

Connell, P. J. (1987a). A comparison of modeling and imitation teaching procedures on language-disordered children. *Journal of Speech and Hearing Research, 30,* 105-113.

Connell, P. J. (1987b). An effect of modeling and imitation teaching procedures on children with and without language impairment. *Journal of Speech and Hearing Research, 30,* 105–113.

Connell, P. J. (1987c). Teaching language rules as solutions to language problems: A baseball analogy. *Language, Speech, and Hearing Services in Schools, 18,* 194–205.

Connell, P. J., Gardner–Gletty, D., Dejewski, J., & Parks–Reinick, L. (1981). Response to Courtright and Courtright. *Journal of Speech and Hearing Research, 24,* 146–148.

Connell, P. J., & Myles-Zitler, C. (1982). An analysis of elicited imitation as a language evaluation procedure. *Journal of Speech and Hearing Disorders, 47,* 390-396.

Connell, P. J., & Stone, C. (1992). Morphene learning of children with specific language impairments under controlled conditions. *Journal of Speech and Hearing Research, 35,* 844-852.

Constable, C. M. (1983). Creating communicative context. In H. Winitz (Ed.), *Treating language disorders: For clinicians by clinicians* (pp. 97–120). Baltimore: University Park Press.

Constable, C. M. (1986). The application of scripts in the organization of language intervention contexts. *Event Knowledge, 10,* 205-230.

Constable, C. M. (1992, March). *What can classroom ethnography do for clinical intervention?* Paper presented at the Conference on Pragmatics: From Theory to Therapy, State University of New York, Buffalo.

Conti-Ramsden, G. (1990). Material recasts and other contingent replies to language-impaired children. *Journal of Speech and Hearing Disorders, 55,* 262-274.

Conti-Ramsden, G., & Friel-Patti, S. (1987). Situational variability in mother-child conversations. In K. E. Nelson & A. van Kleeck (Eds.), *Children's Language*

(Vol. 6, pp. 43–63). Hillsdale, NJ: Lawrence Erlbaum.

Cook–Gumperz, J. (1977). *Situated instructions: Language socialization of school–age children*. New York: Academic Press.

Cook–Gumperz, J., & Corsaro, W. (1976). *Socioecological constraints on children's communicative strategies* (Working Paper 46 on Language and Context). Berkeley, CA: Berkeley Language Behavior Research Laboratory.

Cook-Gumperz, J., & Green, J. L. (1984). A sense of story: Influences on children's story-telling ability. In D. Tannen (Ed.), *Coherence in spoken and written discourse* (pp. 201-218). Norwood, NJ: Ablex.

Cook–Gumperz, J., & Gumperz, J. (1978). Context in children's speech. In N. Waterson & C. Snow (Eds.), *The development of communication* (pp. 3–23). New York: John Wiley.

Cooper, D. C., & Anderson-Inman, L. (1988). Language and socialization. In M. A. Nippold (Ed.), *Later language development: Ages nine through nineteen* (pp. 225-245). Austin, TX: Pro-Ed.

Cooper, J., & Flowers, C. (1987). Children with a history of acquired aphasia: Residual language and academic impairments. *Journal of Speech and Hearing Disorders, 52,* 251–262.

Cooper, J., Moodley, M., & Reynell, J. (1978). *Helping language development.* New York: St. Martin's.

Cooper, J., Moodley, M., & Reynell, J. (1979). The development language programme: Results from a five-year study. *British Journal of Disorders of Communication, 14,* 57-69.

Coplan, J. (1987). Early Language Milestone Scale. Tulsa, OK: Modern Education.

Corrigan, R. (1975). A scalogram analysis of the development of the use and comprehension of "because" in children. *Child Development, 46,* 195–201.

Cosaro, J. (1989). Activities to enhance listening skills. *Language, Speech, and Hearing Services in Schools, 20,* 433–435.

Costello, J. (1983). Generalization across settings: Language intervention with children. In J. Miller, D. Yoder, & R. Schiefelbusch (Eds.), *Contemporary issues in language intervention* (ASHA Report No. 12) (pp. 275–297). Rockville, MD: American Speech–Language–Hearing Association.

Coster, W. J., & Cicchetti, D. (1993). Research on the development of maltreated children: Clinical implications. *Topics in Language Disorders, 13*(4), 25-38.

Coster, W. J., Gersten, M. S., Beeghly, M., & Cicchetti, D. (1989). Communicative functioning in maltreated toddlers. *Developmental Psychology, 25,* 1020-1029.

Courchesne, E. (1988). Hypoplasia of cerebellar vermal lobules VI and VII in autism. *New England Journal of Medicine, 318,* 1349-1354.

Courtright, J., & Courtright, I. (1976). Imitative modeling as a theoretical base for instructing language–disordered children. *Journal of Speech and Hearing Research, 19,* 655–663.

Courtright, J., & Courtright, I. (1979). Imitative modeling as a language intervention strategy: The effects of two mediating variables. *Journal of Speech and Hearing Research, 22,* 389–402.

Cox, M., & Richardson, J. (1985). How do children describe spatial relationships? *Journal of Child Language, 12,* 611–620.

Crago, M., & Annahatak, B. (1985, November). *Evaluation of minority-language children by native speakers.* Paper presented at the Annual Convention of the American Speech-Language-Hearing Association, Washington, DC.

Crago, M. B., & Eriks-Brophy, A. (1992, March). *Culture, conversation, and the co-construction of interaction: Implications for intervention.* Paper presented at Pragmatics From Theory to Therapy, Buffalo, NY.

Craig, H. K. (1979). *A comparison of three–party and two–party conversations of normal children: An examination of increased social complexity.* Unpublished doctoral dissertation, University of Michigan, Ann Arbor.

Craig, H. K. (1983). Applications of pragmatic language models for intervention. In T. Gallagher & C. Prutting (Eds.), *Pragmatic assessment and intervention issues in language* (pp. 101–127). San Diego: College–Hill.

Craig, H. K. (1993). Social skills of children with specific language impairment: Peer relationships. *Language, Speech, and Hearing Services in Schools, 24,* 206–215.

Craig, H. K., & Evans, J. (1989). Turn exchange characteristics of SLI children's simultaneous and nonsimultaneous speech. *Journal of Speech and Hearing Disorders, 54,* 334–347.

Craig, H. K., & Evans, J. (1992). Language sample collection and analysis: Interview compared to freeplay assessment contexts. *Journal of Speech and Hearing Research, 35,* 343-353.

Craig, H. K., & Evans, J. L. (1993). Pragmatics and SLI: Within–group variations in discourse behaviors. *Journal of Speech and Hearing Research, 36,* 777–789.

Craig, H. K., & Washington, J. (1986). Children's turn–taking behaviors: Social–linguistic interactions. *Journal of Pragmatics, 10,* 173–197.

Craig, H. K., & Washington, J. A. (1993). Access behaviors of children with specific language impairment. *Journal of Speech and Hearing Research, 36,* 322-337.

Craik, F. I., & Lockhart, R. S. (1972). Levels of processing: A framework for memory research. *Journal of Verbal Learning and Verbal Behavior, 1,* 671–684.

Crais, E. R. (1987). Fast mapping of novel words in oral story context. *Papers and Reports in Child Language Development, 26,* 40-47.

Crais, E. R. (1990). World knowledge to word knowledge. *Topics in Language Disorders, 10*(3), 45-62.

Crais, E. R. (1991). Moving from "parent involvement" to family-centered services. *American Journal of Speech-Language Pathology, 1*(1), 5–8.

Crais, E. R. (1992, April). *Family-centered assessment and collaborative goal-setting.* Paper presented at the Annual Convention of the New York State Speech-Language-Hearing Association, Kiamesha Lake.

Crais, E. R., & Chapman, R. (1987). Story recall and inferencing skills in language–learning disabled and nondisabled children. *Journal of Speech and Hearing Disorders, 52,* 50–55.

Crais, E. R., & Roberts, J. (1991). Decision making in assessment and early intervention planning. *Language, Speech, and Hearing Services in Schools, 22,* 19-30.

Creaghead, N. A. (1984). Strategies for evaluating and targeting pragmatic behaviors in young children. *Seminars in Speech and Language, 5,* 241–251.

Creaghead, N. A. (1992). Classroom interactional analysis/script analysis. *Best Practices in School Speech Language Pathology, 2,* 65-72.

Creaghead, N. A., & Donnelly, K. (1982). Comprehension of superordinate and subordinate information by good and poor readers. *Language, Speech, and Hearing Services in Schools, 13,* 177–186.

Creech, R. (1989). Incorporating prefixes and suffixes into words strategy. *Fourth Annual Minspeak Conference.* St. Louis, MO: Prentke Romich.

Crittenden, P. M. (1981). Abusing, neglecting, problematic, and adequate dyads: Differentiating by patterns of interaction. *Merrill-Palmer Quarterly, 27,* 201-208.

Crittenden, P. M. (1988). Relationships at risk. In J. Belsky & T. Nazwarski (Eds.), *Clinical implications of attachment* (pp. 136-174). Hillsdale, NJ: Lawrence Erlbaum.

Cross, T. (1977). Mothers' speech adjustments: The contribution of selected listener variables. In C. Snow & C. Ferguson (Eds.), *Talking to children: Language input and acquisition* (pp. 151–188). New York: Cambridge University Press.

Cross, T. (1978). Mothers' speech and its association with rate of language acquisition in young children. In N. Waterson & C. Snow (Eds.), *The development of communication* (pp. 199–216). London: Wiley.

Cross, T. (1981). The linguistic experience of slow language learners. In A. Nesdale, C. Pratt, R. Grieve, J. Field, D. Illingworth, & J. Hogben (Eds.), *Advances in child development.* Proceedings of the First National Conference on Child Development, University of Western Australia, Nedlands.

Cross, T. (1984). Habilitating the language–impaired child: Ideas from studies of parent–child interaction. *Topics in Language Disorders, 4*(4), 1–14.

Crossley, R. (1988, October). *Unexpected communication attainments by persons diagnosed as autistic and intelligently impaired.* Paper presented at the International Society for Augmentative and Alternative Communication, Los Angeles, CA.

Crossley, R., & McDonald, A. (1980). *Annie's coming out.* Melbourne, Australia: Penguin.

Crossley, R., & Remington-Gurney, J. (1992). Getting the words out: Facilitated communication training, *Topics in Language Disorders, 12*(4), 29-45.

Crystal, D. (1982). *Profiling linguistic disability.* London, UK: Edward Arnold.

Crystal, D. (1987). Towards a "bucket" theory of language disability: Taking account of interaction between linguistic levels. *Clinical Linguistics and Phonetics, 1,* 7-22.

Crystal, D., Fletcher, P., & Garman, P. (1976). *The grammatical analysis of language disability.* New York: Elsevier.

Culatta, B. (1992, March). *Replica play, role play, and story enactments: A format for language therapy.* Paper presented at the Conference on Pragmatics: From Theory to Therapy, State University of New York, Buffalo.

Culatta, B., & Horn, D. (1982). A program for achieving generalization of grammatical rules to spontaneous discourse. *Journal of Speech and Hearing Disorders, 47,* 174-181.

Culatta, B., Horn, D., Theadore, G., & Sutherland, D. (1993, November). *Scripted play: Enhancing language and literacy in diverse learners.* Paper presented at the Annual Convention of the American Speech-Language-Hearing Association, Anaheim, CA.

Culatta, B., Page, J., & Ellis, J. (1983). Story retelling as a communicative performance screening tool. *Language, Speech, and Hearing Services in Schools, 14,* 66–74.

Culp, R. E., Watkins, R. V., Lawrence, H., Letts, D., Kelly, D. J., & Rice, M. (1991). Maltreated children's language and speech development: Abused, neglected, and abused and neglected. *First Language, 11,* 337-389.

Cummins, J. (1976). The influence of bilingualism on cognitive growth: A synthesis of research findings and explanatory hypotheses. *Working Papers on Bilingualism, 9,* 1-43.

Cummins, J. (1979a). Language functions and cognitive processing. In J. Das, J. Kirby, & R. Jarman (Eds.), *Simultaneous and successive cognitive processes* (pp. 175–185). New York: Academic Press.

Cummins, J. (1979b). Linguistic interdependence and the educational development of bilingual children. *Review of Educational Research, 49,* 222-251.

Cummins, J. (1980). Psychological assessment of immigrant children: Logic or intuition. *Journal of Multilingual Multicultural Development, 1*(2), 97-111.

Cummins, J. (1981). Empirical and theoretical underpinnings of bilingual education. *Journal of Education, 163,* 16-29.

Cummins, J. (1983). Language proficiency and academic achievement. In J. W. Oller, Jr. (Ed.), *Issues in language testing research* (pp. 108-130). Rowley, MA: Newbury House.

Cummins, J. (1984). *Bilingualism and special education: Issues in assessment and pedagogy.* Austin, TX: Pro-Ed.

Cummins, J. (1986). Empowering minority students: A framework for intervention. *Harvard Educational Review, 58,* 18-39.

Cummins, J., & Das, J. (1978). Simultaneous and successive synthesis and linguistic processes. *International Journal of Psychology, 13,* 129-138.

Cunningham, C., Glenn, S., Wilkinson, P., & Sloper, P. (1985). Mental ability, symbolic play and receptive and expressive language of young children with Down's syndrome. *Journal of Child Psychology and Psychiatry and Applied Disciplines, 26,* 255–265.

Cunningham, C., Reuler, E., Blackwell, J., & Deck, J. (1981). Behavioral and linguistic developments in the interactions of normal and retarded children with their mothers. *Child Development, 52,* 62-70.

Curcio, F. (1978). A study of sensorimotor functioning and communication in mute autistic children. *Journal of Autism and Childhood Schizophrenia, 3,* 281–292.

Curcio, F., & Paccia–Cooper, J. (1982). Strategies in evaluating autistic children's communication. *Topics in Language Disorders, 3*(1), 43–49.

Curtis, M. E. (1987). Vocabulary testing and vocabulary instruction. In M. G. McKeown & M. E. Curtis (Eds.), *The nature of vocabulary acquisition* (pp. 37-51). Hillsdale, NJ: Lawrence Erlbaum.

Curtiss, S., Kutz, W., & Tallal, P. (1992). Delay versus deviance in the language acquisition of language-impaired children. *Journal of Speech and Hearing Research, 35,* 373-383.

Dale, E., & O'Rourke, J. (1981). *The living word vocabulary.* Chicago: World Book-Childcraft.

Dale, P. S. (1980). Is early pragmatic development measurable? *Journal of Child Development, 7,* 1–12.

Dale, P. S. (1991). The validity of a parent report measure of vocabulary and syntax at 24 months. *Journal of Speech and Hearing Research, 34,* 565-571.

Dale, P. S., Bates, E., Reznick, J. S., & Morisset, C. (1989). The validity of a parent report instrument of child language at 20 months. *Journal of Child Language, 16,* 239-249.

Dale, P. S., & Cole, K. (1991). What's normal? Specific language impairment in an individual differences perspective. *Language, Speech, and Hearing Services in Schools, 22,* 80-83.

Dale, P. S., & Henderson, V. (1987). An evaluation of the Test of Early Language Development as a measure of receptive and expressive language. *Language, Speech, and Hearing Services in Schools, 18,* 179–187.

Dalgleish, B. (1975). Cognitive processing and linguistic reference in autistic children. *Journal of Autism and Childhood Schizophrenia, 5,* 353-361.

Damico, J. S. (1985a). Clinical discourse analysis: A functional approach to language assessment. In C. Simon (Ed.), *Communication skills and classroom success* (pp. 165–206). San Diego: College-Hill.

Damico, J. S. (1985b). *The effectiveness of direct observation as a language assessment technique.* Unpublished doctoral dissertation, University of New Mexico, Albuquerque.

Damico, J. S. (1987). Addressing language concerns in the schools: The SLP as a consultant. *Journal of Childhood Communication Disorders, 11*(1), 17–40.

Damico, J. S. (1988). The lack of efficacy in language therapy: A case study. *Language, Speech, and Hearing Services in Schools, 19,* 51–66.

Damico, J. S. (1991a). Clinical Discourse Analysis: A functional language assessment technique. In C. S. Simon (Ed.), *Communication skills and classroom success: Assessment and therapy methodologies for language and learning disabled students* (pp. 125-150). Eau Claire, WI: Thinking Publications.

Damico, J. S. (1991b). Descriptive assessment of communicative ability in LEP students. In E. V. Hamayan & J. S. Damico (Eds.), *Limiting bias in the assessment of bilingual students* (pp. 157-218). Austin, TX: Pro-Ed.

Damico, J. S. (1993). Language assessment in adolescents: Addressing critical issues. *Language, Speech, and Hearing Services in Schools, 24,* 29-35.

Damico, J. S., & Oller, J. W. (1980). Pragmatic versus morphological/systematic criteria for language referrals. *Language, Speech, and Hearing Services in Schools, 11,* 85-94.

Damico, J. S., & Oller, J. (1985). *Spotting language problems.* San Diego: Los Amigos Research Associates.

Damico, J. S., Secord, W. A., & Wiig, E. H. (1992). Descriptive language assessment at school: Characteristics and design. *Best Practices in School Speech Language Pathology, 2,* 1-8.

Daniloff, R., & Moll, K. (1968). Coarticulation of lip rounding. *Journal of Speech and Hearing Research, 11,* 707–721.

Danserean, D. (1987). Transfer from cooperative to individual studying. *Journal of Reading, 30,* 614-619.

Darley, F. (1979). *Evaluation of appraisal techniques in speech and language pathology.* Reading, MA: Addison–Wesley.

Das, J., Kirby, J., & Jarman, R. (1975). Simultaneous and successive synthesis: An alternative model for cognitive abilities. *Psychological Bulletin, 80,* 97-113.

Das, J., Kirby, J., & Jarman, R. (1979). *Simultaneous and successive cognitive processes.* New York: Academic Press.

Davis, A. (1972). *English problems of Spanish speakers.* Urbana, IL: National Council of Teachers of English.

Davis, H., Stroud, A., & Green, L. (1988). Maternal language environment of children with mental retardation. *American Journal of Mental Retardation, 93,* 144-153.

Dawson, G., & Adams, A. (1984). Imitation and social responsiveness in autistic children. *Journal of Abnormal Child Psychology, 12,* 209–226.

Dawson, G., & Galpert, L. (1986). A developmental model for facilitating the social behavior of autistic children. In E. Schopler & G. B. Mesibov (Eds.), *Social behavior in autism* (pp. 237–261). New York: Plenum.

Day, E. C., McCollum, P. A., Cieslak, V. A., & Erickson, J. G. (1981). Discrete point language tests of bilinguals: A review of selected tests. In D. R. Omark & J. G. Erickson (Eds.), *The bilingual exceptional child* (pp. 129-161). Austin, TX: Pro-Ed.

Deal, V., & Rodriguez, V. (1987). *Resource guide to multicultural tests and materials in communicative disorders.* Rockville, MD: American Speech–Language–Hearing Association.

Dean, E. C., Howell, J., Hill, A., & Waters, D. (1990). *Metaphon resource pack.* Windsor, UK: NFER-Nelson.

Dean, E. C., Howell, J., & Waters, D. (1993, November). *Metaphon: An approach to treating children with phonological disorder.* Paper presented at the Annual Convention of the American Speech-Language-Hearing Association, Anaheim, CA.

Dee–Lucas, D., & DiVesta, F. J. (1980). Learner–generated organizational aids: Effects on comprehension. *Journal of Educational Psychology, 72,* 304–311.

DeLemos, C. (1981). International processes in the child's construction of language. In W. Deutsch (Ed.), *The child's construction of language* (pp. 57–76). New York: Academic Press.

DeMaio, L. (1984). Establishing communication networks through interactive play: A method for language programming in the clinic setting. *Seminars in Speech and Language, 5,* 199–211.

DeMyer, M. K. (1975). Research in infantile autism: A strategy and its results. *Biological Psychiatry, 10,* 433-450.

Denckla, M. B., & Rudel, R. G. (1976a). Naming of object drawings by dyslexic and other learning disabled children. *Brain and Language, 3,* 1-15.

Denckla, M. B., & Rudel, R. G. (1976b). Rapid automatized naming (R.A.N.): Dyslexia differentiated from other learning disabilities. *Neuropsychologia, 14,* 471-479.

Denner, P. R., & Pehrsson, R. S. (1987, April). *A comparison of the effects of episodic organizers and traditional notetaking on story recall.* Paper presented at the Annual Meeting of the American Educational Research Association, Washington, DC.

Dennis, M. (1980). Strokes in childhood: Communicative intent, expression, and comprehension after left hemisphere arteriopathy in a right-handed nine-year-old. In R. W. Reiber (Ed.), *Language development and aphasia in children* (pp. 45-67). New York: Academic Press.

Dennis, M. (1992). Word finding in children and adolescents with a history of brain injury. *Topics in Language Disorders, 13*(1), 66-82.

Dennis, M., & Barnes, M. A. (1990). Knowing the meaning, getting the point, bridging the gap, and carrying the message: Aspects of discourse following closed head injury in children and adolescents. *Brain and Language, 39,* 428-446.

Dennis, M., Sugar, J., & Whitaker, H. (1982). The acquisition of tag questions. *Child Development, 53,* 1254–1257.

Derwing, B. (1976). Morpheme recognition and the learning of rules for derivational morphology. *Canadian Journal of Linguistics, 21,* 38-67.

Derwing, B., & Baker, W. (1979). Recent research on the acquisition of English morphology. In P. Fletcher & M. Garman (Eds.), *Language acquisition* (pp. 209-223). Cambridge, UK: Cambridge University Press.

Deshler, D., Alley, G., Warner, M., & Schumaker, J. (1981). Instructional practices for promoting skill acquisition and generalization in severely learning disabled adolescents. *Learning Disability Quarterly, 4,* 145–152.

DeSpain, A., & Simon, C. (1987). Alternative to failure: A junior high school language development–based curriculum. *Journal of Childhood Communication Disorders, 11*(1), 139–179.

Detterman, D. (1979). Memory in the mentally retarded. In N. Ellis (Ed.), *Handbook of mental deficiency: Psychological theory and research* (2nd ed., pp. 727–760). Hillsdale, NJ: Lawrence Erlbaum.

Dever, R. (1978). *Talk: Teaching the American language to kids.* New York: Merrill/Macmillan.

Dever, R., & Gardner, W. (1970). Performance of normal and retarded boys on Berko's Test of Morphology. *Language and Speech, 13,* 162-181.

deVilliers, J., & deVilliers, P. (1978). *Language acquisition.* Cambridge, MA: Harvard University Press.

Dewey, M., & Everard, M. (1974). The near normal autistic adolescent. *Journal of Autism and Childhood Schizophrenia, 4,* 348–356.

Diana v. State Board of Education. (1970). C–70–37 (RFP District N. Calif.).

Diener, C. I., & Dweck, C. S. (1978). An analysis of learned helplessness: Continuous changes in performance, strategy and achievement cognitions following failure. *Journal of Personal and Social Psychology, 25,* 451-462.

Dietrich, K. N., Starr, R. H., & Kaplan, M. G. (1980). Maternal stimulation and care of abused infants. In T. M. Field, S. Goldberg, D. Stern, & A. M. Sostek (Eds.), *High-risk infants and children* (pp. 25–41). New York: Academic Press.

Dik, S. (1980). *Studies in functional grammar.* New York: Academic Press.

Dobe, L. (1989). *A study of interaction styles and patterns of mothers of preverbal children.* Unpublished master's thesis, Ohio State University, Columbus.

Dodge, E., & Mallard, A. (1992). Social skills training using a collaborative service delivery model. *Language, Speech, and Hearing Services in Schools, 23,* 130-135.

Dodge, K. A., Coie, J. D., & Brakke, N. P. (1982). Behavior patterns of socially rejected and neglected preadolescents: The roles of social approach and aggression. *Journal of Abnormal Child Psychology, 10,* 389–409.

Doehring, D., Trites, R., Patel, P., & Fiedorowicz, C. (1981). *Reading disabilities: The interaction of reading, language, and neuropsychological deficits.* New York: Academic Press.

Dollaghan, C. A. (1987a). Comprehension monitoring in normal and language–impaired children. *Topics in Language Disorders, 7*(2), 45–60.

Dollaghan, C. A. (1987b). Fast mapping in normal and language–impaired children. *Journal of Speech and Hearing Disorders, 52,* 218–222.

Dollaghan, C. A., & Campbell, T. F. (1992). A procedure for classifying disruptions in spontaneous language samples. *Topics in Language Disorders, 12*(2), 56-68.

Dollaghan, C. A., Campbell, T., & Tomlin, R. (1990). Video narration as a language sampling context. *Journal of Speech and Hearing Disorders, 55,* 582-590.

Dollaghan, C. A., & Kaston, N. (1986). A comprehension monitoring program for language–impaired children. *Journal of Speech and Hearing Disorders, 51,* 264–271.

Dollaghan, C. A., & Miller, J. (1986). Observational methods in the study of communicative competence. In R. Schiefelbusch (Ed.), *Language competence: Assessment and intervention* (pp. 99–129). San Diego: College–Hill.

Donahue, M. (1983). Language–disabled children as conversational partners. *Topics in Language Disorders, 4,* 15–27.

Donahue, M. (1984). Learning disabled children's conversational competence: An attempt to activate an inactive listener. *Applied Psycholinguistics, 5,* 21–36.

Donahue, M. (1985). Communicative style in learning disabled children: Some implications for classroom discourse. In D. Ropich & F. Spinelli (Eds.), *School discourse problems* (pp. 97–124). San Diego: College–Hill.

Donahue, M., & Bryan, T. (1984). Communicative skills and peer relations of learning-disabled adolescents. *Topics in Language Disorders, 4*(2), 10-21.

Donahue, M., Pearl, R., & Bryan, T. (1980). Learning disabled children's conversational competence: Responses to inadequate messages. *Applied Psycholinguistics, 1,* 387–403.

Donnellan, A. M., & Mirenda, P. L. (1983). A model for analyzing instructional components to facilitate generalization for severely handicapped students. *Journal of Special Education, 17,* 317–331.

Donnellan, A. M., Mirenda, P. L., Mesaros, R., & Fassbender, L. (1984). Analyzing the communicative functions of aberrant behavior. *Journal of the Association for Persons with Severe Handicaps, 9,* 210–222.

Dore, J. (1974). A pragmatic description of early language development. *Journal of Psycholinguistic Research, 3,* 343–350.

Dore, J. (1975). Holophrases, speech acts and language universals. *Journal of Child Language, 2,* 21–40.

Dore, J. (1976). Children's illocutionary acts. In R. Freedle (Ed.), *Discourse production and comprehension* (Vol. 1). Hillsdale, NJ: Lawrence Erlbaum.

Dore, J. (1986). The development of conversational competence. In R. Schiefelbusch (Ed.), *Language competence: Assessment and intervention* (pp. 3–60). San Diego: College–Hill.

Dorval, B., & Eckerman, C. D. (1984). Developmental trends in the quality of conversation achieved by small groups of acquainted peers. *Monographs of the Society for Research in Child Development, 49.*

Douglas, D., & Selinker, L. (1985). Principles for language tests within the "discourse domains" theory of interlanguage. *Language Testing, 2,* 205-226.

Downing, J. (1987). Conversational skills training: Teaching adolescents with mental retardation to be verbally assertive. *Mental Retardation, 25,* 147–155.

Downing, J., & Siegel–Causey, E. (1988). Enhancing the nonsymbolic communicative behavior of children with multiple impairments. *Language, Speech, and Hearing Services in Schools, 19,* 338–348.

Dubois, E., & Bernthal, J. (1978). A comparison of three methods of obtaining articulatory responses. *Journal of Speech and Hearing Disorders, 43,* 295–305.

Duchan, J. F. (1980). The effect of cognitive bias on children's early interpretations of locative commands. *Language Sciences, 2,* 246-259.

Duchan, J. F. (1982a). The elephant is soft and mushy: Problems in assessing children's language. In N.

Lass, L. McReynolds, J. Northern, & D. Yoder (Eds.), *Speech, language, and hearing: Vol. 2. Pathologies of speech and language* (pp. 741–760). Philadelphia: W. B. Saunders.

Duchan, J. F. (1982b). Forward. *Topics in Language Disorders, 3*(1), ix–xiv.

Duchan, J. F. (1983a). Autistic children are non–interactive: Or so we say. *Seminars in Speech and Language, 4,* 53–61.

Duchan, J. F. (1983b). Language processing and geodesic domes. In T. Gallagher & C. Prutting (Eds.), *Pragmatic assessment and intervention issues in language* (pp. 83–100). San Diego: College–Hill.

Duchan, J. F. (1984). Clinical interactions with autistic children: The role of theory. *Topics in Language Disorders, 4*(4), 62–71.

Duchan, J. F. (1986a). Language intervention through sensemaking and fine tuning. In R. Schiefelbusch (Ed.), *Language competence: Assessment and intervention* (pp. 187–212). San Diego: College–Hill.

Duchan, J. F. (1986b). Learning to describe events. *Topics in Language Disorders, 6*(4), 27–36.

Duchan, J. F., & Waltzman, M. M. (1992). *Then* as an indicator of deictic discontinuity in adults' oral descriptions of a film. *Journal of Speech and Hearing Research, 35,* 1367-1375.

Duchan, J. F., & Weitzner–Lin, B. (1987). Nurturant–naturalistic intervention for language–impaired children: Implications for planning lessons and tracking progress. *Asha, 29*(7), 45–49.

Dudley–Marling, C. (1987). The role of SLPs in literacy learning. *Journal of Childhood Communication Disorders, 2*(1), 81–90.

Dudley–Marling, C., & Rhodes, L. (1987). Pragmatics and literacy. *Language, Speech, and Hearing Services in Schools, 18,* 41–52.

Dulay, H. C., & Burt, M. K. (1980). Second language acquisition. In H. C. Dulay, M. Burt, & D. McKeon (Eds.), *Testing and teaching communicatively handicapped Hispanic children: The state of the art in 1980* (pp. 6-50). San Francisco: Bloomsbury West.

Duncan, S. (1974). On the structure of speaker–auditor interaction during speaker turns. *Language and Society, 2,* 161–180.

Duncan, S., & Fiske, D. (1977). *Face–to–face interaction: Research, methods, and theory.* Hillsdale, NJ: Lawrence Erlbaum.

Dunham, J. (1989). The transparency of manual signs in a linguistic and an environmental non–linguistic context. *Augmentative and Alternative Communication, 5,* 214–225.

Dunn, C., & Barron, C. (1982). A treatment program for disordered phonology: Phonetic and linguistic considerations. *Language, Speech, and Hearing Services in Schools, 13,* 100–109.

Dunn, L., & Dunn, L. (1981). Peabody Picture Vocabulary Test—revised. Circle Pines, MN: American Guidance Services.

Dunst, C. (1980). *A clinical and educational manual for use with the Uzgiris and Hunt Scales of Infant Psychological Development.* Austin, TX: Pro–Ed.

Dunst, C., & Lowe, L. (1986). From reflex to symbol: Describing, explaining, and fostering communication competence. *Augmentative and Alternative Communication, 1,* 11-18.

Dunst, C., Lowe, L., & Bartholomew, P. (1990). Contingent social responsiveness, family ecology and infant communicative competence. *NSSLHA Journal, 17,* 39-49.

Durand, J. (1982). Analysis of intervention of self–injurious behavior. *Journal of the Association for Persons with Severe Handicaps, 7,* 44–53.

Durand, V., & Kishi, G. (1986). *Reducing severe behavior problems among persons with dual sensory impairments: An evaluation of a technical assistance model.* Unpublished manuscript, State University of New York, Albany.

Dyer, K., Santarcangelo, S., & Luce, S. (1987). Developmental influences in teaching language forms to individuals with developmental disabilities. *Journal of Speech and Hearing Disorders, 52,* 335–347.

Dyer, K., Williams, L., & Luce, S. (1991). Training teachers to use naturalistic communication strategies in classrooms for students with autism or other severe handicaps. *Language, Speech, and Hearing Services in Schools, 22,* 313-321.

Dyson, A., & Robinson, T. (1987). The effect of phonological analysis procedure on the selection of potential remediation targets. *Language, Speech, and Hearing Services in Schools, 18*(4), 364–377.

Ecklund, S., & Reichle, J. (1987). A comparison of normal children's ability to recall symbols from two logographic systems. *Language, Speech, and Hearing Services in Schools, 18,* 34–40.

Edmaiston, R. (1988). Preschool Literacy Assessment. *Seminars in Speech and Hearing, 9,* 27-36.

Edmonston, N. K., & Thane, N. L. (1990, April). *Children's concept comprehension: Acquisition, assessment, intervention.* Paper presented at the Annual Convention of the New York State Speech Language Hearing Association, Kiamesha Lake.

Edmonston, N. K., & Thane, N. L. (1992). Children's use of comprehension strategies in response to relational words: Implications for assessment. *American Journal of Speech-Language Pathology, 1*(2), 30-35.

Edwards, H. T., & Kallail, K. J. (1977, November). *Ability of learning disabled and regular classroom adolescents to cloze structure and content words.* Paper presented at the National Convention of the American Speech and Hearing Association, Chicago.

Edwards, M. L. (1983). Selection criteria for developing therapy goals. *Journal of Childhood Communication Disorders, 7,* 36–45.

Edwards, M. L. (1984, April). *Phonological analysis.* Presentation for Genesee Valley Speech–Language–Hearing Association, Rochester, NY.

Edwards, M. L. (1992). In support of phonological processes. *Language, Speech, and Hearing Services in Schools, 23,* 233-240.

Eheart, B. (1982). Mother-child interactions with non-retarded and mentally retarded preschoolers. *American Journal of Mental Deficiency, 87,* 20-25.

Ehren, B., & Mullins, B. (1988). *Contextualized adolescent language learning (CALL) curriculum.* West Palm Beach, FL: School Board of Palm Beach County, Florida.

Eisenberg, A. (1982). *Language development in cultural perspective: Talk in three Mexican homes.* Unpublished doctoral dissertation, University of California, Berkeley.

Eisenberg, A. (1985). Learning to describe past experiences in conversation. *Discourse Processes, 8,* 177-204.

Elbert, M. (1992). Consideration of error types: A response to Fey. *Language, Speech, and Hearing Services in Schools, 23,* 241-246.

Elbert, M., Dinnsen, D., Swartzlander, P., & Chin, S. (1990). Generalization to conversational speech. *Journal of Speech and Hearing Research, 55,* 694-699.

Elbert, M., & Gierut, J. (1986). *Handbook of clinical phonology: Approaches to assessment and treatment.* San Diego: College-Hill.

Elbert, M., & McReynolds, L. (1985). The generalization hypothesis: Final consonant deletion. *Language and Speech, 28,* 281-294.

Elbert, M., Rockman, B., & Saltzman, D. (1980). *Contrasts: The use of minimal pairs in articulation training.* Austin, TX: Exceptional Resources.

Ellis, A. W. (1981). Visual and name coding in dyslexic children. *Psychological Research, 43,* 201-218.

Ellis, N., Deacon, J., Harris, L., Poor, A., Angers, D., Diorio, M., Watkins, R., Boyd, B., & Cavalier, A. (1982). Learning, memory, and transfer in profoundly, severely, and moderately mentally retarded persons. *American Journal of Mental Deficiency, 87,* 186-196.

Ellis, N., Deacon, J., & Wooldridge, P. (1985). On the nature of short-term memory deficit in mentally retarded persons. *American Journal of Mental Deficiency, 89,* 393-402.

Ellis, N., Woodley-Zanthos, P., & Dulaney, C. (1989). Memory for spatial location in children, adults, and mentally retarded persons. *American Journal on Mental Retardation, 93,* 521-527.

Ellis, R., & Wells, G. (1980). Enabling factors in adult–child discourse. *First Language, 1,* 46–82.

Ellis Weismer, S. E. (1991). Hypothesis-testing abilities of language-impaired children. *Journal of Speech and Hearing Research, 34,* 1329-1338.

Elshout-Mohr, M., & van Daalen-Kapteijns, M. M. (1987). Cognitive processes in learning word meanings. In M. G. McKeown & M. E. Curtis (Eds.), *The nature of vocabulary acquisition* (pp. 53–71). Hillsdale, NJ: Lawrence Erlbaum.

Emerick, L., & Haynes, W. (1986). *Diagnosis and evaluation in speech pathology* (3rd ed.). Englewood Cliffs, NJ: Prentice–Hall.

Englert, C. S., & Hiebert, E. H. (1984). Children's developing awareness of text structures in expository materials. *Journal of Educational Psychology, 76,* 65-74.

Englert, C. S., & Lichter, A. (1982). Using statement-pie to teach reading and writing skills. *Teaching Exceptional Children, 14,* 164-170.

Englert, C. S., & Thomas, C. C. (1987). Sensitivity to text structure in reading and writing: A comparison of learning disabled and nonhandicapped students. *Learning Disability Quarterly, 10,* 93-105.

Erickson, F. (1984). Rhetoric, anecdote, and rhapsody: Coherence strategies in a conversation among Black American adolescents. In D. Tannen (Ed.), *Coherence in spoken and written discourse* (pp. 81-154). Norwood, NJ: Ablex.

Erickson, J., & Omark, D. (1980). Social perceptions and communicative interactions of handicapped and normal children in a preschool classroom. *Instructional Science, 9,* 253–268.

Erickson, J. G., & Omark, D. R. (Eds.). (1981). *Communication assessment of the bilingual bicultural child.* Austin, TX: Pro-Ed.

Ertmer, D. J. (1986). Language Carnival [Computer program]. Moline, IL: LinguiSystems.

Ervin–Tripp, S. (1966). Language development. In L. Hoffman & M. Hoffman (Eds.), *Review of child development research* (Vol. 2, pp. 55–105). New York: Russell Sage.

Ervin–Tripp, S. (1977). Wait for me roller skate. In S. Ervin–Tripp & C. Mitchell–Kernan (Eds.), *Child discourse* (pp. 165–188). New York: Academic Press.

Espin, C. A., & Sindelar, P. T. (1988). Auditory feedback and writing: Learning disabled and nondisabled students. *Exceptional Children, 55*(1), 45–51.

Evesham, M. (1977). Teaching language skills to children. *British Journal of Disorders of Communication, 12,* 23–29.

Ewing-Cobbs, L., Fletcher, J. M., & Levin, H. S. (1985). In M. Ylvisaker (Ed.), *Head injury rehabilitation: Children and adolescents* (pp. 71-89). Austin, TX: Pro-Ed.

Ewing-Cobbs, L., Levin, H. S., Eisenberg, H. M., & Fletcher, J. M. (1987). Language functions following closed-head injury in children and adolescents. *Journal of Clinical and Experimental Neuropsychology, 9,* 575-592.

Ezell, H., & Goldstein, H. (1991). Comparison of idiom comprehension of normal children and children with mental retardation. *Journal of Speech and Hearing Research, 34,* 812-819.

Faford, M. B., & Haubrich, P. A. (1981). Vocational and social adjustment of learning disabled adults: A follow-up study. *Learning Disability Quarterly, 4,* 122–130.

Falvey, M. A. (1986). *Community-based curriculum: Instructional strategies for students with severe handicaps.* Baltimore: Paul H. Brookes.

Falvey, M. A., Bishop, K., Grenot–Scheyer, M., & Coots, J. (1988). Issues and trends in mental retardation. In S. Calculator & J. Bedrosian (Eds.), *Communication assessment and intervention for adults with mental retardation* (pp. 45–65). San Diego: College–Hill.

Falvey, M. A., McLean, D., & Rosenberg, R. L. (1988). Transition from school to adult life: Communication strategies. *Topics in Language Disorders, 9*(1), 82-86.

Farber, J., Denenberg, M. E., Klyman, S., & Lachman, P. (1992). Language resource room level of service: An urban school district approach to integrative treatment. *Language, Speech, and Hearing Services in Schools, 23,* 293-299.

Farrier, L., Yorkston, K., Marriner, N., & Beukelman, D. (1985). Conversational control in non–impaired speakers using an augmentative communication system. *Augmentative and Alternative Communication, 1,* 65–73.

Fasold, R. W. (1990). *The sociolinguistics of language.* Cambridge, UK: Basil Blackwell.

Fasold, R. W., & Wolfram, W. (1970). Some linguistic features of Negro dialect. In R. Fasold & R. Shuy (Eds.), *Teaching standard English in the inner city* (pp. 41–86). Washington, DC: Center for Applied Linguistics.

Fay, W., & Anderson, D. (1981). Children's echo-reactions as a function of increasing lexical difficulty: A developmental study. *Journal of General Psychology, 138,* 259-267.

Fay, W. H., & Schuler, A. L. (1980). *Emerging language in autistic children.* Baltimore: University Park Press.

Feagans, L., & Short, E. (1986). Referential communication and reading performance in learning disabled children over a 3–year period. *Developmental Psychology, 22,* 177–183.

Felsenfeld, S., Broen, P. A., & McGue, M. (1992). A 23–year follow–up of adults with a history of moderate phonological disorder: Linguistic and personality results. *Journal of Speech and Hearing Research, 35,* 1114–1125.

Felton, R., & Brown, I. S. (1990). Phonological processes as predictors of specific reading skills in children at risk for reading failure. *Reading and Writing: An Interdisciplinary Journal, 2,* 39-59.

Ferguson, C. A. (1978). Learning to pronounce: The earliest stages of phonological development in the child. In F. Minifie & L. Lloyd (Eds.), *Communication and cognitive abilities—Early behavioral assessment* (pp. 273–298). Baltimore: University Park Press.

Ferguson, C. A., Peizer, D., & Weeks, T. (1973). Model–and–replica phonological grammar of a child's first words. *Lingua, 31,* 35–39.

Ferguson, M. L. (1992a). Implementing collaborative consultation: An introduction. *Language, Speech, and Hearing Services in Schools, 23,* 361-362.

Ferguson, M. L. (1992b). The transition to collaborative teaching. *Language, Speech, and Hearing Services in Schools, 23,* 371-372.

Ferrier, E., & Davis, M. (1973). A lexical approach to the remediation of final sound omissions. *Journal of Speech and Hearing Disorders, 38,* 126–130.

Feuerstein, R. (1979). *The dynamic assessment of retarded performers: The learning potential assessment device, theory, instruments, and techniques.* Baltimore: University Park Press.

Feuerstein, R. (1980). *Instrumental enrichment: An intervention program for cognitive modifiability.* Baltimore: University Park Press.

Feuerstein, R., Rand, Y., Jensen, M. R., Kaniel, S., & Tzuriel, D. (1987). Prerequisites for assessment of learning potential: The LPAD model. In C. Schneider Lidz (Ed.), *Dynamic assessment: An interactional approach to evaluating learning potential* (pp. 35–51). New York: Guilford.

Fewell, R., & Langley, M. (1984). Developmental Activities Screening Inventory. Austin, TX: Pro-Ed.

Fey, M. (1986). *Language intervention with young children.* San Diego: College-Hill.

Fey, M. (1988). Generalization issues facing language interventionists: An introduction. *Language, Speech, and Hearing Services in Schools, 19,* 272–281.

Fey, M. (1992a). Articulation and phonetics: An addendum. *Language, Speech, and Hearing Services in Schools, 23,* 277-282.

Fey, M. (1992b). Articulation and phonetics: Inextricable constructs in speech pathology. *Language, Speech, and Hearing Services in Schools, 23,* 225-232.

Fey, M., Cleave, P. L., Long, S. H., & Hughes, D. L. (1993). Two approaches to the facilitation of grammar in children with language impairment: An experimental evaluation. *Journal of Speech and Hearing Research, 36,* 141-157.

Fey, M., & Leonard, L. (1983). Pragmatic skills of specific language impairment. In T. Gallagher & C. Prutting (Eds.), *Pragmatic assessment and intervention issues in language* (pp. 65–82). San Diego: College–Hill.

Fey, M., & Leonard, L. (1984). Partner age as a variable in the conversational performance of specifically language-impaired and normal-language children. *Journal of Speech and Hearing Research, 27*, 413–424.

Fey, M., Leonard, L., & Wilcox, K. (1981). Speech–style modifications of language–impaired children. *Journal of Speech and Hearing Disorders, 46*, 91–97.

Fey, M., & Stalker, C. (1986). A hypothesis–testing approach to treatment of a child with an idiosyncratic (morpho)phonological system. *Journal of Speech and Hearing Disorders, 51*, 324–336.

Fey, M., Warr–Leeper, G., Webber, S., & Disher, L. (1988). Repairing children's repairs: Evaluation and facilitation of children's clarification requests and responses. *Topics in Language Disorders, 8*(2), 63–84.

Figueroa, R. A., Sandoval, J., & Merino, B. (1984). School psychology and limited English-proficient children: New competencies. *Journal of School Psychology, 22*, 131-143.

Fillmore, C. (1968). The case for case. In E. Bach & R. Harmas (Eds.), *Universals in linguistic theory* (pp. 1–90). New York: Holt, Rinehart & Winston.

Fillmore, C., Kempler, D., & Wang, W. (Eds.). (1979). *Individual differences in language ability and language behavior.* New York: Academic Press.

Finegan, E., & Besnier, N. (1989). *Language: Its structure and use.* Orlando, FL: Harcourt Brace Jovanovich.

Fischel, J., Whitehurst, G., Caulfield, M., & DeBaryshe, B. (1988). Language growth in children with expressive language delay. *Pediatrics, 82*, 218-227.

Fish, B., Shapiro, T., & Campbell, M. (1966). Long-term prognosis and the response of schizophrenic children to drug therapy: A controlled study of trifluoperazine. *American Journal of Psychiatry, 123*(1), 32-39.

Fisher, F. W., Shankweiler, D., & Liberman, I. Y. (1985). Spelling proficiency and sensitivity to word structure. *Journal of Memory and Language, 24*, 423-441.

Fisher, H., & Logemann, J. (1987). The Fisher–Logemann Test of Articulation Competence. Boston: Houghton Mifflin.

Fitch, J. L. (1985). Computer Managed Articulation Diagnosis [Computer program]. Tucson, AZ: Communication Skill Builders.

Fitch, J. L. (1986). *Clinical applications of microcomputers in communication disorders.* New York: Academic Press.

Fivush, R. (1984). Learning about school: The development of kindergarteners' school scripts. *Child Development, 55*, 1697-1709.

Fivush, R., & Slackman, E. (1986). The acquisition and development of scripts. In K. Nelson (Ed.), *Event knowledge: Structure and function in development.* Hillsdale, NJ: Lawrence Erlbaum.

Flavell, J. H. (1978). Metacognitive development. In J. M. Scandura & C. J. Brainerd (Eds.), *Structural process theories of human behavior.* Hillsdale, NJ: Lawrence Erlbaum.

Flavell, J. H., & Wellman, H. M. (1977). Metamemory. In R. V. Kail & J. W. Hagen (Eds.), *Perspectives on the development of memory and cognition* (pp. 3–33). Hillsdale, NJ: Lawrence Erlbaum.

Fletcher, P. (1975). Review of D Major: The acquisition of modal auxiliaries in the language of children. *Journal of Child Language, 2*, 318–322.

Fletcher, P. (1978). Review of D. Major, The acquisition of modal auxiliaries in the language of children. *Journal of Child Language, 2*, 318–322.

Fletcher, P. (1979). The development of the verb phrase. In P. Fletcher & M. Garman (Eds.), *Language acquisition* (pp. 261–284). New York: Cambridge University Press.

Flood, J. E. (1978). The effects of first sentences on reader expectations in prose passages. *Reading World, 18*, 306-315.

Fluck, M. (1979). Comprehension of relative clause sentences by children aged five to nine years. *Language and Speech, 21*, 190-201.

Fluharty, N. (1978). Fluharty Preschool Speech and Language Screening Test. Boston: Teaching Resources.

Fokes, J. (1976). Fokes Sentence Builder. Boston: Teaching Resources.

Folger, J., & Chapman, R. (1978). A pragmatic analysis of spontaneous imitations. *Journal of Child Language, 5*, 25–38.

Foster, R., Giddan, J., & Stark, J. (1973). *Assessment of children's language comprehension.* Palo Alto, CA: Consulting Psychologists Press.

Foster, S. (1985). The development of discourse topic skills in infants and young children. *Topics in Language Disorders, 5*(2), 31–45.

Fox, L., Long, S. H., & Langlois, A. (1988). Patterns of language comprehension deficit in abused and neglected children. *Journal of Speech and Hearing Disorders, 53*, 239-244.

Foxx, R., Kyle, M., Faw, G., & Bittle, R. (1988). Cue-pause-point training and simultaneous communication to teach the use of signed labeling repertoires. *American Journal on Mental Retardation, 93*, 305-311.

Francik, E., & Clark, H. (1985). How to make requests that overcome obstacles to compliance. *Journal of Memory and Language, 24*, 560–568.

Frank, H., & Rabinovitch, M. (1974). Auditory short-term memory: Developmental changes in rehearsal. *Child Development, 45*, 397-407.

Frankel, R. (1982). Autism for all practical purposes: A microinteractional view. *Topics in Language Disorders, 3*(1), 33–43.

Fredricks, H., Baldwin, D., & Grove, D. (1974). A home–center based parent–training model. In J. Grim (Ed.), *Training parents to teach: Four models.* Chapel Hill, NC: Technical Assistance Development Systems.

Freeman, B. J., & Ritvo, E. R. (1984). The syndrome of autism: Establishing the diagnosis and principles of management. *Pediatric Annals, 13,* 284-296.

French, L. A., & Nelson, K. N. (1981). Temporal knowledge expressed in preschooler's descriptions of familiar activities. *Papers and Reports on Child Language Development, 20,* 61-69.

French, L. A., & Nelson, K. (1985). *Young children's knowledge of relational terms.* New York: Springer Verlag.

Freston, C. W., & Drew, C. J. (1974). Verbal performance of learning disabled children as a function of input organization. *Journal of Learning Disabilities, 7,* 424-428.

Friedman, P., & Friedman, K. (1980). Accounting for individual differences when comparing the effectiveness of remedial language teaching methods. *Applied Psycholinguistics, 1,* 151-171.

Fried–Oken, M. (1984). *The development of naming skills in normal and language deficient children.* Unpublished doctoral dissertation, Boston University.

Fried–Oken, M. (1987). Qualitative examination of children's naming skills through test adaptations. *Language, Speech, and Hearing Services in Schools, 18,* 206–216.

Friel-Patti, S. (1990). Otitis media: Implications for language learning. *Topics in Language Disorders, 11*(1), 11–22.

Friend, T., & Channell, R. (1987). A comparison of two measures of receptive vocabulary. *Language, Speech, and Hearing Services in Schools, 18,* 231–237.

Frith, U. (1981). Experimental approaches to developmental dyslexia: An introduction. *Psychological Research, 43,* 115–119.

Frome Loeb, D., & Leonard, L. B. (1991). Subject case marking and verb morphology in normally developing and specifically language-impaired children. *Journal of Speech and Hearing Research, 34,* 340-346.

Fromkin, V., & Rodman, R. (1984). *An introduction to language.* New York: Holt, Rinehart & Winston.

Fuchs, D., & Fuchs, L. (1989). Effects of examiner familiarity on black, Caucasian, and Hispanic children: A meta-analysis. *Exceptional Children, 55*(4), 303–308.

Fudala, J. (1970). Arizona Articulation Proficiency Scale: Revised. Los Angeles: Western Psychological Services.

Fujiki, M., & Brinton, B. (1984). Supplementing language therapy: Working with the classroom teacher. *Language, Speech, and Hearing Services in Schools, 15,* 98–109.

Fujiki, M., & Brinton, B. (1987). Elicited imitation revisited: A comparison with spontaneous language production. *Language, Speech, and Hearing Services in Schools, 18,* 301-311.

Fujiki, M., & Willbrand, M. (1982). A comparison of four informal methods of language evaluation. *Language, Speech, and Hearing Services in Schools, 13,* 42–52.

Fuller, C., Vandivers, P., & Kronberg, C. (1987). TALKline: An evaluation of a call-in telephone service for parents. *Journal of the Division of Early Childhood, 11,* 265-270.

Furman, L. N., & Walden, T. A. (1989, April). *The effect of script knowledge on children's communicative interactions.* Paper presented at the meeting of the Society for Research in Child Development, Kansas City, MO.

Furrow, D., Nelson, K., & Benedict, H. (1979). Mothers' speech to children and syntactic development: Some simple relationships. *Journal of Child Language, 6,* 423–442.

Galaburda, A. M. (1989). Ordinary and extraordinary brain development: Anatomical variation in developmental dyslexia. *Annals of Dyslexia, 39,* 67-80.

Galda, L. (1984). Narrative competence: Play, storytelling and comprehension. In A. Pellegrini & T. Yawkey (Eds.), *The development of oral and written language in social context* (pp. 105–118). Norwood, NJ: Ablex.

Gallagher, T. (1977). Revision behaviors in the speech of normal children developing language. *Journal of Speech and Hearing Research, 20,* 303–318.

Gallagher, T. M. (1981). Contingent query sequences within adult–child discourse. *Journal of Child Language, 8,* 51–62.

Gallagher, T. M. (1983). Pre-assessment: A procedure for accommodating language variability. In T. Gallagher & C. Prutting (Eds.), *Pragmatic assessment and intervention issues in language* (pp. 1–28). San Diego: College-Hill.

Gallagher, T. M., & Craig, H. (1982). An investigation of overlap in children's speech. *Journal of Psycholinguistic Research, 11,* 63–75.

Gallagher, T. M., & Craig, H. K. (1984). Pragmatic assessment: Analysis of a highly frequent repeated utterance. *Journal of Speech and Hearing Disorders, 49,* 368-377.

Gallagher, T. M., & Prutting, C. (1983). *Pragmatic assessment and intervention issues in language.* San Diego: College–Hill.

Garcia, E. (1983). *Early childhood bilingualism with special reference to the Mexican-American child.* Albuquerque: University of New Mexico Press.

Garcia, S. B., & Ortiz, A. A. (1988). Preventing inappropriate referrals of language minority students to special education. *New Focus: Occasional Papers in Bilingual Education, 5,* 1-12.

Gardner, H. (1989). An investigation of material interaction with phonologically disabled children as compared to two groups of normally developing children. *British Journal of Disorders of Communication, 24,* 41-59.

Gardner, M. (1979). Expressive One–Word Picture Vocabulary Test. Novato, CA: Academic Therapy.

Gardner, M. (1985). Receptive One–Word Picture Vocabulary Test. Novato, CA: Academic Therapy.

Garfin, D., & Lord, C. (1986). Communication as a social problem in autism. In E. Schopler & G. B. Mesibov (Eds.), *Social behavior in autism* (pp. 133–151). New York. Plenum.

Garnett, K. (1986). Telling tales: Narratives and learning disabled children. *Topics in Language Disorders, 6*(2), 44–56.

Garnett, K. (1986). Telling tales: Narratives and learning-disabled children. *Topics in Language Disorders, 6,* 44-56.

Garnett, K., & Fleischner, J. E. (1983). Automatization and basic fact performance of normal and learning disabled children. *Learning Disability Quarterly, 6,* 223-230.

Garn-Nunn, P. (1992). Using conventional articulation tests with highly unintelligible children: Identification and programming concerns. *Language, Speech, and Hearing Services in Schools, 23,* 52-60.

Garrett, K., & Moran, M. (1992). A comparison of phonetic severity measures. *Language, Speech, and Hearing Services in Schools, 23,* 48-51.

Garrod, S., & Sanford, A. (1983). Topic-dependent effects in language processing. In G. Flores d'Arcais & R. Jarvella (Eds.), *The process of language understanding* (pp. 271–296). New York: John Wiley.

Garvey, C. (1975). Requests and responses in children's speech. *Journal of Child Language, 2,* 41–59.

Garvey, C. (1977). The contingent query: A dependent act in conversation. In M. Lewis & L. Rosenblum (Eds.), *Interaction, conversation, and the development of language* (pp. 63–93). New York: John Wiley.

Gee, J. P. (1986). Units in production of narrative discourse. *Discourse Processes, 9,* 391-422.

Gee, J. P. (1989). Two styles of narrative construction and their linguistic and educational implications. *Discourse Processes, 12,* 287-307.

Gelzheiser, L. M. (1984). Generalization from categorical memory tasks to prose by learning disabled adolescents. *Journal of Educational Psychology, 76,* 1126-1138.

Genesee, F. (1984). The social-psychological significance of bilingual code switching in children. *Applied Psycholinguistics, 5,* 3–20.

Genesee, F. (1987). *Learning through two languages: Studies of immersion and bilingual education.* Cambridge, MA: Newbury House.

Genesee, F. (1988). Bilingual language development in preschool children. In D. Bishop & K. Mogford (Eds.), *Language development in exceptional circumstances* (pp. 62-79). London: Churchill Livingstone.

Gerber, M. M. (1983). Learning disabilities and cognitive strategies. *Journal of Learning Disabilities, 16,* 255-260.

Gerber, M. M. (1984). Investigations of the orthographic problem-solving ability in learning disabled and normally achieving students. *Learning Disability Quarterly, 7,* 157-164.

Gerber, M. M. (1986). Generalization of spelling strategies by LD students as a result of contingent imitation/modeling and mastery criteria. *Journal of Learning Disabilities, 19,* 530-537.

German, D. J. (1982). Word–finding substitutions in children with learning disabilities. *Language, Speech, and Hearing Services in Schools, 13,* 223–230.

German, D. J. (1984). Diagnosis of word-finding disorders in children with learning disabilities. *Journal of Learning Disabilities, 17,* 353-359.

German, D. J. (1986/89). National College of Education Test of Word Finding (TWF). Allen, TX: DLM Teaching Resources.

German, D. J. (1987). Spontaneous language profiles of children with word-finding problems. *Language, Speech, and Hearing Services in Schools, 18,* 217-230.

German, D. J. (1990). National College of Education Test of Adolescent/Adult Word Finding (TAWF). Allen, TX: DLM Teaching Resources.

German, D. J. (1991). Test of Word Finding in Discourse (TWFD). Allen, TX: DLM Teaching Resources.

German, D. J. (1992). Word-finding intervention for children and adolescents. *Topics in Language Disorders, 13*(1), 33-50.

German, D. J., & Simon, E. (1991). Analysis of children's word-finding skills in discourse. *Journal of Speech and Hearing Research, 34,* 309-316.

Gersten, M., Coster, W. J., Schneider-Rosen, K., Carlson, V., & Cicchetti, D. (1986). The socio-emotional basis of communicative functioning: Quality of attachment, language development, and early maltreatment. In M. Lamb, A. L. Brown, & B. Rogoff (Eds.), *Advances in developmental psychology* (Vol. 4, pp. 105-151). Hillsdale, NJ: Lawrence Erlbaum.

Gibbons, J., Anderson, D. R., Smith, R., Field, D. E., & Fischer, C. (1986). Young children's recall and reconstruction of audio and audiovisual narratives. *Child Development, 57,* 1014-1023.

Gibbs, R. W. (1987). Linguistic factors in children's understanding of idioms. *Journal for Child Language, 14,* 569-586.

Gibbs, R. W. (1991). Semantic analyzability in children's understanding of idioms. *Journal of Speech and Hearing Research, 34,* 613-620.

Gierut, J. A. (1989). Maximal opposition approach to phonological treatment. *Journal of Speech and Hearing Disorders, 54,* 9-19.

Gierut, J. A. (1992). The conditions and course of clinically induced phonological change. *Journal of Speech and Hearing Research, 35,* 1049-1063.

Gierut, J. A., Elbert, M., & Dinnsen, D. (1987). A functional analysis of phonological knowledge and generalization learning in children. *Journal of Speech and Hearing Research, 30,* 462-479.

Gillam, R. B., & Johnston, J. R. (1985). Development of print awareness in language-disordered preschoolers. *Journal of Speech and Hearing Research, 28,* 521-526.

Gillam, R. B., & Johnston, J. R. (1992). Spoken and written language relationships in language/learning-impaired and normal achieving school-age children. *Journal of Speech and Hearing Research, 35,* 1303-1315.

Girolometto, L. E. (1988). Improving the social-conversational skills of developmentally delayed children: An intervention study. *Journal of Speech and Hearing Disorders, 53,* 156-167.

Gittelman-Klein, R., & Klein, D. (1976). Methylphenidate effects in learning disabilities. *Archives of General Psychiatry, 33,* 655-664.

Glass, A. L., & Holyoak, S. (1986). *Cognition* (2nd ed.). New York: Random House.

Glenn, C., & Stein, N. (1980). *Syntactic structures and real world themes in stories generated by children* (Technical report). Urbana: University of Illinois, Center for the Study of Reading.

Glennen, S. L., & Calculator, S. N. (1985). Training functional communication board use: A pragmatic approach. *Augmentative and Alternative Communication, 1,* 134-142.

Gobbi, L., Cipani, E., Hudson, C., & Lapenta–Neudeck, R. (1986). Developing spontaneous requesting among children with severe mental retardation. *Mental Retardation, 24,* 357–364.

Godwin, D. C. (1977). The bilingual teacher aide: Classroom asset. *Elementary School Journal, 77,* 265-267.

Goetz, L., Gee, K., & Sailor, W. (1985). Using a behavior chain interruption strategy to teach communication skills to students with severe disabilities. *Journal of the Association for Persons with Severe Handicaps, 10,* 21-30.

Goetz, L., & Sailor, W. (1988). New directions: Communication development in persons with severe disabilities. *Topics in Language Disorders, 8*(4), 41-54.

Goldberg, S. (1977). Social competence in infancy: A model of parent–infant interaction. *Merrill–Palmer Quarterly, 23,* 163–177.

Goldman, R., & Fristoe, M. (1986). The Goldman–Fristoe Test of Articulation. Circle Pines, MN: American Guidance Service.

Goldman, S., & McDermott, R. (1987). The culture of competition in American schools. In G. Spindler (Ed.), *Education and cultural process* (2nd ed., pp. 282-299). Prospect Heights, IL: Waveland.

Goldman-Eisler, F. (1986). *Psycholinguistics: Experiments in spontaneous speech.* New York: Academic Press.

Goldstein, H. (1983). Recombinative generalization: Relationships between environmental conditions and the linguistic repertoire of language learners. *Analysis and Intervention in Development Disorders, 3,* 279-293.

Goldstein, H. (1984). Effects of modeling and corrected practice on generative language learning in preschool children. *Journal of Speech and Hearing Disorders, 49,* 389–398.

Goldstein, H. (1985). Enhancing language generalization using matrix and stimulus equivalence training. In S. F. Warren & A. K. Rogers-Warren (Eds.), *Teaching functional language: Generalization and maintenance of language skills* (pp. 225-250). Baltimore: UPP.

Goldstein, H., Angelo, D., & Mousetis, L. (1987). Acquisition and extension of syntactic repertoires by severely mentally retarded youth. *Research in Developmental Disorders, 8,* 549-574.

Goldstein, H., & Ferrell, D. (1987). Augmenting communicative interaction between handicapped and nonhandicapped preschool children. *Journal of Speech and Hearing Disorders, 52,* 200–211.

Goldstein, H., & Strain, P. S. (1988). Peers as communication intervention agents: Some new strategies and research findings. *Topics in Language Disorders, 9,*(1), 44–59.

Goldstein, H., & Wickstrom, S. (1986). Peer intervention effects on communicative interaction among handicapped and nonhandicapped preschoolers. *Journal of Applied Behavior Analysis, 19,* 209–214.

Goldstein, H., Wickstrom, S., Hoyson, M., Jamieson, B., & Odom, S. (1988). Effects of sociodramatic play training on social and communicative interaction. *Education and Treatment of Children, 11,* 97–117.

Golick, M. (1976). *Language disorders in children: A linguistic investigation.* Unpublished doctoral dissertation, McGill University, Montreal.

Golinkoff, R. (1981). The case for semantic relations. *Journal of Child Language, 8,* 413–437.

Golinkoff, R., Hirsh–Pasek, K., Cauley, K., & Gordon, L. (1987). The eyes have it: Lexical and syntactic comprehension in a new paradigm. *Journal of Child Language, 14,* 23-46.

Gollnick, M., & Chinn, P. (1983). *Multicultural education in a pluralistic society.* St. Louis: C. V. Mosby.

Goodenough-Trepagnier, C., & Prather, P. (1981). Communication systems for the nonvocal based on frequency of phoneme sequences. *Journal of Speech and Hearing Disorders, 24,* 322-329.

Goodenough-Trepagnier, C., Tarry, E., & Prather, P. (1982). Derivation of an efficient nonvocal communication system. *Human Factors, 24,* 163-172.

Goodluck, H. (1986). Children's knowledge of prepositional phrase structure: An experimental test. *Journal of Psycholinguistic Research, 15,* 177-188.

Goodman, J., & Remington, B. (1993). Acquisition of expressive signing: Comparison of reinforcement strategies. *Augmentative and Alternative Communication, 9,* 26-35.

Goodman, K. S. (1969). Analysis of oral reading miscues: Applied psycholinguistics. *Reading Research Quarterly, 5,* 9-30.

Goodman, K. S. (1986a). *What's whole in whole language?* Portsmouth, NH: Heinemann.

Goodman, K. S. (1986b). *What's whole in whole language: A parent-teacher guide.* Portsmouth, NH: Heinemann.

Goodman, Y. M. (1985). Kid-watching: Observing children in the classroom. In A. M. Jaggar & M. T. Smith-Burke (Eds.), *Observing the language learner* (pp. 9–18). Newark, DE: International Reading Association.

Goosens, C. A. (1984). The relative iconicity and learnability of verb referents differentially represented by manual signs, Blissymbols, and Rebus symbols: An investigation with moderately retarded individuals (Doctoral dissertation, Purdue University, West Lafayette, IN). *Dissertation Abstracts International, 45,* 809A.

Goosens, C., & Kraat, A. (1985). Technology as a tool for conversation and language learning for the physically disabled. *Topics in Language Disorders, 6,* 56–70.

Gordon, C., & Braun, C. (1983). Using story schema as an aid to reading and writing. *The Reading Teacher, 37,* 116–121.

Gordon, C., & Braun, C. (1985). Metacognitive processes: Reading and writing narrative discourse. In D. Forrest–Pressley, G. MacKinnon, & T. Waller (Eds.), *Metacognition, cognition, and human performance* (Vol. 2, pp. 1–75). New York: Academic Press.

Gordon-Brannan, M. (1994). Assessing intelligibility: Children's expressive phonologies. *Topics in Language Disorders, 14*(2), 17–25.

Gottesleben, R., Tyack, D., & Buschini, G. (1974). Three case studies in language learning: Applied linguistics. *Journal of Speech and Hearing Disorders, 39,* 213–224.

Gottesman, R. L. (1979). Follow–up of learning disabled children. *Learning Disability Quarterly, 2,* 60–69.

Graham, J., & Graham, L. (1971). Language behavior of the mentally retarded: Syntactic characteristics. *American Journal of Mental Deficiency, 73,* 623-629.

Graham, L. (1976). Language programming and intervention. In L. Lloyd (Ed.), *Communication assessment and intervention strategies* (pp. 371–422). Baltimore: University Park Press.

Graves, D. (1981). Research update: Writing research for the 80's: What is needed? *Language Arts, 58,* 197–206.

Graves, M. F. (1987). The roles of instruction in fostering vocabulary development. In M. G. McKeown & M. E. Curtis (Eds.), *The nature of vocabulary acquisition* (pp. 165–184). Hillsdale, NJ: Lawrence Erlbaum.

Gray, B., & Ryan, B. (1973). *A language program for the non–language child.* Champaign, IL: Research Press.

Graybeal, C. M. (1981). Memory for stories in language-impaired children, *Applied Psycholinguistics, 2,* 269-283.

Greenberg, J. (1966). *Language universals.* The Hague: Mouton.

Greene, L., & Jones–Bamman, L. (1985). *Getting smarter: Simple strategies for better grades.* Belmont, CA: David S. Lake.

Greenspan, S. (1979). Social intelligence in the retarded. In N. Ellis (Ed.), *Handbook of mental deficiency: Psychological theory and research* (2nd ed., pp. 483–531). Hillsdale, NJ: Lawrence Erlbaum.

Greenspan, S. (1988). Fostering emotional and social development in infants with disabilities. *Zero to Three, 8,* 8–18.

Greenwald, C., & Leonard, L. (1979). Communicative and sensorimotor development of Down's syndrome children. *American Journal of Mental Deficiency, 84,* 296-303.

Grice, H. P. (1975). Logic and conversation. In P. Cole & J. Morgan (Eds.), *Syntax and semantics: Speech acts* (Vol. 3, pp. 41-59). New York: Academic Press.

Grieve, R., Hoogenraad, R., & Murray, D. (1977). On the young child's use of lexis and syntax in understanding locative instructions. *Cognition, 5,* 235-250.

Griffith, P. L., Ripich, D. N., & Dastoli, S. L. (1986). Story structure, cohesion, and propositions in story recalls by learning-disabled and nondisabled children. *Journal of Psycholinguistic Research, 15*(6), 539-555.

Griffith, P. L., & Sanford, A. (1975). Learning Accomplishment Profile for Infants. Winston–Salem, NC: Kaplan School Supply Corp.

Grimm, H. (1982). *On the interrelation of internal and external factors in the development of language structures in normal and dysphasic preschoolers: A longitudinal study.* Paper presented at the Kamehameha Educational Research Institute, Hawaii.

Groher, M. (1983). Communication disorders. In M. Rosenthal, E. R. Griffith, M. R. Bond, & J. D. Miller (Eds.), *Rehabilitation of the head injured adult.* Philadelphia: F. A. Davis.

Grossman, H. (1983). *Classification in mental retardation.* Washington, DC: American Association on Mental Deficiency.

Gruenewald, L., & Pollak, S. (1984). *Language interaction in teaching and learning.* Baltimore: University Park Press.

Grunwell, P. (1982). *Clinical phonology.* Rockville, MD: Aspen.

Grunwell, P. (1985). *Phonological assessment in child speech.* Austin, TX: Pro-Ed.

Grunwell, P. (1987). *Clinical phonology.* Baltimore: Williams & Wilkins.

Guess, D., Benson, H., & Siegel–Causey, E. (1985). Concepts and issues related to choice–making and autonomy among persons with severe disabilities. *Journal of the Association for Persons with Severe Handicaps, 10,* 79–86.

Guess, D., & Helmsteter, E. (1986). Skill cluster instruction and individualized curriculum sequencing model. In R. Horner, L. Meyers, & H. Fredericks (Eds.), *Education of learners with severe handicaps: Exemplary service strategies* (pp. 221–248). Baltimore: Paul H. Brookes.

Guess, D., Keogh, W., & Sailor, W. (1978). Generalization of speech and language behavior: Measurement and training tactics. In R. L. Schiefelbusch (Ed.), *Bases of language intervention* (pp. 373–395). Austin, TX: Pro-Ed.

Guess, D., Sailor, W., & Baer, D. (1974). To teach language to retarded children. In R. L. Schiefelbusch & L. L. Lloyd (Eds.), *Language perspectives: Acquisition, retardation, and intervention* (pp. 529–563). Baltimore: University Park Press.

Guess, D., & Siegel–Causey, E. (1985). Behavioral control education of severely handicapped students: Who's doing what to whom? Why? In D. Bricker & J. Filler (Eds.), *Severe mental retardation: From theory to practice* (pp. 230–244). Reston, VA: Division on Mental Retardation of the Council for Exceptional Children.

Guevremont, D., Osnes, R., & Stokes, T. (1986a). Preparation for effective self–regulation: The development of generalized verbal control. *Journal of Applied Behavior Analysis, 19,* 99–104.

Guevremont, D., Osnes, R., & Stokes, T. (1986b). Programming maintenance after correspondence training interventions with children. *Journal of Applied Behavior Analysis, 19,* 215–219.

Guilford, A. M., & Nawojczyk, D. C. (1988). Standardization of the Boston Naming Test at the kindergarten and elementary school levels. *Language, Speech, and Hearing Services in Schools, 19,* 395-400.

Gulland, D. M., & Hinds-Howell, D. G. (1986). *The Penguin dictionary of English idioms.* London: Penguin.

Gullo, F., & Gullo, J. (1984). An ecological language intervention approach with mentally retarded adolescents. *Language, Speech, and Hearing Services in Schools, 15,* 182-191.

Gumperz, J. J., Kaltman, H., & O'Connor, M. C. (1984). Cohesion in spoken and written discourse: Ethnic style and the transition to literacy. In D. Tannen (Ed.), *Coherence in spoken and written discourse* (pp. 3-20). Norwood, NJ: Ablex.

Gunderson, L., & Shapiro, J. (1987). Some findings on whole language instruction. *Reading-Canada-Lecture, 5,* 22-26.

Gundlach, R. A. (1981). On the nature and development of children's writing. In C. H. Fredericksen & J. F. Dominic (Eds.), *Writing: The nature, development, and teaching of written communication* (Vol. 2, pp. 133–151). Hillsdale, NJ: Lawrence Erlbaum.

Guralnick, M. J. (1990). Peer interactions and the development of handicapped children's social and communicative competence. In H. C. Foot, M. J. Morgan, & R. H. Shute (Eds.), *Children helping children* (pp. 275-305). New York: John Wiley.

Gutierrez-Clellan, V. F., & Heinrichs-Ramos, L. (1993). Referential cohesion in the narratives of Spanish-speaking children: A developmental study. *Journal of Speech and Hearing Research, 36,* 559-567.

Gutierrez-Clellan, V. F., & Iglesias, A. (1992). Causal coherence in the oral narratives of Spanish-speaking children. *Journal of Speech and Hearing Research, 35,* 363-372.

Gutierrez-Clellan, V. F., & McGrath, A. (1991, November). *Syntactic complexity in Spanish narratives: A developmental study.* Paper presented at the Annual Convention of the American Speech-Language-Hearing Association, Atlanta.

Gutierrez-Clellan, V. F., & Quinn, R. (1993). Assessing narratives of children from diverse cultural/lingual groups. *Language, Speech, and Hearing Services in Schools, 24,* 2-9.

Gutowski, W., & Chechile, R. (1987). Encoding, storage, and retrieval components of associative memory deficits of mildly mentally retarded adults. *American Journal of Mental Deficiency, 92,* 85-93.

Haas, A., & Owens, R. (1985, November). *Preschoolers' pronoun strategies: You and me make us.* Paper presented at the Annual Convention of the American

Speech-Language-Hearing Association, Washington, DC.

Hadley, P. A., & Rice, M. L. (1991). Conversational responsiveness of speech- and language-impaired preschoolers. *Journal of Speech and Hearing Research, 34,* 1308-1317.

Haelsig, P., & Madison, C. (1986). A study of phonological processes exhibited by 3-, 4-, and 5-year-old children. *Language, Speech, and Hearing Services in Schools, 17,* 107–114.

Hagen, C. (1984). Language disorders in head trauma. In A. Holland (Ed.), *Language disorders in adults* (pp. 245-282). San Diego: College-Hill.

Hale-Benson, J. E. (1986). *Black children: Their roots, culture, and learning styles* (rev. ed.). Baltimore: Johns Hopkins University Press.

Hale-Benson, J. E. (1990a). Visions for children: Afro-American early childhood education programs. *Early Childhood Research Quarterly, 5,* 199-213.

Hale-Benson, J. E. (1990b). Visions for children: Educating Black children in the context of their culture. In K. Lomotry (Ed.), *Going to school: The Afro-American experience* (pp. 209-222). Albany: State University of New York.

Hale–Haniff, M., & Siegel, G. (1981). The effect of context on verbal elicited imitation. *Journal of Speech and Hearing Disorders, 45,* 27–30.

Hall, P., & Tomblin, J. (1978). A follow-up study of children with articulation and language disorders. *Journal of Speech and Hearing Disorders, 43,* 227-241.

Hall, R. (1984). *Sniglets (Snig'lit): Any word that doesn't appear in the dictionary, but should.* New York: Macmillan.

Halle, J. W. (1987). Teaching language in the natural environment: An analysis of spontaneity. *Journal of the Association of Persons with Severe Handicaps, 12,* 28-37.

Halle, J. W. (1988). Adopting the natural environment as the context of training. In S. Calculator & J. Bedrosian (Eds.), *Communication assessment and intervention for adults with mental retardation* (pp. 155-185). San Diego: College-Hill.

Halle, J. W., Baer, D. M., & Spradlin, J. E. (1981). An analysis of teachers' generalized use of delay in helping children. *Journal of Applied Behavior Analysis, 14,* 389-409.

Halle, J. W., Marshall, A., & Spradlin, J. (1979). Time delay: A technique to increase language use and facilitate generalization in retarded children. *Journal of Applied Behavior Analysis, 12,* 431–439.

Halliday, M. (1975). *Learning how to mean: Explorations in the development of language.* New York: Arnold.

Halliday, M. A. K. (1974). *Language and social man* (Schools Council Programme in Linguistics and English Teaching, Papers Series II, Vol. 3). London: Longman.

Halliday, M. A. K. (1978). *Language as social semiotic.* Austin, TX: Pro-Ed.

Halliday, M. A. K., & Hasan, R. (1976). *Cohesion in English.* London: Longman.

Hamayan, E., & Damico, J. (1991). Developing and using a second language. In E. Hamayan & J. Damico (Eds.), *Limiting bias in the assessment of bilingual students* (pp. 40–75). Austin, TX: Pro-Ed.

Hammill, D., Brown, V., Larsen, S., & Wiederholt, J. (1980). *Test of Adolescent Language: A multidimensional approach to assessment.* Austin, TX: Pro-Ed.

Hammill, D., Brown, V., Larsen, S., & Wiederholt, J. L. (1987). Test of Adolescent Language. Austin, TX: Pro-Ed.

Hammill, D., Brown, V., Larsen, S., & Wiederholt, J. L. (1989). Test of Adolescent Language Development—2. Austin, TX: Pro-Ed.

Hammill, D., & Newcomer, P. (1982). The Test of Language Development—Primary. Austin, TX: Empiric.

Handekman, J., Harris, S., Kristoff, B., Fuentes, F., & Alessandri, M. (1991). A specialized program for preschool children with autism. *Language, Speech, and Hearing Services in Schools, 22,* 107-110.

Hanf, M. B. (1971). Mapping: A technique for translating reading into thinking. *Journal of Reading, 14,* 225-230.

Hanna, R., Lippert, E., & Harris, A. (1982). *Developmental Communication Curriculum Inventory.* San Antonio: Psychological Corp.

Hansen, C. (1978). Story retelling used with average and learning disabled readers as a measure of reading comprehension. *Learning Disabilities Quarterly, 1,* 62-69.

Haring, T., Neetz, J., Lovinger, L., Peck, C., & Semmel, M. (1988). Effects of four modified incidental teaching procedures to create opportunities for communication. *Journal of the Association for Persons with Severe Handicaps, 12,* 218-226.

Haring, T., Roger, B., Lee, M., Breen, C., & Gaylord-Ross, R. (1986). Teaching social language to moderately handicapped students. *Journal of Applied Behavior Analysis, 19,* 159-171.

Harris, P., & Folch, L. (1985). Decrement in the understanding of *big* among English- and Spanish-speaking children. *Journal of Child Language, 12,* 685–690.

Harris, P., Morris, J., & Terwogt, M. (1986). The early acquisition of spatial adjectives: A cross-linguistic study. *Journal of Child Language, 13,* 335-352.

Harris, S. (1975). Teaching language to nonverbal children with emphasis on problems of generalization. *Psychological Bulletin, 28,* 565-580.

Hart, B. (1985). Naturalistic language training techniques. In S. Warren & A. Rogers-Warren (Eds.),

Teaching functional language (pp. 63–88). Baltimore: University Park Press.

Hart, B., & Risley, T. (1968). Establishing the use of descriptive adjectives in the spontaneous speech of disadvantaged preschool children. *Journal of Applied Behavior Analysis, 1,* 109–120.

Hart, B., & Risley, T. (1974). Using preschool materials to modify the language of disadvantaged children. *Journal of Applied Behavior Analysis, 7,* 243–256.

Hart, B., & Risley, T. (1975). Incidental teaching of language in the preschool. *Journal of Applied Behavior Analysis, 8,* 411-420.

Hart, B., & Risley, T. (1980). In vivo language training: Unanticipated and general effects. *Journal of Applied Behavior Analysis, 12,* 407–432.

Hart, B., & Risley, T. (1986). Incidental strategies. In R. Schiefelbusch (Ed.), *Language competence: Assessment and intervention* (pp. 213–226). San Diego: College-Hill.

Hart, B., & Rogers-Warren, A. (1978). A milieu approach to teaching language. In R. Schiefelbusch (Ed.), *Language intervention strategies* (pp. 193–236). Baltimore: University Park Press.

Hartup, W. (1983). Peer relations. In E. M. Hetherington (Ed.), *Handbook of child psychology* (Vol. 4). New York: John Wiley.

Hasenstab, M., & Laughton, J. (1982). *Reading, writing, and the exceptional child: A psycho-socio-linguistic approach.* Rockville, MD: Aspen.

Haslett, B. J. (1983). Children's strategies for maintaining cohesion in their written and oral stories. *Communication Education, 32,* 91-105.

Haviland, S., & Clark, H. (1974). What's new: Acquiring new information as a process in comprehension. *Journal of Verbal Learning and Verbal Behavior, 13,* 512-521.

Haynes, W., Haynes, M., & Jackson, J. (1982). The effects of phonetic context and linguistic complexity on /s/ misarticulation in children. *Journal of Communication Disorders, 15,* 287–297.

Haynes, W., & Moran, M. (1989). A cross-sectional developmental study of final consonant production in southern Black children from preschool through third grade. *Language, Speech, and Hearing Services in Schools, 20,* 400–406.

Haynes, W., & Steed, S. (1987). Multiphonemic scoring of articulation in imitative sentences: Some preliminary data. *Language, Speech, and Hearing Services in Schools, 18,* 4–14.

Hazel, E. (1990). Peer-assisted carryover alternatives. *Language, Speech, and Hearing Services in Schools, 21,* 185-187.

Hazen, N. L., & Black, B. (1989). Preschool peer communication skills: The role of social status and interaction context. *Child Development, 60,* 867-876.

Heath, S. B. (1982). What no bedtime story means: Narrative skills at home and at school. *Language in Society, 11*(1), 49-76.

Heath, S. B. (1983). *Ways with words: Language, life, and work in communities and classrooms.* London: Cambridge University Press.

Heath, S. B. (1986a). Separating "things of the imagination" from life: Learning to read and write. In W. Teale & E. Sulzby (Eds.), *Emergent literacy* (pp. 156–172). Norwood, NJ: Ablex.

Heath, S. B. (1986b). Taking a cross-cultural look at narratives. *Topics in Language Disorders, 7*(1), 84–94.

Heberle, D. (1992, April). *Effective instructional strategies.* Paper presented at LEP/ESL Conference, State University of New York, Geneseo.

Hecaen, H. (1983). Acquired aphasia in children: Revised. *Neuropsychologia, 21,* 581-587.

Hedberg, N. L., & Fink, R. (1985, November). *Surface and deep structure characteristics of language disordered children's narratives.* Paper presented at the Annual Convention of the American Speech-Language-Hearing Association, Washington, DC.

Hedberg, N. L., & Stoel-Gammon, C. (1986). Narrative analysis: Clinical procedures. *Topics in Language Disorders, 7,* 58-69.

Hegde, M. (1980). An experimental-clinical analysis of grammatical and behavioral distinctions between verbal auxiliary and copula. *Journal of Speech and Hearing Research, 23,* 864–877.

Hegde, M., Noll, M., & Pecora, R. (1979). A study of some factors affecting generalization of language training. *Journal of Speech and Hearing Disorders, 44,* 301–320.

Heifetz, L. (1980). From consumer to middleman: Emerging roles for parents in the network of services for retarded children. In R. Abidin (Ed.), *Parent education and intervention handbook* (pp. 349–384). Springfield, IL: Charles C. Thomas.

Heimlich, J., & Pittelman, S. (1986). *Semantic mapping: Classroom applications.* Newark, DE: International Reading Association.

Helmstetter, E., & Guess, D. (1987). Application of individualized curriculum sequencing model to learners with severe sensory impairments. In L. Goetz, D. Guess, & K. Stremel-Campbell (Eds.), *Innovative program design for individuals with sensory impairments* (pp. 255–282). Baltimore: Paul H. Brookes.

Helton, J. (1974). *The value of occupation, education, and income in predicting PPVT scores of preschool-aged children: Some comments on criteria commonly utilized for social class stratification.* Unpublished master's thesis, University of Tennessee, Knoxville.

Hendrick, D., Prather, E., & Tobin, A. (1975). The Sequenced Inventory of Communication Development. Seattle: University of Washington Press.

Henry, M. (1990). *Words*. Los Gatos, CA: Lex.

Hermelin, B. (1978). Images and language. In M. Rotter & E. Schopler (Eds.), *Autism: A reappraisal of concepts and treatment* (pp. 141–154). New York: Plenum.

Hermelin, B., & O'Connor, N. (1967). Remembering of words by psychotic and subnormal children. *British Journal of Psychology, 58*, 213-218.

Hess, C., Haug, H., & Landry, R. (1989). The reliability of type-token ratios for the oral language of school age children. *Journal of Speech and Hearing Research, 32*, 536–540.

Hess, C., Sefton, K., & Landry, R. (1986). Sample size and type-token ratios for oral language of preschool children. *Journal of Speech and Hearing Research, 29*, 129–134.

Hester, P., & Hendrickson, J. (1977). Training functional expressive language: The acquisition and generalization of five-element syntactic response. *Journal of Applied Behavior Analysis, 10*, 316.

Hewitt, L. E., (1992, March). *Facilitating narrative comprehension: The importance of subjectivity.* Paper presented at the Conference on Pragmatics: From Theory to Therapy, State University of New York, Buffalo.

Higginbothom, D. (1992). Evaluation of keystroke savings across five assistive communication technologies. *Augmentative and Alternative Communication, 8*, 258-272.

Higginbotham, D., & Yoder, D. (1982). Communication within natural conversational interaction: Implications for severely communicatively impaired persons. *Topics in Language Disorders, 2*, 1–19.

Hill, S., & Haynes, W. (1992). Language performance in low-achieving elementary school students. *Language, Speech, and Hearing Services in Schools, 23*, 169-175.

Hirst, W., & Weil, J. (1982). Acquisition of epistemic and deontic meanings of modals. *Journal of Child Language, 9*, 659–666.

Hixson, P. K. (1985). DSS Computer Program [Computer program]. Omaha, NE: Computer Language Analysis.

Hoag, L., & Bedrosian, J. (1992). Effects of speech output type, message length, and reauditorization on perceptions of the communicative competence of an adult AAC user. *Journal of Speech and Hearing Research, 35*, 1363-1366.

Hobbs, M., & Bacharach, V. (1990). Children's understanding of big buildings and big cars. *Child Study Journal, 20*, 1-18.

Hodson, B. (1980). The Assessment of Phonological Processes. Danville, IL: Interstate.

Hodson, B. (1985). Computerized Assessment of Phonological Processes (CAPP) [Computer program]. Danville, IL: Interstate.

Hodson, B. (1992). Applied phonology: Constructs, contributions, and issues. *Language, Speech, and Hearing Services in Schools, 23*, 247-253.

Hodson, B., & Paden, E. (1981). Phonological processes which characterize unintelligible speech and intelligible speech in early childhood. *Journal of Speech and Hearing Disorders, 46*, 369–373.

Hodson, B., & Paden, E. (1983). *Targeting intelligible speech: A phonological approach to remediation.* San Diego: College-Hill.

Hodson, B., & Paden, E. (1991). *Teaching intelligible speech: A phonological approach to remediation* (2nd ed.). Austin, TX: Pro-Ed.

Hoffman, L. P. (1993, May). Language in the school context: What is least restrictive. *Proceedings of contemporary issues in language and learning: Toward the year 2000* (pp. 16-18). Rockville, MD: American Speech-Language-Hearing Association.

Hoffman, P. R. (1992). Synergistic development of phonetic skill. *Language, Speech, and Hearing Services in Schools, 23*, 254-260.

Hoffman, P. R., Norris, J. A., & Monjure, J. (1990). Comparison of process targeting and whole language treatments for phonologically delayed preschool children. *Language, Speech, and Hearing Services in Schools, 21*, 102-109.

Hoffman, P. R., Schuckers, G., & Daniloff, R. (1989). *Children's phonetic disorders: Theory and treatment.* San Diego: College-Hill.

Holdaway, D. (1979). *Foundations of literacy.* Aukland, New Zealand: Ashton-Scholastic.

Holland, A. (1975). Language therapy for children: Some thought on context and content. *Journal of Speech and Hearing Disorders, 40*, 514-523.

Holton, J. (1987). *Parent interaction strategies with handicapped children: Evaluation of a new assessment scale through measurement over intervention.* Unpublished master's thesis, Ohio State University, Columbus.

Holzhauser-Peters, L., & Andrin-Husemann, D. (1990). Alternate service delivery: What are our options? *Hearsay: Journal of the Ohio Speech and Hearing Association*, Fall/Winter, 91-96.

Hood, L., & Bloom, L. (1979). What, when, and how about why: A longitudinal study of expressions of causality in the language development of two-year-old children. *Monographs of the Society for Research in Child Development, 6*(Serial No. 181).

Horner, R., & Budd, C. (1983). *Teaching manual sign language to a nonverbal student: Generalization of sign use and collateral reduction of maladaptive behavior.* Eugene: University of Oregon, Center on Human Development.

Horner, R., & Budd, C. (1985, March). Acquisition of manual sign use: Collateral reduction of maladaptive behavior, and factors limiting generalization. *Education and Training of the Mentally Retarded, 20,* 39–47.

Horstmeier, D., & MacDonald, J. (1978a). *Ready, set, go—Talk to me.* San Antonio: Psychological Corp.

Horstmeier, D., & MacDonald, J. (1978b). Environmental Prelanguage Battery. San Antonio: Psychological Corp.

Hoskins, B. (1979, November). *A story of hypothesis testing behavior in language-impaired children.* Paper presented at the Annual Convention of the American Speech-Language Association, Atlanta.

Hoskins, B. (1987). *Conversations: Language intervention for adolescents.* Allen, TX: DLM Teaching Resources.

Houghton, J., Bronicki, G., & Guess, D. (1987). Opportunities to express preferences and make choices among students with severe disabilities in classroom settings. *Journal of the Association for Persons with Severe Handicaps, 12,* 18–27.

House, L., & Rogerson, B. (1984). *Comprehensive screening tool for determining the optimal communication mode.* East Aurora, NY: United Educational Services.

Howell, J., & Dean, E. C. (1991). *Treating phonological disorders in children: Metaphon—Theory to practice.* San Diego, CA: Singular.

Hresko, W., Reid, D., & Hammill, D. (1981). Test of Early Language Development. Los Angeles: Western Psychological Services.

Hughes, D., Fey, M., & Long, S. (1992). Developmental sentence scoring: Still useful after all these years. *Topics in Language Disorders, 12*(2), 1-12.

Hughes, D., Low, W., Fey, M. E., & Alsop, W. (1990). Computer-Assisted Tutorial for Learning Developmental Sentence Scoring, Version 2.0 [Computer program]. Mt. Pleasant: Central Michigan University, Department of Communication Disorders.

Hunt, J. (1961). *Intelligence and experience.* New York: Ronald Press.

Hunt, K. W. (1970). Syntactic maturity in school children and adults. *Monologues of the Society for Research in Child Development, 35*(Serial No. 134).

Hunt, P., Alwell, M., & Goetz, L. (1988). Acquisition of conversational skills and the reduction of inappropriate social interactional behaviors. *Journal of the Association of Persons with Severe Handicaps, 13*(1), 20-27.

Hunt, P., Alwell, M., & Goetz, L. (1991). Interacting with peers through conversation turntaking with a communication book adaptation. *Augmentative and Alternative Communication, 7,* 117-126.

Hunt, P., & Goetz, L. (1988). Teaching spontaneous communication in natural settings through interrupted behavior chains. *Topics in Language Disorders, 9*(1), 58-71.

Hunt, P., Goetz, L., Alwell, M., & Sailor, W. (1986). Using an interrupted behavior chain strategy to teach generalized communication responses. *Journal of the Association for Persons with Severe Handicaps, 11,* 196-204.

Hurlbut, B., Iwata, B., & Green, J. (1982). Non-vocal language acquisition in adolescents with severe physical disabilities: Blissymbols versus iconic stimulus formats. *Journal of Applied Behavior Analysis, 15,* 241-258.

Huttenlocker, J., Smiley, P., & Charney, R. (1983). The emergence of action categories in the child: Evidence of verb meanings. *Psychological Review, 90,* 72–93.

Hyde, J. P. (1982). Rat talk: The special vocabulary of some teenagers. *English Journal, 71,* 98-101.

Hyltenstam, K. (1985). Second language variable output and language teaching. In K. Hyltenstam & M. Pienemann (Eds.), *Modeling and assessing second language acquisition* (pp. 113–136). Clevedon, Avon: Multilingual Matters.

Hyman, C. A., Parr, R., & Browne, K. (1979). An observational study of mother-infant interaction in abusing families. *Child Abuse and Neglect, 3,* 241-246.

Hymes, D. (1974). *Foundations in sociolinguistics: An ethnographic approach.* Philadelphia: University of Pennsylvania Press.

Hynd, G. W., Marshall, R., & Gonzalez, J. (1991). Learning disabilities and presumed central nervous system dysfunction. *Learning Disabilities Quarterly, 14,* 283-296.

Iacono, T., Mirenda, P., & Beukelman, D. (1993). Comparison of unimodal and multimodal AAC techniques for children with intellectual disabilities. *Augmentative and Alternative Communication, 9,* 83-94.

Iglesias, A. (1986, May). *The cultural-linguistic minority student in the classroom: Management decisions.* Workshop presented at the State University College at Buffalo, NY.

Iglesias, A., Gutierrez-Clellan, V. F., & Marcano, M. (1986, November). *School discourse: Cultural variations.* Short course presented to the American Speech-Language-Hearing Association, Detroit, MI.

Ingalls, R. (1978). *Mental retardation: The changing outlook.* New York: John Wiley.

Ingram, D. (1972). Transivity in children. *Language, 47,* 888-910.

Ingram, D. (1976). *Phonological disabilities in children.* New York: Elsevier.

Ingram, D. (1981). *Procedures for the phonological analysis of children's language.* Baltimore: University Park Press.

Ingram, D. (1983). The analysis and treatment of phonological disorders. *Seminars in Speech and Language, 4,* 375–388.

Ingram, D. (1991). Toward a theory of phoneme acquisition. In J. Miller (Ed.), *Research on child language disorders: A decade of progress* (pp. 55-72). Austin, TX: Pro-Ed.

Irwin, J. W. (1980a). The effects of explicitness and clause order on the comprehension of reversible causal relationships. *Reading Research Quarterly, 15,* 477-488.

Irwin, J. W. (1980b). The effects of linguistic cohesion on prose comprehension. *Journal of Reading Behavior, 12,* 325-332.

Irwin, J. W. (1986). *Teaching reading comprehension processes.* Englewood Cliffs, NJ: Prentice-Hall.

Irwin, J. W. (1988). Linguistic cohesion and the developing reader/writer. *Topics in Language Disorders, 8*(3), 14-23.

Irwin, J. W., & Moe, A. (1986). Cohesion, coherence, and comprehension. In J. W. Irwin (Ed.), *Understanding and teaching cohesion comprehension.* Newark, DE: International Reading Association.

Irwin, J. W., & Pulver, C. (1984). The effects of explicitness, clause order, and reversibility on children's comprehension of causal relationships. *Journal of Educational Psychology, 76,* 399-407.

Isaacson, S. (1987). Effective instruction in written language. *Focus on Exceptional Children, 19,* 1-12.

Iwata, B., Dorsey, M., Slifer, K., Bauman, K., & Richman, G. (1982). Toward a functional analysis of self-injury. *Analysis and Intervention in Developmental Disabilities, 2,* 3–20.

Jacobson, R. (1985). Uncovering the covert bilingual: How to retrieve the hidden home language. In E. E. Garcia & R. V. Padilla (Eds.), *Advances in bilingual education research* (pp. 150–180). Tucson: University of Arizona Press.

Jaeger, J. J. (1984). Assessing the status of the vowel shift rule. *Journal of Psycholinguistic Research, 13,* 13-36.

Jaggar, A. M. (1985). On observing the language learner: Introduction and overview. In A. M. Jaggar & M. T. Smith-Burke (Eds.) *Observing the language learner* (pp. 1–7). Newark, DE: International Reading Association.

James, S. (1989). Assessing children with language disorders. In D. Bernstein & E. Tiegerman (Eds.), *Language and communication disorders in children* (2nd ed., pp. 157–207). New York: Merrill/Macmillan.

Jarman, R. (1978). Patterns of cognitive ability in retarded children: A reexamination. *American Journal of Mental Deficiency, 82,* 344-348.

Jarman, R., & Das, J. (1977). Simultaneous and successive synthesis and intelligence. *Intelligence, 1,* 151-169.

Jenkins, R., & Bowen, L. (1994). Facilitating development of preliterate children's phonological abilities. *Topics in Language Disorders, 14*(2), 26–39.

Jimenez, B., & Iseyama, D. (1987). A model for training and using communication assistants. *Language, Speech, and Hearing Services in Schools, 18,* 168–171.

Johnson, A., Johnston, E., & Weinrich, B. (1981, November). *I say yes—but I mean no: Pragmatic therapy ideas.* Paper presented at the Annual Convention of the American Speech-Language-Hearing Association, Los Angeles.

Johnson, A., Johnston, E., & Weinrich, B. (1984). Assessing pragmatic skills in children's language. *Language, Speech, and Hearing Services in Schools, 15,* 2–9.

Johnson, B., McGonigel, M., & Kaufman, R. (1989). *Guidelines and recommended practices for the individualized family service.* Chapel Hill, NC: Frank Porter Graham Child Development Center.

Johnson, D., Johnson, R., Roy, P., & Holubee, E. (1984). *Circles of learning: Cooperation in the classroom.* Alexandria, VA: Association for Supervision and Curriculum Development.

Johnson, D. D., & Pearson, P. D. (1984). *Teaching reading comprehension* (2nd ed.). New York: Holt, Rinehart & Winston.

Johnson, D. J., & Myklebust, H. (1967). *Learning disabilities: Educational principles and practices.* New York: Grune & Stratton.

Johnson, H., & Hood, S. (1988). Teaching chaining to unintelligible children: How to deal with open syllables. *Language, Speech, and Hearing Services in Schools, 19,* 211–220.

Johnson, J., Winney, B., & Pederson, O. (1980). Single word versus connected speech articulation testing. *Language, Speech, and Hearing Services in Schools, 11,* 169–174.

Johnston, J. (1982a). Interpreting the Leiter IQ: Performance profiles of young normal and language-impaired children. *Journal of Speech and Hearing Research, 25,* 291-296.

Johnston, J. (1982b). Narratives: A new look at communication problems in older language disordered children. *Language, Speech, and Hearing Services in Schools, 13,* 144–145.

Johnston, J. (1983). What is language intervention? The role of theory. In J. Miller, D. Yoder, & R. Schiefelbusch (Eds.), *Contemporary issues in language intervention* (pp. 52–57). Rockville, MD: American Speech-Language-Hearing Association.

Johnston, J. (1984). Acquisition of locative meanings: *Behind* and *in front of. Journal of Child Language, 11,* 407-422.

Johnston, J. (1988a). Generalization: The nature of change. *Language, Speech, and Hearing Services in Schools, 19,* 314–329.

Johnston, J. (1988b). Specific language disorders in the child. In N. Lass, L. McReynolds, J. Northern, & D.

Yoder (Eds.), *Handbook of speech-language pathology and audiology* (pp. 685-715). Philadelphia: B. C. Decker.

Johnston, J. (1991). The continuing relevance of cause: A reply to Leonard's "Specific language impairment as a clinical category." *Language, Speech, and Hearing Services in Schools, 22*, 75-79.

Johnston, J., & Kamhi, A. (1984). The same can be less: Syntactic and semantic aspects of the utterances of language impaired children. *Merrill-Palmer Quarterly, 30*, 65-86.

Johnston, J., & Schery, T. (1976). The use of grammatical morphemes by children with communication disorders. In D. Morehead & A. Morehead (Eds.), *Normal and deficient child language* (pp. 239–258). Baltimore: University Park Press.

Johnston, J., & Slobin, D. (1979). The development of locative expressions in English, Italian, Serbo-Croatian and Turkish. *Journal of Child Language, 6*, 353-357.

Johnston, J., & Smith, L. (1989). Dimensional thinking in language impaired children. *Journal of Speech and Hearing Research, 32*, 33-38.

Johnston, J., Trainor, M., Casey, P., & Hagler, P. (1981, November). *Effect of interview style and materials on language samples.* Paper presented at the Annual Convention of the American Speech-Language-Hearing Association, Los Angeles.

Johnston, P. H. (1987). Teachers as evaluation experts. *The Reading Teacher, 40*, 744-748.

Johnston, P. H., & Winograd, P. N. (1985). Passive failure in reading. *Journal of Reading Behavior, 4*, 279-301.

Jones, C., & Adamson, L. (1987). Language used in mother-child and mother-child-sibling interactions. *Child Development, 58*, 356-366.

Jones, D. (1978). A comparative study of mother-child communication with Down's syndrome and normal infants. In H. Schaffer & J. Dunn (Eds.), *The first year of life: Psychological and medical implications of early experience* (pp. 175-195). New York: John Wiley.

Jordan, F., Murdock, B., & Buttsworth, D. (1991). Closed-head injured children's performance on narrative tasks. *Journal of Speech and Hearing Research, 34*, 572-582.

Jordan, F. M., Ozanne, A. O., & Murdoch, B. E. (1988). Long-term speech and language disorders subsequent to closed head injury in children. *Brain Injury, 2*, 179-185.

Jorm, A. (1983). *The psychology of reading and spelling disabilities.* Boston: Routledge & Kegan Paul.

Kahn, J. (1975). A comparison of manual and oral language training. *Mental Retardation, 15*, 21-23.

Kahn, J. (1982, May). *Cognitive training and its relationship to language of profoundly retarded children.* Paper presented at the Annual Convention of the American Association on Mental Deficiency, Boston.

Kahn, M. L., & Lewis, N. (1986). Khan–Lewis Phonological Analysis (KLPA). Circle Pines, MN: American Guidance Service.

Kail, R. (1984). *The development of memory in children* (2nd ed.). San Francisco: Freeman.

Kail, R., Hale, C., Leonard, L., & Nippold, M. (1984). Lexical storage and retrieval in language-impaired children. *Applied Psycholinguistics, 5*, 37-50.

Kail, R., & Leonard, L. B. (1986). Word-finding abilities in language-impaired children. *ASHA Monographs Number 25.* Rockville, MD: American Speech-Language-Hearing Association.

Kail, R., & Marshall, C. (1978). Reading skill and memory scanning. *Journal of Educational Psychology, 70*, 808–814.

Kameenui, E. J., Dixon, R. C., & Carnine, D. W. (1987). Issues in the design of vocabulary instruction. In M. G. McKeown & M. E. Curtis (Eds.), *The nature of vocabulary acquisition* (pp. 129–146). Hillsdale, NJ: Lawrence Erlbaum.

Kamhi, A. G. (1981). Developmental vs. difference theories of mental retardation: A new look. *American Journal of Mental Deficiency, 86*, 1-7.

Kamhi, A. G. (1984). Problem solving in child language disorders: The clinician as clinical scientist. *Language, Speech, and Hearing Services in Schools, 15*, 226–234.

Kamhi, A. G. (1987). Metalinguistic abilities in language-impaired children. *Topics in Language Disorders, 7*(2), 1-12.

Kamhi, A. G. (1988). A reconceptualization of generalization and generalization problems. *Language, Speech, and Hearing Services in Schools, 19*, 304–313.

Kamhi, A. G. (1992). The need for a broad-based model of phonological disorders. *Language, Speech, and Hearing Services in Schools, 23*, 261-268.

Kamhi, A. G. (1993). Assessing complex behaviors: Problems with reification, quantification, and ranking. *Language, Speech, and Hearing Services in Schools, 24*, 110-113.

Kamhi, A. G., & Catts, H. W. (1989). Language and reading: Convergences, divergences, and development. In A. G. Kamhi & H. W. Catts (Eds.), *Reading disorders: A developmental language perspective* (pp. 1-34). San Diego: College-Hill.

Kamhi, A. G., Catts, H., & Davis, M. (1984). The management of sentence processing demands. *Journal of Speech and Hearing Research, 27*, 329–338.

Kamhi, A. G., Catts, J., Koenig, L., & Lewis, B. (1984). Hypothesis-testing and nonlingual symbolic abilities in language-impaired children. *Journal of Speech and Hearing Disorders, 49*, 169-176.

Kamhi, A. G., Gentry, B., Mauer, D., & Gholson, B. (1990). Analogical learning and transfer in language-impaired children. *Journal of Speech and Hearing Disorders, 55,* 140-148.

Kamhi, A. G., Minor, J., & Mauer, D. (1990). Content analysis and intratest performance profiles on the Columbia and the TONI. *Journal of Speech and Hearing Research, 33,* 375-379.

Kamhi, A. G., & Nelson, L. (1988). Early syntactic development: Simple clause types and grammatical morphology. *Topics in Language Disorders, 8*(2), 26–43.

Kangas, K., & Lloyd L. (1988). Early cognitive skills as prerequisites to augmentative and alternative communication use: What are we waiting for? *Augmentative and Alternative Communication, 4,* 211–221.

Kaplan, E., Goodglass, H., & Weintraub, N. (1983). The Boston Naming Test. Philadelphia: Lea & Febiger.

Karlan, G., & Lloyd, L. L. (1983). Considerations in the planning of communication intervention: Selecting a lexicon. *Journal of the Association for Persons with Severe Handicaps, 8,* 13-25.

Karmiloff-Smith, A. (1981). The grammatical marking of thematic structure in the development of language production. In W. Deutsch (Ed.), *The child's construction of language* (pp. 121–148). New York: Academic Press.

Karmiloff-Smith, A. (1983). Language acquisition as a problem-solving process. *Stanford Papers and Reports on Child Development, 22,* 1–22.

Karrar, R., Nelson, M., & Galbraith, G. (1979). Psychophysiological research with the mentally retarded. In N. Ellis (Ed.), *Handbook of mental deficiency: Psychological theory and research* (2nd ed., pp. 231–288). Hillsdale, NJ: Lawrence Erlbaum.

Kaye, K. (1979). Thickening thin data: The maternal role in developing communication and language. In M. Bullowa (Ed.), *Before speech* (pp. 191–206). New York: Cambridge University Press.

Kaye, K., & Charney, R. (1981). Conversational asymmetry between mothers and children. *Journal of Child Language, 8,* 35–49.

Keefe, K., Feldman, H., & Holland, A. (1989). Lexical learning and language abilities in pre-schoolers with perinatal brain damage. *Journal of Speech and Hearing Disorders, 54,* 395–402.

Keenan, E. O. (1976). Towards a universal definition of "subject." In C. N. Li (Ed.), *Subject and topic* (pp. 303–333). New York: Academic Press.

Keenan, E. O., & Schieffelin, B. B. (1976). Topic as a discourse notion: A study of topic in the conversation of children and adults. In C. N. Li (Ed.), *Subject and topic* (pp. 335-384). New York: Academic Press.

Kellas, G., Ashcroft, M., & Johnson, N. (1973). Rehearsal processes in the short-term memory performance of mildly retarded adolescents. *American Journal of Mental Deficiency, 77,* 670-679.

Keller-Cohen, D. (1987). Context and strategy in acquiring temporal connectives. *Journal of Psycholinguistic Research, 16,* 165-183.

Kelly, C., & Dale, P. (1989). Cognitive skills associated with the onset of multiword utterances. *Journal of Speech and Hearing Research, 32,* 645–656.

Kelly, D., & Rice, M. (1986). A strategy for language assessment of young children: A combination of two approaches. *Language, Speech, and Hearing Services in Schools, 17,* 83–94.

Kemper, S. (1984). The development of narrative skills: Explanations and entertainments. In S. Kuczaj (Ed.), *Discourse development: Progress in cognitive development research* (pp. 99–124). New York: Springer Verlag.

Kemper, S., & Edwards, L. (1986). Children's expression of causality and their construction of narratives. *Topics in Language Disorders, 7*(1), 11–20.

Keogh, J., & Sugden, D. (1985). *Motor skill development.* New York: Macmillan.

Keogh, W. J., & Reichle, J. (1985). Communication and intervention for the "difficult-to-teach" severely handicapped. In S. Warren & A. Rogers-Warren (Eds.), *Teaching functional language: Generalization and maintenance of language skills* (pp. 157–194). Baltimore: University Park Press.

Kernan, K. (1990). Comprehension of syntactically indicated sequence by Down's syndrome and other mentally retarded adults. *Journal of Mental Deficiency Research, 34,* 169-178.

Kessler, C. (1984). Language acquisition in bilingual children. In N. Miller (Ed.), *Bilingualism and language disability: Assessment and remediation* (pp. 26-54). San Diego: College–Hill.

Khan, L., & James, S. (1983). Grammatical morpheme development in three language disordered children. *Journal of Childhood Communication Disorders, 6,* 85-100.

Kieras, D. E. (1981). Topicalization effects in cued recall of technical prose. *Memory and Cognition, 9,* 541-549.

Kieras, D. E. (1985). Thematic processes in the comprehension of expository prose. In B. Britton & J. Black (Eds.), *Understanding expository text* (pp. 89–107). Hillsdale, NJ: Lawrence Erlbaum.

Kiernan, B., & Swisher, L. (1990). The initial learning of novel English words: Two single-subject experiments with minority-language children. *Journal of Speech and Hearing Research, 33,* 707-716.

Kiernan, C. (1983). The use of nonvocal communication techniques with autistic individuals. *Journal of Child Psychology and Psychiatry, 24,* 339-375.

Kiernan, C. (1984). Imitation and learning of hand postures. In J. Berg (Ed.), *Perspectives and progress in mental retardation.* Baltimore: University Park Press.

Kim, Y., & Lombardino, L. (1991). The efficacy of script contexts in language comprehension intervention with children who have mental retardation. *Journal of Speech and Hearing Research, 34,* 845-857.

King, D. (1976). An innovative language habilitative program for preschool age children. In S. Adler (Ed.), *Early identification and intensive remediation of language retarded children* (pp. 133–162). Springfield, IL: Charles C. Thomas.

King, D. F., & Goodman, K. S. (1990). Whole language: Cherish learners and their language. *Language, Speech, and Hearing Services in Schools, 21,* 221-227.

King, R., Jones, D., & Lasky, E. (1982). In retrospect: A fifteen year follow-up of speech-language–disordered children. *Language, Speech, and Hearing Services in Schools, 13,* 24-32.

King, T. (1991). A signalling device for non-oral communicators. *Language, Speech, and Hearing Services in Schools, 22,* 277-282.

Kinsbourne, M. (1981). The development of cerebral dominance. In S. D. Filskov & T. J. Boll (Eds.), *Handbook of clinical neuropsychology* (Vol. 2, pp. 399–417). New York: John Wiley.

Kintsch, W., & van Dijk, T. (1978). Toward a model of text comprehension and productions. *Psychological Review, 85,* 363-394.

Kintsch, W., & Vipond, D. (1977, June) *Reading comprehension and readability in educational practice and psychological theory.* Paper presented at the Conference on Memory, University of Uppsala, Sweden.

Kirk, S., McCarthy, J., & Winfield, K. (1968). Illinois Test of Psycholinguistic Abilities. Urbana: University of Illinois Press.

Kirkpatrick, E. M., & Schwarz, C. M. (Eds.). (1982). *Chambers idioms.* Edinburgh, Scotland: Chambers.

Klecan-Aker, J. (1984, November). *The syntax of normal and learning disabled school-age children.* Paper presented at the Annual Convention of the American Speech-Language-Hearing Association, San Francisco.

Klecan-Aker, J. (1985). Syntactic abilities in normal and language deficient middle school children. *Topics in Language Disorders, 5*(3), 46–54.

Klecan-Aker, J. S., & Carrow-Woolfolk, E. (1987). Elicited imitation and spontaneous language sampling as tools in language assessment and intervention. *Tejas, XIII,* 34-39.

Klecan-Aker, J., & Hamburg, E. (1991). *An investigation of the stories of normal and language-disordered second- and fourth-grade children.* Unpublished manuscript.

Klecan-Aker, J. S., Swank, P. R., & Johnson, D. L. (1991, November). *A reliability and validity study of children's stories.* Paper presented at the Annual Convention of the American Speech-Language-Hearing Association, Atlanta.

Klee, T. (1992). Developmental and diagnostic characteristics of quantitative measures of children's language production. *Topics in Language Disorders, 12*(2), 28–41.

Klee, T., & Fitzgerald, M. (1985). The relation between grammatical development and mean length of utterance in morphemes. *Journal of Child Language, 12,* 251-269.

Klee, T., Schaffer, M., May, S., Membrino, I., & Mougey, K. (1989). A comparison of the age-MLU relationship in normal and specifically language impaired preschool children. *Journal of Speech and Hearing Disorders, 54,* 226-233.

Klein, H. (1981). Productive strategies for the pronunciation of early polysyllabic lexical items. *Journal of Speech and Hearing Research, 24,* 389–405.

Klein, H. (1984). Procedure for maximizing phonological information from single-word responses. *Language, Speech, and Hearing Services in Schools, 15,* 267–274.

Klein, M. D., & Briggs, M. H. (1987). *Observation of communicative interactions.* Los Angeles: California State University, Mother-Infant Communication Project.

Klein, M. D., Wulz, S., Hall, M., Walso, L., Carpenter, S., Lathan, D., Meyers, S., Fox, T., & Marshall, A. (1981). *Comprehensive communication curriculum guide* (ECI Document No. 902). Lawrence: University of Kansas, Kansas Early Childhood Institute.

Klima, E., & Bellugi, U. (1973). Syntactic regularities in the speech of children. In C. Ferguson & D. Slobin (Eds.), *Studies in child language* (pp. 333–353). New York: Holt, Rinehart & Winston.

Klink, M., Gerstman, L., Raphael, L., Schlanger, B., & Newsome, L. (1986). Phonological process usage by young EMR children and nonretarded preschool children. *American Journal of Mental Deficiency, 91,* 190-195.

Knight-Arest, I. (1984). Communicative effectiveness of learning disabled and normally achieving 10-to-13-year-old boys. *Learning Disability Quarterly, 7,* 237–245.

Knoblauch, C. (1980). Intentionality in the writing process: A case study. *College Composition and Communication, 31,* 153–159.

Koegel, R., Dyer, K., & Bell, L. (1987). The influence of child-preferred activities on autistic children's social behavior. *Journal of Applied Behavior Analysis, 20,* 243-252.

Koegel, R., & Johnson, J. (1989). Motivating language use in autistic children. In G. Dawson (Ed.), *Autism: Nature, diagnosis, and treatment.* New York: Guilford.

Koegel, R., & Rincover, A. (1977). Research on the difference between generalization and maintenance in extra-therapy responding. *Journal of Applied Behavior Analysis, 10,* 1-12.

Koegel, R. L., Rincover, A., & Egel, A. L. (1982). *Educating and understanding autistic children.* San Diego: College-Hill.

Koegel, R., & Williams, J. (1980). Direct vs. indirect response-reinforcer relationships in teaching autistic children. *Journal of Abnormal Child Psychology, 8,* 537-547.

Koenig, L., & Biel, C. (1989). A delivery system of comprehensive language services in a school district. *Language, Speech, and Hearing Services in Schools, 20,* 338-365.

Kohl, F. (1981). Effects of motoric requirements on the acquisition of manual sign responses by severely handicapped students. *American Journal of Mental Deficiency, 85,* 396-403.

Kohl, F. L., Beckman, P. J., & Swenson-Pierce, A. (1984). The effects of directed play on functional toy use and interaction of handicapped preschoolers. *Journal of the Division for Early Childhood, 8,* 114-118.

Kohler, F., & Fowler, S. (1985). Training prosocial behaviors to young children: An analysis of reciprocity with untrained peers. *Journal of Applied Behavior Analysis, 18,* 187-200.

Kopchick, G., & Lloyd, L. (1976). Total communication for the severely language impaired: A 24-hour approach. In L. Lloyd (Ed.), *Communication assessment and intervention strategies* (pp. 501-521). Baltimore: University Park Press.

Kouri, T. (1989). How manual sign acquisition relates to the development of spoken language: A case study. *Language, Speech, and Hearing Services in Schools, 20,* 50-62.

Kouri, T. A. (1994). Lexical comprehension in young children with developmental delays. *American Journal of Speech-Language Pathology, 3*(1), 79-87.

Kovarsky, D. (1992). Ethnography and language assessment: Toward the contextualized description and interpretation of communicative behavior. *Best Practices in School Speech-Language Pathology, 2,* 115-122.

Kozleski, E. S. (1991). Expectant delay procedure for teaching requests. *Augmentative and Alternative Communication, 7,* 11-19.

Kraat, A. W. (1985). *Communicative interaction between aided and natural speakers: An IPCAS study report.* Toronto: Canadian Rehabilitation Council for the Disabled.

Krashen, S. D. (1981). *Second language acquisition and second language learning.* Oxford: Pergamon.

Krashen, S. D. (1982). *Principles and practice in second language acquisition.* New York: Pergamon.

Krashen, S. D. (1983). Newmark's "ignorance hypothesis" and current second language acquisition theory. In S. Gass & L. Selinker (Eds.), *Language transfer in language learning* (pp. 135-153). Rowley, MA: Newbury House.

Krashen, S. D., & Biber, D. (1988). *On course.* Sacramento: California Association for Bilingual Education.

Krashen, S. D., Long, M., & Scarcella, R. (1979). Age, rate, and eventual attainment in second language acquisition. *TESOL Quarterly, 13,* 573-582.

Kresheck, J., & Nicolosi, L. (1973). A comparison of black and white children's scores on the Peabody Picture Vocabulary Test. *Language, Speech, and Hearing Services in Schools, 4,* 37-40.

Kuczaj, S. (1982). Old and new forms, old and new meanings: The form-function hypotheses revisited. *First Language, 3,* 55-61.

Kuczaj, S., & Lederberg, A. (1977). Height, age, and function: Differing influences on children's comprehension of *younger* and *older. Journal of Child Language, 4,* 395-416.

Kuczaj, S., & Maratsos, M. (1975). On the acquisition of front, back, and side. *Journal of Child Language, 46,* 395-416.

Kuhn, D., & Phelps, H. (1976). The development of children's comprehension of causal direction. *Child Development, 47,* 248-251.

Kunze, L., Lockhart, S., Didow, S., & Caterson, M. (1983). Interactive model for the assessment and treatment of the young child. In H. Winits (Ed.), *Treating language disorders: For clinicians by clinicians* (pp. 19-96). Baltimore: University Park Press.

Kurth, R. J. (1988, April). *Process variables in writing instruction using word processing, word processing with voice synthesis, and no word processing in second grade.* Paper presented at the Annual Meeting of the American Educational Research Association, New Orleans.

Kwiatkowski, J., & Shriberg, L. D. (1992). Intelligibility assessment in developmental phonological disorders: Accuracy of caregiver gloss. *Journal of Speech and Hearing Research, 35,* 1095-1104.

Kysela, G., Hillyard, A., McDonald, L., & Ahlsten-Taylor, J. (1981). Early intervention: Design and evaluation. In R. Schiefelbusch & D. Bricker (Eds.), *Early language: Acquisition and intervention* (pp. 341-388). Baltimore: University Park Press.

Labato, D., Barrera, R., & Feldman, R. (1981). Sensorimotor functioning and prelinguistic communication of severely and profoundly retarded individuals. *American Journal of Mental Deficiency, 85,* 489-496.

Labov, W. (1972). Language in the inner city. *Studies in the Black English vernacular* (pp. 354-396). Philadelphia: University of Pennsylvania Press.

Lackner, J. (1968). A developmental study of language behavior in retarded children. *Neuropsychologia, 6,* 301-320.

Lahey, M. (1988). *Language disorders and language development.* New York: Macmillan.

Lahey, M. (1990). Who shall be called language disordered? Some reflections and one perspective. *Journal of Speech and Hearing Disorders, 55,* 612-620.

Lahey, M. (1992). Lingual and cultural diversity: Further problems for determining who shall be called language disordered. *Journal of Speech and Hearing Research, 35,* 638-639.

Lahey, M., & Bloom, L. (1977). Planning a first lexicon: Which words to teach first. *Journal of Speech and Hearing Disorders, 42,* 340-350.

Lahey, M., Launer, P., & Schiff-Myers, N. (1983). Prediction of production: Elicited imitation and spontaneous speech productions of language-disordered children. *Applied Psycholinguistics, 4,* 317-343.

Lahey, M., & Silliman, E. (1987, April). *In other words, how do you put it? Narrative development and disorders.* Paper presented at the Annual Convention of the New York State Speech-Language-Hearing Association, Kiamesha Lake.

Lakoff, G. (1987). *Women, fire, and dangerous things: What categories reveal about the mind.* Chicago: University of Chicago Press.

Lakoff, R. (1973). The logic of politeness: Or minding your p's and q's. In C. Corum, T. Smith-Stark, & A. Weiser (Eds.), *Papers from the Ninth Regional Meeting of the Chicago Linguistic Society.* Chicago: University of Chicago, Department of Linguistics.

LaMarre, J., & Holland, J. (1985). The functional independence of mands and tacts. *Journal of Experimental Analysis of Behavior, 43,* 5–19.

Lambert, W. E. (1981). Bilingualism and language acquisition. In H. Winitz (Ed.), *Native language and foreign language acquisition* (Annals of the New York Academy of Sciences, Vol. 379, pp. 9-22). New York: New York Academy of Sciences.

Lamberts, F. (1981). Sign and symbol in children's processing of familiar auditory stimuli. *American Journal of Mental Deficiency, 86,* 300-308.

Landry, S. H., & Chapieski, M. L. (1990). Joint attention of six-month-old Down syndrome and preterm infants: I. Attention to toys and mother. *American Journal of Mental Retardation, 94,* 488-498.

Langdon, H. W. (1989). Language disorder or difference? Assessing the language skills of Hispanic students. *Exceptional Children, 56,* 37-45.

Lange, G. (1978). Organization-related processes in children's recall. In P. Ornstein (Ed.), *Memory development in children* (pp. 101–128). Hillsdale, NJ: Lawrence Erlbaum.

Langenfield, K. K., & Coltrane, C. (1991, November). *Preschool phonological classroom: A pilot program.* Paper presented at the Annual Convention of the American Speech-Language-Hearing Association, Atlanta.

Langer, J. A., & Applebee, N. (1986). Reading and writing instruction: Toward a theory of teaching and learning. In *Review of research in education.* Washington, DC: American Educational Research Association.

Lapadat, J. C. (1991). Pragmatic language skills of students with language and/or learning disabilities: A quantitative synthesis. *Journal of Learning Disabilities, 24,* 147-158.

Larry P. v. Riles. (1972, June 21). USLW 2033 (US).

Larson, V. L., & McKinley, N. L. (1987). *Communication assessment and intervention strategies for adolescents.* Eau Claire, WI: Thinking Publications.

Larson, V. L., & McKinley, N. L. (1993). Adolescent language: An introduction. *Language, Speech, and Hearing Services in Schools, 24,* 19-20.

Larson, V. L., McKinley, N. L., & Boley, D. (1993). Service delivery models for adolescents with language disorders. *Language, Speech, and Hearing Services in Schools, 24,* 36-42.

Lasky, E. Z. (1984). Introduction of microcomputers for specialists in communication disorders. In A. H. Schwartz (Ed.), *The handbook of microcomputer applications in communication disorders* (pp. 1-15). San Diego: College–Hill.

Lau v. Nichols, 411 U.S. 563 (1974).

Laughton, J., & Hasenstab, M. (1986). *The language learning process: Implications for management of disorders.* Rockville, MD: Aspen.

Launer, P., & Lahey, M. (1981). Passages: From the fifties to the eighties in language assessment. *Topics in Language Disorders, 1*(3), 11–29.

Lawrence, C. (1992). Assessing the use of age-equivalent scores in clinical management. *Language, Speech, and Hearing Services in Schools, 23,* 6-8.

Layton, T., & Sharifi, H. (1979). Meaning and structure of Down's syndrome and nonretarded children's spontaneous speech. *American Journal of Mental Deficiency, 83,* 439-445.

Lazar, R. T., Warr-Leeper, G. A., Nicholson, C. B., & Johnson, S. (1989). Elementary school teachers' use of multiple meaning expressions. *Language, Speech, and Hearing Services in Schools, 20,* 420-430.

Lee, L. (1971). Northwestern Syntax Screening Test. Evanston, IL: Northwestern University Press.

Lee, L. (1974). Developmental Sentence Analysis. Evanston, IL: Northwestern University Press.

Lee, L., Koenigsknecht, R., & Mulhern, S. (1975). *Interactive language development teaching.* Evanston, IL: Northwestern University Press.

Lee, R. F., & Kamhi, A. G. (1990). Metaphoric competence in children with learning disabilities. *Journal of Learning Disabilities, 23,* 476-482.

Lee, R. F., Kamhi, A. G., & Nelson, L. (1983, November). *Communicative sensitivity in language-impaired children.* Paper presented at the Annual Convention of the American Speech-Language-Hearing Association, Cincinnati.

Legarreta, D. (1979). The effects of program models on language acquisition by Spanish-speaking children. *TESOL Quarterly, 13,* 521-534.

Lehnert, W., & Vine, E. (1987). The role of affect in narrative structure. *Cognition and Emotion, 1,* 299–322.

Lehr, E. (1989). Community integration after traumatic brain injury: Infants and children. In P. Bach-y-Rita (Ed.), *Traumatic brain injury.* New York: Demos.

Leifer, J., & Lewis, M. (1984). Acquisition of conversational response skills by young Down syndrome and nonretarded children. *American Journal of Mental Deficiency, 88,* 610-618.

Lemme, M., Hedberg, N., & Bottenberg, D. (1984). Cohesion in narratives of aphasic adults. In R. Brookshire (Ed.), *Proceedings of Clinical Aphasiology Conference.* Minneapolis: BRK.

Lempers, J., & Elrod, M. (1983). Children's appraisal of different sources of referential communicative inadequacies. *Child Development, 54,* 509–515.

Leona, M. H. (1978). An examination of adolescent clique language in a suburban secondary school. *Adolescence, 13,* 495-502.

Leonard, L. (1982). The nature of specific language impairment in children. In S. Rosenberg (Ed.), *Handbook of applied psycholinguistics* (pp. 295-327). Hillsdale, NJ: Lawrence Erlbaum.

Leonard, L. B. (1972). What is deviant language? *Journal of Speech and Hearing Disorders, 37,* 315-340.

Leonard, L. B. (1975). Modeling as a clinical procedure in language training. *Language, Speech, and Hearing Services in Schools, 6,* 72–85.

Leonard, L. B. (1979). Language impairment in children. *Merrill-Palmer Quarterly, 25,* 205-232.

Leonard, L. B. (1980). The speech of language-disabled children. *Bulletin of the Orton Society, 30,* 141-152.

Leonard, L. B. (1981). Facilitating language skills in children with specific language impairment: A review. *Applied Psycholinguistics, 2,* 89–118.

Leonard, L. B. (1985). The contribution of phonetic context to an unusual phonological pattern: A case study. *Language, Speech, and Hearing Services in Schools, 16,* 110–118.

Leonard, L. B. (1986). Conversational replies in children with specific language impairment. *Journal of Speech and Hearing Research, 29,* 114-119.

Leonard, L. B. (1987). Is specific language impairment a useful construct? In S. Rosenberg (Ed.), *Advances in applied psycholinguistics* (Vol. 1, pp. 1-39). Cambridge, UK: Cambridge University Press.

Leonard, L. B. (1988). Lexical development and processing in specific language impairment. In R. L. Schiefelbusch & L. L. Lloyd (Eds.), *Language perspectives: Acquisition, retardation, and intervention* (2nd ed., pp. 69–87). Austin, TX: Pro-Ed.

Leonard, L. B. (1989). Language learnability and specific language impairment in children. *Applied Psycholinguistics, 10,* 179-202.

Leonard, L. B. (1990). Language disorders in preschool children. In G. H. Shames & E. H. Wiig (Eds.), *Human communication disorders: An introduction* (3rd ed., pp. 159-192). New York: Merrill/Macmillan.

Leonard, L. B. (1991). Specific language impairment as a clinical category. *Language, Speech, and Hearing Services in Schools, 22,* 66-68.

Leonard, L. B., Bolders, J., & Miller, J. (1976). An examination of the semantic relations reflected in the language usage of normal and language-disordered children. *Journal of Speech and Hearing Research, 19,* 371–392.

Leonard, L. B., McGregor, K. K., & Allen, G. D. (1992). Grammatical morphology and speech perception in children with specific language impairments. *Journal of Speech and Hearing Research, 35,* 1076-1085.

Leonard, L. B., Nippold, M. A., Kail, R., & Hale, C. (1983). Picture naming in language-impaired children. *Journal of Speech and Hearing Research, 26,* 609-615.

Leonard, L. B., Prutting, C. A., Perozzi, J., & Berkley, R. (1978). Non-standardized approaches to the assessment of language behaviors. *American Speech and Hearing Association, 20,* 371–379.

Leonard, L. B., Sabbadini, L., Leonard, J., & Volterra, V. (1987). Specific language impairments in children: A cross-lingual study. *Brain and Language, 32,* 233-252.

Leonard, L. B., Sabbadini, L., Volterra, V., & Leonard, J. (1988). Some influences on the grammar of English and Italian-speaking children with specific language impairments. *Applied Psycholinguistics, 9,* 39-57.

Leonard, L. B., Schwartz, R., Allen, G., Swanson, L., & Loeb, D. (1989). Unusual phonological behavior and the avoidance of homonymy in children. *Journal of Speech and Hearing Research, 32,* 583–590.

Leonard, L. B., Schwartz, R., Chapman, K., Rowan, L., Prelock, P., Terrell, B., Weiss, A., & Merrick, C. (1982). Early lexical acquisition in children with specific language impairments. *Journal of Speech and Hearing Research, 25,* 554-559.

Leonard, L. B., Steckol, D., & Panther, K. (1983). Returning meaning to semantic relations: Some clinical implications. *Journal of Speech and Hearing Disorders, 48,* 25–35.

Levin, H. S., Benton, A. L., & Grossman, R. G. (1982). *Neurobehavioral consequences of closed head injury.* New York: Oxford University Press.

Levin, H. S., & Eisenberg, H. M. (1979a). Neuropsychological impairment after closed head injury in children and adolescents. *Journal of Pediatric Psychology, 4,* 389-402.

Levin, H. S., & Eisenberg, H. M. (1979b). Neuropsychological outcome of closed head trauma in children and adolescents. *Child's Brain, 5,* 281-292.

Levin, H. S., Eisenberg, H. M., Wigg, N., & Kobayoski, K. (1982). Memory and intellectual ability after head injury in children and adolescents. *Neurosurgery, 11,* 668-673.

Levin, H. S., Ewing-Cobbs, L., & Benton, A. L. (1984). Age and recovery from brain damage: A review of clinical studies. In S. W. Scheff (Ed.), *Aging and recovery of function in the central nervous system* (pp. 169-205). New York: Plenum.

Levin, H. S., Grossman, R. G., & Kelly, P. (1976). Aphasic disorders in patients with closed head injury. *Journal of Neurology, Neurosurgery, and Psychiatry, 39,* 1062-1070.

Levin, J. R., Johnson, D. D., Pittelman, S. D., Hayes, B. L., Levine, K. M., Shriberg, L. K., & Toms-Bronowski, S. (1984). A comparison of semantic- and mnemonic-based vocabulary-learning strategies. *Reading Psychology, 5,* 1-15.

Levine, K. (1986). *The social context of literacy.* London: Routledge & Kegan Paul.

Levine, M. (1987). *Developmental variation and learning disorders.* Cambridge, MA: Educators Publishing Service.

Levinson, S. (1978). Activity types and language. *Pragmatics Microfiche, 3,* D1–G5.

Lewis, L., Duchan, J., & Lubinski, R. (1985, November). *Assessing aspect through videotape procedures.* Paper presented at the Annual Convention of the American Speech-Language-Hearing Association, Washington, DC.

Lewis, M., & Michalson, L. (1983). *Children's moods and emotions.* New York: Plenum.

Li, C., & Thompson, S. (1976). Subject and topic: A new typology of language. In C. Li (Ed.), *Subject and topic* (pp. 457–490). New York: Academic Press.

Liberman, I. Y. (1983). A language-oriented view of reading and its disorders. In H. Myklebust (Ed.), *Progress in learning disabilities* (Vol. 5, pp. 81–102). New York: Grune & Stratton.

Liberman, I. Y., & Liberman, A. M. (1990). Whole language versus code emphasis: Underlying assumptions and their implications for reading instruction. *Annals of Dyslexia, 40,* 51-76.

Liberman, I. Y., Rubin, H., Duques, S., & Carlisle, J. (1985). Linguistic abilities and spelling proficiency in kindergartners and adult poor spellers. In D. B. Gray & J. F. Kavanaugh (Eds.), *Biobehavioral measures of dyslexia* (pp. 163-176). Parkton, MD: York.

Liberman, I. Y., & Shankweiler, D. (1985). Phonology and problems of learning to read and write. *RASE Remedial and Special Education, 6,* 8–17.

Lidz, C. S. (1987). Historical perspectives. In C. S. Lidz (Ed.), *Dynamic assessment: An interactional approach to evaluating learning potential* (pp. 3-34). New York: Guilford.

Lieberman, P., Meskill, R. H., Chatillon, M., & Schupack, H. (1985). Phonetic speech perception deficits in dyslexia. *Journal of Speech and Hearing Research, 20,* 480-486.

Lieberman, R., Heffron, A., West, S., Hutchinson, E., & Swem, T. (1987). A comparison of four adolescent language tests. *Language, Speech, and Hearing Services in Schools, 18,* 250–266.

Lieberman, R., & Michael, A. (1986). Content relevance and content coverage in tests of grammatical ability. *Journal of Speech and Language Disorders, 51,* 71–81.

Lieven, E. (1978). Conversations between mothers and young children: Individual differences and their possible implications for the study of language learning. In C. Snow & C. Ferguson (Eds.), *Talking to children: Language input and acquisition* (pp. 173–187). Cambridge, UK: Cambridge University Press.

Lieven, E. (1982). Context, process and progress in young children's speech. In M. Beveridge (Ed.), *Children thinking through language* (pp. 7–26). London: Edward Arnold.

Lieven, E. (1984). Interactional style and children's language learning. *Topics in Language Disorders, 4*(4), 15–23.

Light, J. (1988). Interaction involving individuals using augmentative and alternative communication systems: State of the art and future directions. *Augmentative and Alternative Communication, 2,* 98-107.

Light, J., Collier, B., & Parnes, P. (1985). Communication interaction between young nonspeaking physically disabled children and their caregivers: Part 1—Discourse patterns. *Augmentative and Alternative Communication, 1,* 74–83.

Light, J., Dattilo, J., English, J., Gutierrez, L., & Hartz, J. (1992). Instructing facilitators to support the communication of people who use augmentative communication systems. *Journal of Speech and Hearing Research, 35,* 865-875.

Light, L., & Anderson, P. (1983). Memory for scripts in young and older adults. *Memory and Cognition, 11,* 435-444.

Light, P., Remington, B., Clarke, S., & Watson, J. (1989). Signs of language? In I. Leudar, M. Beveridge, & G. Conti-Ramsden (Eds.), *Language and communication in the mentally handicapped* (pp. 56-79). London: Chapman & Hall.

Liles, B. (1985a). Cohesion in the narratives of normal and language disordered children. *Journal of Speech and Hearing Research, 28,* 1213-133.

Liles, B. (1985b). Production and comprehension of narrative discourse in normal and language disordered children. *Journal of communication disorders, 18,* 409-427.

Liles, B. (1987). Episode organization and cohesive conjunctives in narratives of children with and without language disorder. *Journal of Speech and Hearing Research, 30,* 185-196.

Liles, B. (1990, April). *Clinical implications for narrative production.* Paper presented at the Annual Convention of the New York State Speech-Language-Hearing Association, Kiamesha Lake.

Liles, B., Coelho, C., Duffy, R., & Zalagens, M. (1989). Effects of elicitation procedures on the narratives of normal and closed-head-injured adults. *Journal of Speech and Hearing Disorders, 54,* 356-366.

Liles, B., & Watt, J. (1984). On the meaning of language delay. *Folia Phaniatrica, 36,* 40-48.

Lindamood, C., & Lindamood, P. (1979). Lindamood Auditory Conceptualization Test. Allen, TX: DLM Teaching Resources.

Lipson, M. Y., & Wixson, K. K. (1986). Reading disability research: An interactionist perspective. *Review of Educational Research, 56,* 111-136.

Litt, M. D., & Schreibman, L. (1982). Stimulus-specific reinforcement in the acquisition of receptive labels by autistic children. *Journal of Analysis and Intervention in Developmental Disabilities, 1,* 171-186.

Lively, M. (1984). Developmental sentence scoring: Common scoring errors. *Language, Speech, and Hearing Services in Schools, 15,* 154–168.

Livesley, W. S., & Bromley, D. B. (1973). *Person perception in childhood and adolescence.* London: John Wiley.

Lloyd, P., Baker, E., & Dunn, J. (1984). Children's awareness of communication. In C. Garvey, L. Feagans, & R. Golinkoff (Eds.), *The origins and growth of communication* (pp. 281–296). Norwood, NJ: Ablex.

Loban, W. (1976). *Language development: Kindergarten through grade twelve* (Research Report No. 18). Urbana, IL: National Council of Teachers of English.

Loban, W. (1979). Relationships between language and literacy. *Language Arts, 56,* 485–486.

Lobato, D., Barrera, R., & Feldman, R. (1981). Sensorimotor functioning and prelinguistic communication of severely and profoundly mentally retarded individuals. *American Journal of Mental Deficiency, 85,* 489-496.

Lockhart, R., & Craik, F. (1990). Levels of processing: A retrospective commentary on a framework for memory research. *Canadian Journal of Psychology, 44,* 87-112.

Loeb, D., & Leonard, L. B. (1988). Specific language impairment and parameter theory. *Clinical linguistics and phonetics, 2,* 317-327.

Long, S. H. (1991). Integrating microcomputer applications into speech and language assessment. *Topics in Language Disorders, 11*(2), 1-17.

Long, S. H., & Fey, M. E. (1988). Computerized Profiling Version 6.1 (Apple II series) [Computer program]. Ithaca, NY: Ithaca College.

Long, S. H., & Fey, M. E. (1989). Computerized Profiling Version 6.2 (Macintosh and MS-DOS series) [Computer program]. Ithaca, NY: Ithaca College.

Long, S. H., & Fey, M. E. (1991). Computerized Profiling, Version 1.0 (Macintosh) [Computer program]. Ithaca, NY: Ithaca College, Department of Speech Pathology and Audiology.

Long, S. H., & Masterson, J. J. (1993). Computer technology: Use in language analysis. *Asha, 35*(8), 40-41, 51.

Longacre, R. (1983). *The grammar of discourse.* New York: Plenum.

Longhurst, T. (1984). The scope of normative language assessment. In K. Ruder & M. Smith (Eds.), *Developmental language intervention: Psycholinguistic applications* (pp. 21–55). Baltimore: University Park Press.

Longhurst, T., & Grubb, S. (1974). A comparison of language samples collected in four situations. *Language, Speech, and Hearing Services in Schools, 5,* 71–78.

Lord, C. (1984). Language comprehension and cognitive disorder in autism. In L. Siegel & F. Morrison (Eds.), *Cognitive development in atypical children* (pp. 67–82). New York: Springer Verlag.

Lord, C. (1985). Autism and the comprehension of language. In E. Schopler & G. Mesibov (Eds.), *Communication problems in autism* (pp. 257–282). New York: Plenum.

Lord, C. (1988). Enhancing communication in adolescents with autism. *Topics in Language Disorders, 9*(1), 72-81.

Lord, C., & Magill, J. (1988). Observing social behavior in an asocial population: Methodological and clinical issues. In G. Dawson (Ed.), *Autism: New perspectives on diagnosis, nature, and treatment* (pp. 46–66). New York: Guilford.

Lord, C., & O'Neill, P. J. (1983). Language and communication needs of adolescents with autism. In E. Schopler & G. Mesibov (Eds.), *Autism through adolescents* (pp. 57-77). New York: Plenum.

Lord, C., Rutter, M. L., Goode, S., Heemsbergen, J., Jordan, H., & Mawhood, L. (in press). Autism Diagnostic Observation Schedule: A standardized method of observing social and communicative behavior in persons with autism and other severe social deficits. *Journal of Autism and Developmental Disabilities.*

Louko, L., & Edwards, M. (1990, April). *Enhancing generalization for more efficient and effective phonological remediation.* Paper presented at the Annual Convention of the New York State Speech-Language-Hearing Association, Kiamesha Lake.

Lovaas, O. (1977). *The autistic child: Language development through behavior modification.* New York: John Wiley.

Lovaas, O. I., & Schreibman, L. (1971). Stimulus over-selectivity of autistic children in a two-stimulus situation. *Behavior Research and Therapy, 9,* 305-310.

Lovaas, O. I., Schreibman, L., Koegel, R., & Rehm, R. (1971). Selective responding by autistic children to multiple sensory input. *Journal of Olinormal Psychology, 71,* 211-222.

Love, R. J., & Webb, W. G. (1986). *Neurology for the speech-language pathologist.* Stoneham, MA: Butterworth.

Loveland, K., Landry, S., Hughes, S., Hall, S., & McEvoy, R. (1988). Speech acts and the pragmatic deficits of autism. *Journal of Speech and Hearing Research, 31,* 593–604.

Lovett, M., Dennis, M., & Newman, J. (1986). Making reference: The cohesive use of pronouns in the narrative discourse of hemidecorticate adolescents. *Brain and Language, 29,* 224–251.

Lovinger, S. (1974). Socio-dramatic play and language development in preschool disadvantaged children. *Psychology in the Schools, 11,* 313–320.

Low, G., Newman, P., & Ravsten, M. (1989). Pragmatic considerations in treatment: Communication-centered instruction. In N. Craighead, P. Newman, & W. Secord (Eds.), *Assessment and remediation of articulatory and phonological disorders* (pp. 217–242). New York: Merrill/Macmillan.

Lowe, R. (1986). Phonological process analysis using three position tests. *Language, Speech, and Hearing Services in Schools, 17,* 72–79.

Lucariello, J. (1990). Freeing talk from the here-and-now: The role of event knowledge and maternal scaffolds. *Topics in Language Disorders, 10*(3), 14-29.

Lucariello, J., Kyratzis, A., & Engel, S. (1986). Event representations, context, and language. *Event Knowledge, 7,* 136-160.

Lucas, E. (1980). *Semantic and pragmatic language disorders.* Rockville, MD: Aspen.

Lund, N. J., & Duchan, J. F. (1983). *Assessing children's language in naturalistic contexts.* Englewood Cliffs, NJ: Prentice-Hall.

Lund, N. J., & Duchan, J. F. (1988). *Assessing children's language in naturalistic contexts.* Englewood Cliffs, NJ: Prentice-Hall.

Luria, A. (1975). Basic problems of language in the light of psychology and neurolinguistics. In E. Lenneberg & E. Lenneberg (Eds.), *Foundations of language development: A multidisciplinary approach* (pp. 49–73). New York: Academic Press.

Lust, B., & Mervis, C. (1980). Development of coordination in the natural speech of young children. *Journal of Child Language, 7,* 279–304.

Lutzer, V. D. (1988). Comprehension of proverbs by average children and children with learning disorders. *Journal of Learning Disabilities, 21,* 104-108.

Lynch, E. W., & Hanson, M. J. (1992). *Developing cross–cultural competence: A guide for working with young children and their families.* Baltimore: Paul H. Brookes.

Lynch, M. A., & Roberts, J. (1982). *The consequences of child abuse.* New York: Academic Press.

Lyngaas, K., Nyberg, B., Hoekenga, R., & Gruenewald, L. (1983). Language intervention in the multiple contexts of the public school setting. In J. Miller, D. Yoder, & R. Schiefelbusch (Eds.), *Contemporary issues in language intervention* (pp. 239-252). Rockville, MD: ASHA.

Macarthur, C. A. (1988). The impact of computers on the writing process. *Exceptional Children, 54,* 536–542.

MacArthur Communicative Development Inventory: Infants. San Diego: San Diego State University, Center for Research in Language.

MacDonald, J. (1978a). Environmental Language Inventory. San Antonio: Psychological Corp.

MacDonald, J. (1978b). OLIVER: Parent-Administered Communication Inventory. San Antonio: Psychological Corp.

MacDonald, J. (1985). Language through conversation: A model for intervention with language-delayed persons. In S. Warren & A. Rogers-Warren (Eds.), *Teaching functional language* (pp. 89–122). Baltimore: University Park Press.

MacDonald, J. (1989). *Becoming partners with children: From play to conversation.* Chicago: Riverside.

MacDonald, J., Blott, J., Gordon, K., Spiegel, B., & Hartmann, M. (1974). An experimental parent-assisted treatment program for preschool language-delayed children. *Journal of Speech and Hearing Disorders, 39,* 395-415.

MacDonald, J., & Carroll, J. (1992a). Communication with young children: An ecological model for clinicians, parents, collaborative professionals. *American Journal of Speech-Language Pathology, 1*(4), 39-48.

MacDonald, J., & Carroll, J. (1992b). A social partnership model for assessing early communication development: An interaction model for preconversational children. *Language, Speech, and Hearing Services in Schools, 23,* 113-124.

MacDonald, J., & Gillette, Y. (1982). *A conversational approach to language delay: Problems and solutions.* Columbus, OH: Nisonger Center.

MacDonald, J., & Gillette, Y. (1986). Communicating with persons with severe handicaps: Roles of parents and professionals. *Journal of the Association for Persons with Severe Handicaps, 11,* 255–265.

MacDonald, J., & Gillette, Y. (1988). Ecological Communication System (ECO). San Antonio: Psychological Corp.

Mackay, D. G. (1978). Derivational rules and the internal lexicon. *Journal of Verbal Learning and Verbal Behavior, 17,* 61-71.

Mackie, B. C. (1982). *The effects of a sentence-combining program on the reading comprehension and written composition of fourth-grade students.* Unpublished doctoral dissertation, Hofstra University, Hempstead, NY.

MacLachlan, B. G., & Chapman, R. S. (1988). Communication breakdowns in normal and language-learning-disabled children's conversation and narration. *Journal of Speech and Hearing Disorders, 53,* 2-9.

MacWhinney, B. (Ed.). (1978). Acquisition of morphophonology. *Chicago: Social Research Child Development Monographs, 43,*(1-2, Serial No. 174).

Madrid, D. L., & Garcia, E. E. (1985). The effect of language transfer on bilingual proficiency. In E. E. Garcia & R. V. Padilla (Eds.), *Advances in bilingual education research* (pp. 53–70). Tucson: University of Arizona Press.

Magill, J. (1986). *The nature of social deficits of children with autism.* Unpublished doctoral dissertation, University of Alberta, Edmonton.

Mahoney, G., & Powell, A. (1986). *Transactional intervention program: Teacher's guide.* Farmington: University of Connecticut, Health Center, Pediatric Research and Training Center.

Mahoney, G., & Weller, E. (1980). An ecological approach to language intervention. *New Directions for Exceptional Children, 2,* 17–32.

Major, D. (1974). *The acquisition of modal auxiliaries in the language of children.* The Hague: Mouton.

Maltz, A. (1981). Comparison of cognitive deficits among autistic and retarded children on the Arthur Adaptation of the Leiter International Performance Scales. *Journal of Autism and Developmental Disabilities, 11,* 413-426.

Mandler, J. M., & Johnson, N. S. (1977). Remembrance of things parsed: Story structure and recall. *Cognitive Psychology, 9,* 111-151.

Mann, V. (1984). Review: Reading skill and language skill. *Developmental Review, 4,* 1-15.

Manolson, A. (1979). Parent training: A means of implementing pragmatics in early language remediation. *Human Communication, 4,* 275-281.

Manolson, A. (1985). *It takes two to talk: Hanen early language parent guidebook.* Toronto: Hanen Resource Center.

Marcell, M., & Armstrong, V. (1982). Auditory and visual sequential memory of Down syndrome and nonretarded children. *American Journal of Mental Deficiency, 87,* 86-95.

Marcell, M., & Weeks, S. (1988). Short-term memory difficulties and Down's syndrome. *Journal of Mental Deficiency Research, 32,* 153-162.

Marion, K. (1983). Data-based language programs: A closer look. In H. Winits (Ed.), *Treating language disorders* (pp. 11–24). Baltimore: University Park Press.

Markman, E. (1981). Comprehension monitoring. In W. P. Dickson (Ed.), *Children's oral communication skills* (pp. 61-84). New York: Academic Press.

Marr, M. K., Natter, R., & Wilcox, C. B. (1980, November). *Testing a child in a language you don't speak.* Paper presented at the Annual Convention of the American Speech-Language-Hearing Association, Detroit.

Marsh, H. W., Cairns, L., Relich, J., Barnes, J., & Debus, R. L. (1984). The relationship between dimensions of self–attribution and dimensions of self–concept. *Journal of Educational Psychology, 76,* 3-32.

Marshall, G., & Herbert, M. (1981). *Recorded telephone messages: A way to link teachers and parents.* Evaluation Report by CEMREL, Inc., for the Department of Education, Washington, DC.

Marshall, N., & Glock, D. (1978). Comprehension of connected discourse: A study into the relationships between the structure of text and information recalled. *Reading Research Quarterly, 11,* 10-56.

Marshall, N., Hegrenes, J., & Goldstein, S. (1973). Verbal interactions: Mothers and their retarded children vs. mothers and their nonretarded children. *American Journal of Mental Deficiency, 77,* 415–419.

Marslen-Wilson, W., & Tyler, L. (1980). The temporal structure of spoken understanding. *Cognition, 8,* 1–71.

Martin, J. (1972). Rhythmic (hierarchical) versus serial structure in speech and other behaviors. *Psychological Review, 79,* 487–509.

Martlew, M., Connolly, K., & McLeod, C. (1976). Language use, role, and context in a five-year-old. *Journal of Child Language, 5,* 81-99.

Marvin, C. (1987). Consultation services: Changing roles for SLP's. *Journal of Childhood Communication Disorders, 11*(1), 1–16.

Masterson, J. J. (1993a). Classroom-based phonological intervention. *American Journal of Speech-Language Pathology, 2*(1), 5-10.

Masterson, J. J. (1993b). The performance of children with language learning disabilities on two types of cognitive tasks. *Journal of Speech and Hearing Research, 36,* 1026–1036.

Masterson, J. J., Evans, L. H., & Aloia, M. (1993). Verbal analogical reasoning in children with language-learning disorders. *Journal Speech and Hearing Research, 36,* 76-82.

Masterson, J. J., & Kamhi, A. G. (1991). The effects of sampling conditions on sentence production in normal, reading-disabled, and language-learning-disabled children. *Journal of Speech and Hearing Research, 34,* 549-558.

Masterson, J. J., & Pagan, F. (1989). Interactive System for Phonological Analysis (ISPA) [Computer program]. University: University of Mississippi.

Matsuda, M. (1989). Working with Asian parents: Some communication strategies. *Topics in Language Disorders, 9*(3), 45–53.

Mattes, L. (1982). The elicited language analysis procedure: A method for scoring sentence imitation tasks. *Language, Speech, and Hearing in Schools, 13,* 37–41.

Mattes, L. J., & Omark, D. R. (1984). *Speech and language assessment for the bilingual handicapped.* Austin, TX: Pro-Ed.

Mattingly, I. (1972). Reading, the linguistic process, and linguistic awareness. In J. Kavanagh & I. Mattingly (Eds.), *Language by ear and eye* (pp. 133–147). Cambridge: MIT Press.

Maurer, H., & Sherrod, K. (1987). Context of directives given to young children with Down syndrome and nonretarded children: Development over two years. *American Journal on Mental Deficiency, 91,* 579-590.

Maxwell, S. E., & Wallach, G. P. (1984). The language-learning disabilities connection: Symptoms of early language disability change over time. In G. Wallach & K. Butler (Eds.), *Language learning disabilities in school-age children* (pp. 15-34). Baltimore: Williams & Wilkins.

McAfee, D. C. (1980). *Effect of sentence-combining instruction on the reading and writing achievement of fifth-grade children in a suburban school district.* Unpublished doctoral dissertation, Texas Women's University, Denton.

McCabe, A., & Peterson, C. (1985). A naturalistic study of the production of causal connectives by children. *Journal of Child Language, 12,* 145–160.

McCabe, A., & Peterson, C. (1990). *Keep them talking: Parental styles of interviewing and subsequent child narrative skill.* Paper presented at the 5th International Congress for the Study of Child Language, Budapest.

McCabe, A., & Rollins, P. R. (1994). Assessment of preschool narrative skills. *American Journal of Speech-Language Pathology, 3*(1), 45–56.

McCaleb, P., & Prizant, B. (1985). Encoding of new versus old information by autistic children. *Journal of Speech and Hearing Disorders, 50,* 230–240.

McCartney, K. A., & Nelson, K. (1981). Children's use of scripts in story recall. *Discourse Processes, 4,* 59-70.

McCauley, R., & Demetras, M. J. (1990). The identification of language impairments in the selection of specifically language-impaired subjects. *Journal of Speech and Hearing Disorders, 55,* 468-475.

McCauley, R., & Swisher, L. (1983, November). *Uses and misuses of norm-referenced tests in language assessment.* Paper presented at the Annual Convention of the American Speech-Language-Hearing Association, Cincinnati.

McCauley, R., & Swisher, L. (1984a). Psychometric review of language and articulation tests for preschool children. *Journal of Speech and Hearing Disorders, 49,* 34–42.

McCauley, R., & Swisher, L. (1984b). Use and misuse of norm-referenced tests in clinical assessment: A hypothetical case. *Journal of Speech and Hearing Disorders, 49,* 338–348.

McCauley, R., & Swisher, L. (1987). Are maltreated children at risk for speech and language impairment? An unanswered question. *Journal of Speech and Hearing Disorders, 52,* 301-303.

McClure, E. (1981). Formal and functional aspects of the code-switching discourse of bilingual children. In R. Duran (Ed.), *Latino language and communicative behavior* (pp. 69–94). Norwood, NJ: Ablex.

McConkey, R., Jeffree, D., & Hewson, S. (1979). Involving parents in extending the language development of their young mentally handicapped children. *British Journal of Disorders of Communication, 14,* 203-218.

McConkey, R., & O'Connor, M. (1982). A new approach to parental involvement in language intervention programmes. *Child: Care, Health, and Development, 8,* 163–176.

McCormick, L. (1986). Keeping up with language intervention trends. *Teaching Exceptional Children, 18,* 123–129.

McCormick, L., & Goldman, R. (1984). Designing an optimal learning program. In L. McCormick & R. Schiefelbusch (Eds.), *Early language intervention: An introduction* (pp. 201–242). New York: Merrill/Macmillan.

McCune-Nicolich, L., & Carroll, S. (1981). Development of symbolic play: Implications for the language specialist. *Topics in Language Disorders, 2,* 1–16.

McCutchen, D. (1982). *Development of local coherence in children's writing.* Unpublished manuscript.

McCutchen, D., & Perfetti, C. A. (1982). Coherence and connectedness in the development of discourse production. *Text, 2,* 113-139.

McDade, H. L., & Adler, S. (1980). Down syndrome and short-term memory impairment: A storage or retrieval deficit. *American Journal of Mental Deficiency, 84,* 561-567.

McDade, H. L., & Varnedoe, D. (1987). Training parents to be language facilitators. *Topics in Language Disorders, 7*(3), 19–30.

McDermott, R., Gospodinoff, K., & Aram, L. (1976). *Criteria for an ethnographically adequate description of activities and their contexts.* Paper presented at the Annual Meeting of the American Anthropological Association, Washington, DC.

McDermott, R., & Hood, L. (1982). Institutionalized psychology and the ethnography of schooling. In P. Gilmore & A. Glatthorn (Eds.), *Children in and out of school* (pp. 232–249). Washington, DC: Center for Applied Linguistics.

McDonald, L., & Pien, D. (1982). Mother conversational behavior as a function of interactional intent. *Journal of Child Language, 9,* 337–358.

McGee, G., Krantz, P., Mason, D., & McClanahan, L. (1983). A modified incidental-teaching procedure for autistic youth: Acquisition and generalization of receptive object labels. *Journal of Applied Behavior Analysis, 16,* 329–338.

McGee, G. G., Krantz, P. J., & McClannahan, L. E. (1984). Conversational skills for autistic adolescents: Teaching assertiveness in naturalistic game settings. *Journal of Autism and Developmental Disorders, 14,* 319–330.

McGhee-Bidlack, B. (1991). The development of noun definitions: A metalinguistic analysis. *Journal of Child Language, 18,* 417–434.

McGregor, G., Young, J., Gerak, J., Thomas, B., & Vogelsberg, R. T. (1992). Increasing functional use of an assistive communication device by a student with severe disabilities. *Augmentative and Alternative Communication, 8,* 243-250.

McGregor, K., & Leonard, L. (1989). Facilitating word-finding skills of language-impaired children. *Journal of Speech and Hearing Disorders, 54,* 141-147.

McKeown, M. G., & Curtis, M. E. (Eds.). (1987). *The nature of vocabulary acquisition.* Hillsdale, NJ: Lawrence Erlbaum.

McKinley, N., & Lord-Larson, V. (1985). Neglected language-disordered adolescent: A delivery model. *Language, Speech, and Hearing Services in Schools, 16,* 2–15.

McKinley, N., & Schwartz, L. (1987). *Referential communication: Barrier activities for speakers and listeners, Part 2.* Eau Claire, WI: Thinking Publications.

McLaughlin, B. (1977). *Second language learning in children: Vol. I. Preschool children.* Hillsdale, NJ: Lawrence Erlbaum.

McLean, J. E., & Snyder-McLean, L. K. (1978). *A transactional approach to early language training: Derivation of a model system.* New York: Merrill/Macmillan.

McLean, J. E., & Snyder-McLean, L. K. (1987). Form and function of communicative behaviour among persons with severe developmental disabilities. *Australia and New Zealand Journal of Developmental Disabilities, 13*(2), 83-98.

McLean, J. E., & Snyder-McLean, L. K. (1988a). Applications of pragmatics to severely mentally retarded children and youth. In R. L. Schiefelbusch & L. L. Lloyd (Eds.), *Language perspectives: Acquisition, retardation, and intervention* (pp. 255-288). Austin, TX: Pro-Ed.

McLean, J. E., & Snyder-McLean, L. K. (1988b, September). *Assessment and treatment of communicative competencies among clients with severe/profound developmental disabilities.* Workshop presented for Craig Developmental Disabilities Service Office and State University of New York, Geneseo.

McLean, J. E., Snyder-McLean, L. K. (in press). Communication intent and its realizations among persons with severe intellectual deficits. In N. Krasnegor, R. Schiefelbusch, & D. Rumbaugh (Eds.), *Biobehavioral foundations of language development.* Hillsdale, NJ: Lawrence Erlbaum.

McLean, J. E., Snyder-McLean, L. K., Brady, N. C., & Etter, R. (1991). Communication profiles of two types of gesture using nonverbal persons with severe to profound mental retardation. *Journal of Speech and Hearing Research, 34,* 294-308.

McLeavey, B., Toomey, J., & Dempsey, P. (1982). Nonretarded and mentally retarded children's control over syntactic structures. *American Journal of Mental Deficiency, 86,* 485-494.

McLoughlin, C., & Gullo, D. (1984). Comparison of three formal methods of preschool language assessment. *Language, Speech, and Hearing Services in Schools, 15,* 146–153.

McMorrow, M., Fox, R., Faw, G., & Bittle, E. (1987). Cues-pause-point language training: Teaching echolalics functional use of their verbal labeling repertoires. *Journal of Applied Behavior Analysis, 20,* 11-22.

McNaughton, D., & Light, J. (1989). Teaching facilitators to support the communication skills of an adult with severe cognitive disabilities: A case study. *Augmentative and Alternative Communication, 5,* 35–41.

McNutt, J. C., & Hamayan, E. (1984). Subgroups of older children with articulation disorders. In R. G. Daniloff (Ed.), *Articulation assessment and treatment issues* (pp. 51-70). San Diego: College–Hill.

McWilliams, P. J., & Winton, P. (1990). *Brass tacks: A self-rating of family-focused practices in early intervention. Part II: Individual interactions.* Chapel Hill, NC: Frank Porter Graham Child Development Center.

Mecham, M., Jex, J., & Jones, J. (1967). Utah Test of Language Development. Salt Lake City: Communication Research Associates.

Mehrabian, A. (1972). *Nonverbal communication.* Chicago: Aldine & Atherton.

Mele-McCarthy, J. (1990, April). *What's the meta with phonology?* Paper presented at the Annual Convention of the New York State Speech-Language-Hearing Association, Kiamesha Lake.

Meline, T., & Brackin, S. (1987). Language-impaired children's awareness of inadequate messages. *Journal of Speech and Hearing Disorders, 52,* 263–270.

Menn, L. (1971). Phonotactic rules in beginning speech. *Lingua, 26,* 225–251.

Mentis, M., & Prutting, C. A. (1987). Cohesion in the discourse of normal and head-injured adults. *Journal of Speech and Hearing Research, 30,* 88-98.

Mentis, M., & Prutting, C. A. (1991). Analysis of topic as illustrated in a head-injured and a normal adult. *Journal of Speech and Hearing Research, 34,* 583-595.

Menyuk P., Chesnick, M., Liebergott, J., Korngold, B., D'Agostino, R., & Belanger, A. (1991). Predicting reading problems in at-risk children. *Journal of Speech and Hearing Research, 34,* 893-903.

Menyuk, P., & Looney, P. (1972). A problem of language disorder: Length vs. structure. *Journal of Speech and Hearing Research, 15,* 264-279.

Mercer, C., & Snell, M. (1977). *Learning theory research in mental retardation.* New York: Merrill/Macmillan.

Mercer, J. R., & Lewis, J. P. (1975). *System of Multicultural Pluralistic Assessment. Technical manual.* Unpublished manuscript, University of California, Riverside.

Merrill, E. (1985). Differences in semantic processing speed of mentally retarded and nonretarded persons. *American Journal of Mental Deficiency, 90,* 71-80.

Merrill, E., & Bilsky, L. (1990). Individual differences in the representation of sentences in memory. *American Journal on Mental Retardation, 95,* 68-76.

Merritt, D., & Liles, B. (1985, November). *Story recall and comprehension in older language disordered children.* Paper presented at the Annual Convention of the American Speech-Language-Hearing Association, San Francisco.

Merritt, D., & Liles, B. (1987). Story grammar ability in children with and without language disorder: Story generation, story retelling, and story comprehension. *Journal of Speech and Hearing Research, 30,* 539-552.

Merritt, D., & Liles, B. (1989). Narrative analysis: Clinical applications of story generation and story retelling. *Journal of Speech and Hearing Disorders, 54,* 438–447.

Mervis, C. B. (1988). Early lexical development: Theory and application. In L. Nadel (Ed.), *The psychobiology of Down's syndrome* (pp. 104-144). Cambridge: MIT Press.

Mervis, C. B. (1990). Early conceptual development of children with Down syndrome. In D. Cicchetti & M. Beeghly (Eds.), *Children with Down syndrome: A developmental perspective* (pp. 252-301). Cambridge, UK: Cambridge University Press.

Mesibov, G. B. (1984). Social skills training with verbal autistic adolescents and adults: A program model. *Journal of Autism and Developmental Disorders, 14,* 395–404.

Messick, C. (1988). Ins and outs of the acquisition of spatial terms. *Topics in Language Disorders, 8*(2), 14–25.

Messick, S. (1980). Test validity and the ethics of assessment. *American Psychologist, 35,* 1012–1027.

Meyer, A., & Rose, D. (1987, October). Word processing: A new route around old barriers. *The Exceptional Parent,* pp. 26–29.

Meyer, B. (1975). *The organization of prose and its effects on memory.* Amsterdam: North-Holland.

Meyer, B. (1987). Follow the author's top-level organization: An important skill for reading comprehension. In R. Tierney, P. Anders, & J. Mitchell (Eds.), *Understanding reader's understanding* (pp. 59-76). Hillsdale, NJ: Lawrence Erlbaum.

Meyer, L. F., & Evans. (1986). Modification of excess behavior: An adaptive and functional approach for educational and community settings. In R. Horner, L. Meyer, & H. Fredericks (Eds.), *Education of learners with severe handicaps* (pp. 315–350). Baltimore: Paul H. Brookes.

Meyers, L. F., & Fogel, P. (1985). Representational Play [Computer program]. Santa Monica, CA: Peal Software.

Meyerson, R. F. (1978). Children's knowledge of selected aspects of *Sound Pattern of English.* In R. Campbell & P. Smith (Eds.), *Recent advances in psychology of language: Formal and experimental approaches* (pp. 377-402). New York: Plenum.

Miall, D. (1989). Beyond the schema given: Affective comprehension of literary narratives. *Cognition and Emotion, 3,* 55–78.

Michaels, S. (1981). "Sharing time": Children's narrative styles and differential access to literacy. *Language in Society, 10,* 423-442.

Michaels, S. (1986). Narrative presentations: An oral preparation for literacy with first graders. In J. Cook-Gumperz (Ed.), *The social construction of literacy* (pp. 94–116). Cambridge, UK: Cambridge University Press.

Michel, P. A. (1990). What first graders think about reading. In R. W. Blake (Ed.), *Whole language: Explorations and applications* (pp. 41–46). Schenectady: New York State English Council.

Middleton, J. (1989). Annotation: Thinking about head injuries in children. *Journal of Child Psychology and Psychiatry, 30,* 663-670.

Milianti, F., & Culliman, W. (1974). Effects of age and word frequency on object recognition and naming in children. *Journal of Speech and Hearing Research, 17,* 373-385.

Miller, G. A., & Gildea, P. M. (1987). How children learn words. *Scientific American, 257,* 94-99.

Miller, J. F. (1978). Assessing children's language behavior: A developmental process approach. In R. Schiefelbusch (Ed.), *Bases of language intervention* (pp. 269–318). Baltimore: University Park Press.

Miller, J. F. (1981). *Assessing language production in children: Experimental procedures.* Baltimore: University Park Press.

Miller, J. F. (1991). Quantitative productive language disorders. In J. Miller (Ed.), *Research on child language disorders: A decade of progress.* Austin, TX: Pro-Ed.

Miller, J. F., & Chapman, R. (1983). *SALT: Systematic Analysis of Language Transcripts: User's manual.* Madison: University of Wisconsin Press.

Miller, J. F., & Chapman, R. (1984). Disorders of communication: Investigating the development of language of mentally retarded children. *American Journal of Mental Deficiency, 88,* 536–545.

Miller, J. F., & Chapman, R. (1985). Systematic Analysis of Language Transcripts (SALT) Version 1.3 (MS-DOS) [Computer program]. Madison, WI: Language Analysis Laboratory, Waisman Center on Mental Retardation and Human Development.

Miller, J. F., Chapman, R., & MacKenzie, H. (1981). Individual differences in the language acquisition of mentally retarded children. *Proceedings from the Second Wisconsin Symposium on Research in Child Language.* Madison: University of Wisconsin.

Miller, J. F., Freiberg, C., Rolland, M., & Reeves, M. A. (1992). Implementing computerized language sample analysis in the public school. *Topics in Language Disorders, 12*(2), 69-82.

Miller, J. F., & Yoder, D. (1974). An ontogenetic language teaching strategy for retarded children. In R. L. Schiefelbusch & L. L. Lloyd (Eds.), *Language perspectives: Acquisition, retardation, and intervention* (pp. 505–528). Baltimore: University Park Press.

Miller, L. (1984). Problem solving and language disorders. In G. P. Wallach & K. G. Butler (Eds.), *Language learning disabilities in school–age children* (pp. 199-229). Baltimore: Williams & Wilkins.

Miller, L. (1989). Classroom-based language intervention. *Language, Speech, and Hearing Services in Schools, 20,* 153-169.

Miller, L. (1993). Testing and the creation of disorder. *American Journal of Speech-Language Pathology, 2*(1), 13-16.

Miller, N. (1984). Some observations concerning formal tests in cross-cultural settings. In N. Miller (Ed.), *Bilingualism and language disability: Assessment and remediation* (pp. 107-114). Austin, TX: Pro-Ed.

Miller, P. (1982). *Amy, Wendy, and Beth.* Austin: University of Texas Press.

Millford, R., & Hecht, B. F. (1980). Learning to speak without an accent: Acquisition of a second language phonology. *Papers Representing Child Language Development, 18,* 16–74.

Milosky, L. (1990). The role of world knowledge in language comprehension and language intervention. *Topics in Language Disorders, 10*(3), 1–13.

Milosky, L., & Wilkinson, L. (1984, November). *Requests for information and responses obtained in classroom learning groups.* Paper presented at the Annual Convention of the American Speech-Language-Hearing Association, San Francisco.

Minami, M., & McCabe, A. (1991). Haiku as a discourse regulation device: A stanza analysis of Japanese children's personal narratives. *Language in Society, 20,* 577–599.

Mineo, B. A., & Goldstein, H. (1990). Generalized learning of receptive and expressive action-object responses by language-delayed preschoolers. *Journal of Speech and Hearing Disorders, 55,* 665-678.

Miniutti, A. (1991). Language deficiencies in inner-city children with learning and behavioral problems. *Language, Speech, and Hearing Services in Schools, 22,* 31-38.

Minner, S., & Prater, G. (1987). Parental use of telephone answering equipment to assist handicapped children: Techniques. *American Journal for Remedial Education and Counseling, 3,* 51-56.

Mire, S., & Chisholm, R. (1990). Functional communication goals for adolescents and adults who are severely and moderately mentally handicapped. *Language, Speech, and Hearing Services in Schools, 21,* 57–58.

Mirenda, P., & Donnellan, A. (1986). Effects of adult interaction style on conversational behavior in students with severe communication problems. *Language, Speech, and Hearing Services in Schools, 17,* 126–141.

Mirenda, P., & Locke, P. (1989). A comparison of symbol transparency in nonspeaking persons with intellectual disabilities. *Journal of Speech and Hearing Disorders, 54,* 131–140.

Mirenda, P., & Schuler, A. L. (1988). Augmentative communication for persons with autism: Issues and strategies. *Topics in Language Disorders, 9*(1), 24-43.

Mishler, E. (1975). Studies in dialogue and discourse: Types of discourse initiated by and sustained through questioning. *Journal of Psycholinguistic Research, 4,* 99–121.

Mishler, E. (1979). Meaning in context: Is there any other kind? *Harvard Educational Review, 49,* 1–19.

Mistry, J., & Lange, G. (1985). Children's organization and recall of information in scripted narratives. *Child Development, 56,* 953–961.

Mizuko, M. (1987). Transparency and ease of learning of symbols represented by Blissymbolics, PCS, and Picsyms. *Augmentative and Alternative Communications, 3,* 129–136.

Moats, L. C., & Smith, C. (1992). Derivational morphology: Why it should be included in language assessment and instruction. *Language, Speech, and Hearing Services in Schools, 23,* 312-319.

Moberly, P. C. (1978). *Elementary children's understanding of anaphoric relationship in connected discourse.* Unpublished doctoral dissertation, Northwestern University, Evanston, IL.

Moeller, M., & McConkley, A. (1984). Language intervention with preschool deaf children: A cognitive/linguistic approach. In W. Perkins (Ed.), *Current therapy of communication disorders: Hearing disorders* (pp. 11–25). New York: Thieme-Stratton.

Moeller, M., Osberger, M., & Eccarius, M. (1986). Cognitively based strategies for use with hearing-impaired students with comprehension deficits. *Topics in Language Disorders, 6*(4), 37–50.

Moerk, E. (1977). *Pragmatic and semantic aspects of early language development.* Baltimore: University Park Press.

Monahan, D. (1984). *Remediation of common phonological processes.* Tigard, OR: C. C. Publications.

Monahan, D. (1986). Remediation of common phonological processes: Four case studies. *Language, Speech, and Hearing Services in Schools, 17,* 199–206.

Monson, D. (1982, May). *Effect of type and distance on comprehension of anaphoric relationships.* Paper presented at the International Reading Association WORD Research Conference, Seattle, WA.

Montgomery, J. (1992a, May). *Collaborating within the classroom: Using whole language to remediate speech and language disorders in school–age children.* Genesee Valley Speech-Language-Hearing Association Spring Workshop, Rochester, NY.

Montgomery, J. (1992b). Perspectives from the field: Language, speech, and hearing services in schools. *Language, Speech, and Hearing Services in Schools, 23,* 363-364.

Montgomery, J. K., & Bonderman, I. R. (1989). Serving preschool children with severe phonological disorders. *Language, Speech, and Hearing Services in Schools, 20,* 76-84.

Mooney, M. (1988). *Developing life-long readers.* Wellington, New Zealand: Department of Education.

Moore-Brown, B. (1991). Moving in the direction of change: Thoughts for administrators and speech-language pathologists. *Language, Speech, and Hearing Services in Schools, 22,* 148-149.

Moran, M. (1993). Final consonant deletion in African American children speaking Black English: A closer look. *Language, Speech, and Hearing Services in Schools, 24,* 161-166.

Moran, M., Money, S., & Leonard, D. (1984). Phonological process analysis of the speech of mentally retarded adults. *American Journal of Mental Deficiency, 89,* 304-306.

Moran, M. R., & Bryne, M. C. (1977). Mastery of verb tense markers by normal and learning disabled children. *Journal of Speech and Hearing Research, 20,* 529-542.

Moran, M. R., Schumaker, J. B., & Vetter, A. F. (1981). *Teaching a paragraph organization strategy to learning disabled adolescents* (Research Report No. 54). Lawrence: University of Kansas, Institute for Research in Learning Disabilities.

Mordecai, D. R., Palin, M. W., & Palmer, C. B. (1985). Lingquest 1 [Computer program]. Columbus, OH: Macmillan.

Morehead, D., & Ingram, D. (1976). The development of base syntax in normal and linguistically deviant children. In D. Morehead & A. Morehead (Eds.), *Normal and deficient child language* (pp. 209–238). Baltimore: University Park Press.

Morris, S. (1982). Pre-Speech Assessment Scale. Clifton, NJ: Preston.

Morris, S., & Klein, M. (1987). Pre-Feeding Skills. Tucson, AZ: Therapy Skill Builders.

Morrison, J. A., & Shriberg, L. D. (1992). Articulation testing versus conventional speech sampling. *Journal of Speech and Hearing Research, 35,* 259-273.

Morrow, D. R., Mirenda, P., Beukelman, D. P., & Yorkston, K. M. (1993). Vocabulary selection for augmentative communication systems: A comparison of three techniques. *American Journal of Speech-Language Pathology, 2*(2), 19-30.

Moses, N., & Maffei, L. (1989, April). *Classroom language intervention for communication–oriented preschools.* Paper presented at the Annual Convention of the New York State Speech-Language-Hearing Association, Liberty.

Mosisset, C. E., Barnard, K. E., Greenberg, M. T., Booth, C. L., & Spicker, S. J. (1990). Environmental influences on early language development: The context of social risk. *Development and Psychopathology, 2,* 127-149.

Mulac, A., & Tomlinson, C. (1977). Generalization of an operant remediation program for syntax with language-delayed children. *Journal of Communication Disorders, 10,* 231–244.

Muma, J. R. (1978). *Language handbook: Concepts, assessment, and intervention.* Englewood Cliffs, NJ: Prentice-Hall.

Muma, J. (1983). Speech-language pathology: Emerging clinical expertise in language. In T. Gallagher &

C. Prutting (Eds.), *Pragmatic assessment and intervention issues in language* (pp. 195–205). San Diego: College-Hill.

Muma, J. (1986). *Language acquisition: A functional perspective.* Austin, TX: Pro-Ed.

Muma, J., Lubinski, R., & Pierce, S. (1982). A new era in language assessment: Data or evidence. In N. Lass (Ed.), *Speech and language advances in basic research and practice* (Vol. 7, pp. 135–147). New York: Academic Press.

Muma, J., & Pierce, S. (1981). Language intervention: Data or evidence? *Topics in Learning and Learning Disabilities, 1*(2), 1–12.

Muma, J., Pierce, D., & Muma, D. (1983). Language training in speech-language pathology. *ASHA, 26*(6), 35–42.

Mundell, C., & Lucas, E. (1978). *A parent–conducted pragmatic language program for Down's syndrome children.* Unpublished manuscript, Washington State University, Pullman.

Murray-Branch, J., Udarari-Solner, A., & Bailey, B. (1991). Textural communication systems for individuals with severe intellectual and dual sensory impairments. *Language, Speech, and Hearing Services in Schools, 22,* 260-268.

Musselwhite, C. (1983). Pluralistic assessment in speech-language pathology: Use of dual norms in the placement process. *Language, Speech, and Hearing Services in Schools, 14,* 29–37.

Musselwhite, C., & St. Louis, K. (1982). *Communication programming for the severely handicapped: Vocal and nonvocal strategies.* San Diego: College-Hill.

Nagy, W. E., & Anderson, R. C. (1984). How many words are there in printed English? *Reading Research Quarterly, 24,* 262-282.

Nagy, W. E., Anderson, R. C., & Herman, P. A. (1987). Learning word meanings from context during normal reading. *American Educational Research Journal, 24,* 237-270.

Nagy, W. E., Anderson, R. C., Schommer, M., Scott, J. A., & Stallman, A. C. (1989). *Reading Research Quarterly, 24,* 262-283.

Nagy, W. E., & Herman, P. A. (1987). Breadth and depth of vocabulary knowledge: Implications for acquisition and instruction. In M. G. McKeown & M. E. Curtis (Eds.), *The nature of vocabulary acquisition* (pp. 19-35). Hillsdale, NJ: Lawrence Erlbaum.

Nagy, W. E., Herman, P. A., & Anderson, R. C. (1985). Learning words from context. *Reading Research Quarterly, 20,* 233-253.

Naiman, N., Frohlich, M., & Stern, H. H. (1975). *The good language learner.* Toronto: Ontario Institute for Studies in Education.

Nakamura, P., & Newhoff, M. (1982, November). *Clinical speech adjustments to normal and language-disordered*

children. Paper presented at the Annual Convention of the American Speech-Language-Hearing Association, Toronto.

Nakayama, M. (1987). Performance factors in subject-auxiliary inversion in children. *Journal of Child Language, 14,* 113–127.

Naremore, R., & Dever, R. (1975). Language performance of educable mentally retarded and normal children at five age levels. *Journal of Speech and Hearing Research, 18,* 82-95.

Narrol, H., & Giblon, S. (1984). *The fourth "R"—Uncovering hidden learning potential.* Baltimore: University Park Press.

National Council of Teachers of English. (1976). *Language development: Kindergarten through grade twelve.* Urbana, IL: Author.

National Joint Committee on Learning Disabilities. (1991). Learning disabilities: Issues on definition (A position paper). *Asha, 33,*(Suppl. 5), 18–20.

Nelsen, E. A., & Rosenbaum, E. (1972). Language patterns within the youth subculture: Development of slang vocabulary. *Merrill-Palmer Quarterly, 18,* 273-285.

Nelson, C. D. (1991). *Practical procedures for children with language disorders.* Austin, TX: Pro-Ed.

Nelson, K. (1973). *Structure and strategy in learning to talk. Society for Research in Child Development Monographs.* Chicago: University of Chicago Press.

Nelson, K. (1977). The syntagmatic-paradigmatic shift revisited: A review of research and theory. *Psychological Bulletin, 84,* 93-116.

Nelson, K. (1981a). Acquisition of words by first-language learners. *Annals of the New York Academy of Sciences, 379,* 148–159.

Nelson, K. (1981b). Social cognition in a script framework. In L. Ross & J. Flavell (Eds.), *The development of social cognition in children.* Cambridge, UK: Cambridge University Press.

Nelson, K. (1981c). Toward a rare-event cognitive comparison theory of syntax acquisition. In P. Dale & D. Ingram (Eds.), *Child language—An international perspective* (pp. 229–240). Baltimore: University Park Press.

Nelson, K. (1985). *Making sense: The acquisition of shared meaning.* New York: Academic Press.

Nelson, K. (Ed.) (1986). *Event knowledge: Structure and function in development.* Hillsdale, NJ: Lawrence Erlbaum.

Nelson, K., & Brown, A. (1978). The semantic-episodic distinction in memory development. In P. Ornstein (Ed.), *Memory development in children* (pp. 233–242). Hillsdale, NJ: Lawrence Erlbaum.

Nelson, K., & Denninger, M. (1977). *The shadow technique in the investigation of children's acquisition of new syntactic forms.* Unpublished manuscript, New School for Social Research, New York.

Nelson, K., Fivush, R., Hudson, J., & Lucariello, J. (1983). Scripts and the development of memory. In M. T. Chi (Ed.), *Contributions to human development: Trends in memory development research* (Vol. 9). New York: Karger.

Nelson, K., & Gruendel, J. (1979). At morning it's lunchtime: A scriptal view of children's dialogues. *Discourse Processes, 2,* 73-94.

Nelson, K., & Gruendel, J. (1981). Generalized event representations: Basic building blocks of cognitive development. In M. E. Lamb & A. L. Brown (Eds.), *Advances in developmental psychology* (Vol. 1, pp. 131–158). Hillsdale, NJ: Lawrence Erlbaum.

Nelson, K., & Lucariello, J. (1983). The development of meaning in first words. In M. Barrett (Ed.), *Children's single-word speech* (pp. 59–86). New York: John Wiley.

Nelson, L., Kamhi, A. G., & Apel, K. (1987). Cognitive strengths and weaknesses in language-impaired children: One more look. *Journal of Speech and Hearing Disorders, 52,* 36-43.

Nelson, L., & Weber-Olsen, M. (1980). The Elicited Language Inventory and the influence of contextual cues. *Journal of Speech and Hearing Disorders, 45,* 549–563.

Nelson, N. W. (1984). Beyond information processing: The language of teachers and textbooks. In G. Wallach & K. Butler (Eds.), *Language learning disabilities in school-age children* (pp. 154–178). Baltimore: Williams & Wilkins.

Nelson, N. W. (1985). Teachers talk and children listen—Fostering a better match. In C. Simon (Ed.), *Communication skills and classroom success: Assessment of language-learning disabled students* (pp. 65–104). San Diego: College-Hill.

Nelson, N. W. (1986a). Individual processing in classroom settings. *Topics in Language Disorders, 6*(2), 13–27.

Nelson, N. W. (1986b). What is meant by meaning (and how can it be taught)? *Topics in Language Disorders, 6*(4), 1–14.

Nelson, N. W. (1988a). The consultant model. *ASHA Audioteleconference.* Rockville, MD: ASHA.

Nelson, N. W. (1988b). *Planning individualized speech and language intervention programs: Objectives for infants, children, and adolescents.* Tucson, AZ: Communication Skill Builders.

Nelson, N. W. (1989). Curriculum-based language assessment and intervention. *Language, Speech, and Hearing Services in Schools, 20,* 170-184.

Nelson, N. W. (1992). Targets of curriculum-based language assessment. *Best Practices in School Speech-Language Pathology, 2,* 73-86.

Nelson, N. W. (1993). *Childhood language disorders in context: Infancy through adolescence.* New York: Macmillan.

Nelson, N. W., & Hyter, D. (1990). *Black English Sentence Scoring: Development and use as a tool for nonbiased assessment.* Unpublished manuscript, Western Michigan University, Kalamazoo.

Nelson, N. W., & Schwentor, B. A. (1990). Reading and writing. In D. R. Beukelman & K. M. Yorkston (Eds.), *Communication disorders following traumatic brain injury: Management of cognitive, language, and motor impairments* (pp. 191-249). Austin, TX: Pro-Ed.

Nestheide, C., & Culatta, B. (1980, November). *Incorporating language training into daily activities.* Paper presented at the Annual Convention of the American Speech-Language-Hearing Association, Detroit.

Newcomer, P., & Hammill, D. (1977). The Test of Language Development. Austin, TX: Empiric.

Newcomer, P., & Hammill, D. (1988). Test of Language Development—2 Primary. Austin, TX: Pro-Ed.

Newell, A. F., Arnott, J. L., Booth, L., Beattie, W., Brophy, B., & Ricketts, I. W. (1992). Effect of the "PAL" word prediction system on the quality and quantity of text generation. *Augmentative and Alternative Communication, 8,* 304-311.

Newfield, M. (1966). *A study of the acquisition of English morphology by normal and EMR children.* Unpublished master's thesis, Ohio State University, Columbus.

Newfield, M. & Schlanger, B. (1968). The acquisition of English morphology in normal and educable mentally retarded children. *Journal of Speech and Hearing Research, 11,* 693-706.

Newhoff, M., & Leonard, L. (1983). Diagnosis of developmental language disorders. In I. Meitus & B. Weinberg (Eds.), *Diagnosis in speech-language pathology* (pp. 71–112). Baltimore: University Park Press.

Newman, J., Lovett, M., & Dennis, M. (1986). The use of discourse analysis in neurolinguistics: Some findings from the narratives of hemidecorticate adolescents. *Topics in Language Disorders, 7*(1), 31–44.

Newman, J. M. (1985). *Whole language: Theory in use.* Portsmouth, NH: Heinemann.

Newport, E., Gleitman, H., & Gleitman, L. (1977). Mother, I'd rather do it myself: Some effects and non-effects of maternal speech style. In C. Snow & C. Ferguson (Eds.), *Talking to children: Language input and acquisition* (pp. 109–150). Cambridge, UK: Cambridge University Press.

Newson, J. (1979). The growth of shared understandings between infant and caregiver. In N. Bullowa (Ed.), *Before speech* (pp. 207–222). New York: Cambridge University Press.

Nicholas, M., Obler, L. K., Albert, M. L., & Helm-Estabrooks, N. (1985). Empty speech in Alzheimer's disease and fluent aphasia. *Journal of Speech and Hearing Research, 28*, 405–410.

Nicholls, J. G. (1979). Development of perception of own attainment and causal attributions for success and failure in reading. *Journal of Educational Psychology, 71*, 94-99.

Nietupski, J., Hamre-Nietupski, S., Clancy, P., & Veerhusen, K. (1986). Guidelines for making simulation an effective adjunct to in vivo community instruction. *Journal of the Association for Persons with Severe Handicaps, 11*, 12–18.

Nietupski, J., Scheutz, G., & Ockwood, L. (1980). The delivery of communication therapy services to severely handicapped students: A plan for change. *Journal of the Association for the Severely Handicapped, 5*, 13-23.

Ninio, A., & Bruner, J. (1978). The achievements and antecedents of labeling. *Journal of Child Language, 5*, 1–15.

Ninio, A., & Wheeler, P. (1983). Functions of speech in mother–infant interactions. In L. Feagans, C. Garvey, & R. Golinkoff (Eds.), *The origins and growth of communication* (pp. 196–207). Norwood, NJ: Ablex.

Nippold, M. (1985). Comprehension of figurative language in youth. *Topics in Language Disorders, 5*(3), 1-20.

Nippold, M. A. (1988a). Figurative language. In M. A. Nippold (Ed.), *Later language development: Ages nine through nineteen* (pp. 179-210). Austin, TX: Pro-Ed.

Nippold, M. A. (1988b). The literate lexicon. In M. Nippold (Ed.), *Later language development* (pp. 29-47). San Diego: College-Hill.

Nippold, M. A. (1990). *Idioms in textbooks for kindergarten through eighth grade students.* Unpublished manuscript.

Nippold, M. A. (1991). Evaluating and enhancing idiom comprehension in language-disordered students. *Language, Speech, and Hearing Services in Schools, 22*, 100-106.

Nippold, M. A. (1992). The nature of normal and disordered word finding in children and adolescents. *Topics in Language Disorders, 13*(1), 1-14.

Nippold, M. A. (1993). Developmental markers in adolescent language: Syntax, semantics, and pragmatics. *Language, Speech, and Hearing Services in Schools, 24*, 21-28.

Nippold, M. A., Erskine, B., & Freed, D. (1988). Proportional and functional analogical reasoning in normal and language-impaired children. *Journal of Speech and Hearing Disorders, 53*, 440-449.

Nippold, M. A., & Fey, S. H. (1983). Metaphoric understanding in preadolescents having a history of language acquisition difficulties. *Language, Speech, and Hearing Services in Schools, 14*, 171-180.

Nippold, M. A., & Martin, S. T. (1989). Idiom interpretation in isolation versus context: A developmental study with adolescents. *Journal of Speech and Hearing Research, 32*, 59-66.

Nippold, M. A., & Rudzinski, M. (1993). Familiarity and transparency in idiom explanation: A developmental study of children and adolescents. *Journal of Speech and Hearing Research, 36*, 728–737.

Nippold, M. A., Schwarz, I. E., & Lewis, M. (1992). Analyzing the potential benefit of the microcomputer use for teaching figurative language. *American Journal of Speech-Language Pathology, 1*(2), 36-43.

Nippold, M. A., Schwarz, I. E., & Undlin, R. A. (1992). Use and understanding of adverbial conjuncts: A developmental study of adolescents and young adults. *Journal of Speech and Hearing Research, 35*, 108-118.

Nippold, M. A., Scott, C. M., Norris, J. A., & Johnson, C. J. (1993, November). *School-age children and adolescents: Establishing language norms, Part 2.* Paper presented at the Annual Convention of the American Speech–Language–Hearing Association, Anaheim, CA.

Nippold, M. A., Stephens, M. I., & Fey, S. H. (1983, June). *Sentential ambiguity as a probe for comprehension deficits in preadolescents.* Paper presented at the Symposium on Research in Child Language Disorders, Madison, WI.

Noel, M. (1980). Referential communication abilities of learning disabled children. *Learning Disability Quarterly, 3*, 70–75.

Norris, J. (1989). Providing language remediation in the classroom: An integrated language-to-reading intervention model. *Language, Speech, and Hearing Services in Schools, 20*, 205–218.

Norris, J. A. (1992). Some questions and answers about whole language. *American Journal of Speech-Language Pathology, 1*(4), 11-14.

Norris, J. A., & Bruning, R. (1988). Cohesion in the narratives of good and poor readers. *Journal of Speech and Hearing Disorders, 53*, 416–424.

Norris, J. A., & Damico, J. S. (1990). Whole language in theory and practice: Implications for language intervention. *Language, Speech, and Hearing Services in Schools, 21*, 212-220.

Norris, J. A., & Hoffman, P. R. (1990a). Comparison of adult-initiated vs. child-initiated interaction styles with handicapped prelanguage children. *Language, Speech, and Hearing Services in Schools, 21*, 28–36.

Norris, J. A., & Hoffman, P. R. (1990b). Language intervention within naturalistic environments. *Language, Speech, and Hearing Services in Schools, 21*, 72-84.

Norris, M., Juarez, M., & Perkins, M. (1989). Adaptation of a screening test for bilingual and bidialectal populations. *Language, Speech, and Hearing Services in Schools, 20,* 381–390.

Nugent, P., & Mosley, J. (1987). Mentally retarded and nonretarded individuals' attention allocation and capacity. *American Journal of Mental Deficiency, 91,* 598-605.

Nye, C., Foster, S., & Seaman, D. (1987). Effectiveness of language intervention with the language/learning disabled. *Journal of Speech and Hearing Disorders, 52,* 348–357.

Oakhill, J. (1984). Inferential and memory skills in children's comprehension of stories. *British Journal of Educational Psychology, 54,* 31–39.

Oates, R. K., Peacock, A., & Forrest, D. (1984). The development of abused children. *Developmental Medicine and Child Neurology, 26,* 649-656.

O'Brien, M., & Nagel, K. (1987). Parents' speech to toddlers: The effect of play context. *Journal of Child Language, 14,* 269-279.

Ochs, E. (1982). Talking to children in Western Samoa. *Language in Society, 11,* 77–104.

O'Connor, L, & Schery, T. K. (1989). *Using microcomputers to develop communication skills in young severely handicapped children* (Unpublished final project report, Grant No. Goo87300283). Washington, DC: U. S. Department of Education.

Odom, S. (1983). The development of social interchanges in infancy. In S. Garwood & R. Rewell (Eds.), *Educating handicapped infants: Issues in development and intervention* (pp. 215–254). Rockville, MD: Aspen.

Odom, S., Hoyson, M., Jamieson, B., & Strain, P. (1985). Increasing handicapped preschoolers' peer social interactions: Cross-setting and component analysis. *Journal of Applied Behavior Analysis, 18,* 3-16.

O'Donnell, R., Griffin, W., & Norris, R. (1967). *Syntax of kindergarten and elementary school children: A transformational analysis* (Research Report No. 8). Champaign, IL: National Council of Teachers of English.

Ogletree, W. (1993, April). *Communication assessment and intervention for persons with severe-to-profound mental retardation.* Paper presented at the Annual Convention of the New York State Speech-Language-Hearing Association, Rochester.

Oliver, C., & Halle, J. (1982). Language training in the everyday environment: Teaching functional sign use to a retarded child. *Journal of the Association for Persons with Severe Handicaps, 8,* 50–62.

Oller, D. (1974). Simplification as the goal of phonological processes in child speech. *Language Learning, 24,* 299–303.

Oller, J. W. (1983). *Issues in language testing research.* Rowley, MA: Newbury House.

Oller, J. W., Jr. (1979). *Language tests at school: A pragmatic approach.* London: Longman.

Oller, J. W., Jr., Baca, L., & Vigil, A. (1978). Attitudes and attained proficiency in ESL: A sociolinguistic study of Mexican Americans in the Southwest. *TESOL Quarterly, 11,* 173–183.

Olsen-Fulero, L. (1982). Style and stability in mother conversational behavior: A study of individual differences. *Journal of Child Language, 9,* 543–564.

Olson, D. (1970). Language and thought: Aspects of a cognitive theory of semantics. *Psychological Review, 77,* 257–273.

Olson, D. (1984). "See! Jumping!" Some oral antecedents of literacy. In H. Goelman, A. Oberg, & F. Smith (Eds.), *Awakening to literacy* (pp. 185-192). Portsmouth, NH: Heinemann.

Olswang, L., & Bain, B. (1991). Intervention issues for toddlers with specific language impairment. *Topics in Language Disorders, 11*(4), 69-84.

Olswang, L., Bain, B., & Johnson, G. (1990). Using dynamic assessment with children with language disorders. In S. Warren & J. Reichle (Eds.), *Causes and effects in communication and language intervention* (pp. 187–215). Baltimore: Paul H. Brookes.

Olswang, L., Kriegsmann, E., & Mastergeorge, A. (1982). Facilitating functional requesting in pragmatically impaired children. *Language, Speech, and Hearing Services in Schools, 13,* 202–222.

Olswang, L., Stoel-Gammon, C., Coggins, T., & Carpenter, R. (1987). *Assessing prelinguistic behaviors in developmentally young children.*

Orazi, D., & Wilcox, M. (1982, November). *The modification of spontaneous communicative behaviour in language-disordered children.* Paper presented at the convention of the American Speech and Hearing Association, Toronto.

Orelove, F., & Sobsey, D. (1987). *Educating children with multiple disabilities: A transdisciplinary approach.* Baltimore: Paul H. Brookes.

Ornitz, E., Guthrie, D., & Farley, A. (1977). The early development of autistic children. *Journal of Autism and Childhood Schizophrenia, 7,* 207-229.

Orum, L. (1986). *The education of Hispanics: Status and implications.* Washington, DC: National Council of La Raza.

Owens, R. (1978). *Speech acts in the early language of nondelayed and retarded children: A taxonomy and distributional study.* Unpublished doctoral dissertation, Ohio State University, Columbus.

Owens, R. (1982a). Caregiver Interview and Environmental Observation. San Antonio: Psychological Corp.

Owens, R. (1982b). Developmental Assessment Tool. San Antonio: Psychological Corp.

Owens, R. (1982c). Diagnostic Interactional Survey (DIS). San Antonio: Psychological Corp.

Owens, R. (1982d). *Program for the acquisition of language with the severely impaired (PALS)*. San Antonio: Psychological Corp.

Owens, R., Haney, M., Giesow, V., Dooley, L., & Kelly, R. (1983). Language test content: A comparative study. *Language, Speech, and Hearing Services in Schools, 14*, 7–21.

Owens, R., & House, L. (1984). Decision-making processes in augmentative communication. *Journal of Speech and Hearing Disorders, 49*, 18–25.

Owens, R., & MacDonald, J. (1982). Communicative uses of the early speech of nondelayed and Down syndrome children. *American Journal of Mental Deficiency, 86*, 503-510.

Owens, R., McNerney, C., Bigler-Burke, L., & Lepre-Clark, C. (1987, June). Language facilitators with residential retarded populations. *Topics in Language Disorders, 7*(3), 47–63.

Owens, R., & Rogerson, B. (1988). Adults at the presymbolic level. In S. Calculator & J. Bedrosian (Eds.), *Communication assessment and intervention for adults with mental retardation* (pp. 189–230). San Diego: College-Hill.

Paccia-Cooper, J., and Curcio, F. (1982). Language processing and forms of immediate echolalia in autistic children. *Journal of Speech and Hearing Research, 25*, 42-47.

Pacheco, R. (1983). Bilingual mentally retarded children: Language confusion or real deficits? In D. R. Omark & J. G. Erickson (Eds.), *The bilingual child* (pp. 232-253). San Diego: College–Hill.

Paden, E., & Moss, S. (1985). Comparison of three phonological analysis procedures. *Language, Speech, and Hearing Services in Schools, 16*, 103–109.

Page, J. (1982, May). *The communication game: Pragmatics and early communication training for severely/profoundly retarded individuals*. Paper presented at the Annual Convention of the American Association on Mental Deficiency, Boston.

Page, J., & Horn, D. (1987). Comprehension in developmentally delayed children. *Language, Speech, and Hearing Services in Schools, 18*, 63–71.

Palermo, D. (1982). Theoretical issues in semantic development. In S. Kuczaj (Ed.), *Language development: Vol. 1. Syntax and semantics* (pp. 335–396). Hillsdale, NJ: Lawrence Erlbaum.

Palin, M., & Mordecai, D. (1985). Lingquest 2 [Computer program]. Columbus, OH: Macmillan.

Palincsar, A. S., & Brown, A. L. (1983). *Reciprocal teaching of comprehension-monitoring activities* (Technical Report No. 269). Champaign: University of Illinois, Center for the Study of Reading.

Palincsar, A. S., & Brown, A. L. (1984). Reciprocal teaching of comprehension fostering and comprehension monitoring activities. *Cognition and Instruction, 1*, 117-175.

Palincsar, A. S., & Brown, A. L. (1986). Interactive teaching to promote independent learning from text. *The Reading Teacher, 39*, 771-777.

Palmatier, R. A., & Ray, H. L. (1989). *Sports talk: A dictionary of sports metaphors*. New York: Greenwood.

Paluszek, S., & Feintuch, F. (1979). Comparing imitation and comprehension training in two language impaired children. *Working Papers in Experimental Speech-Language Pathology and Audiology, 8*, 72–91.

Paluszny, M. A. (1979). *Autism: A practical guide for parents and professionals*. Syracuse, NY: Syracuse University Press.

Panagos, J., & Prelock, P. (1982). Phonological constraints on the sentence productions of language-disordered children. *Journal of Speech and Hearing Disorders, 26*, 23-31.

Panagos, J., Quine, H., & Klich, P. (1979). Syntactic and phonological influences in children's articulations. *Journal of Speech and Hearing Research, 22*, 841–848.

Papanicolaon, A. C., DiScenna, A., Gillespie, L., & Aram, D. M. (1990). Probe–evoked potential findings following unilateral left hemisphere lesions in children. *Archives of Neurology, 47*, 562-566.

Paris, S. G., & Oka, E. (1986). Children's reading strategies, metacognition, and motivation. *Developmental Review, 6*, 25-56.

Paris, S. G., & Upton, L. R. (1976). Children's memory for inferential relationships in prose. *Child Development, 4*, 660-668.

Parnell, M., & Amerman, J. (1983). Answers to *wh-* questions: Research and application. In T. Gallagher & C. Prutting (Eds.), *Pragmatic assessment and intervention issues in language* (pp. 129–150). San Diego: College-Hill.

Parnell, M., Amerman, J., & Harting, R. (1986). Responses of language-disordered children to *wh-* questions. *Language, Speech, and Hearing Services in Schools, 17*, 95–106.

Parnell, M., Patterson, S., & Harding, M. (1984). Answers to *wh-* questions: A developmental study. *Journal of Speech and Hearing Research, 27*, 297–305.

Paul, R. (1989a, June). *Outcomes of early expressive language delay: Age three*. Paper presented at the Symposium for Research in Child Language Disorders, University of Wisconsin, Madison.

Paul, R. (1989b). *Profiles of toddlers with delayed expressive language development*. Paper presented at the Biennial Meeting of the Society for Research in Child Development, Kansas City, MO.

Paul, R. (1990). Comprehension strategies: Interactions between world knowledge and the development of sentence comprehension. *Topics in Language Disorders, 10*(3), 63-75.

Paul, R. (1991). Profiles of toddlers with slow expressive language development. *Topics in Language Disorders, 11*(4), 1-13.

Paul, R., & Alforde, S. (1993). Grammatical morpheme acquisition in 4–year–olds with normal, impaired, and late–developing language. *Journal of Speech and Hearing Research, 36,* 1271-1275.

Paul, R., Fisher, M., & Cohen , D. (1988). Comprehension strategies in children with autism and specific language disorders. *Journal of Autism and Developmental Disorders, 18,* 669-679.

Paul, R., & Jennings, P. (1992). Phonological behavior in toddlers with slow expressive language development. *Journal of Speech and Hearing Research, 35,* 99-107.

Paul, R., Looney, S., & Dahm, P. (1991). Communication and socialization skills at age 2 and 3 in "late-talking" young children. *Journal of Speech and Hearing Research, 34,* 858-865.

Paul, R., Lynn, T., & Lohr-Flanders, M. (1990, November). *Otitis media and speech/language development in late-talkers.* Paper presented at the Annual Convention of the American Speech-Language-Hearing Association, Seattle.

Paul, R., & Shriberg, L. (1982). Associations between phonology and syntax in speech-delayed children. *Journal of Speech and Hearing Research, 25,* 536-547.

Paul, R., & Smith, R. (1991). *Narrative skills in four year olds with normal, impaired, and late-developing language.* Paper presented at the Biennial Meeting of the Society for Research in Child Development, Seattle.

Paul, R., & Smith, R. L. (1993). Narrative skills in 4-year-olds with normal, impaired, and late developing language. *Journal of Speech and Hearing Research, 36,* 592-598.

Paynter, E., & Bumpas, T. (1977). Imitative and spontaneous articulatory assessment of 3-year-old children. *Journal of Speech and Hearing Disorders, 42,* 119–125.

Pearson, D. (1988). A group therapy idea for new clinicals in the school setting: Keep little hands busy. *Language, Speech, and Hearing Services in Schools, 19,* 432.

Pease, D. M., Gleason, J. B., & Pan, B. A. (1989). Gaining meaning: Semantic development. In J. B. Gleason (Ed.), *The development of language* (2nd ed., pp. 101-134). New York: Merrill/Macmillan.

Peck, C., & Schuler, A. (1987). Assessment of social/communicative behavior for students with autism and severe handicaps: The importance of asking the right questions. In T. Layton (Ed.), *Language and treatment of autistic and developmentally disordered children.* Springfield, IL: Charles C. Thomas.

Pecyna, P. (1984). *The use of nonspeech communication systems to facilitate language acquisition in severely handicapped preschool children.* Unpublished doctoral dissertation, Kent State University, Kent, OH.

Pecyna, P. (1988). Rebus symbol communication training with a severely handicapped preschool child: A case study. *Language, Speech, and Hearing Services in Schools, 19,* 128–143.

Pecyna-Rhyner, P., Lehr, D., & Pudlas, K. (1990). An analysis of teacher responsiveness to communicative initiations of preschool children with handicaps. *Language, Speech, and Hearing Services in Schools, 21,* 91–97.

Pehrsson, R. S. (1982). *An investigation of comprehension during the process of silent reading: The op-in procedure* (Final Report, Grant No. 486). Pocatello: Idaho State University.

Pehrsson, R. S., & Denner, P. R. (1985). *Assessing silent reading during the process: An investigation of the op-in procedure.* Paper presented at the Annual Meeting of the Northern Rocky Mountain Educational Research Association, Jackson, WY.

Pehrsson, R. S., & Denner, P. R. (1988). Semantic organizers: Implications for reading and writing. *Topics in Language Disorders, 8*(3), 24-37.

Pehrsson, R. S., & Mook, J. E. (1983). *A model of curriculum development in rural schools.* Unpublished manuscript.

Pehrsson, R. S., & Robinson, H. A. (1985). *The semantic organizer approach to writing and reading instruction.* Rockville, MD: Aspen.

Pellegrini, A., & Galda, L. (1982). The effect of thematic-fantasy play training on the development of children's story comprehension. *American Educational Research Journal, 19,* 443–452.

Pellegrini, A. D. (1983). Sociolinguistic contexts of the preschool. *Journal of Applied Developmental Psychology, 4,* 397-405.

Pellegrini, A. D. (1985). Relations between symbolic play and literate behavior. In L. Galda & A. Pellegrini (Eds.), *Play, language, and stories: The development of children's literate behavior* (pp. 79–97). Norwood, NJ: Ablex.

Pellegrini, A. D., & Galda, L. (1990). Children's play, language, and early literacy. *Topics in Language Disorders, 10*(3), 76-88.

Pellegrini, A. D., & Perlmutter, J. (1989). Classroom contextual effects on children's play. *Developmental Psychology, 25,* 289-296.

Pena, E., & Iglesias, A. (1989, November). *System for dynamic scoring.* Paper presented to the American Speech-Language-Hearing Association, St. Louis, MO.

Penalosa, F. (1981). *Introduction to a sociology of language.* Rowley, MA: Newbury House.

Perera, K. (1986a). Grammatical differentiation between speech and writing in children aged 8 to 12. In A. Wilkinson (Ed.), *The writing of writing* (pp. 90–108). New York: Open University Press.

Perera, K. (1986b). Language acquisition and writing. In P. Fletcher & M. Garman (Eds.), *Language acquisi-*

tion (2nd ed., pp. 494–533). Cambridge, UK: Cambridge University Press.

Perlman, R. (1984). Bilingual teacher aids: Diagnosis and assessment. *IABBE Forum, 2.*

Perozzi, J. (1985). A pilot study of bilingual language facilitation: Theoretical and intervention implications. *Journal of Speech and Hearing Disorders, 50,* 403-406.

Perozzi, J. A., & Chavez Sanchez, M. L. (1992). The effect of instruction in L₁ on receptive acquisition of L₂ for bilingual children with language delay. *Language, Speech, and Hearing Services in Schools, 23,* 348-352.

Peters, A. (1984) *The units of language acquisition.* New York: Cambridge University Press.

Peterson, C., & McCabe, A. (1983). *Developmental psycholinguistics: Three ways of looking at a child's narrative.* New York: Plenum.

Peterson, P., & Swing, S. (1985). Students' cognitions as mediators of the effectiveness of small-group learning. *Journal of Educational Psychology, 77,* 299–312.

Petrey, S. (1977). Word associations and the development of lexical memory. *Cognition, 5,* 55-71.

Pflaum, S. W., & Pascarella, E. T. (1980). Interactive effects of prior reading achievement and training in context on the reading of learning disabled children. *Reading Research Quarterly, 16,* 138-158.

Phelps–Terasaki, D., & Phelps–Gunn, T. (1992). Test of Pragmatic Language. Austin, TX: Pro–Ed.

Phillips, J., & Balthazar, E. (1979). Some correlates of language deterioration in severely and profoundly retarded long-term institutionalized residents. *American Journal of Mental Deficiency, 83,* 402–408.

Phillips, S. U. (1982). *The invisible culture: Communication in classroom and community on the Warm Springs Indian Reservation.* New York: Longman.

Piaget, J., & Inhelder, B. (1969). *The psychology of the child.* New York: Basic Books.

Piche–Cragoe, L., Reichle, J., & Sigafoos, J. (1986). *Requesting validity intervention.* Unpublished manuscript, University of Minnesota, Minneapolis.

Pidek, C. (1987). *The assignment book.* Schaumburg, IL: Communication Concepts.

Pinsleur, P. (1980). *How to learn a foreign language.* Boston: Heinle & Heinle.

Plante, E., & Vance, R. (1994). Selection of preschool language tests: A data–based approach. *Language, Speech, and Hearing Services in Schools, 25,* 15–24.

Platt, J., & Coggins, T. (1990). Comprehension of social-action games in prelinguistic children. *Journal of Speech and Hearing Disorders, 55,* 315-326.

Polk, X., Schilmoeller, G., Emboy, L., Holman, J., & Baer, D. (1976, May). *Prompted generalization through experimenters' instructions: A parent training study.*

Paper presented at the Annual Meeting of the Midwestern Association of Behavior Analysis, Chicago.

Pollack, M. D. (1980). *The effects of testwiseness language of test administration, and language competence on readiness test performance of low socio-economic level, Spanish speaking children.* Ann Arbor: University of Michigan.

Pollio, H., Barlow, J., Fine, H., & Pollio, M. (1977). *Psychology and the poetics of growth.* Hillsdale, NJ: Lawrence Erlbaum.

Poplack, S. (1982). Sometimes I'll start a sentence in Spanish y termino en espanol: Toward a typology of code-switching. In J. Amastae & L. Elias-Olivares (Eds.), *Spanish in the United States: Sociolinguistic aspects* (pp. 230–263). New York: Cambridge University Press.

Poplin, M., Gray, R., Larsen, S., Banikowski, A., & Mehring, T. (1980). A comparison of components of written expression abilities in learning disabled and non-learning disabled students at three grade-levels. *Learning Disability Quarterly, 3,* 46-53.

Powell, T. (1991). Planning for phonological generalization: An approach to treatment target selection. *American Journal of Speech-Language Pathology, 1*(3), 21-27.

Powell, T., & Elbert, M. (1984). Generalization following the reduction of early- and later-developing consonant clusters. *Journal of Speech and Hearing Disorders, 49,* 211-218.

Powell, T., Elbert, M., & Dinnsen, D. (in press). Stimulability as a factor in the phonological generalization of misarticulating preschool children. *Journal of Speech and Hearing Research.*

Prater, R. (1982). Functions of consonant assimilation and reduplication in early word productions of mentally retarded children. *American Journal of Mental Deficiency, 86,* 399-404.

Prather, E., Breecher, S., Stafford, M., & Wallace, E. (1980). Screening Test of Adolescent Language. Seattle: University of Washington Press.

Preece, A. (1987). The range of narrative forms conversationally produced by young children. *Journal of Child Language, 14,* 353–373.

Preferred practice patterns for the professions of speech-language pathology and audiology. (1993, March). *Asha, 35,*(Suppl. 11).

Prelock, P., Messick, C., Schwartz, R., & Terrell, B. (1981). Mother-child discourse during the one-word stage. *Proceedings from the Second Wisconsin Symposium on Research in Child Language Disorders.* Madison: University of Wisconsin, Department of Communicative Disorders.

Prelock, P., & Panagos, J. (1980). Minicry versus imitative production in the speech of the retarded. *Journal of Psycholinguistic Research, 9,* 565–578.

Price, P. (1984). A study of mother-child interaction strategies with mothers of young developmentally delayed children. In J. Berg (Ed.), *Perspectives and progress in mental retardation*. Sixth Congress of the International Association for the Scientific Study of Mental Deficiency. Baltimore: University Park Press.

Prizant, B. M. (1983a). Echolalia in autism: Assessment and intervention. *Seminars in Speech and Language, 4,* 63–67.

Prizant, B. M. (1983b). Language acquisition and communicative behavior in autism: Toward an understanding of the "whole" of it. *Journal of Speech and Hearing Disorders, 46,* 241-249.

Prizant, B. M. (1984). Assessment and intervention of communication problems in children with autism. *Communication Disorders, 9,* 127–142.

Prizant, B. M., & Duchan, J. F. (1981). The functions of immediate echolalia in autistic children. *Journal of Speech and Hearing Disorders, 46,* 241-249.

Prizant, B. M., & Rentschler, G. (1983). Language-impaired children's use of language across three conversational situations. *Australian Journal of Human Communication Disorders, 11,* 5–16.

Prizant, B. M., & Rydell, P. (1984). An analysis of the functions of delayed echolalia in autistic children. *Journal of Speech and Hearing Disorders, 27,* 183–192.

Prizant, B. M., & Schuler, A. (1987). Facilitating communication: Language approaches. In D. Cohen & A. Donnellan (Eds.), *Handbook of autism and pervasive developmental disorders.* New York: John Wiley.

Prizant, B. M., & Wetherby, A. M. (1985). Intentional communicative behavior of children with autism: Theoretical and practical issues. *Australian Journal of Human Communication Disorders, 13* 23–59.

Prizant, B. M., & Wetherby, A. M. (1988a). Providing services to children with autism (ages 0 to 2 years) and their families. *Topics in Language Disorders, 9*(1), 1-23.

Prizant, B. M., & Wetherby, A. M. (1988b, October). *Toward early detection of communication problems in infants and toddlers.* Paper presented at the conference of the International Association of Infant Mental Health, Providence, RI.

Pruess, J., Vadasy, P., & Fewell, R. (1987). Language development in children with Down syndrome: An overview of recent research. *Education and Training of the Mentally Retarded, 22,* 44-55.

Prutting, C. A. (1979). Process \prâ\,ses\n: the action of moving forward progressively from one point to another on the way to completion. *Journal of Speech and Language Disorders, 44,* 3–30.

Prutting, C. A. (1982). Pragmatic and social competence. *Journal of Speech and Hearing Disorders, 42,* 123–134.

Prutting, C. A. (1983). Scientific inquiry and communicative disorders: An emerging paradigm across six decades. In T. Gallagher & C. Prutting (Eds.), *Prag-matic assessment and intervention issues in language* (pp. 247–267). San Diego: College-Hill.

Prutting, C. A., Bagshaw, N., Goldstein, H., Juskowitz, S., & Umen, I. (1978). Clinician-child discourse: Some preliminary questions. *Journal of Speech and Hearing Disorders, 43,* 123–139.

Prutting, C. A., & Connolly, J. (1976). Imitation: A closer look. *Journal of Speech and Hearing Disorders, 41,* 412–422.

Prutting, C. A., & Kirchner, D. M. (1983). Applied pragmatics. In T. M. Gallagher & C. A. Prutting (Eds.), *Pragmatic assessment and intervention issues in language* (pp. 29-64). Austin, TX: Pro-Ed.

Prutting, C. A., & Kirchner, D. M. (1987). A clinical appraisal of the pragmatic aspects of language. *Journal of Speech and Hearing Disorders, 52,* 105-119.

Purcell, S., & Liles, B. (1992). Cohesion repairs in the narratives of normal-language and language-impaired school-aged children. *Journal of Speech and Hearing Research, 35,* 354-362.

Pye, C. (1987). Pye Analysis of Language (PAL) [Computer program]. Lawrence: University of Kansas.

Randall-David, E. (1989). *Strategies for working with culturally diverse communities and clients.* Washington, DC: Association for the Care of Children's Health.

Raphael, T. S., & Englert, C. S. (1990). Reading and writing: Partners in constructing meaning. *The Reading Teacher, 43,* 388-400.

Rapin, I., & Allen, D. A. (1983). Developmental language disorders: Nosologic consideration. In U. Kirk (Ed.), *Neuropsychology of language, reading, and spelling* (pp. 155-184). New York: Academic Press.

Rapin, I., & Wilson, B. (1978). Children with developmental language disabilities: Neurological aspects and assessment. In M. Wyke (Ed.), *Developmental dysphasia* (pp. 13-41). New York: Academic Press.

Ratner, N., & Bruner, I. (1978). Games, social exchange and the acquisition of language. *Journal of Child Language, 5,* 391–402.

Ravn, K., & Gelman, S. (1984). Rule usage in children's understanding of "big" and little." *Child Development, 55,* 2141–2150.

Ray, S. (1989). Context and psychoeducational assessment of hearing impaired children. *Topics in Language Disorders, 9*(4), 33–44.

Reason, J., & Mycielska, K. (1982). *Absent-minded? The psychology of mental lapses and everyday errors.* Englewood Cliffs, NJ: Prentice-Hall.

Records, N. L., & Tomblin, J. B. (1994). Clinical decision making: Describing the decision rules of practicing speech–language pathologists. *Journal of Speech and Hearing Research, 37,* 144–156.

Reed, V. A. (1986). An overview of children's language disorders. In V. A. Reed (Ed.), *An introduction to chil-*

dren with language disorders (pp. 65-79). New York: Macmillan.

Rees, N. (1974). The speech pathologist and the reading process. *ASHA, 16,* 255–258.

Rees, N. (1978). Art and science of diagnosis in hearing, language, and speech. In S. Singh & J. Lynch (Eds.), *Diagnostic procedures in hearing, language, and speech* (pp. 3–22). Baltimore: University Park Press.

Rees, N., & Wollner, S. (1981, April). *PAPER'S TITLE?* Paper presented at the Annual Convention of the New York State Speech-Language-Hearing Association, Liberty.

Reich, P. (1986). *Language development.* Englewood Cliffs, NJ: Prentice-Hall.

Reichle, J. (1990, April). *Intervention with presymbolic clients: Setting up an initial communication system.* Paper presented at the Annual Convention of the New York State Speech-Language-Hearing Association, Kiamesha Lake.

Reichle, J., Busch, C., & Doyle, S. (1986). The topical relationship among adjacent utterances in productively delayed children's language addressed to their mothers. *Journal of Communication Disorders, 19,* 63–74.

Reichle, J., & Karlan, G. (1985). The selection of an augmentative system in communication intervention: A critique of decision rules. *Journal of the Association for Persons with Severe Handicaps, 10,* 146-156.

Reichle, J., Piche-Cragoe, L., Sigafoos, J., & Doss, S. (1988). Optimizing functional communication for persons with severe handicaps. In S. Calculator & J. Bedrosian (Eds.), *Communication assessment and intervention for adults with mental retardation* (pp. 239–264). San Diego: College-Hill.

Reichle, J., Rogers, N., & Barrett, C. (1984). Establishing pragmatic discriminations among the communicative functions of requesting, rejecting, and commenting in an adolescent. *Journal of the Association for Persons with Severe Handicaps, 9,* 31–36.

Reichle, J., & Yoder, D. (1985). Communication board use in severely handicapped learners. *Language, Speech, and Hearing Services in Schools, 16,* 58–63.

Reid, G. (1980). Overt and covert rehearsal in short-term motor memory of mentally retarded and nonretarded persons. *American Journal of Mental Deficiency, 85,* 69-77.

Rein, R., & Kernan, C. (1989). The functional use of verbal perseveratives by adults who are mentally retarded. *Education and Training in Mental Retardation, 24,* 381-389.

Remington, B., & Clarke, S. (1983). Acquisition of expressive signing by autistic children: An evaluation of the relative effects of simultaneous communication and sign-alone training. *Journal of Applied Behavior Analysis, 16,* 315-328.

Remington, B., & Clarke, S. (1993a). Simultaneous communication and speech comprehension. Part I: Comparison of two methods of teaching expressive signing and speech comprehension skills. *Augmentative and Alternative Communication, 9,* 36-48.

Remington, B., & Clarke, S. (1993b). Simultaneous communication and speech comprehension. Part II: Comparison of two methods of overcoming selective attention during expressive sign training. *Augmentative and Alternative Communication, 9,* 49-60.

Rentel, V. M., & King, M. L. (1983). Present at the beginning. In P. Mosenthal, L. Tamor, & S. A. Walmsley (Eds.), *Research on writing: Principles and methods* (pp. 139–176). New York: Longman.

Rescorla, L. (1989). The Language Development Survey: A screening tool for delayed language in toddlers. *Journal of Speech and Hearing Disorders, 54,* 587-599.

Rescorla, L. (1990, June). *Outcomes of expressive language delay.* Paper presented at the Symposium for Research in Child Language Disorders, Madison, WI.

Rescorla, L. (1991). Identifying expressive language delay at age two. *Topics in Language Disorders, 11*(4), 14-20.

Rescorla, L., & Goossens, M. (1992). Symbolic play development in toddlers with expressive specific language impairment (SLI-E). *Journal of Speech and Hearing Research, 35,* 1290-1302.

Rescorla, L., & Schwartz, E. (1988). *Outcome of specific expressive language delay (SELD).* Paper presented at the Sixth International Conference on Infant Studies, Washington, DC.

Restak, R. M. (1979). *The brain: The last frontier.* New York: Warner.

Reutzel, D. R. (1985). Story maps improve comprehension. *The Reading Teacher, 38,* 400-404.

Reutzel, D. R., & Hollingsworth, P. M. (1988). Whole language and the practitioner. *Academic Therapy, 23,* 405-416.

Rhodes, L. K., & Dudley-Marling, C. (1988). *Readers and writers with a difference: A holistic approach to teaching learning disabled and remedial students.* Portsmouth, NH: Heinemann.

Ribowsky, H. (1986). *The comparative effects of a code emphasis approach and a whole language approach upon emerging literacy of kindergarten children.* Unpublished doctoral dissertation, New York University, New York.

Rice, M. L. (1983). Contemporary accounts of the cognitive/language relationship: Implications for speech-language clinicians. *Journal of Speech and Hearing Disorders, 48,* 347–359.

Rice, M. L. (1984). Cognitive aspects of communication development. In R. Schiefelbusch & J. Pickar (Eds.),

The acquisition of communicative competence (pp. 141–189). Baltimore: University Park Press.

Rice, M. L. (1986). Mismatched premises of the communicative competence model and language intervention. In R. Schiefelbusch (Ed.), *Language competence: Assessment and intervention* (pp. 261–281). San Diego: College-Hill.

Rice, M. L., Buhr, J. C., & Nemeth, M. (1990). Fast-mapping word-learning abilities of language-delayed preschoolers. *Journal of Speech and Hearing Disorders, 55,* 33-42.

Rice, M. L., Buhr, J., & Oetting, J. B. (1992). Speech-language-impaired children's quick incidental learning of words: The effect of a pause. *Journal of Speech and Language Research, 35,* 1040-1048.

Rice, M. L., & Oetting, J. B. (1993). Morphological deficits of children with SLI: Evaluation of number marking and agreement. *Journal of Speech and Hearing Research, 36,* 1249–1257.

Rice, M. L., Oetting, J. B., Marquis, J., Bode, J., & Pae, S. (1994). Frequency of input effects on word comprehension of children with specific language impairment. *Journal of Speech and Hearing Research, 37,* 106–122.

Rice, M. L., Sell, M. A., & Hadley, P. A. (1990). The Social Interactive Coding System (SICS): An on-line, clinically relevant descriptive tool. *Language, Speech, and Hearing Services in Schools, 21,* 2–14.

Rice, M. L., Snell, M. H., & Hadley, P. A. (1991). Social interactions of speech and language-impaired children. *Journal of Speech and Hearing Research, 34,* 1299-1307.

Richards, M. (1979). Sorting out what's in a word from what's not: Evaluating Clark's semantic feature acquisition theory. *Journal of Experimental Child Psychology, 27,* 1–47.

Richgels, D., McGee, D., Lomax, R., & Sheard, C. (1987). Awareness of four text structures: Effects on recall of expository text. *Reading Research Quarterly, 22,* 177-196.

Rie, E., & Rie, H. (1977). Recall, retention, and Ritalin. *Journal of Consulting and Clinical Psychology, 45,* 967-972.

Rie, H., Rie, E., & Stewart, S. (1976). Effects of methylphenidate on underachieving children. *Journal of Consulting and Clinical Psychology, 44,* 250–260.

Rieke, J., & Lewis, J. (1984). Preschool intervention strategies: The communication base. *Topics in Language Disorders, 5*(1), 41–57.

Riley, A. (1984). *Evaluating acquired skills in communication.* Tucson, AZ: Communication Skill Builders.

Rinehart, S. D., Stahl, S. A., & Erickson, L. G. (1986). Some effects of summarization training on reading and studying. *Reading Research Quarterly, 12,* 422-438.

Ripich, D., & Griffith, P. (1985, November). *Story structure, cohesion, and propositions in learning disabled children.* Paper presented at the Annual Convention of the American Speech-Language-Hearing Association, Washington, DC.

Ripich, D., & Panagos, J. (1985). Assessing children's knowledge of sociolinguistic rules for speech therapy lessons. *Journal of Speech and Hearing Disorders, 50,* 335–345.

Ripich, D., & Spinelli, F. (1985). *School discourse strategies.* San Diego: College-Hill.

Ritvo, E. R., & Freeman, B. J. (1978). National Society for Autistic Children definition of the syndrome of autism. *Journal of Autism and Childhood Schizophrenia, 8,* 162-167.

Rizzo, J. M., & Stephens, M. I. (1981). Performance of children with normal and impaired oral language production on a set of auditory comprehension tests. *Journal of Speech and Hearing Disorders, 46,* 150-159.

Roberts, K. (1983). Comprehension and production of word order in stage I. *Child Development, 54,* 443-449.

Roberts, K., & Horowitz, F. (1986). Basic level categorization in seven- and nine-month-old infants. *Journal of Child Language, 13,* 191–208.

Robertson, S., & Suci, G. (1980). Event perception by children in the early stage of language production. *Child Development, 51,* 89–96.

Robinson, L. A., & Owens, R. E. (in press). Functional augmentative communication and positive behavior change: A case study. *Augmentative and Alternative Communication.*

Rodgon, M., Jankowski, W., & Alenskas, L. (1977). A multi-functional approach to single-word usage. *Journal of Child Language, 4,* 23–43.

Rodino, A. M., Gimbert, C., Perez, C., Craddock-Willis, K., & McCabe, A. (1992, October). *"Getting your point across": Contractive sequencing in low-income African American and Latino children's personal narratives.* Paper presented at the 16th Annual Boston University Conference on Language Development, Boston.

Rodriguez, R., Prieto, A., & Rueda, R. (1984). Issues in bilingual multicultural special education. *NABE Journal, 8,* 55–66.

Rogers, S., D'Eugenio, D., Brown, S., Donovan, C., & Lynch, E. (1978). Early Intervention Developmental Profile. Ann Arbor: University of Michigan Press.

Rogers-Warren, A., & Warren, S. (1985). Mands for verbalization: Facilitating the display of newly trained language in children. *Behavior Modification, 4,* 361-382.

Roller, E., Rodriguez, T., Warner, J., & Lindahl, P. (1992). Integration of self-contained children with severe speech-language needs into the regular education classroom. *Language, Speech, and Hearing Services in Schools, 23,* 365-366.

Rom, A., & Leonard, L. B. (1990). Interpreting deficits in grammatical morphology in specific language-impaired children: Preliminary evidence from Hebrew. *Clinical Linguistics and Phonetics, 4,* 95-105.

Romer, L., & Schoenberg, B. (1991). Increasing requests made by people with developmental disabilities and deaf-blindness through the use of behavior interruption strategies. *Education and Training in Mental Retardation, 26,* 70-78.

Romski, M., & Sevcik, R. (1989). An analysis of visual-graphic symbol meanings for two non-speaking adults with severe mental retardation. *Augmentative and Alternative Communication, 5,* 109–144.

Romski, M., Sevcik, R., & Joyner, S. (1984). Nonspeech communication systems: Implications for language intervention with mentally retarded children. *Topics in Language Disorders, 5,* 66–81.

Romski, M., Sevcik, R., & Pate, J. (1988). Establishment of symbolic communication in persons with severe retardation. *Journal of Speech and Hearing Disorders, 53,* 94–107.

Romski, M., White, R., Millen, C., & Rumbaugh, D. (1984). Effects of computer-keyboard teaching in symbolic communication of severely retarded persons: Five case studies. *The Psychological Record, 34,* 39–51.

Rondal, J. (1978). Maternal speech to normal and Down's syndrome children matched for mean length of utterances. In C. Meyers (Ed.), *Quality of life in severely and profoundly mentally retarded people* (pp. 193–265). Washington, DC: American Association on Mental Deficiency.

Rondal, J., Ghiotto, M., Bredart, S., & Bachelet, J. (1987). Age-relation, reliability, and grammatical validity of measures of utterance length. *Journal of Child Language, 14,* 433–446.

Rondal, J., Ghiotto, M., Bredart, S., & Bachelet, J. (1988). Mean length of utterance of children with Down syndrome. *American Journal of Mental Deficiency, 93,* 64-66.

Roseberry, C., & Connell, P. (1991). The use of an invented language rule in the differentiation of normal and language–impaired Spanish–speaking children. *Journal of Speech and Hearing Research, 34,* 596–603.

Rosegrant, T. J. (1985). Using the microcomputer as a tool for learning to read and write. *Journal of Learning Disabilities, 18,* 113–115.

Rosegrant, T. J., & Cooper, W. (1987). Talking Text Writer [Computer program]. New York: Scholastic.

Rosen, C. & Gerring, J. (1986). *Head trauma: Educational reintegration.* San Diego: College-Hill.

Rosenthal, J. H. (1970). A preliminary psycholinguistic study of children with learning disabilities. *Journal of Learning Disabilities, 3,* 391–395.

Rosier, P., & Farella, M. (1976). Bilingual education at Rock Point—Some early results. *TESOL Quarterly, 10,* 379-388.

Rosin, M., Swift, E., Bless, D., & Vetter, D. (1988). Communication profiles of adolescents with Down syndrome. *Journal of Childhood Communication Disorders, 12,* 49-64.

Rosinski-McClendon, M., & Newhoff, M. (1987). Conversational responsiveness and assertiveness in language-impaired children. *Language, Speech, and Hearing Services in Schools, 18,* 53–62.

Ross, B. L. (1989). *The impact of individual differences in scripts memory for script-related stories.* Unpublished master's thesis, University of Utah, Salt Lake City.

Ross, B. L., & Berg, C. A. (1989). *The use of personal scripts in remembering new events across adulthood.* Paper presented at the meeting of the Society for Research in Child Development, Kansas City, MO.

Ross, B. L., & Berg, C. A. (1990). Individual differences in script reports: Implications for language assessment. *Topics in Language Disorders, 10*(3), 30-44.

Ross, D., & Ross, S. (1979). Cognitive training for the EMR child: Language skills prerequisite to relevant-irrelevant discrimination tasks. *Mental Retardation, 17,* 3-7.

Rossetti, L. M. (1990). Rossetti Infant–Toddler Language Scale. East Moline, IL: LinguiSystems.

Roth, F. (1986). Oral narrative abilities of learning-disabled students. *Topics in Language Disorders, 7*(1), 1–30.

Roth, F., & Spekman, N. (1984a). Assessing the pragmatic abilities of children: Part 1. Organizational framework and assessment parameters. *Journal of Speech and Hearing Disorders, 49,* 2–11.

Roth, F., & Spekman, N. (1984b). Assessing the pragmatic abilities of children: Part 2. Guidelines, considerations, and specific evaluation procedures. *Journal of Speech and Hearing Disorders, 49,* 12–17.

Roth, F., & Spekman, N. (1985, June). *Story grammar analysis of narratives produced by learning disabled and normally achieving students.* Paper presented at the Symposium on Research in Child Language Disorders, Madison, WI.

Roth, F., & Spekman, N. (1986). Narrative discourse: Spontaneously generated stories of learning-disabled and normally achieving students. *Journal of Speech and Hearing Disorders, 51,* 8–23.

Roth, F., & Spekman, N. (1989a). Higher order language processing and reading disabilities. In A. Kamhi & H. Catts (Eds.), *Reading disabilities: A developmental language perspective.* San Diego: College-Hill.

Roth, F., & Spekman, N. (1989b). The oral syntactic proficiency of learning disabled students: A spontaneous story sampling analysis. *Journal of Speech and Hearing Research, 32,* 67–77.

Roth, F. P., & Clark, D. M. (1987). Symbolic play and social participation abilities of language-impaired and normally developing children. *Journal of Speech and Hearing Disorders, 52,* 17-29.

Roth, P. (1987). Temporal characteristics of maternal verbal styles. In K. E. Nelson & A. van Kleeck (Eds.), *Children's language* (Vol. 6). Hillsdale, NJ: Lawrence Erlbaum.

Rotholz, D. A., Berkowitz, S. F., & Burberry, J. (1989). Functionality of two modes of communication in the community by students with developmental disabilities: A comparison of signing and communication books. *Journal of the Association for Persons with Severe Handicaps, 14,* 227-233.

Rowland, C., & Schweigert, P. (1989a). Tangible symbols: Symbolic communication for individuals with multisensory impairments. *Augmentative and Alternative Communication, 5,* 226–234.

Rowland, C., & Schweigert, P. (1989b). *Tangible symbol systems for individuals with multisensory impairments* [Videotape and manual]. Tucson, AZ: Communication Skill Builders.

Rubin, H. (1988). Morphological knowledge and early writing ability. *Language and Speech, 31,* 337-355.

Rubin, H., Patterson, P. A., & Kantor, M. (1991). Morphological development and writing ability in children and adults. *Language, Speech, and Hearing Services in Schools, 22,* 228-235.

Rudel, R., Denckla, M., Broman, M., & Hirsch, S. (1980). Word-finding as a function of stimulus context: Children compared with aphasic adults. *Brain and Language, 10,* 111-119.

Ruder, K., Smith, J., & Hermann, P. (1974). Effect of verbal imitation and comprehension on verbal production of lexical items. *ASHA Monographs, 18,* 15–29.

Rumelhart, D. (1975). Notes on a schema for stories. In D. Bobrow & A. Collins (Eds.), *Representation and understanding: Studies in cognitive science* (pp. 211–236). New York: Academic Press.

Rumelhart, D. E. (1984). Understanding understanding. In J. Flood (Ed.), *Understanding reading comprehension: Cognition, language, and the structure of prose* (pp. 1–20). Newark, DE: International Reading Association.

Rumelhart, D. E., McClelland, J., & PDP Research Group. (1986). *Parallel distributed processing: Explorations in the microstructure of cognition.* Cambridge: MIT Press.

Rumelhart, D. E., & Ortony, A. (1977). The representation of knowledge in memory. In R. C. Anderson, R.

J. Spiro, & W. E. Montague (Eds.), *Schooling and the acquisition of knowledge* (pp. 99–135). Hillsdale, NJ: Lawrence Erlbaum.

Rumsey, J. M., Rapoport, M. D., & Sceery, W. R. (1985). Autistic children as adults: Psychiatric, social, and behavioral outcomes. *Journal of the American Academy of Child Psychiatry, 24,* 465-473.

Ruscello, D. M., St. Louis, K. O., & Mason, N. (1991). School-aged children with phonologic disorders: Coexistence with other speech-language disorders. *Journal of Speech and Hearing Research, 34,* 236-242.

Russell, N. (1993). Educational considerations in traumatic brain injury: The role of the speech-language pathologist. *Language, Speech, and Hearing Services in Schools, 24,* 67-75.

Russell, S. C., & Kaderavek, J. N. (1993). Alternative models for collaboration. *Language, Speech, and Hearing Services in Schools, 24,* 76–78.

Russo, J., & Owens, R. (1982). Development of an objective observation tool for parent-child interaction. *Journal of Speech and Hearing Disorders, 47,* 165–173.

Rutherford, D., & Tesler, E. (1971). *The Word Literacy Test.* Paper presented to the Association for Children and Adults with Learning Disabilities, Chicago.

Rutter, M. (1985). Infantile autism and other pervasive disorders. In M. Rutter & L. Hersov (Eds.), *Child and adolescent psychiatry: Modern approaches* (pp. 545–566). London: Blackwell.

Sabin, E., Clemmer, E., O'Connell, D., & Kowal, S. (1979). A pausological approach to speech development. In A. Siegman & S. Feldstein (Eds.), *Of speech and time* (pp. 35–55). Hillsdale, NJ: Lawrence Erlbaum.

Sachs, J. (1983). Talking about the there and then: The emergence of displaced reference in parent-child discourse. In K. Nelson (Ed.), *Children's language* (Vol. 4). Hillsdale, NJ: Lawrence Erlbaum.

Sacks, H., Schegloff, E., & Jefferson, G. (1974). A simplest systematics for the organization of turn-taking in conversation. *Language, 50,* 696–735.

Sacks, J., & Young, E. (1982). Infant Scale of Communication Intent. *Pediatrics Update, 7,* 1–5.

Salvia, J., & Ysseldyke, J. (1988). *Assessment in special and remedial education* (4th ed.). Boston: Houghton Mifflin.

Salzberg, C., & Villani, T. (1983). Speech training by parents of Down syndrome toddlers: Generalization across settings and instructional contexts. *Journal of Mental Deficiency, 87,* 403–413.

Salzinger, S., Feldman, R. S., Hammer, M., & Rosario, M. (1991). Risk for physical child abuse and the personal consequences for its victims. *Criminal Justice and Behavior, 18,* 64-81.

Sameroff, A., & Chandler, M. (1975). Reproductive risk and the continuum of caretaking causality. In F. Horowitz, M. Hetherington, F. Scarr-Salapatek, & G. Siegel (Eds.), *Review of child development research* (Vol. 4, pp. 187–244). Chicago: University of Chicago Press.

Sameroff, A., & Feise, B. (1990). Transactional regulation and early intervention. In S. Meisels & P. Shonkoff (Eds.), *Early intervention: Handbook of early childhood intervention.* New York: Cambridge University Press.

Samuels, S. (1983). Diagnosing reading problems. *Journal of Learning and Learning Disabilities, 2*(4), 1–11.

Sanchez, R. (1983). *Chicano discourse.* Rowley, MA: Newbury House.

Sanders, J. (1986). *Microcomputer applications for speech-language services in the schools.* San Diego: College-Hill.

Sandoval-Martinez, S. (1982). Findings from the Head Start Bilingual Curriculum Development and Evaluation Report. *National Association for Bilingual Education Journal, 7,* 1-12.

Sarno, M. T. (1980). Nature of verbal impairment after closed head injury. *Journal of Nervous and Mental Disorders, 160,* 685-692.

Sarno, M. T., Buonaguro, A., & Levita, E. (1986). Characteristics of verbal impairment in closed head injured patients. *Archives of Physical Medicine and Rehabilitation, 67,* 400-405.

Sattler, J. M. (1988). *Assessment of children* (3rd ed.). San Diego: Author.

Satz, P., & Bullard-Bates, C. (1981). Acquired aphasia in children. In M. T. Sarno (Ed.), *Acquired aphasia* (pp. 399-426). New York: Academic Press.

Saunders, K., & Spradlin, J. (1989). Conditional discrimination in mentally retarded adults: The effect of training the component simple discriminations. *Journal of the Experimental Analysis of Behavior, 52,* 1-12.

Saunders, R., & Sailor, W. (1979). A comparison of three strategies of reinforcement on two-choice learning problems with severely retarded children. *AAESPH Review, 4,* 323-333.

Savage, R. (1991). Identification, classification, and placement issues for students with traumatic brain injury. *Journal of Head Trauma Rehabilitation, 6,* 1-9.

Savage, R., & Wolcott, G. (1988). *An educator's manual: What educators need to know about students with traumatic brain injury.* Southborough, MA: National Head Injury Foundation.

Saville-Troike, M. (1986). Anthropological considerations in the study of communication. In O. L. Taylor (Ed.), *Nature of communication disorders in culturally and lingually diverse populations* (pp. 47-72). San Diego: College-Hill.

Sawyer, D. (1981). The relationship between selected auditory abilities and beginning reading achievement. *Language, Speech, and Hearing Services in Schools, 12,* 95–99.

Sawyer, D. (1987). Test of Awareness of Language Segments. Rockville, MD: Aspen.

Sawyer, D. J. (1991). Whole language in context: Insights into the current great debate. *Topics in Language Disorders, 11*(3), 1-13.

Sawyer, J. (1973). Social aspects of bilingualism in San Antonio, Texas. In R. Bailey & J. Robinson (Eds.), *Varieties of present-day English* (pp. 226–235). New York: Macmillan.

Scarborough, H., & Dobrich, W. (1990). Development of children with early language delay. *Journal of Speech and Hearing Research, 33,* 70-83.

Scarborough, H., Wycokoff, J., & Davidson, R. (1986). A reconsideration of the relationship between age and mean utterance length. *Journal of Speech and Hearing Research, 29,* 394–399.

Schank, R. C., & Abelson, R. (1977). *Scripts, plans, goals, and understanding.* Hillsdale, NJ: Lawrence Erlbaum.

Schegloff, E. A., & Sacks, H. (1973). Opening up closings. *Semiotica, 4,* 289-327.

Scherer, N., & Olswang, L. (1989). Using structured discourse as a language intervention technique with autistic children. *Journal of Speech and Hearing Disorders, 54,* 383–394.

Scherer, N., & Owings, N. (1982, November). *Mothers' role in conversational exchanges with retarded children.* Paper presented at the Annual Convention of the American Speech-Language-Hearing Association, Toronto.

Schery, T., & O'Connor, L. (1992). The effectiveness of school-based computer language intervention with severely handicapped children. *Language, Speech, and Hearing Services in Schools, 23,* 43-47.

Schetz, K. (1989). Computer-aided language/concept enrichment in kindergarten: Consultation program model. *Language, Speech, and Hearing Services in Schools, 20,* 2–10.

Schieffelin, B. B., & Eisenberg, A. R. (1984). Cultural variations in children's conversations. In R. L. Schiefelbusch & J. Pickar (Eds.), *The acquisition of communicative competence* (pp. 377-422). Baltimore: University Park Press.

Schiff-Myers, N. (1992). Considering arrested language development and language loss in the assessment of second language learners. *Language, Speech, and Hearing Services in Schools, 23,* 28-33.

Schiff-Myers, N., Coury, J., & Perez, D. (1989, May). *A "bilingual" evaluation of a bilingual child: How necessary is it?* Paper presented at the Annual Convention of the New Jersey Speech-Language-Hearing Association, Parsippany.

Schmauch, V., Panagos, J., & Klich, P. (1978). Syntax influences and accuracy of consonant production in language-disordered children. *Journal of Communication Disorders, 11,* 315–323.

Schmidt, H. D., & Rodgers-Rhyme, A. (1988). *Strategies: Effective practices for teaching all children.* Madison: Wisconsin State Department of Public Instruction, Bureau of Exceptional Children.

Schober-Peterson, D., & Johnson, C. (1989). Conversational topics of 4-year-olds. *Journal of Speech and Hearing Research, 32,* 857–870.

Schodorf, J. (1982). A comparative analysis of parent-child interactions of language-delayed and linguistically normal children. *Dissertation Abstracts International, 42*(5), 1838B.

Schopler, E., & Mesibov, G. (1987). *Neurobiological issues in autism.* New York: Plenum.

Schreibman, L. (1988). *Developmental clinical psychology and psychiatry. Vol. 15: Autism.* Newbury Park, CA: Sage.

Schreibman, L., & Carr, E. (1978). Elimination of echolalic responding to questions through the training of a generalized verbal response. *Journal of Applied Behavioral Analysis, 11,* 453–463.

Schubel, R., & Erickson, J. (1992). Model programs for increasing parent involvement through telephone technology. *Language, Speech, and Hearing Services in Schools, 23,* 125-129.

Schuler, A. L., & Goetz, C. (1981). The assessment of severe language disabilities: Communicative and cognitive considerations. *Analysis and Intervention in Developmental Disabilities, 1,* 333–346.

Schuler, A. L., & Prizant, B. M. (1987). Facilitating language: Prelanguage approaches. In D. J. Cohen & A. M. Donnellan (Eds.), *Handbook of autism and pervasive developmental disorders* (pp. 301-315). New York: John Wiley.

Schultz, M. M. (1986). *The semantic organizer: A prewriting strategy for first grade students.* Unpublished doctoral dissertation, University of Connecticut, Storrs.

Schumaker, J., & Deshler, D. (1984). Setting demand variables. *Topics in Language Disorders, 4*(2), 22–40.

Schumaker, J., & Deshler, D. (1988). Implementing the Regular Education Initiative in secondary schools: A different ball game. *Journal of Learning Disabilities, 21,* 36-42.

Schumaker, J., Deshler, D., Alley, G., Warner, M., & Denton, P. (1984). Multipass. A learning strategy for improving reading comprehension. *Learning Disability Quarterly, 5,* 295-304.

Schwartz, L., & McKinley, N. (1984). *Daily communication: Strategies for the language disordered adolescent.* Eau Claire, WI: Thinking Publications.

Schwartz, R. (1992). Clinical applications of recent advances in phonetics theory. *Language, Speech, and Hearing Services in Schools, 23,* 269-276.

Schwartz, R., Chapman, K., Terrell, B., Prelock, P., & Rowan, L. (1985). Facilitating word combination in language-impaired children in discourse structure. *Journal of Speech and Hearing Disorders, 50,* 31–39.

Schwejda, P. (1986). Predictive Linguistic Program: Development Copy. Version 1. 6.86 [Computer program]. Adaptive Peripherals.

Scollon, R. (1979). A real early stage: An unzipped condensation of a dissertation on child language. In E. Ochs & V. Schiesselin (Eds.), *Developmental pragmatics* (pp. 215–227). New York: Academic Press.

Scollon, R., & Scollon, S. B. K. (1979). *Linguistic convergence: An ethnography of speaking at Fort Chipewyan.* Alberta, Canada: Academic Press.

Scollon, R., & Scollon, S. B. K. (1981). *Narrative, literacy, and face in interethnic communication.* Norwood, NJ: Ablex.

Scott, C. M. (1984a). Adverbial connectivity in conversations of children 6 to 12. *Journal of Communication and Language, 11,* 423-452.

Scott, C. M. (1984b, November). *What happened in that: Structural characteristics of school children's narratives.* Paper presented at the Annual Convention of the American Speech-Language-Hearing Association, San Francisco.

Scott, C. M. (1987). *Summarizing text: Context effects in language disordered children.* Paper presented at the First International Symposium, Specific Language Disorders in Children, University of Reading, England.

Scott, C. M. (1988a). Producing complex sentences. *Topics in Language Disorders, 8*(2), 44–62.

Scott, C. M. (1988b). A perspective on the evaluation of school children's narratives. *Speech, Language, and Hearing Services in Schools, 19,* 67–82.

Scott, C. M., & Erwin, D. L. (1992). Descriptive assessment of writing: Process and products. *Best Practices in School Speech-Language Pathology, 2,* 87-98.

Scott, C. M., Nippold, M. A., Norris, J. A., & Johnson, C. J. (1992, November) *School-age children and adolescents: Establishing language norms.* Paper presented at the Annual Convention of the American Speech-Language-Hearing Association, San Antonio.

Scott, C. M., & Rush, D. (1985). Teaching adverbial connectivity: Implications from current research. *Child Language Teaching and Therapy, 1,* 264-280.

Scoville, R. (1983). Development of the intention to communicate: The eye of the beholder. In L. Feagans, C. Garvey, & R. Golinkoff (Eds.), *The origins and growth of communication* (pp. 109–122). Norwood, NJ: Ablex.

Segal, E., Duchan, J., & Scott, P. (1991). The role of interclausal connectives in narrative structuring: Evidence from adults' interpretations of simple stories. *Discourse Processes, 14,* 27-54.

Seidenberg, P. L. (1988). Cognitive and academic instructional intervention for learning disabled adolescents. *Topics in Language Disorders, 8*(3), 56-71.

Seidenberg, P. L. (1989). Relating text-processing research to reading and writing instruction for learning disabled students. *Learning Disabilities Focus, 5,* 4-12.

Seidenberg, P. L., & Bernstein. D. K. (1986). The comprehension of similes and metaphors by learning-disabled and nonlearning-disabled children. *Language, Speech, and Hearing Services in Schools, 17,* 219-229.

Seitz, S. (1975). Language intervention—Changing the language environment of the retarded child. In R. Koch, F. de la Cruz, & F. Menolascino (Eds.), *Down's syndrome: Research, prevention and management* (pp. 157–179). New York: Bruner/Mazel.

Seitz, S., & Reidell, G. (1974). Parent-child interactions as the therapy target. *Journal of Communication Disorders, 7,* 295-304.

Seliger, H. W. (1982). Testing authentic language: The problem of meaning. *Language Testing, 2,* 60-73.

Seligman, M. E. (1975). *Helplessness: On depression, development, and death.* New York: Freeman.

Selinker, L., Swain, M., & Dumas, G. (1975). The interlanguage hypothesis extended to children. *Language Learning, 25,* 139–152.

Selman, R. L., Beardslee, W., Schultz, L. H., Krupa, M., & Podorefsky, D. (1986). Assessing adolescent interpersonal negotiation strategies: Toward the integration of structural and functional models. *Developmental Psychology, 22,* 450-459.

Selman, R. L., & Bryne, D. F. (1976). A structural-developmental analysis of levels of role taking in middle childhood. *Child Development, 45,* 803-806.

Semel, E., & Wiig, E. (1980). *Clinical evaluation of language functions.* San Antonio: Psychological Corp.

Semel, E., Wiig, E., & Secord, W. (1987). Clinical Evaluation of Language Fundamentals—Revised. San Antonio: Psychological Corp.

Semmel, M. (1967). Language behavior of mentally retarded and culturally disadvantaged children. In J. Magary & R. McIntyre (Eds.), *Distinguished lectures in special education.* Berkeley: University of California.

Semmel, M., & Herzog, B. (1966). The effects of grammatical form class on the recall of Negro and Caucasian educable retarded children. *Studies of Language and Language Behavior, 3,* 1-9.

Semmel, M., Peck, C., Haring, T., & Theimer, K. (1984, April). *Assessment and training of social/communicative skills for children with autism and severe handicaps.* Paper presented at the Annual Convention of the Council for Exceptional Children, Washington, DC.

Sena, R., & Smith, L. (1990). New evidence on the development of the *big. Child Development, 61,* 1034-1052.

Sevcik, R. A., & Romski, M. A. (1986). Representational matching skills of persons with severe retardation. *Augmentative and Alternative Communication, 2,* 160–164.

Sevcik, R. A., Romski, M. A., & Wilkinson, K. M. (1991). Roles of graphic symbols in the language acquisition process for persons with severe cognitive disabilities. *Augmentative and Alternative Communication, 7,* 161-170.

Sewell, T. E. (1987). Dynamic assessment as a nondiscriminatory procedure. In C. Schneider Lidz (Ed.), *Dynamic assessment: An interactional approach to evaluating learning potential* (pp. 426–443). New York: Guilford.

Seymour, H. (1992). The invisible children: A reply to Lahey's perspective. *Journal of Speech and Hearing Research, 35,* 640-641.

Seymour, H., Ashton, N., & Wheeler, L. (1986). The effect of race on language elicitation. *Language, Speech, and Hearing Services in Schools, 17,* 146–151.

Seymour, S. (1981). Cooperation and competition: Some issues and problems in cross cultural analysis. In R. Monroe & B. Whiting (Eds.), *Handbook of cross cultural human development* (pp. 717–738). New York: Garland.

Shadden, B. B. (1992, March). *Discourse analysis procedures used with adults.* Paper presented at the Conference on Pragmatics: From Theory to Therapy, State University of New York, Buffalo.

Shaffer, D., Bijur, P., Chadwick, O. F., & Rutter, M. (1980). Head injury and later reading disability. *Journal of the American Academy of Child Psychiatry, 19,* 592-610.

Shane, H., & Bashir, A. (1980). Election criteria for the adoption of an augmentative communication system: Preliminary considerations. *Journal of Speech and Hearing Disorders, 45,* 408–414.

Shane, H., Lipshultz, R., & Shane, C. (1982). Facilitating the communicative interaction of non-speaking persons in large residential settings. *Topics in Language Disorders, 2,* 73–84.

Shantz, C. U., & Wilson, K. (1972). Training communication skills in young children. *Child Development, 43,* 118–122.

Shapiro, H. R. (1992). Debatable issues underlying whole-language philosophy: A speech-language pathologist's perspective. *Language, Speech, and Hearing Services in Schools, 23,* 308-311.

Shatz, M. (1978). The relationship between cognitive processes and the development of communication skills. In B. Keasey (Ed.), *Nebraska Symposium on Motivation, 1977* (pp. 1–42). Lincoln: University of Nebraska Press.

Shearer, W. M. (1984). Academic and instructional applications for microcomputers. In A. H. Schwartz

(Ed.), *The handbook of microcomputer applications in communication disorders* (pp. 193-218). San Diego: College-Hill.

Shelton, B., Gast, D., Wolery, M., & Winterling, V. (1991). The role of small group instruction in facilitating observational and incidental learning. *Language, Speech, and Hearing Services in School, 22,* 123-133.

Shelton, R., Spier, C., & Lewis, M. (1984). Misunderstanding of children's speech: Its relationship to articulatory change. *Human Communication, 8,* 1-11.

Shevin, M., & Klein, M. (1984). The importance of choice-making skills for students with severe disabilities. *Journal of the Association for Persons with Severe Handicaps, 9,* 159–166.

Shewan, C. (1988). 1988 omnibus survey: Adaptation and progress in times of change. *Asha, 30*(8), 27–30.

Shewan, C., & Malm, K. (1987). The status of multilingual/multicultural service issues among ASHA members. *Asha, 31,*(9), 78.

Shipley, K., & Banis, C. (1989). *Teaching morphology developmentally* (rev. ed.). Tucson, AZ: Communication Skill Builders.

Shipley, K., Maddox, M., & Driver, J. (1991). Children's development of irregular past tense verb forms. *Language, Speech, and Hearing Services in Schools, 22,* 115-122.

Shohamy, E., & Reves, T. (1982). Authentic language tests: Where from and where to? *Language Testing, 2,* 48-59.

Shriberg, L. D. (1983). Natural phonologic process approach. In W. Perkins (Ed.), *Current therapy of communication disorders: Phonologic-articulatory disorders* (pp. 3–10). New York: Thieme-Stratton.

Shriberg, L. D. (1986). Program to Examine Phonetic and Phonologic Evaluation Records (PEPPER) Version 4.0 [Computer program]. Madison: University of Wisconsin.

Shriberg, L. D. (1993). Four new speech and prosody-voice measures for genetics research and other studies of developmental phonological disorders. *Journal of Speech and Hearing Research, 36,* 105-140.

Shriberg, L. D., & Kwiatkowski, J. (1980). *Natural process analysis: A procedure for phonological analysis of continuous speech samples.* New York: John Wiley.

Shriberg, L. D., & Kwiatkowski, J. (1982). Phonological disorders III: A procedure for assessing severity of involvement. *Journal of Speech and Hearing Disorders, 47,* 256-270.

Shriberg, L. D., & Kwiatkowski, J. (1985). Continuous speech sampling for phonologic analysis of speech-delayed children. *Journal of Speech and Hearing Disorders, 50,* 323–334.

Shriberg, L. D., Kwiatkowski, J., Best, S., Hengst, J., & Terselic-Weber, B. (1986). Characteristics of children with speech delays of unknown origin. *Journal of Speech and Hearing Disorders, 51,* 140-161.

Shriberg, L. D., Kwiatkowski, J., & Snyder, T. (1989). Tabletop versus microcomputer-assisted speech management: Stabilization phase. *Journal of Speech and Hearing Disorders, 54* 233–248.

Shriberg, L. D., & Widder, C. (1990). Speech and prosody characteristics of adults with mental retardation. *Journal of Speech and Hearing Research, 33,* 627-653.

Shriner, T. H., Holloway, M. S., & Daniloff, R. C. (1969). The relationship between articulatory deficits and syntax in speech-defective children. *Journal of Speech and Hearing Research, 12,* 213-325.

Shultz, J., Florio, S., & Erickson, F. (1982). Where's the floor? Aspects of the cultural organization of social relationships in communication at home and at school. In P. Gilmore & A. Glatthorn (Eds.), *Children in and out of school* (pp. 88–123). Washington, DC: Center for Applied Linguistics.

Shuy, R. W. (1981a). A holistic view of language. *Research in the Teaching of English, 15,* 101-111.

Shuy, R. W. (1981b). Toward a developmental theory of writing. In C. H. Fredericksen & J. F. Dominic (Eds.), *Writing: The nature, development, and teaching of written communication* (Vol. 2, pp. 119–132). Hillsdale, NJ: Lawrence Erlbaum.

Siegel, G. (1975). The use of language tests. *Language, Speech, and Hearing Services in Schools, 6,* 211–217.

Siegel, G. (1979). Appraisal of language development. In F. Darely (Ed.), *Evaluation of appraisal techniques in speech and language pathology.* Reading, MA: Addison-Wesley.

Siegel, G., & Broen, P. (1976). Language assessment. In L. Lloyd (Ed.), *Communication assessment and intervention strategies* (pp. 73–122). Baltimore: University Park Press.

Siegel, L., Cunningham, C., & van der Spuy, H. (1979, April). *Interactions in language-delayed and normal preschool children and their mothers.* Paper presented to the Conference of the Society for Research in Child Development, San Francisco.

Siegel, R., Winitz, H., & Conkey, H. (1963). The influence of testing instruments on articulatory responses of children. *Journal of Speech and Hearing Disorders, 28,* 67–76.

Siegel-Causey, E., & Downing, J. (1987). Nonsymbolic communication development: Theoretical concepts and educational strategies. In L. Goetz, D. Guess, & K. Stremel-Campbell (Eds.), *Innovative program design for individuals with sensory impairments* (pp. 15–48). Baltimore: Paul H. Brookes.

Siegel-Causey, E., Ernst, B., & Guess, D. (1987). Elements of nonsymbolic communication and early interaction processes. In M. Ballis (Ed.), *Communication development in young children with deaf-blindness: Literature review III* (pp. 57-102). Monmouth, OR: Communication Skills Center for Young Children with Deaf-Blindness, Teaching Research Division.

Siegel–Causey, E., & Guess, D. (1989). *Enhancing nonsymbolic communication interactions among learners with severe disabilities.* Baltimore: Paul H. Brookes.

Sigman, M., & Ungerer, J. (1984). Cognitive and language skills in autistic, mentally retarded, and normal children. *Developmental Psychology, 20,* 293–302.

Silliman, E. R. (1984). Interactional competencies in the instructional context: The role of teaching discourse in learning. In G. Wallach & K. Butler (Eds.), *Language learning disabilities in school-age children* (pp. 288–317). Baltimore: Williams & Wilkins.

Silliman, E. R. (1993, June). *Integrating language and literacy programming: Building collaborative partnerships.* Paper presented at the Conference of the Rochester City School District, Rochester, NY.

Silliman, E. R., & Leslie, S. P. (1983). Social and cognitive aspects of fluency in the instructional setting. *Topics in Language Disorders, 3,* 61-74.

Silliman, E. R., Wilkinson, L. C., & Hoffman, L. P. (1993). Documenting authentic progress in language and literacy learning: Collaborative assessment in classrooms. *Topics in Language Disorders, 14*(1), 58–71.

Silverman, F. (1989). *Communication for the speechless* (2nd ed.). Englewood Cliffs, NJ: Prentice-Hall.

Simeonsson, R. J., Olley, J. G., & Rosenthal, S. L. (1987). Early intervention for children with autism. In M. Guralnick & F. Bennett (Eds.), *The effectiveness of early intervention for at-risk and handicapped children* (pp. 275–296). New York: Academic Press.

Simmons, J. Q., & Baltaxe, C. (1975). Language patterns of adolescent autistics. *Journal of Autism and Childhood Schizophrenia, 5,* 333-351.

Simmons-Miles, R. (1983, November). *Assessment of phonological disorders and single-word picture naming.* Paper presented at the Annual Convention of the American Speech-Language-Hearing Association, Cincinnati.

Simner, M. (1983). The warning signs of school failure: An updated profile of the at-risk kindergarten child. *Topics in Early Childhood Special Education, 3*(4), 17–28.

Simon, C. S. (1979). *Communicative competence: A functional-pragmatic approach to language therapy.* Tucson, AZ: Communication Skill Builders.

Simon, C. S. (1984). *Evaluating communicative competence: A functional-pragmatic procedure.* Tucson, AZ: Communication Skill Builders.

Simon, C. S. (1985). *Communication skills and classroom success: Therapy methodologies for language-learning disabled students.* San Diego: College-Hill.

Simon, C. S. (1987). *Classroom Communication Screening Procedure for Early Adolescents: A handbook for assessment and intervention.* Tempe, AZ: Communi-Cognitive Publications.

Sininger, Y., Klatzky, R., & Kirchner, D. (1989). Memory scanning speed in language-disordered children. *Journal of Speech and Hearing Research, 32,* 289–297.

Skarakis-Doyle, E., & Mullin, K. (1990). Comprehension monitoring in language disordered children: A preliminary investigation of cognitive and linguistic factors. *Journal of Speech and Hearing Disorders, 55,* 700-705.

Skarakis-Doyle, E., & Prutting, C. (1988). Characteristics of symbolic play in language disordered children. *Human Communication Canada, 12*(1), 7-17.

Skutnabb–Kangas, T., & Toukomas, T. (1976). *Teaching migrant children's mother tongue and learning the language of the host country in the context of the sociocultural situation of the migrant family.* Helsinki: Finnish National Commission for UNESCO.

Slackman, E., Hudson, J., & Fivush, R. (1986). Actions, actors, links, and goals: The structure of children's event representations. In K. Nelson (Ed.), *Event knowledge: Structure and function in development.* Hillsdale, NJ: Lawrence Erlbaum.

Sleight, C., & Prinz, P. (1985). Use of abstracts, orientations, and codes in narratives by language-disordered and nondisordered children. *Journal of Speech and Hearing Disorders, 50,* 361–371.

Sleight, M., & Niman, C. (1984). *Gross motor and oral motor development in children with Down syndrome: Birth through three years.* St. Louis, MO: St. Louis Association for Retarded Citizens.

Slobin, D. (1971). On the learning of morphological rules: A reply to Palerino and Eberhart. In D. Slobin (Ed.), *The ontogenesis of grammar* (pp. 215-233). New York: Academic Press.

Slobin, D. (1973). Cognitive prerequisites for the acquisition of grammar. In C. Ferguson & D. Slobin (Eds.), *Studies in child language development* (pp. 175–208). New York: Holt, Rinehart.

Smeets, P. M., & Striefel, S. (1976). Acquisition and cross-modal generalization of receptive and expressive signing skills in a retarded deaf girl. *Journal of Mental Deficiency Research, 20,* 251-260.

Smilansky, S. (1968). *The effects of sociodramatic play on disadvantaged preschool children.* New York: John Wiley.

Smit, A. B., & Bernthal, J. E. (1983). Performance of articulation-disordered children on language and perception measures. *Journal of Speech and Hearing Research, 26,* 123-136.

Smith, C. R. (1991). *Learning disabilities: The interaction of learner, task, and setting.* Newton, MA: Allyn & Bacon.

Smith, F. (1973). Twelve easy ways to make learning to read difficult. In F. Smith (Ed.), *Psycholinguistics and reading* (pp. 183–196). New York: Holt, Rinehart & Winston.

Smith, F. (1982a). *Understanding reading*. New York: Holt, Rinehart & Winston.

Smith, F. (1982b) *Writing and the reader.* New York: Holt, Rinehart & Winston.

Smith, F. (1988). *Understanding reading* (4th ed.). Hillsdale, NJ: Lawrence Erlbaum.

Smith, L., & von Tetzchner, S. (1986). Communicative, sensorimotor, and language skills of young children with Down's syndrome. *American Journal of Mental Deficiency, 91*(1), 57-66.

Smith, M. (1985). Managing the aggressive and self-injurious behavior of adults disabled by autism. *Journal of the Association for Persons with Severe Handicaps, 4*, 228–232.

Smith-Burke, M. T., Deegan, D., & Jaggar, A. M. (1991). Whole language: A viable alternative to special education and remedial education. *Topics in Language Disorders, 11*(3), 58-68.

Smitherman, G. (1985). What go round come round: Keep in perspective. In C. Brookes (Ed.), *Tapping potential: English and language arts for the black learner* (pp. 41–62). Urbana, IL: Black Caucus of the National Council of Teachers of English.

Snell, M., & Browder, D. (1986). Community-referenced instruction: Research and issues. *Journal of the Association for Persons with Severe Handicaps, 11*, 1-11.

Snell, M., & Gast, D. (1981). Applying time delay procedure to the instruction of the severely handicapped. *Journal of the Association for the Severely Handicapped, 6*(3), 3–14.

Snell, M., & Zirpoli, T. (1987). Intervention strategies. In M. Snell (Ed.), *Systematic instruction of persons with severe handicaps* (pp. 110–150). New York: Merrill/Macmillan.

Snow, C. E. (1977a). Mothers' speech research: From input to interaction. In C. Snow & C. Ferguson (Eds.), *Talking to children: Language input and acquisition* (pp. 31–50). Cambridge, UK: Cambridge University Press.

Snow, C. E. (1977b). The development of conversation between mothers and babies. *Journal of Child Language, 4*, 1-22.

Snow, C. E. (1979). The role of social interaction in language acquisition. In A. Collins (Ed.), *Children's language and communication* (pp. 157–182). Hillsdale, NJ: Lawrence Erlbaum.

Snow, C. E. (1989). Imitativeness: A trait or a skill? In G. E. Speidel & K. E. Nelson (Eds.), *The many faces of imitation in language learning* (pp. 73-90). New York: Springer Verlag.

Snow, C. E. (1990). The development of definitional skill. *Journal of Child Language, 17*, 697-710.

Snow, C. E., & Goldfield, B. A. (1983). Turn the page please; Situation-specific language acquisition. *Journal of Child Language, 10*, 551-569.

Snow, C. E., & Hoefnagel–Hohe, M. (1978). The critical period for language acquisition: Evidence from second language meaning. *Child Development, 49*, 1114–1128.

Snow, C. E., Midkiff-Borunda, S., Small, A., & Proctor, A. (1984). Therapy as social interaction: Analyzing the contexts for language remediation. *Topics in Language Disorders, 4*(4), 72–85.

Snow, C. E., Perlman, R., & Nathan, D. (1987). Why routines are different: Toward a multiple-factors model of the relation between input and language acquisition. In K. E. Nelson & A. van Kleeck (Eds.), *Children's language* (Vol. 6). Hillsdale, NJ: Lawrence Erlbaum.

Snyder, L., Apolloni, T., & Cooke, T. (1977). Integrated settings at the early childhood level: The role of nonretarded peers. *Exceptional Children, 43*, 262–266.

Snyder, L. S. (1984). Developmental language disorders: Elementary school age. In A. L. Holland (Ed.), *Language disorders in children: Recent advances* (pp. 129-158). San Diego: Singular.

Snyder, L. S., Bates, E., & Bretherton, I. (1981). Content and context in early lexical development. *Journal of Child Language, 8*, 565-582.

Snyder, L. S., & Downey, D. (1983). Pragmatics and information processing. *Topics in Language Disorders, 4*(1), 75–86.

Snyder. L. S., & Godley, D. (1992). Assessment of word-finding disorders in children and adolescents. *Topics in Language Disorders, 13*(1), 15-32.

Snyder-McLean, L., Etter-Schroeder, R., & Rogers, N. (1986, November). *Issues in Piagetian cognitive assessment of severely/profoundly retarded individuals.* Paper presented at the Annual Convention of the American Speech-Language-Hearing Association, Detroit.

Snyder-McLean, L., & McLean, J. (1978). Verbal information gathering strategies: The child's use of language to acquire language. *Journal of Speech and Hearing Disorders, 43*, 306-325.

Snyder-McLean, L., & McLean, J. (1987). Effectiveness of early intervention for children with language and communication disorders. In M. Guaralnick & J. Bennett (Eds.), *The effectiveness of early intervention for at-risk and handicapped children* (pp. 213-274). New York: Academic Press.

Sobsey, D., & Reichle, J. (1986). *Components of reinforcement for attention signal switch activation.* Unpublished manuscript, University of Minnesota, Minneapolis.

Sommers, R., & Starkey, K. (1977). Dichotic verbal processing in Down's syndrome children having qualitatively different speech and language skills. *American Journal of Mental Deficiency, 82,* 44-53.

Song, A., Jones, S., Lippert, J., Metzger, K., Miller, J., & Borreca, C. (1980). Wisconsin Behavior Rating Scale, Revised. Madison: Central Wisconsin Center for Developmental Disabilities.

Sonnenmeier, R. M. (1992, March). *Script-based language intervention: Learning to participate in life events.* Paper presented at the Conference on Pragmatics: From Theory to Therapy, State University of New York, Buffalo.

Sonnenschein, S., & Whitehurst, C. (1984). Developing referential communication: A hierarchy of skills. *Child Development, 55,* 1936–1945.

Sparks, S. N. (1989). Speech and language in maltreated children: Response to McCauley & Swisher (1987). *Journal of Speech and Hearing Disorders, 54,* 124-126.

Spector, C. (1990). Linguistic humor comprehension of normal and language-impaired adolescents. *Journal of Speech and Hearing Disorders, 55,* 533-541.

Spekman, N. (1981). Dyadic verbal communication abilities of learning disabled and normally achieving fourth and fifth grade boys. *Learning Disability Quarterly, 4,* 139–151.

Spekman, N. (1983). Discourse and pragmatics. In C. Wren (Ed.), *Language learning disabilities: Diagnosis and remediation* (pp. 53–120). Rockville, MD: Aspen.

Spiegel, B. (1983). The effect of context on language learning by severely retarded young adults. *Language, Speech, and Hearing Services in Schools, 14,* 252–259.

Spinelli, F., & Terrell, B. (1984). Remediation in context. *Topics in Language Disorders, 5*(1), 29–40.

Spitz, H. (1966). The role of input organization in the learning and memory of mental retardates. In N. Ellis (Ed.), *International review of research in mental retardation* (Vol. 2, pp. 29–56). New York: Academic Press.

Spitz, H. (1979). Beyond field theory in the study of mental deficiency. In N. Ellis (Ed.), *Handbook of mental deficiency: Psychological theory and research* (2nd ed.). Hillsdale, NJ: Lawrence Erlbaum.

Spradlin, J., & Siegel, G. (1982). Language training in natural and clinical environments. *Journal of Speech and Hearing Disorders, 47,* 2–6.

Spragle, D., & Micucci, S. (1990). Signs of the week: A functional approach to manual sign training. *Augmentative and Alternative Communication, 6,* 29–37.

Spring, C., & Farmer, R. (1975). Perception span of poor readers. *Journal of Reading Behavior, 7,* 297-305.

Sprott, R. A., & Kemper, S. (1987). The development of children's code-switching: A study of six bilingual children across two situations. In E. F. Pemberton,

M. A. Sell, & G. B. Simpson (Eds.), *Working papers in language development: 1987, 2,* 116–134.

Squire, J. R. (1983). Composing and comprehending: Two sides of the same basic process. *Language Arts, 60,* 581-589.

Staab, C. (1983). Language functions elicited by meaningful activities: A new dimension in language programs. *Language, Speech, and Hearing Services in Schools, 14,* 164–170.

Stafford, M., Sundberg, M., & Braam, S. (1978, April). *An experimental analysis of mands and tacts.* Paper presented at the Annual Convention of the Midwest Association of Behavior Analysis, Chicago.

Stainback S., & Stainback, W. (Eds.). (1992). *Curriculum considerations in inclusive classrooms: Facilitating learning for all students.* Baltimore: Paul H. Brookes.

Stainback W., & Stainback, S. (Eds.). (1990). *Support network for inclusive schooling: Interdependent integrated education.* Baltimore: Paul H. Brookes.

Stallnaker, L., & Creaghead, N. (1982). An examination of language samples obtained under three experimental conditions. *Language, Speech, and Hearing Services in Schools, 13,* 121–128.

Stanovich, K. E. (1991). Discrepancy definitions of reading disability: Has intelligence led us astray? *Reading Research Quarterly, 26,* 7-29.

Stark, J. (1985, April). *Learning disabilities and reading: Myths and realities.* Paper presented at the Annual Convention of the New York State Speech-Language-Hearing Association, Kiamesha Lake.

Stark, R. E., & Tallal, P. (1981) Perceptual and motor deficits in language impaired children. In R. Keith (Ed.), *Central auditory and language disorders in children* (pp. 121–144). San Diego: College-Hill.

Stark, R. E,, & Tallal, P. (1988). *Language, speech, and reading disorders in children: Neuropsychological studies.* San Diego: College-Hill.

Steffensen, M. (1986). Register, cohesion, and cross-cultural reading comprehension. *Applied Linguistics, 7,* 71-85.

Stein, N. (1982). What's in a story: Interpreting the interpretations of story grammars. *Discourse Processes, 5,* 319–335.

Stein, N., & Glenn, C. (1979). An analysis of story comprehension in elementary school children. In R. Freedle (Ed.), *New directions in discourse processing* (Vol. 2, pp. 53–120). Norwood, NJ: Ablex.

Stein, N., & Policastro, M. (1984). The concept of story: A comparison between children's and teachers' viewpoints. In H. Mandl, N. Stein, & T. Trabasso (Eds.), *Learning and comprehension of text* (pp. 113–155). Hillsdale, NJ: Lawrence Erlbaum.

Steiner, S., & Larson, V. L. (1991). Integrating microcomputers into language intervention with children. *Topics in Language Disorders, 11*(2), 18-30.

Steinmann, M. (1982). Speech act theory and writing. In M. Nystrand (Ed.), *What writers know: The language, process, and structure of written discourse* (pp. 291–323). New York: Academic Press.

Stephens, B., & McLaughlin, J. (1974). Two-year gains in reasoning by retarded and nonretarded persons. *American Journal of Mental Deficiency, 77*, 311-313.

Stephens, I., Dallman, W., & Montgomery, A. (1988, November). *Developmental sentence scoring through age nine.* Paper presented at the Annual Convention of the American Speech-Language-Hearing Association, Boston.

Stephens, M., & Montgomery, A. (1985). A critique of recent relevant standardized tests. *Topics in Language Disorders, 5*(3), 21–45.

Sterling, C. M. (1983). Spelling errors in context. *British Journal of Psychology, 74*, 353-364.

Stern, D. (1971). A microanalysis of mother-infant interaction. *Journal of the American Academy of Child Psychiatry, 10*, 501–517.

Stern, D., Jaffee, J., Beebe, B., & Bennett, S. (1975). Vocalizing in unison and in alternation: Two modes of communication within the mother-infant dyad. *Annals of the New York Academic of Sciences, 263*, 89–100.

Sternat, J., Nietupski, J., Messina, R., Lyon, S., & Brown, L. (1977). Occupational and physical therapy services for severely handicapped students: Towards a naturalized public school service delivery model. In E. Sontag, J. Smith, & N. Certo (Eds.), *Educational programming for the severely and profoundly handicapped* (pp. 263–278). Reston, VA: Council for Exceptional Children, Division on Mental Retardation.

Sternberg, L. (1984, May). *Prelanguage communication programming techniques.* Workshop at State University of New York, Geneseo.

Sternberg, L., McNerney, C., & Pegnatore, L. (1985). Developing co-active imitation behaviors with profoundly mentally handicapped students. *Education and Training of the Mentally Retarded, 20*, 260–267.

Sternberg, L., Pegnatore, L., & Hill, C. (1983). Establishing interactive communication behaviors with profoundly mentally handicapped students. *Journal of the Association for Persons with Severe Handicaps, 8*, 39–46.

Sternberg, R. J. (1987). Most vocabulary is learned from context. In M. G. McKeown & M. E. Curtis (Eds.), *The nature of vocabulary acquisition* (pp. 89-105). Hillsdale, NJ: Lawrence Erlbaum.

Sternberg, R. J., & Powell, J. S. (1983) Comprehending verbal comprehension. *American Psychologist, 38*, 878-893.

Sternberg, R. J., & Wagner, R. K. (1982). Automatization failure in learning disabilities. *Topics in Learning and Learning Disabilities, 2*(2), 1–11.

Stevens, S. (1975). *Psychophysics.* New York: John Wiley.

Stevick, E. (1976). *Memory, meaning, and method.* Rowley, MA: Newbury House.

Stice, C. F., & Betrand, N. P. (1989, December). *The text and textures of literacy learning in whole language vs. traditional/skills classrooms.* Paper presented at the meeting of the International Reading Association, Tucson, AZ.

Stice, C. F., & Betrand, N. P. (1990). *Whole language and the emergent literacy of at-risk children: a two-year comparative study.* Nashville: Tennessee State University Center of Excellence.

Stickler, K. R. (1987). *Guide to analysis of language transcripts.* Eau Claire, WI: Thinking Publications.

Stillman, R. (1978). Callier–Azusa Scale. Dallas: University of Texas, Callier Center for Communication Disorders.

Stillman, R., & Battle, C. (1984). Developing pre-language communication in the severely handicapped: An interpretation of the VanDijk method. *Seminars in Speech and Language, 5*, 159–170.

Stockman, I., & Vaughn-Cooke, F. (1982). A re-examination of research on the language of black children: The need for a new framework. *Journal of Education, 164*, 157–172.

Stockman, I., & Vaughn-Cooke, F. (1986). Implications of semantic category research for the language assessment of nonstandard speakers. *Topics in Language Disorders, 6*(4), 15–25.

Stokes, T., & Baer, D. (1977). An implicit technology of generalization. *Journal of Applied Behavior Analysis, 10*, 349–367.

Stone, C. A., & Wertsch, J. V. (1984). A social interactional analysis of learning disabilities remediation. *Journal of Learning Disabilities, 17*, 194-199.

Stowe, L. (1988). Thematic structures and sentence comprehension. In G. Carlson & M. Tanenhaus (Eds.), *Linguistic structure in language processing* (pp. 319–358). Dordrecht, The Netherlands: Reidel.

Street, B. (1984). *Literacy in theory and practice.* New York: Cambridge University Press.

Stremel-Campbell, K., & Campbell, C. (1985). Training techniques that may facilitate generalization. In S. Warren & A. Rogers-Warren (Eds.), *Teaching functional language: Generalization and maintenance of language skills* (pp. 309-339). Baltimore: University Park Press.

Stremel-Campbell, K., Johnson-Dorn, N., Guida, J., & Udell, T. (1984). *Communication curriculum.* Monmouth, OR: Teaching Research Integration Project for Children and Youth with Severe Handicaps.

Strominger, A., & Bashir, A. (1977, November). *A nine-year follow-up of language-delayed children.* Paper presented at the Annual Convention of the American Speech-Language-Hearing Association, Chicago.

Sturner, R. A., Heller, J. H., Funk, S. G., & Layton, T. L. (1993). The Fluharty Preschool Speech and Language Screening Test: A population–based validation study using sample–independent decision rules. *Journal of Speech and Hearing Research, 36,* 738–745.

Sturner, R. A., Layton, T. L., Evans, A. W., Heller, J. H., Funk, S. G., & Machon, M. W. (1994). Preschool speech and language screening: A review of currently available tests. *American Journal of Speech–Language Pathology, 3,* 25–36.

Sulzby, E. (1982). "Text" as an object of metalinguistic knowledge: A study in literacy development. *First Language, 3,* 181–199.

Summers, J. A., Brotherson, M. J., & Turnbull, A. P. (1988). The impact of handicapped children on families. In E. W. Lynch & R. B. Lewis (Eds.), *Exceptional children and adults* (pp. 504–544). Glenview, IL: Scott, Foresman.

Sutton-Smith, B. (1981). *The folkstories of children.* Philadelphia: University of Pennsylvania Press.

Sutton-Smith, B. (1986). The development of fictional narrative performances. *Topics in Language Disorders, 7*(1), 1–10.

Swank, L. K. (1994). Phonological coding abilities: Identification of impairments related to phonologically based reading problems. *Topics in Language Disorders, 14*(2), 56–71.

Swiffin, A. L., Arnott, J. L., Pickering, J. A., & Newell, A. F. (1987). Adaptive and predictive techniques in a communication prothesis. *Augmentative and Alternative Communication, 3,* 181-191.

Swisher, L., & Demetras, M. J. (1985). The expressive language characteristics of autistic children compared with mentally retarded or specific language-impaired children. In E. Schopler & G. B. Mesibov (Eds.), *Communication problems in autism* (pp. 147-162). New York: Plenum.

Switzy, H., Rotatori, A., Miller, T., & Freagon, S. (1979). The developmental model and its implications for assessment and instruction for the severely/profoundly handicapped. *Mental Retardation, 17,* 167–170.

Tager–Flusberg, H. (1981a). Linguistic functioning in autism. *Journal of Autism and Developmental Disorders, 11,* 45–56.

Tager-Flusberg, H. (1981b). On the nature of linguistic functioning in early infantile autism. *Journal of Autism and Developmental Disabilities, 11,* 45-56.

Tager-Flusberg, H. (1981c). Sentence comprehension in autistic children. *Applied Psycholinguistics, 2,* 3-24.

Tager-Flusberg, H. (1985). The conceptual basis for referential word meaning in children with autism. *Child Development, 56,* 1167-1178.

Tager-Flusberg, H. (1989). Putting words together: Morphology and syntax in the preschool years. In J.

Gleason (Ed.), *Language development* (pp. 139–171). Columbus, OH: Macmillan.

Tallal, P., & Piercy, M. (1973a). Defects of non-verbal auditory perception in children with developmental aphasia. *Nature, 241,* 468-469.

Tallal, P., & Piercy, M. (1973b). Developmental aphasia: Impaired rate of non-verbal processing as a function of sensory modality. *Neuropsychologia, 11,* 389-398.

Tallal, P., & Piercy, M. (1974). Developmental aphasia: Rate of auditory processing and selective impairment of consonant perception. *Neuropsychologia, 12,* 83-93.

Tallal, P., & Piercy, M. (1975). Developmental aphasia: The perception of brief vowels and extended stop consonants. *Neuropsychologia, 13,* 69-74.

Tallal, P., Stark, R. (1981). Speech acoustic-cue discrimination abilities of normally developing and language-impaired children. *Journal of the Acoustical Society of America, 69,* 568-574.

Tallal, P., Stark, R., Kallman, C., & Mellitis, D. (1981). A reexamination of some perceptual abilities of language impaired and normal children as a function of age and sensory modality. *Journal of Speech and Hearing Research, 24,* 351-357.

Tannen, D. (1982). The oral/literate continuum in discourse. In D. Tannen (Ed.), *Spoken and written language. Exploring orality and literacy* (pp. 1-16). Norwood, NJ: Ablex.

Tannock, R. (1988a). Control and reciprocity in mothers' interactions with Down syndrome and normal children. In K. Marfo (Ed.), *Parent-child interaction and developmental disorders: Theory, research, and intervention* (pp. 163-180). New York: Praeger.

Tannock, R. (1988b). Mothers' directiveness in their interactions with their children with and without Down syndrome. *American Journal on Mental Deficiency, 93,* 154-165.

Tannock, R., Girolametto, L., & Siegel, L. (1990). Are the social-communicative and linguistic skills of developmentally delayed children enhanced by a conversational model of language intervention? In L. B. Olswang, C. K. Thompson, S. F. Warren, & N. J. Minghetti (Eds.), *Treatment efficacy research in communication disorders* (pp. 115-123). Rockville, MD: ASHA Foundation.

Tanz, C. (1980). *Studies in the acquisition of deictic terms.* Cambridge, UK: Cambridge University Press.

Tapajna, M., & Finn-Scardine, L. (1981, November). *Comprehensive program planning for non-speech communication.* Paper presented at the Annual Convention of the American Speech-Language-Hearing Association, Los Angeles.

Tarone, E. (1988). *Variation in interlanguage.* London: Edward Arnold.

Tattershall, S. (1987). Mission impossible: Learning how a classroom works before it's too late. *Journal of Childhood Communication Disorders, 2*(1), 181–184.

Taylor, A., & Turnure, J. (1979). Imagery and verbal elaboration with retarded children: Effects on learning and memory. In N. Ellis (Ed.), *Handbook of mental deficiency: Psychological theory and research* (2nd ed., pp. 659–698). Hillsdale, NJ: Lawrence Erlbaum.

Taylor, B. M. (1980). Children's memory for expository text after reading. *Reading Research Quarterly, 15,* 399-411.

Taylor, M. B., & Williams, J. P. (1983). Comprehension of learning disabled readers: Task and text variations. *Reading Research Quarterly, 75,* 743-751.

Taylor, O. (in press). Clinical practice as a social occasion. In L. Cole & V. Deal (Eds.), *Communication disorders in multicultural populations.* Rockville, MD: American Speech-Language-Hearing Association.

Taylor, O. L. (1986a). Language differences. In G. Shames & E. Wiig (Eds.), *Human communication* (2nd ed., pp. 385–413). New York: Merrill/Macmillan.

Taylor, O. L. (1986b). Teaching Standard English as a second dialect. In O. L. Taylor (Ed.), *Treatment of communication disorders in culturally and lingually diverse populations* (pp. 153–178).San Diego: College-Hill.

Taylor, O. L. (1989). Old wine in new bottles: Some things change yet remain the same. *Asha, 31*(9), 72-73.

Taylor, O. L. (1990). Cross-cultural communication: An essential of effective communication. (ERIC Document Reproduction Service No. ED 325 593)

Taylor, O. L. (in press). Clinical practice as a social occasion. In L. Cole & V. Deal (Eds.), *Communication disorders in multicultural populations.* Rockville, MD: American Speech–Language–Hearing Association.

Taylor, O. L., Payne, K., & Anderson, N. (1987). Distinguishing between communication disorders and communication differences. *Seminars in Speech and Language, 8,* 415-427.

Teale, W. H., & Sulzby, E. (1986). Emergent literacy as a perspective for examining how young children become writers and readers. In W. H. Teale & E. Sulzby (Eds.), *Emergent literacy: Writing and reading* (pp. vii-xxv). Norwood, NJ: Ablex.

Templeton, S. (1980). Spelling, phonology, and the older student. In E. H. Henderson & J. W. Beers (Eds.), *Developmental and cognitive aspects of learning to spell: A reflection of word knowledge* (pp. 85-96). Newark, DE: International Reading Association.

Templin, M. (1957). *Certain language skills in children.* Minneapolis: University of Minnesota Press.

Templin, M., & Darley, F. (1969). The Templin-Darley Tests of Articulation. Iowa City: University of Iowa, Bureau of Educational Research and Services.

Terdal, L., Jackson, R., & Garner, A. (1976). Mother-child interactions: A comparison between normal and developmentally delayed groups. In E. Mash, L. Hamerlynck, & L. Handy (Eds.), *Behavioral modification and families* (pp. 249-264). New York: Bruner/Mazel.

Terrell, B. Y., & Hale, J. E. (1992). Serving a multicultural population: Different learning styles. *American Journal of Speech-Language Pathology, 1*(2), 5-9.

Terrell, B. Y., Schwartz, R. G., Prelock, P. A., & Messick, C. K. (1984). Symbolic play in normal and language-impaired children. *Journal of Speech and Hearing Research, 27,* 424-429.

Terrell, S. L., Arensberg, K., & Rosa, M. (1992). Parent-child comparative analysis: A criterion-referenced method for the nondiscriminatory assessment of a child who spoke a relatively uncommon dialect of English. *Language, Speech, and Hearing Services in Schools, 23,* 34-42.

Terrell, S. L., & Terrell, F. (1983). Distinguishing linguistic differences from disorders: The past, present and future of nonbiased assessment. *Topics in Language Disorders, 3*(3), 1-7.

Thal, D. J. (1989). *Language and gestures in late talkers.* Paper presented at the Biennial Meeting of the Society for Research in Child Development, Kansas City, MO.

Thal, D. J., & Bates, E. (1988). Language and gesture in late talkers. *Journal of Speech and Hearing Research, 31,* 115-123.

Thal, D. J., & Tobias, S. (1992). Communicative gestures in children with delayed onset of oral expressive vocabulary. *Journal of Speech and Hearing Research, 35,* 1281-1289.

Thal, D. J., Tobias, S., & Morrison, D. (1991). Language and gesture in late talkers: A one-year follow-up. *Journal of Speech and Hearing Research, 34,* 604-612.

Theadore, G., Maher, S. R., & Prizant, B. M. (1990). Early assessment and intervention with emotional and behavioral disorders and communication disorders. *Topics in Language Disorders, 10*(4), 42-56.

Thomas, A. (1979). Learned helplessness and expectancy factors: Implications for research in learning disabilities. *Review of Educational Research, 49,* 208-221.

Thomas, J. (1989). A standardized method for collecting and analyzing language samples of pre-school and primary children in the public schools. *Language, Speech, and Hearing Services in Schools, 20,* 85–92.

Thorndyke, P. (1977). Cognitive structures in comprehension and memory of narrative discourse. *Cognitive Psychology, 9,* 77–110.

Thorum, A. R. (1986). The Fullerton Language Test for Adolescents. Palo Alto: Consulting Psychologists Press.

Tiegerman, E., & Siperstein, M. (1982, April). *Communication training: Changing mother-child interaction.* Paper presented at the Annual Convention of the New York State Speech and Hearing Association, Ellenville.

Tiegerman, E., & Siperstein, M. (1984). Individual patterns of interaction in the mother-child dyad: Implications for parent intervention. *Topics in Language Disorders, 4*(4), 50-61.

Tierney, R. S., & Pearson, P. D. (1983). Toward a composing model of reading. *Language Arts, 60,* 568-580.

Tizard, B., Cooperman, D., Joseph, A., & Tizard, J. (1972). Environmental effects on language development: A study of young children in long stay residential nurseries. *Child Development, 43,* 705–728.

Tomasello, M. (1987). Learning to use prepositions: A case study. *Journal of Child Language, 14,* 79-98.

Tomasello, M., & Farrar, M. J. (1986). Joint attention and early language. *Child Development, 57,* 1454-1463.

Tomasello, M., Farrar, J., & Dines, J. (1984). Children's speech revisions for a familiar and an unfamiliar adult. *Journal of Speech and Hearing Research, 27,* 359–363.

Tomasello, M., & Todd, M. (1983). Joint attention and lexical acquisition style. *First Language, 4,* 197-212.

Tomblin, J. B. (1991). Examining the cause of specific language impairment. *Language, Speech, and Hearing Services in Schools, 22,* 69-74.

Torgesen, J. K. (1977). The role of nonspecific factors in the task performance of learning disabled children. *Journal of Learning Disabilities, 12,* 514–521.

Torgesen, J. K. (1980). Conceptual and educational implications of the use of efficient task strategies by learning disabled children. *Journal of Learning Disabilities, 13,* 19-26.

Torgesen, J. K. (1982). The study of short–term memory in learning disabled children. In K. Gadow & I. Bialer (Eds.), *Advances in learning and behavioral disabilities* (Vol. 1). Greenwich, CT: JAI.

Torgeson, J. (1985). Memory processes in reading disordered children. *Journal of Learning Disabilities, 18,* 350–357.

Torrance, N., & Olson, D. (1984). Oral language competence and the acquisition of literacy. In A. Pelligrini & T. Yawkey (Eds.), *The development of oral and written language in social contexts.* Norwood, NJ: Ablex.

Tosi, A. (1984). Bilingual education. Problems and practices. In N. Miller (Ed.), *Bilingualism and language disability* (pp. 199-219). San Diego: College–Hill.

Tough, J. (1973). *Focus on meaning: Talking to some purpose with young children.* London: Allen & Unwin.

Tough, J. (1977). *The development of meaning.* New York: John Wiley.

Tough, J. (1979). *Talk for teaching and learning.* Portsmouth, NH: Heinemann.

Trabasso, T., & Van Den Broek, P. (1985). Causal thinking and the representation of narrative events. *Journal of Memory and Language, 24,* 612–630.

Trantham, C., & Pedersen, J. (1976). *Normal language development.* Baltimore: Williams & Wilkins.

Trickett, P. K., Aber, J. L., Carlson, V., & Cicchetti, D. (1991). Relationship of socioeconomic status to the etiology and developmental sequelae of physical child abuse. *Developmental Psychology, 27,* 148-158.

Tronick, E., Als, H., & Adamson, L. (1979). Structure of early face-to-face communicative interactions. In M. Bullowa (Ed.), *Before speech* (pp. 249–372). New York: Cambridge University Press.

Trosborg, A. (1982). Children's comprehension of before and after reinvestigated. *Journal of Child Language, 9,* 381-402.

Tucker, G. R., Hamayan, E., & Genesee, F. (1976). Affective, cognitive, and social factors in second language acquisition. *Canadian Modern Language Review, 23,* 214–226.

Tucker, J. (1985). Curriculum-based assessment: An introduction. *Exceptional Children, 52,* 199–204.

Turnbull, A. P., Summers, J. A., & Brotherson, M. J. (1983). *Family life cycle: Theoretical and empirical implications and future directions for families with mentally retarded members.* Paper presented at the NICHD Conference on Families with Retarded Children, Washington, DC.

Turner, L., & Bray, N. (1985). Spontaneous rehearsal by mildly mentally retarded children and adolescents. *American Journal of Mental Deficiency, 78,* 640-648.

Turner, R. L. (1989). The great debate—Can both Carbo and Chall be right? *Phi Delta Kappan, 71,* 276-283.

Tyack, D. (1981). Teaching complex sentences. *Language, Speech, and Hearing Services in Schools, 12,* 49–56.

Tyack, D., & Gottsleben, R. (1977). *Language sampling, analysis, and training: A handbook for teachers and clinicians.* Palo Alto: Consulting Psychologists Press.

Tyack, D., & Gottsleben, R. (1986). Acquisition of complex sentences. *Language, Speech, and Hearing Services in Schools, 17,* 160–174.

Tyler, A., Edwards, M., & Saxman, J. (1987). Clinical application of two phonologically based treatment procedures. *Journal of Speech and Hearing Disorders, 52,* 393–409.

Tyler, A., & Nagy, W. (1987). *The acquisition of English derivational morphology* (Technical Report No. 407). Urbana, IL: Center for the Study of Reading.

Udwin, O., & Yule, W. (1983). Imaginative play in language disordered children. *British Journal of Communication, 18,* 197-205.

U.S. Bureau of the Census. (1990). *The Hispanic population in the United States: March 1990.* Washington, DC: Author.

U.S. Department of Health and Human Services. (1981). *Study findings of the National Study of the Incidence and Severity of Child Abuse and Neglect* (DHHS Publication No. OHDS 82-30325). Washington, DC: Government Printing Office.

Uzgiris, I., & Hunt, J. (1975). *Assessment in infancy: Ordinal scales of psychological development.* Urbana: University of Illinois Press.

Vanderheiden, G. C., & Kelso, D. P. (1987). Comparative analysis of fixed-vocabulary communication acceleration techniques. *Augmentative and Alternative Communication, 3,* 196-206.

Vanderheiden, G. C., & Lloyd, L. L. (1986). Communication systems and their components. In S. Blackstone (Ed.), *Augmentative communication* (pp. 49–162). Rockville, MD: American Speech-Language-Hearing Association.

van der Lely, H. K., & Harris, M. (1990). Comprehension of reversible sentences in specifically language-impaired children. *Journal of Speech and Hearing Disorders, 55,* 101-117.

van der Lely, H. K., & Howard, D. (1993). Children with specific language impairment: Linguistic impairment or short–term memory deficit? *Journal of Speech and Hearing Research, 36,* 1193–1207.

vanDijk, J. (1985). An educational curriculum for deaf-blind multihandicapped persons. In D. Ellis (Ed.), *Sensory impairments in mentally handicapped people* (pp. 374–382). San Diego: College-Hill.

Van Dijk, T. A. (1979). Relevance assignment in discourse comprehension. *Discourse Processes, 2,* 113-126.

van Kleeck, A. (1984). Metalinguistic skills: Cutting across spoken and written language and problem-solving skills. In G. Wallach & K. Butler (Eds.), *Language learning disabilities in school age children* (pp. 128-153). Baltimore: Williams & Wilkins.

van Kleeck, A. (1994). Potential cultural bias in training parents as conversational partners with their children who have delays in language development. *American Journal of Speech-Language Pathology, 3*(1), 67–78.

Vaughn-Cooke, F. (1983). Improving language assessment in minority children. *Asha, 25,* 29-34.

Vellutino, F. R. (1977). Alternative conceptualization of dyslexia: Evidence in support of a verbal deficit hypothesis. *Harvard Educational Review, 47,* 334-354.

Vellutino, F. R. (1979). *Dyslexia: Theory and research.* Cambridge: MIT Press.

Venn, M. L., Wolery, M., Fleming, L. A., DeCesare, L. D., Morris, A., & Cuffs, M. S. (1993). Effects of teaching preschool peers to use the mand-model procedure during snack activities. *American Journal of Speech-Language Pathology, 2*(1), 38-46.

Vetter, D. (1982). Language disorders and schooling. *Topics in Language Disorders, 2*(4), 13–19.

Vicker, B. (1985). *Recognizing and enhancing the communication skills of your group home clients.* Bloomington: Indiana Developmental Training Center.

Vigil, N. A., & Oller, J. W. (1976). Rule fossilization: A tentative model. *Language Learning, 26,* 218–295.

Vihman, M. (1978). Consonant harmony: Its scope and function in child language. In J. Greenberg (Ed.), *Universals in human language: Vol. 2. Phonology* (pp. 281–334). Stanford, CA: Stanford University.

Violette, J., & Swisher, L. (1992). Echolalic responses by a child with autism to four experimental conditions of sociolinguistic input. *Journal of Speech and Hearing Research, 35,* 139-147.

Visch-Brink, E. G., & van de Sandt-Koenderman, M. (1984).The occurrence of paraphrasias in the spontaneous speech of children with an acquired aphasia. *Brain and Language, 23,* 258-271.

Vogel, S. (1983). A qualitative analysis of morphological development in learning disabled and achieving children. *Journal of Learning Disabilities, 6,* 457-465.

Vogel, S. A. (1975). *Syntactic abilities in normal and dyslexic children.* Baltimore: University Park Press.

Vonnegut, K. (1974). Afterword. In C. Hart, L. Pogrebin, M. Rodgers, & M. Thomas (Eds.), *Free to be . . . you and me.* New York: McGraw-Hill.

Vorih, L., & Rosier, P. (1978). Rock Point Community School: An example of a Navajo-English bilingual elementary school program. *TESOL Quarterly, 12,* 263-269.

Wagner, J. R., & Rice, M. L. (1988, November). *The acquisition of verb-particle constructions: How do children figure them out?* Paper presented at the Annual Convention of the American Speech-Language-Hearing Association, Boston.

Wagner, R. E., & Torgeson, J. (1987). The nature of phonological processing and its causal role in the acquisition of reading skills. *Psychological Bulletin, 101,* 192–212.

Wales, R. (1986). Deixis. In P. Fletcher & M. Garman (Eds.), *Language acquisition* (pp. 401–428). Cambridge, UK: Cambridge University Press.

Wallach, G. (1980). So you want to know what to do with language disabled children above the age of six. *Topics in Language Disorders, 1*(1), 99–113.

Wallach, G., & Butler, K. (1984). *Language learning disabilities in school-age children.* Baltimore: Williams & Wilkins.

Wallach, G., & Liebergott, J. W. (1984). Who shall be called "learning disabled"?: Some new directions. In G. Wallach & K. Butler (Eds.), *Language learning disabilities in school age children* (pp. 1-14). Baltimore: Williams & Wilkins.

Wallach, G., & Miller, L. F. (1988). *Language intervention and academic success.* San Diego: College-Hill.

Waltz, D., & Pollack, J. (1985). Massively parallel parsing: A strongly interactive model of natural language interpretation. *Cognitive Science, 9,* 51–74.

Wanska, S., Bedrosian, J., & Pohlman, J. (1986). Effects of play materials on the topic performance of preschool children. *Language, Speech, and Hearing Services in Schools, 17,* 152–159.

Warden, D. A. (1976). The influence of context on children's use of identifying expressions and reference. *British Journal of Psychology, 67*(1), 101-112.

Warren, S. F. (1985). Clinical strategies for the measurement of language generalization. In S. Warren & A. Rogers-Warren (Eds.), *Teaching functional language* (pp. 197–224). Baltimore: University Park Press.

Warren, S. F. (1988). A behavioral approach to language generalization. *Language, Speech, and Hearing Services in Schools, 19,* 292–303.

Warren, S. F., & Bambara, L. (1989). An experimental analysis of milieu language intervention: Teaching the action-objective form. *Journal of Speech and Hearing Disorders, 54,* 448-461.

Warren, S. F., & Kaiser, A. (1986a). Generalization of treatment effects by young language-delayed children: A longitudinal analysis. *Journal of Speech and Language Disorders, 51,* 239–251.

Warren, S. F., & Kaiser, A. (1986b). Incidental language teaching: A critical review. *Journal of Speech and Hearing Disorders, 47,* 42–52.

Warren, S. F., McQuarter, R., & Rogers-Warren, A. (1984). The effects of mands and models on the speech of unresponsive socially isolated children. *Journal of Speech and Hearing Disorders, 47,* 42–52.

Warren, S. F., & Rogers-Warren, A. (1980). Current perspectives in language remediation: A special monograph. *Education and Treatment in Children, 5,* 133–153.

Warren, S. F., & Rogers-Warren, A. (1985). Teaching functional language: An introduction. In S. Warren & A. Rogers-Warren (Eds.), *Teaching functional language* (pp. 3–24). Baltimore: University Park Press.

Warren, S. F., Rogers-Warren, A., Baer, D., & Guess, D. (1980). Assessment and facilitation of generalization. In W. Sailor, B. Wilcox, & L. Brown (Eds.), *Methods of instruction for severely handicapped students.* Baltimore: Paul H. Brookes.

Warren, S. F., Yoder, P. J., Gazdag, G. E., Kim, K., & Jones, H. A. (1993). Facilitating prelingual communication skills in young children with developmental delay. *Journal of Speech and Hearing Research, 36,* 83-97.

Washington, D., & Naremore, R. (1978). Children's use of spatial prepositions in two- and three-dimensional tasks. *Journal of Speech and Hearing Research, 21,* 151–165.

Washington, J. A., & Craig, H. K. (1992). Performances of low-income, African-American preschool and kindergarten children on the Peabody Picture Vocabulary Test—Revised. *Language, Speech, and Hearing Services in Schools, 23,* 329-333.

Wasserman, G. A., Green, A., & Allen, R. (1983). Going beyond abuse: Maladaptive patterns of interaction in abusing mother-child pairs. *Journal of the American Academy of Child Psychiatry, 22,* 245-252.

Waterson, N. (1978). Growth of complexity in phonological development. In N. Waterson & C. Snow (Eds.), *The development of communication* (pp. 415–442). New York: John Wiley.

Waterson, N., & Snow, C. (1978). *The development of communication.* New York: John Wiley.

Watkins, O., & Watkins, M. (1980). The modality effect and echoic persistence. *Journal of Experimental Psychology General, 109,* 251-278.

Watkins, R. V., & Pemberton, E. F. (1987). Clinical applications of recasting: Review and theory. *Child Language Teaching and Therapy, 3,* 311-328.

Watkins, R. V., & Rice, M. L. (1989, November). *Verb particle acquisition in language-impaired and normally developing children.* Paper presented at the Convention of the American Speech-Language-Hearing Association, St. Louis.

Watkins, R. V., & Rice, M. L. (1991). Verb particle and preposition acquisition in language-impaired preschoolers. *Journal of Speech and Hearing Research, 34,* 1130-1141.

Watson, D., Omark, D., Gronell, S., & Heller, B. (1986). *Nondiscriminatory assessment: A practitioner's handbook.* Sacramento: California State Department of Education.

Watson, L. (1977, November). *Conversational participation by language deficient and normal children.* Paper presented at the Annual Convention of the American Speech and Hearing Association, Chicago.

Watson, L., & Bassinger, J. (1974). Parent training technology: A potential service delivery system. *Mental Retardation, 12,* 3–10.

Watson-Gego, K. A., & Boggs, S. T. (1977). From verbal play to talk story: The role of routines in speech events among Hawaiian children. In S. Ervin-Tripp & C. Mitchell-Kernan (Eds.), *Child discourse* (pp. 67-90). New York: Academic Press.

Watzlawick, P., Beavin, J., & Jackson, D. (1967). *Pragmatics of human communication.* New York: Norton.

Wayman, K. I., Lynch, E. W., & Hanson, M. J. (1990). Home-based early childhood services: Cultural sensitivity in a family systems approach. *Topics in Early Childhood Special Education, 10*(4), 56-75.

Weaver, C. (1991). Whole language and its potential for developing readers. *Topics in Language Disorders, 11*(3), 28-44.

Weaver, P., & Dickinson, D. (1982). Scratching below the surface structure: Exploring the usefulness of story grammars. *Discourse Processes, 5,* 225–243.

Weaver, R., & Dickenson, D. (1979). Story comprehension and recall in dyslexic students. *Bulletin of the Orton Society, 29,* 157-171.

Webber, B. L. (1978). *A formal approach to discourse anaphora.* New York: Garland.

Weber-Olsen, M., Putnam-Sims, P., & Gannon, J. (1983). Elicited imitation and the Oral Language Sentence Imitation Screening Test (OLS-IST): Content or context. *Journal of Speech and Hearing Disorders, 48,* 368–378.

Weeks, T. (1971). Speech registers in young children. *Child Development, 42,* 1119–1131.

Weiner, F. (1979). *Phonological process analysis.* Baltimore: University Park Press.

Weiner, F. (1981). Treatment of phonological disability using the method of meaningful minimal contrast: Two case studies. *Journal of Speech and Hearing Disorders, 46,* 97-103.

Weiner, F. (1985). Process Analysis 2.0 [Computer program]. State College. PA: Parrot Software.

Weiner, F. (1988). Parrot Easy Language Sample Analysis (PELSA) [Computer program]. State College, PA: Parrot Software.

Weiner, F., & Lewnau, L. (1979, November). *Nondiscriminatory speech and language testing of minority children: Linguistic interferences.* Paper presented at the Annual Convention of the American Speech-Language-Hearing Association, Atlanta.

Weiner, F., & Ostrowski, A. (1979). Effects of listener uncertainty on articulatory inconsistency. *Journal of Speech and Hearing Disorders, 44,* 487-493.

Weiner, P., & Hoock, W. (1973). The standardization of tests: Criteria and criticisms. *Journal of Speech and Hearing Research, 16,* 616–626.

Weinrich, B., Glaser, A., & Johnston, E. (1987). *A sourcebook of adolescent pragmatic activities.* Tucson, AZ: Communication Skill Builders.

Weinstein, G. (1984). Literacy and second language acquisition: Issues and perspectives. *TESOL Quarterly, 18,* 471–484.

Weismer, S., & Hesketh, L. J. (1993). The influence of prosodic and gestural cues on novel word acquisition by children with specific language impairment. *Journal of Speech and Language Research, 36,* 1013–1025.

Weismer, S., & Murray-Branch, J. (1989). Modeling versus modeling plus evoked production training: A comparison of two language intervention methods. *Journal of Speech and Hearing Disorders, 54,* 269–281.

Weiss, A., & Nakamura, M. (1992). Children with normal language skills in preschool classrooms for children with language impairments: Differences in modeling style. *Language, Speech, and Hearing Services in Schools, 23,* 64-70.

Weiss, B., Weisz, J., & Bromfield, R. (1986). Performance of retarded and nonretarded persons on information-processing tasks: Further tests of the similar structure hypothesis. *Psychological Bulletin, 100,* 157-175.

Weistuch, L., & Brown, B. B. (1987). Motherese as therapy: A programme and its dissemination. *Child Language Teaching and Therapy, 3,* 57-71.

Weistuch, L., & Lewis, M. (1986). *Effect of maternal language intervention strategies on the language of delayed two to five year olds.* Paper presented at the Conference of the Eastern Psychological Association, New York.

Welch, S. (1981). Teaching generative grammar to mentally retarded children: A review and analysis of a decade of behavioral research. *Mental Retardation, 19,* 277–284.

Wellman, H. (1985). The origins of metacognition. In D. Forest-Pressley, G. MacKinnon, & T. Waller (Eds.), *Metacognition, cognition, and human performance* (pp. 1-31). New York: Academic Press.

Wells, G. (1981). *Language through interaction.* New York: Cambridge University Press.

Wells, G. (1985). *Language development in the pre-school years.* New York: Cambridge University Press.

Werner, E. (1984). *Child care: Kith, kin, and hired hands.* Baltimore: University Park Press.

Westby, C. E. (1984). Development of narrative language abilities. In G. Wallach & K. Butler (Eds.), *Language learning disabilities in school-age children* (pp. 103-127). Baltimore: Williams & Wilkins.

Westby, C. E. (1985). Learning to talk—Talking to learn: Oral-literate language differences. In C. Simon (Ed.), *Communication skills and classroom success: Therapy methodologies for language-learning disabled students.* San Diego: College-Hill.

Westby, C. E. (1988). Children's play: Reflections of social competence. *Seminars in Speech and Language, 9*(1), 1–14.

Westby, C. E. (1990). The role of the speech-language pathologist in whole language. *Language, Speech, and Hearing Services in Schools, 21,* 228-237.

Westby, C. E. (1992). Narrative assessment. *Best Practices in School Speech-Language Pathology, 2,* 53-64.

Westby, C. E. & Costlow, L. (1991). Implementing a whole language program in a special education class. *Topics in Language Disorders, 11*(3), 69-84.

Westby, C. E., Van Dongen, R., & Maggart, Z. (1989). Assessing narrative competence. *Seminars in Speech and Language, 10,* 63-76.

Wetherby, A. K., Cain, D. H., Yonclas, D. G., & Walker, V. G. (1988). Analysis of intentional communication of normal children from the prelinguistic to the multiword stage. *Journal of Speech and Hearing Research, 31,* 240-252.

Wetherby, A. K., & Prizant, B. M. (1989). The expression of communicative intent: Assessment issues. *Seminars in Speech and Language, 10,* 77-94.

Wetherby, A. K., & Prizant, B. M. (1990). Communication and Symbolic Behavior Scales—Experimental edition. San Antonio, TX: Special Press.

Wetherby, A. K., & Prizant, B. M. (1991a). Communication and Symbolic Behavior Scales. Chicago: Riverside.

Wetherby, A. K., & Prizant, B. M. (1991b). Profiling young children's communicative competence. In S. Warren & J. Reichle (Eds.), *Causes and effects in language assessment and intervention* (pp. 217–253). Baltimore: Paul H. Brookes.

Wetherby, A. K., & Prutting, C. A. (1984). Profiles in communicative and cognitive-social abilities in autistic children. *Journal of Speech and Hearing Disorders, 27,* 364-377.

Wetherby, A. K., & Rodriguez, G. (1992). Measurement of communicative intentions in normally developing children during structured and unstructured contexts. *Journal of Speech and Hearing Research, 35,* 130-138.

Wetherby, A. K., Yonclas, D., & Bryan, A. (1989). Communicative profiles in preschool children with handicaps: Implications for early identification. *Journal of Speech and Hearing Disorders, 54,* 148-158.

Wetherby, A. M. (1986). Ontogeny of communicative functions in autism. *Journal of Autism and Developmental Disorders, 16,* 295–316.

Wexler, K., Blau, A., Dore, J., & Leslie, S. (1982, April). *A pragmatic view of how nonverbal and vocal persons communicate.* Paper presented at the Annual Convention of the New York State Speech-Language-Hearing Association, West Liberty.

Whaley, J. (1981). Readers' expectation for story structure. *Reading Research Quarterly, 17,* 90–114.

Whitacre, J. D., Luper, H. L., & Pollio, H. R. (1970). General language deficits in children with articulation problems. *Language, and Speech, 13,* 231-239.

White, T. G., Power, M. A., & White, S. (1989). Morphological analysis: Implications for teaching and understanding vocabulary growth. *Reading Research Quarterly, 24,* 283-304.

Whitehurst, G. L., Fischel, J. E., & Arnold, D. S. (1989). *Correlates and discriminants of developmental expressive disorder.* Paper presented to the Society for Research in Child Development, Kansas City, MO.

Whitehurst, G. L., Fischel, J. E., Lonigan, C. J., Valdez-Menchaca, M. C., Arnold, D. S., & Smith, M. (1991). Treatment of early expressive language delay: If, when, and how. *Topics in Language Disorders, 11*(4), 55-68.

Wiegel-Crump, C. A., & Dennis, M. (1986). Development of word-finding. *Brain and Language, 27,* 1-23.

Wiig, E. H. (1982a). *Let's talk: Developing prosocial communication skills.* San Antonio: Psychological Corp.

Wiig, E. H. (1982b). Let's Talk Inventory for Adolescents. San Antonio: Psychological Corp.

Wiig, E. H. (1984). Language disabilities in adolescents: A question of cognitive strategies. *Topics in Language Disorders, 4*(2), 41–58.

Wiig, E. H. (1990). Language disabilities in school-age children and youth. In G. H. Shames & E. H. Wiig (Eds.), *Human communication disorders: An introduction* (3rd ed., pp. 193-220). New York: Merrill/Macmillan.

Wiig, E. H., & Roach, M. A. (1975). Immediate recall of semantically varied "sentences" by learning disabled adolescents. *Perceptual and Motor Skills, 40,* 119-125.

Wiig, E. H., & Semel, E. M. (1973). Comprehension of linguistic concepts requiring logical operations by learning disabled children. *Journal of Speech and Hearing Research, 16,* 627-636.

Wiig, E. H., & Semel, E. M. (1974). Logico-grammatical sentence comprehension by learning disabled adolescents. *Perceptual Motor Skills, 38,* 1331-1334.

Wiig, E. H., & Semel, E. M. (1975). Productive language abilities in learning disabled adolescents. *Journal of Learning Disabilities, 8,* 578-586.

Wiig, E. H., & Semel, E. M. (1976). *Language disabilities in children and adolescents.* New York: Merrill/Macmillan.

Wiig, E. H., & Semel, E. M. (1984). *Language assessment and intervention for the learning disabled* (2nd ed.). New York: Merrill/Macmillan.

Wiig, E. H., Semel, E. M., & Crouse, M. A. (1973). The use of English morphology by high risk and learning disabled children. *Journal of Learning Disabilities, 6,* 457-465.

Wiig, E. H., Semel, E. M., & Nystrom, L. (1982). Comparison of rapid naming abilities in language-learning disabled and academically achieving eight-year-olds. *Language, Speech, and Hearing Services in Schools, 13,* 11-22.

Wilbur, R. (1983). Where do we go from here. In J. Miller, D. Yoder, & R. Schiefelbusch (Eds.), *Contemporary issues in language intervention* (pp. 137–143). Rockville, MD: American Speech-Language-Hearing Association.

Wilbur, R. (1987). *American Sign Language: Linguistic and applied dimensions* (2nd ed.). San Diego: College-Hill.

Wilcox, K., & McGuinn-Aasby, S. (1988). The performance of monolingual and bilingual Mexican children on the TACL. *Language, Speech, and Hearing Services in Schools, 19*, 34–40.

Wilcox, M., & Leonard, L. (1978). Experimental acquisition of *wh-* questions in language-disordered children. *Journal of Speech and Hearing Research, 21*, 220–239.

Wilcox, M. J. (1984). Developmental language disorders: Preschoolers. In A. Holland (Ed.), *Language disorders in children* (pp. 101–128). San Diego: College-Hill.

Wilcox, M. J., & Campbell, P. (1983, November). *Assessing communication in low-functioning multi-handicapped children.* Paper presented at the Annual Convention of the American Speech-Language-Hearing Association, Cincinnati.

Wilcox, M. J., Kouri, T., & Caswell, S. (1990). Partner sensitivity to communication behavior of young children with development disorders. *Journal of Speech and Hearing Disorders, 55*, 679-693.

Wilcox, M. J., Kouri, T., & Caswell, S. (1991). Early language intervention: A comparison of classroom and individual treatment. *American Journal of Speech-Language Pathology, 1*(3), 49-62.

Wilkinson, I., & Milosky, I. (1987). School-age children's metapragmatic knowledge of requests and responses in the classroom. *Topics in Language Disorders, 7*(2), 61–70.

Willbrand, M. L. (1977). Psycholinguistic theory and therapy for initiating two-word utterances. *British Journal of Disorders of Communication, 12*, 37-46.

Williams, A. L. (1993). Phonological reorganization: A qualitative measure of phonological improvement. *American Journal of Speech-Language Pathology, 2*(2), 44-51.

Williams, F., Cairns, H., & Cairns, C. (1971). *An analysis of the variations from standard English pronunciation in the phonetic performance of two groups of nonstandard-English-speaking children.* Austin: University of Texas, Center for Communication Research.

Williams, J. P. (1984). Categorization, macrostructure, and finding the main idea. *Journal of Educational Psychology, 76*, 874-879.

Williams, J. P. (1986, August). *Reading comprehension: Categorization, macrostructures, and finding the main idea.* Paper presented to the American Psychological Association, Washington, DC.

Williams, J. P. (1988). Identifying main ideas: A basic aspect of reading comprehension. *Topics in Language Disorders, 8*(3), 1-13.

Williams, J. P., Taylor, M. B., & Granger, S. (1981). Text variations at the level of the individual sentence and the comprehension of simple expository paragraphs. *Journal of Educational Psychology, 73*, 851-865.

Williams, R., & Wolfram, W. (1977). *Social dialects: Differences vs. disorders.* Washington, DC: American Speech-Language-Hearing Association.

Williams, T. (1989). A social skills group for autistic children. *Journal of Autism and Developmental Disorders, 19*, 143–156.

Wilson, M., & Fox, B. (1983). Microcomputer Language Assessment and Development Systems (Micro-LADS) [Computer program]. Burlington, VT: Laureate Learning Systems.

Wimmer, H. (1979). Processing of script deviation by young children. *Discourse Processes, 2*, 301–310.

Wing, C. (1990). A preliminary investigation of generalization to untrained words following two treatments of children's word-finding problems. *Language, Speech, and Hearing Services in Schools, 21*, 151-156.

Winitz, H. (1973). Problem solving and the delay of speech as strategies in the teaching of language. *ASHA, 15*, 583–586.

Winitz, H. (1983). Use and abuse of the developmental approach. In H. Winitz (Ed.), *Treating language disorders: For clinicians by clinicians* (pp. 25-42). Baltimore: University Park Press.

Winner, E. (1988). *The point of words.* Cambridge, MA: Harvard University Press.

Winograd, P. N. (1984). Strategic difficulties in summarizing texts. *Reading Research Quarterly, 19*, 404-425.

Winograd, P. N., & Niquette, G. (1988). Assessing learned helplessness in poor readers. *Topics in Language Disorders, 8*(3), 38-55.

Winogron, H. W., Knights, R. M., & Bawden, H. N. (1984). Neuropsychological deficits following head injury in children. *Journal of Clinical Neuropsychology, 6*, 269-286.

Winton, P., & Bailey, D. (in press). Communicating with families: Examining practices and facilitating change. In R. Fewell, D. Saxton, & M. Lobman (Eds.), *Families of young children with special needs: A primer for services.* Austin, TX: Pro-Ed.

Wixson, K., Bosky, A., Yochum, M., & Alvermann, D. (1984). An interview for assessing students' perceptions of classroom reading tasks. *The Reading Teacher, 37*, 346-352.

Wolf, M. (1978). Social validity: The case for subjective measurement or how applied behavior analysis is finding its heart. *Journal of Applied Behavior Analysis, 11*, 203-214.

Wolf, M. (1979). *The relationship of disorders of word-finding and reading in children and aphasics.* Unpublished doctoral dissertation. Harvard University, Cambridge, MA.

Wolf, M. (1982). The word-retrieval process and reading in children and aphasia. In K. Nelson (Ed.), *Chil-*

dren's language (Vol. 3, pp. 437-493). Hillsdale, NJ: Lawrence Erlbaum.

Wolf, M. (1984). Naming, reading, and the dyslexias: A longitudinal overview. *Annals of Dyslexia, 34,* 87-115.

Wolf, M., Bally, H., & Morris, R. (1986). Automaticity, retrieval processes, and reading: A longitudinal study in average and impaired readers. *Child Development, 57,* 988-1000.

Wolf, M., & Segal, D. (1992). Word finding and reading in the developmental dyslexias. *Topics in Language Disorders, 13*(1), 51-65.

Wolfram, W. (1983). Test interpretation and sociolinguistic differences. *Topics in Language Disorders, 3*(3), 21-24.

Wolfram, W. (1985). The phonologic system: Problems of second language acquisition. In J. M. Costelli (Ed.), *Speech disorders in adults* (pp. 59–76). Austin, TX: Pro-Ed.

Wolfram, W., & Christian, D. (1976). *Appalachian speech.* Arlington, VA: Center for Applied Linguistics.

Wolk, L. (1990). *An investigation of young children who stutter and exhibit phonological difficulties.* Unpublished doctoral dissertation, Syracuse University, Syracuse, NY.

Woltosz, W. (1988). *Words+, Inc.* Pittsburgh, PA: Adaptive Communication Systems.

Wong, B. Y. (1979). Increasing retention of main ideas through questioning strategies. *Learning Disability Quarterly, 2,* 42-47.

Wong, B. Y. (1986). A cognitive approach to teaching spelling. *Exceptional Children, 53,* 169-173.

Wong, B. Y., & Jones, W. (1982). Increasing metacomprehension in learning disabled and normally achieving students through self-questioning training. *Learning Disability Quarterly, 5,* 228-246.

Wood, D. (1983). Teaching: Natural and contrived. *Child Development Society Newsletter, 32,* 2–8.

Woods, T. (1984). Generality on the verbal tacting of autistic children as a function of "naturalness" in antecedent control. *Journal of Behavior Therapy and Experimental Psychiatry, 15,* 27–32.

Work, R. S., Cline, J. A., Ehren, B. J., Keiser, D. L., & Wujek, C. (1993). Adolescent language programs. *Language, Speech, and Hearing Services in Schools, 24,* 43-53.

Wren, C. (1981). Identifying patterns of syntactic disorder in six-year-old children. *British Journal of Disorders of Communication, 16,* 101–109.

Wren, C. (1982). Identifying patterns of processing disorder in six-year-old children with syntax problems. *British Journal of Disorders of Communication, 17,* 83–92.

Wren, C. (1985). Collecting language samples from children with syntax problems. *Language, Speech, and Hearing Services in Schools, 16,* 83–102.

Wulz, S., Hall, M., & Klein, M. (1983). A home-centered instructional communication strategy for severely handicapped children. *Journal of Speech and Hearing Disorders, 48,* 2–10.

Wysocki, K., & Jenkins, J. R. (1987). Deriving word meanings through morphological generalization. *Reading Research Quarterly, 22,* 66-81.

Ylvisaker, M. (1986). Language and communication disorders following pediatric head injury. *Journal of Head Trauma Rehabilitation, 1,* 48-56.

Ylvisaker, M., & Szekeres, S. (1989). Metacognitive and executive impairments in head-injured children and adults. *Topics in Language Disorders, 9,* 34-49.

Yoder, D. (1984). *Conversational interaction of augmentative system's users: What does our research tell us?* Paper presented at the Third International Conference on Augmentative and Alternative Communication, Boston.

Yoder, D. (1985, June). *Communication and the severely-profoundly retarded.* Paper presented at the Conference on Communication and the Developmentally Disabled: The State of the Art in 1985, Buffalo, NY.

Yoder, P. J. (1987). The relationship between degree of infant handicap and the clarity of infant cues. *American Journal of Mental Deficiency, 91,* 639-641.

Yoder, P. J., & Davies, B. (1990). Do parents' questions and topic continuations elicit replies from developmentally delayed children? A sequential analysis. *Journal of Speech and Hearing Research, 33,* 563-573.

Yoder, P. J., Davies, B., Bishop, K., & Munson, L. (1994). Effect of adult continuing *wh-* questions on conversational participation in children with developmental disabilities. *Journal of Speech and Hearing Research, 37,* 193–204.

Yoder, P. J., & Feagans, L. (1988). Mothers' attributions of communication to prelinguistic behavior of infants with developmental delays and mental retardation. *American Journal of Mental Retardation, 93,* 36-43.

Yoder, P. J., Kaiser, A. P., & Alpert, C. L. (1991). An exploratory study of the interaction between language teaching methods and child characteristics. *Journal of Speech and Hearing Research, 34,* 155-167.

Yoder, P. J., Kaiser, A. P., Alpert, C., & Fischer, R. (1993). Following the child's lead when teaching nouns to preschoolers with mental retardation. *Journal of Speech and Hearing Research, 36,* 158–167.

Yorkston, K., & Dowden, P. (1984). Nonspeech language and communication systems. In A. Holland (Ed.), *Language disorders in adults* (pp. 283–312). San Diego: College-Hill.

Yorkston, K., Honsinger, M., Dowden, P., & Marriner, N. (1989). Vocabulary selection: A case report. *Augmentative and Alternative Communication, 5,* 101–108.

Yorkston, K., Smith, K., & Beukelman, D. (1990). Extended communication samples of augmented communicators: I. A comparison of individualized versus standard single-word vocabularies. *Journal of Speech and Hearing Disorders, 55,* 217–224.

Yoshinaga-Itano, C., & Snyder, L. (1985). Form and meaning in the written language of hearing impaired children. *Volta Review, 87*(5), 75-90.

Young, E. C. (1983). A language approach to treatment of phonological process problems. *Language, Speech, and Hearing Services in Schools, 14,* 47–53.

Young, E. C. (1987). The effects of treatment on consonant cluster and weak syllable reduction processes in misarticulating children. *Language, Speech, and Hearing Services in Schools, 18,* 23–33.

Young, E. C., & Sacks, G. (1982, June). *Remediation of developmental speech disorders with treatment of phonological processes.* Paper presented at the Regional Convention of the American Speech-Language-Hearing Association, Philadelphia.

Young, J. (1988). *Developing social conversational skills: An intervention study of preverbal handicapped children with their parents.* Unpublished master's thesis, Ohio State University, Columbus.

Young, L. W. L. (1982). Inscrutability revisited. In J. J. Gumperz (Ed.), *Language and social identify* (pp. 72–84). Cambridge, UK: Cambridge University Press.

Youniss, J. (1980). *Parents and peers in social development.* Chicago: University of Chicago Press.

Zachman, L., Huisingh, R., Jorgensen, C., & Barrett, M. (1978a). Oral Language Sentence Imitation Diagnostic Inventory. Moline, IL: LinguiSystems.

Zachman, L., Huisingh, R., Jorgensen, C., & Barrett, M. (1978b). Oral Language Sentence Imitation Screening Test. Moline, IL: LinguiSystems.

Zametkin, A. J., & Rapoport, J. L. (1987). Neurobiology of attention deficit disorder with hyperactivity: Where have we come in 50 years? *Journal of the American Academy of Child and Adolescent Psychiatry, 66,* 246-253.

Zeaman, D., & House, B. (1979). A review of attention theory. In N. Ellis (Ed.), *Handbook of mental deficiency: Psychological theory and research* (2nd ed., pp. 63–120). Hillsdale, NJ: Lawrence Erlbaum.

Zimmerman, I., Steiner, V., & Pond, R. (1979). Preschool Language Scale—Revised. San Antonio: Psychological Corp.

Zwitman, D., & Sonderman, J. (1979). A syntax program designed to present base linguistic structures to language-disordered children. *Journal of Communicative Disorders, 13,* 232–237.

Author Index

Subject Index